MELANOMA – CURRENT CLINICAL MANAGEMENT AND FUTURE THERAPEUTICS

Edited by **Mandi Murph**

Melanoma – Current Clinical Management and Future Therapeutics
http://dx.doi.org/10.5772/58516
Edited by Mandi Murph

Contributors

Monica Neagu, Carolina Constantin, Estelle Leclerc, Carlo Riccardo Rossi, John D'Orazio, Erin Wolf Horrell, Kalin Wilson, Paola Savoia, Paolo Fava, Isabel Pires, Luis Resende, Felisbina Luisa Queiroga, Joana Moreira, Justina Prada, Rolland Gyulai, Zsuzsanna Lengyel, Zsolt Kádár, Mandi Murph, Duane Miller, Yasuhiro Nakamura, Miriam Jasiulionis, Ana Carolina Monteiro, Mariana Mariana Toricelli, Hinrich Abken, Jennifer Makalowski, Norma E. Herrera, Corina-Daniela Ene, Ilinca Nicolae

Published by InTech
Janeza Trdine 9, 51000 Rijeka, Croatia

Publishing Process Manager Iva Simcic
Technical Editor InTech DTP team
Cover InTech Design team

First published April, 2015
Printed in Croatia

Additional hard copies can be obtained from orders@intechopen.com

Melanoma – Current Clinical Management and Future Therapeutics , Edited by Mandi Murph
p. cm.
ISBN 978-953-51-2036-0

Meet the editor

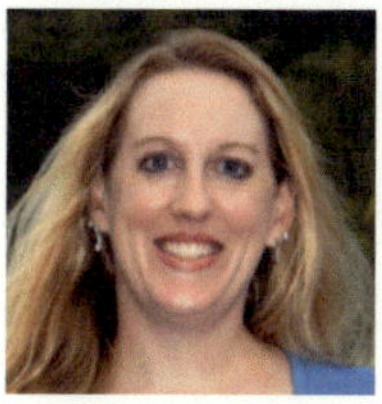

Mandi M. Murph is an Associate Professor in the Department of Pharmaceutical and Biomedical Sciences in the College of Pharmacy at the University of Georgia. She holds an American Cancer Society Research Scholar award for research on melanoma. Her laboratory works on pre-clinical testing of novel therapeutic compounds for use against BRAF wild-type V600 melanoma and researches molecular means to exploit melanoma signaling pathways. She has grant funding from the Georgia Research Alliance and the National Cancer Institute, which is part of the National Institutes of Health. Before becoming a professor at the University of Georgia, Murph received training at the University of Texas M.D. Anderson Cancer Center in Houston. She teaches cancer therapy courses to University of Georgia students.

Contents

Preface

There has never been a more rapid period of formulary expansion for melanoma treatment than what has transpired in recent years. This rapid expansion comprises various choices for monoclonal antibody immunotherapy, or immune system checkpoint therapy, and targeted, small molecule inhibitors against BRAF and MEK. Since these options have entered the clinic, the entire melanoma research landscape and disease management has undergone restructuring. Other types of cancers have even followed suit with immunotherapy indication expansions that were initially intended for melanoma.

Thus, Melanoma – Current Clinical Management and Future Therapeutics offers readers an advanced course on revamped melanoma, but it can also function as an addendum to polish expertise on this changing field. The first section of the book includes a thorough introduction to melanoma, with a chapter that describes disease epidemiology, intrinsic versus extrinsic risk factors and the role of pigmentation genetics in incidence. In addition to cutaneous superficial spreading melanoma, the most common type of melanoma, a separate introductory chapter discusses acral lentiginous melanoma, which is more common among individuals with dark pigmentation, and provides visual clinical presentations of disease. The last introductory chapter provides a molecular primer of signaling mechanisms driving melanoma progression.

Othersections of the book deal with clinical management and therapeutic treatment of melanoma. For example, clinical chapters discuss melanoma surgery and staging of disease among cutaneous and acral melanoma, including canine melanocytic tumors, and include a plethora of surgical images. Among these chapters, surgical removal of extensive disease and skin grafting for facial reconstruction are visually depicted in numerous figures. In addition, sentinel lymph node biopsy and lymphadenectomy are portrayed in a detailed clinical chapter, which exhibits multiple photographs of the surgical excision technique performed among those with advanced disease.

Immunotherapy is the major therapeutic approach discussed in this book, with several chapters outlining the applications for immune system checkpoints in melanoma. Clinical trial data is discussed combining small molecule inhibitors of MAPK, PI3K or mTOR, with and without immunotherapy, reflecting the successes and challenges with this approach, as well as with inhibitors of angiogenesis Adverse events and treatment side effects have a chapter devoted to this topic, since toxicities are an unfortunate but integral component of treatment. Finally, emerging research about potential targets in melanoma comprises the last section where readers will find chapters on autotaxin, gangliosides and RAGE.

This book would not have been possible without the help of Iva Simcic, whose help guided me through this process. I thank her for her time, energy and patience. I hope that the readership enjoys this collection of work as much as I did.

Prof. Mandi Murph
University of Georgia
USA

Section 1

Introduction to Melanoma

Chapter 1

Melanoma — Epidemiology, Risk Factors, and the Role of Adaptive Pigmentation

Erin M. Wolf Horrell, Kalin Wilson and
John A. D'Orazio

Additional information is available at the end of the chapter

http://dx.doi.org/10.5772/58994

1. Introduction

Malignant cutaneous melanoma is an aggressive form of skin cancer that affects well over 100,000 individuals world-wide each year. Melanoma results from uncontrolled proliferation of melanocytes and can occur throughout the body including skin, mucosal surfaces, and the retina. This chapter will focus on cutaneous melanoma because it is the most common site of the disease. Cutaneous melanoma has a high association with exposure to UV radiation and is most commonly found on sun exposed surfaces [5]. If diagnosed in its early stages, resection of cutaneous melanoma is associated with favorable five-year survival rates. As melanoma progresses, however, it has a tendency to metastasize beyond its primary site. It expands both radially and vertically through the skin and eventually spreads throughout the body via hematogenous or lymphatic routes. Long-term prognosis correlates strongly with the stage of disease, and after melanoma metastasizes, survival rates markedly decline. In general, five-year survival rates for metastatic melanoma are under 20%. Thus, early identification and treatment are essential clinical tools to minimize mortality.

For a variety of reasons, the incidence of melanoma has increased faster than any other cancer over the last several decades [6] (Figure 1), and the estimated healthcare cost in 2020 is predicted to be 4.58 billion dollars [7]. Considering the deadly nature of metastatic melanoma along with the steady increase in incidence throughout the past century, appropriate measures to prevent the development of the disease are important and will require a more complete knowledge of the risk factors associated with this disease. This chapter reviews the epidemiologic and genetic risk factors associated with the development of malignant cutaneous melanoma, with an emphasis on mechanisms of melanocyte resistance to UV damage in the skin.

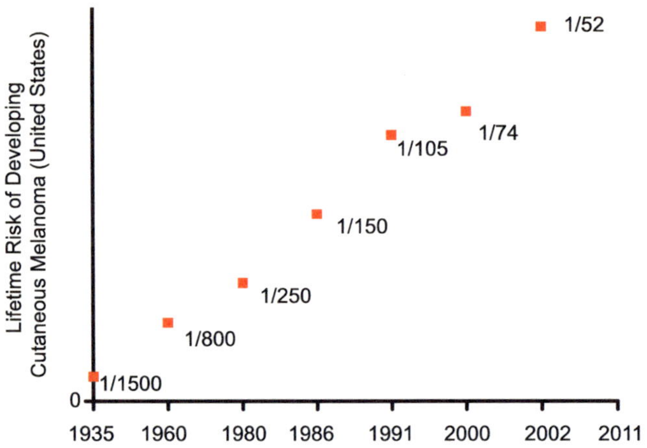

Figure 1. Lifetime risk of melanoma has increased in the United States from 1935-2011. (Adapted from [4]).

2. Epidemiology

This section will address the epidemiology of melanoma in reference to risk factors, incidence and mortality, gender differences, and variations between ethnicities.

2.1. Incidence and mortality

The Surveillance, Epidemiology, and End Results (SEER) database predicts a diagnosis of melanoma in over 76,000 individuals in the United States for 2014. Though it can affect patients of any age, melanoma traditionally affects older individuals with an average age at diagnosis and death of 62 and 69 years respectively. While many cancer incidence rates have plateaued over the last century, the incidence of melanoma has steadily increased [6]. In the early 1930's, the lifetime risk of developing melanoma for an American was 1 in 1500, while in 2002, it was reported to be 1 in 68 [8]. The melanoma incidence rate increased an additional 1.8% per year between 2002 and 2012, such that 21.3 per 100,000 individuals were diagnosed with melanoma between 2007 and 2011 [1]. Though some portion of this rise is due to enhanced awareness and improvements in diagnosis, the causes underlying the increased incidence may be diverse. An important factor may be that life span has increased during this time period. As melanoma incidence correlates with age, we would expect more cases in a population of individuals that live longer [9]. However, chief among the potential contributive factors is increased exposure to ultraviolet (UV) radiation, either solar or artificial. The popularization of a tanned physique in Western cultures beginning the early 1900's has led to intentional exposures to UV. Many individuals believe they look better, feel healthier, appear younger and are happier with tanned skin [10]. The desire for UV exposure coupled with increased recreational and occupational opportunities, results in significantly more time devoted to sun exposure or in artificial tanning beds.

Although incidence rates have been increasing steadily, melanoma mortality rates have stabilized over the past 20 years due to advances in medical, surgical and supportive care [11]. The overall five-year survival rate is currently above 90%, likely related to diagnosis at curable stages for the majority of cases [1]. From 1975 until the 1990's, the mortality rate climbed 1.9% per year. From 2006-2010, there were 2.7 deaths per 100,000 individuals, and 9,700 individuals are predicted to die from melanoma in 2014 [1] (Figure 2). The mortality rate for women has actually decreased by 0.6% from 1989-2007. The mortality rate for men has increase 0.2% during the same time frame [1].

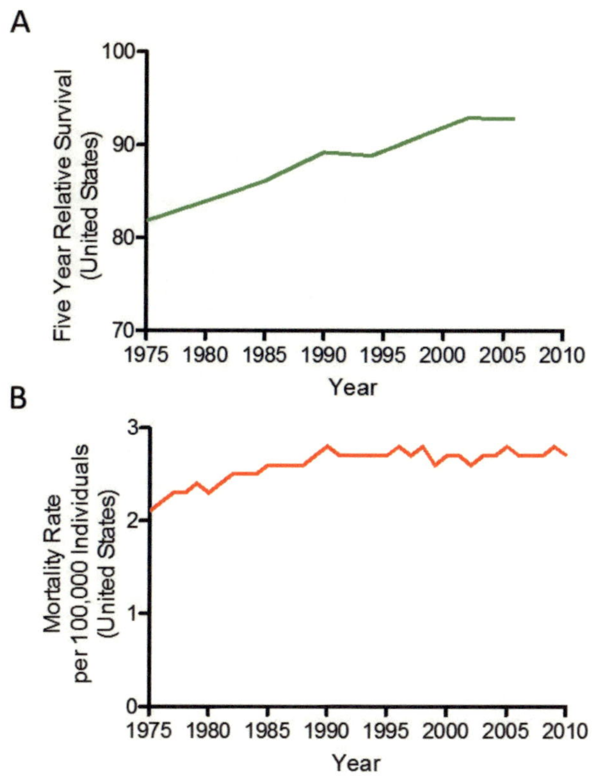

Figure 2. A. Five year relative survival rate for melanoma in the United States from 1975-2009. B. Mortality rate for melanoma in the United States from 1975-2009 (Adapted from [1]).

2.2. Gender

Melanoma affects men and women differently. Before the age of 40, women are more susceptible to melanoma (1 in 391 women versus 1 in 691 men diagnosed each year), however, after the age of 40, the rates reverse, and 1 in 35 men will develop melanoma versus 1 in 54 women [12]. Overall men are more susceptible to melanoma, with 27.7 new cases per 100,000 men versus 16.7 new cases per 100,000 women [1]. While the mortality rate for women is decreasing, it is actually increasing for men [13]. Men account for 60% of deaths due to melanoma [14]. Although both genders are experiencing a rise in melanoma rates, there has been a massive increase in the incidence rate for women under 40, presumably due to recreational UV exposure and the popularization of having a tanned complexion [15]. In women between the ages of 20-29, melanoma is the 2nd most common cancer, trailing behind breast cancer [16]. In fact, there has been a 50% increase in melanoma incidence in young adult women since 1980 such that it is now the leading cause of cancer death among women ages 20 – 25 years old. Melanoma also is the second-most common cancer in adolescents and young adults (men and women) between the ages of 15 and 29 years. Melanoma presentation appears to differ somewhat between genders. In women, melanoma often presents on the extremities while in men, it most frequently presents on the trunk [17].

2.3. Ethnicity

The incidence, mortality rates, and presentation for melanoma differ markedly by ethnicity (Figure 3). Caucasians are the most likely to develop melanoma, however the overall five year survival is lower for African Americans than Caucasians (77% and 91% respectively) [13]. The initial diagnosis is generally at a later stage in individuals with darker skin pigmentation than in Caucasians [18] and tends to be a different subtype. Caucasians frequently present with superficial spreading melanoma while individuals with darker pigmentation often present with acral lentigenous melanoma[19]. In African Americans, Asians, Filipinos, Indonesians, and Native Hawaiians, melanoma often presents on areas that are not sun exposed including the palms and soles of hands and feet respectively, mucous membranes, and nail beds while melanoma in Caucasians generally presents on sun-exposed areas [20].

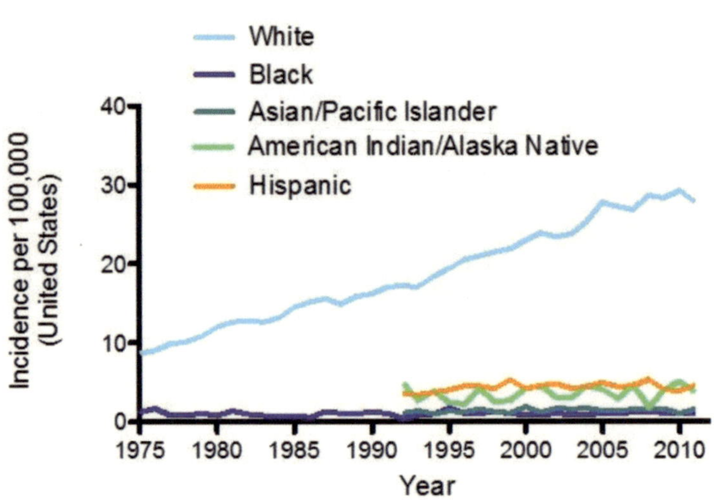

Figure 3. Melanoma incidence rate by ethnicity in the United States from 1975-2011. There is a discrepancy in the incidence rate between the different ethnicities. Ethnicities with fairer complexions have a higher incidence rate than ethnicities with darker complexions (Adapted from [1]).

http://dx.doi.org/10.5772/58994

3. Risk factors

Risk factors for the development of melanoma can be divided into extrinsic and intrinsic factors and include exposure to UV radiation either via sunlight or indoor tanning salons, medications, chemical exposures, presence of nevi, family history of cancer, and pigment of skin [21] (Table 1).

Extrinsic Risk Factors		Intrinsic Risk Factors	
Ultraviolet Radiation	UV exposure, especially blistering sunburns in childhood, correlates with melanoma risk.	History of Skin Cancer	A family and personal history of melanoma and non-melanoma skin cancer increases risk of melanoma
	Countries located closer to the equator with increased sun exposure have a higher melanoma incidence rate	Nevi	A large number of congenital nevi, nevi with large diameter, and dysplastic nevi are all associated with an increased risk
	Indoor tanning bed use increases incidence and mortality rate of melanoma	Medical History	Immunosuppressive states and a past medical history of non-cutaneous skin cancer increase the risk of melanoma
Medication	Psoralen, UVA light therapy and neonatal blue light phototherapy are associated with an increased risk of melanoma	Defective DNA Repair	Individuals diagnosed with xeroderma pigmentosum cannot repair UV induced DNA damage
Environmental Exposure	Polyvinyl chloride, heavy metals and pesticides are associated with an increased risk of melanoma	Skin Complexion	Fair skin, inability to tan, and increased susceptibility to UV induced sunburn increase risk for melanoma

Table 1. Major melanoma risk factors.

3.1. Extrinsic

3.1.1. Ultraviolet radiation

Ultraviolet radiation, probably the single-most important environmental carcinogen with respect to melanoma, is found in natural sunlight and in artificial tanning sources. UV energy is conventionally divided into three wavelengths: UVA (320-400 nm), UVB (290-320 nm), and UVC (100-280 nm). Each type of UV energy has its own distinctive energy profile, biophysical characteristics, and effects on biologic tissue. Although solar energy contains all three UV subtypes, absorption of the higher-energy UV components by atmospheric ozone results in ambient sunlight being mainly (>90%) UVA and the remainder UVB. Both UVA and UVB are bioactive and cause DNA damage and cellular injury that contribute to carcinogenesis. In fact, exposure to UV radiation may be responsible for over 80% of all melanomas [22].

UVA and UVB contribute to the pathogenesis of melanoma via distinct but overlapping mechanisms [23]. UVA (and to a lesser extent UVB) causes DNA damage indirectly through the generation of highly reactive free radicals and oxidative injury [24, 25]. Free radicals change DNA in ways that ultimately affect base-pairing, which can lead to mutation. Oxidation of

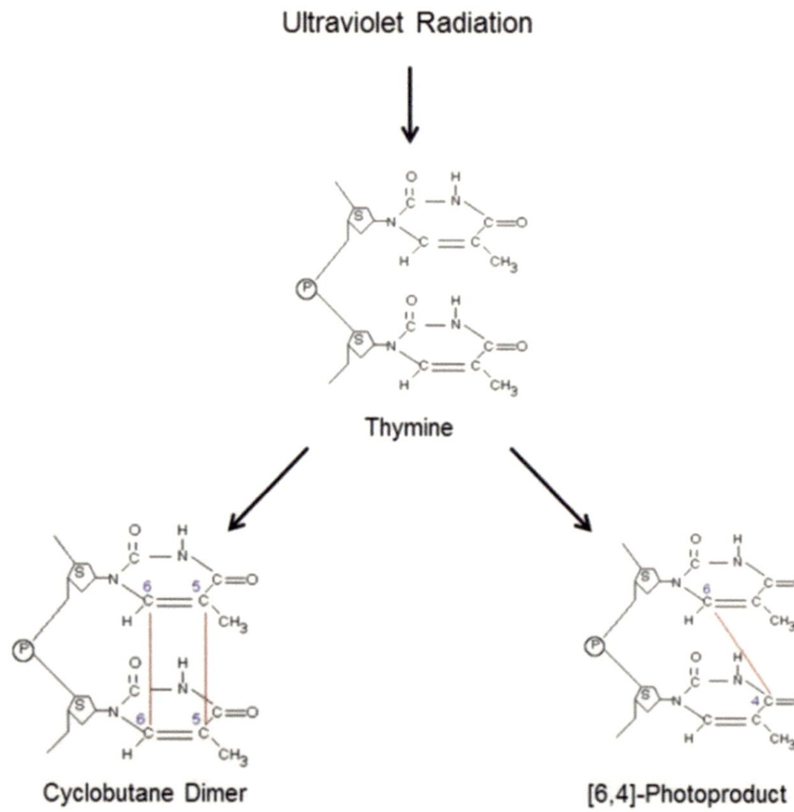

Figure 4. Generation of 6,4-photoproducts and cyclobutane dimers from adjacent pyrimidines. UVB radiation is absorbed by thymine and cytosine residues, resulting in the formation of mutagenic photoproducts that contribute to malignancy.

guanine, for example, is well-known to cause formation of 8-oxo-dG which base pairs with A instead of C; this change leads to transversion point mutations if not repaired in a timely manner. Indeed, some estimate that up to 80% of malignant cutaneous melanomas may result from indirect DNA damage, highlighting the importance of "lower UV energy" in the pathogenesis of melanoma [26]. UVB radiation, in contrast, is higher in energy and directly affects adjacent pyrimidines in the double helix to cause a photochemical reaction. Through direct absorption of UVB energy by pyrimidines, two major types of photoproducts are generated: cyclopyrimidine dimers (CPD's) and 6,4 photoproducts (6,4-PP) [27-30] (Figure 4). Both lesions distort the DNA double helix and, if left unrepaired, lead to characteristic "UV signature" transition mutations (G →T and G→C mutations) [30]. It is largely through the identification of these UV signature mutations that we know that UV is a major risk factor for skin cancer and melanoma [31]. Although UVC, the UV component with the highest energy per photon, can cause substantial damage to cells, the ozone layer absorbs the majority of UVC emitted by the sun, therefore this component is not thought to be a significant contributor to most cases of melanoma. Melanomas classically occur on sun exposed skin [32], and exposure to UV radiation correlates with not only the risk for melanoma [33] but also mortality rates [34]. The correlation between melanoma risk is particularly strong with the UVA component, providing further evidence that UVA may be a significant causative factor in melanomagenesis [35].

3.1.1.1. Geographic factors

The global distribution of melanoma also demonstrates the importance of UV radiation in the pathogenesis of this disease. Countries that are located on latitudes closer to the equator have increased UV intensity and higher rates of melanoma among fair-skinned persons [4, 36]. Australia and New Zealand, which are near the equator, have the highest incidence of melanoma in the world with a risk of 1 in 50 individuals [21]. The World Heath Organization reports that Australia and New Zealand have an age adjusted incidence rate of 35.1 individuals per 100,000 individuals [2]. The incidence of melanoma in Australia has doubled from 1986-2006 [37]. Norway, despite also having a fair-skinned, UV-sensitive population predominantly of Scandinavian descent, has a relatively low incidence of melanoma, presumably due to its high latitude (with comparatively weak ambient solar energy) and low UV exposure [38]. High altitudes are also a risk factor for development of melanoma, presumably because UV strength is higher due to less interference between solar energy and particulate matter present in the atmosphere [39, 40] (Figure 5).

Although latitude and altitude do play a major role in melanoma risk, skin complexion is also an important component to explain the variations in melanoma incidence throughout the world. Central America, despite being closer to the equator than North America has a significantly lower age adjusted incidence rates (1.5 and 13.8 individuals per 100,000 individuals) presumably due to having a predominantly dark-skinned complexion [2].

3.1.1.2. UV exposure patterns

Intermittent sun exposure confers a higher risk for developing melanoma than continual exposure [41-43], but the age at which the exposure causes the greatest damage is still controversial. Some studies suggest that sun exposure for a younger individual is more likely to be associated with the development of melanoma [44], while others suggest age of exposure is less important than the cumulative dose of UV [45]. Regardless of age, sunburn is a major risk factor in the development of melanoma, and the risk doubles with more than 5 sunburns [45, 46] or one or more blistering sunburns [43].

3.1.1.3. Sunscreen

The effect of sunscreen on melanoma prevalence is also controversial for a variety of reasons. The widespread use of broad-spectrum sunscreen has not decreased the incidence despite blocking both UVA and UVB radiation. Early sunscreens were designed to prevent sunburn and only blocked UVB radiation. Individuals who used UVB blocking sunscreen were able to stay out in the sun for longer periods of time and were exposed to greater doses of UVA radiation. A delay may exist between the advent of broad-spectrum sunscreen and its effect on melanoma incidence due to the latency between sun exposure and development of

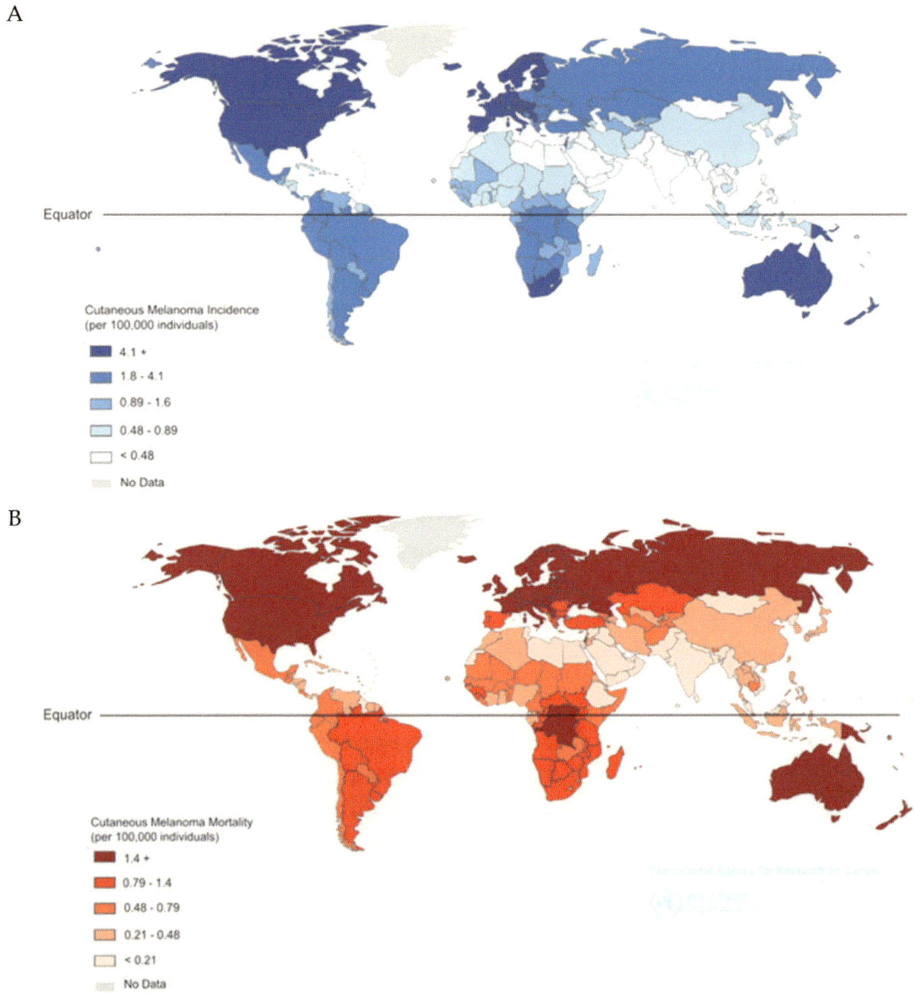

Figure 5. Geographical variation in melanoma incidence (A) and mortality (B). Melanoma incidence is highest in countries populated by fair-skinned persons living in high-UV environments (adapted with permission from [2]).

melanoma. In addition, the use of sunscreen can also promote cellular damage by increasing the reactive oxygen species [47] and if absorbed past the epidermis, can cause photosensitization in melanocytes [48]. Despite some negative effects, the American Society for Clinical Oncology states that the use of broad-spectrum sunscreen with an SPF of 15 or greater decreases an individual's risk of melanoma by up to 50% and should be worn daily to prevent damage from UV radiation [45, 49].

3.1.1.4. Indoor tanning bed use

There has been an explosive increase in the widespread use of indoor tanning beds since their invention in the early 1970's. Over 30 million individuals use indoor tanning salons [50] and over 70% are female [51]. Overall, 2-3 million of salon-users are teenagers [52]. At age 17, 35% of American females admit to use of an artificial tanning device [53]. The prevalence of artificial tanning is concerning, especially among young adolescents. The earlier tanning begins, the more potential risk there is for carcinogenesis and malignant transformation. In individuals between 18-29 years of age, 76% diagnosed with malignant melanoma had previously used artificial tanning devices [54]. There is a strong positive correlation not only between the use of indoor tanning beds and the development of melanoma [55] but also with death due to melanoma [56]. One tanning session increases the chance an individual will develop melanoma by 20%, and each additional session per year increases risk by another 2% [54]. The International Agency for Research on Cancer classifies UV tanning devices in Group1, most dangerous oncogenic substances [57]. Among salon establishments, artificial tanning beds vary in their delivered dose, and the amount of UVA and UVB radiation is unregulated [10] making artificial tanning incredibly dangerous. State legislative statues vary as to whether minors have restricted access. Many experts hypothesize that the burgeoning use of artificial tanning salons over the last three decades may be a major contributing factor to the continued increase in melanoma incidence.

3.1.2. Medications

Many medications that have great benefit for disease treatment also increase patient susceptibility to cancer. Psoralen and ultraviolet A radiation (PUVA) is an effective treatment for psoriasis and other dermatologic conditions. Psoralen increases reactivity to UV radiation, therefore the combination of psoralen and UVA causes a substantial degree of cellular damage. Patients who receive PUVA have a 10 fold increase in risk of developing melanoma 15 years after treatment, and the risk increases with number of treatment sessions (>250) and time following treatments [58].

Neonatal blue light phototherapy (NBLP) is another example of light therapy that may lead to an increased risk for the development of melanoma. NBLP is a treatment for neonates with elevated bilirubin levels and risk of kernicterus. The therapy is associated with short term side effects that are treatable and/or reversible; however, it may also increase the risk of development of melanoma in later years. The blue lamps used for treatment generally emit a combination of blue light and wavelengths in the UVA region of the spectrum [59]. UVA is known to cause DNA damage as explained above, and some studies have demonstrated that visual light can also cause damage through increased activity along the cytokine and oxidant signaling pathways [60]. Reports disagree as to whether exposure to NBLP causes an increase in nevi number and melanoma susceptibility. Bauer et al. assessed 8112 Caucasian children and showed no correlation between nevi number and exposure to NBLP [61]. However, Matichard et al. and Csoma et al. demonstrated that treatment with NBLP correlated with size of nevus (nevi > 2mm in diameter significantly correlated with exposure to NBLP) [62] or with presence of atypical nevi respectively [63]. A study of twins in 2011 demonstrated that NBLP treatment correlated with a higher prevalence of both clinically normal and dysplastic nevi [64] suggesting that NBLP does increase the risk of development of melanoma in adulthood, and children who receive NBLP should be monitored throughout life.

3.1.3. Heavy metals and chemical exposure

Exposure to heavy metals and certain chemicals are associated with an increased risk of melanoma, presumably through mutagenic changes to DNA in melanocytes. Fortes and de Vries suggest that exposure to polycyclic hydrocarbons (for example, individuals who work in industries associated with petroleum, printing, and electronics), ionizing radiation, polyvinyl chloride (a substance present in clothing dye), heavy metals, and pesticides all increase the risk of developing melanoma [65]. Both polycyclic aromatic hydrocarbons [66] and heavy metals [67] react with UVA to generate free radicals which can subsequently damage DNA, but a variety of molecular mechanisms may be involved in carcinogenesis with these agents.

3.2. Intrinsic

3.2.1. History of skin cancer

Personal or family history of skin cancers is associated with higher melanoma risk. UV-initiated malignancies such as squamous cell carcinoma, basal cell carcinoma or actinic keratosis [68, 69] may indicate cumulative UV exposure, however other skin malignancies not thought to be UV-related (e.g. mycosis fungoides) also increase risk of melanoma [70]. Increased risk from skin cancers such as mycosis fungoides may be due to the immunosuppression associated with the disease (immunodeficiency discussed below). First degree relatives of an individual with melanoma also have a higher risk of developing melanoma than the general population [71], and if a first degree relative has had multiple melanomas, the relative risk of an individual developing melanoma is increased to 61.78 [72]. A past medical history of cutaneous melanoma also substantially increases the risk of subsequently developing another [73, 74]. Although the majority of melanomas are sporadic, 10% of diagnoses are in the setting of familial syndromes [75]. For example, individuals diagnosed with Dysplastic Nevus Syndrome, also known as the Familial Atypical Multiple-Mole Melanoma Syndrome, have a 48.9% risk of developing melanoma by age 50 and an 82% risk by age 72 [76]. One of the most common causes of a familial melanoma syndrome is a mutation in the cyclin dependent kinase inhibitor 2A (*CDKN2A*) gene [75] which regulates cell cycle progression. However it is important to note that increased melanoma prevalence within a family may also represent shared environmental factors such as geography and chemical exposure rather than genetic mutations.

3.2.2. Nevi

Nevi can foreshadow the development of melanoma [77-79]. In 1978 two independent studies reported an association between nevi and melanoma for individuals with familial melanoma syndromes. Reimer et al. reported there was "a syndrome of pigmented lesions in melanoma-prone families" [80] while Lynch et al. described melanomas that were linked to individuals with a large number of "moles of variable size and color" [81]. A majority of benign nevi and melanomas share a common mutation in the BRAF gene (V600E) which results in a gain of function in BRAF signaling [26, 82-84]. This mutation activates the mitogen activated protein kinase cascade leading to the deregulation of the cell cycle and an increase in cell division.

http://dx.doi.org/10.5772/58994

While the BRAF mutation may be sufficient for the formation of a benign nevus, additional mutations are needed (e.g. PTEN loss) for the nevus to convert to a malignant melanoma.

The number of nevi, the presence of atypical or large nevi, and the development of new nevi all correlate with melanoma risk [85, 86]. *De novo* nevi formation is a result of exposure to UV radiation, and sunscreen may not influence this process [87-89]. While the risk of melanoma rises with an increased number of total body nevi, malignant degeneration of any particular nevus is rare. Rather, melanomas generally arise from dysplastic nevi, [90], and the risk of a normal nevus converting to melanoma is very low [91]. The presence of only one dysplastic nevus increases risk by 2 fold, however, >10 dysplastic nevi can increase the risk up to 12 fold [92] [93]. Dysplastic nevi are present in 34-56% of melanoma cases [94].

Risk associated with congenital nevi varies with size and quantity. Small congenital nevi are not associated with an increase in risk [92] while large congenital nevi covering over 5% of the body surface area confers an increased risk [95]. Individual large congenital nevi >20 cm in diameter increase an individual's lifetime risk of melanoma to 10% [96]. Reports suggest that if a melanoma is going to arise from a congenital nevi, most will occur by the age of 10 pointing to the importance for screening the pediatric population [97].

3.2.3. Medical history

Medical conditions associated with immunodeficiency or that use immunosuppressive therapies can trigger melanoma. Patients diagnosed with human immunodeficiency virus/acquired immunodeficiency syndrome have an increased prevalence of melanoma with a 50% increased risk of the disease [98] [99]. Because antiretroviral treatment for HIV/AIDS has increased patient's lifespan, these individuals should be closely monitored and obtain regular screening throughout their life. Patients who receive an organ transplant not only have 2.4 greater risk of developing melanoma [100], they also have a more aggressive cancer [101] and a worse prognosis [102] than the general population. Transfer of melanoma from donor to recipient is possible if the donor was previously afflicted with the condition [103].

A previous medical history of noncutaneous skin cancer is also associated with an increased risk of developing melanoma. Individuals who were previously diagnosed with Kaposi sarcoma, breast cancer, lymphoma, prostate cancer, thyroid cancer, and leukemia had an increased risk of subsequently developing melanoma [104]. Childhood cancer survivors have a 2.5 fold increased risk of developing melanoma [105] and are diagnosed at a younger age than the general population (32 years) [106]. Studies speculate that the increased risk following malignancy may be due to either germline mutations in oncogenes or due to the chemotherapy and radiation to treat the prior malignancy [105].

Although melanoma is associated with the production of female hormones, no increased risk of melanoma-associated pathogenesis can be attributed to pregnancy [107]. A majority of women who are pregnant experience a phenomenon known as melasma, an increase in pigment due to increases in melanocyte activity [108]; however, the increase in pigment is not associated with an increase in melanoma incidence.

3.2.4. Nucleotide excision repair

Nucleotide excision repair (NER) is the molecular process by which bulky DNA lesions are recognized, excised, and repaired by the coordinated actions of multiple factors [109-111]. As described above, UVB radiation and to a lesser extent UVA radiation promote the formation of photoproducts that distort the double helix and prevent transcription [112, 113]. Without accurate repair, these photoproducts may cause transition mutations and lead to unregulated cellular proliferation and carcinogenesis.

There are two primary mechanisms of NER, global genome NER (GGR) and transcription coupled NER (TCR), which differ in their initiation site (Figure 6). GGR recognizes damage in non-transcribed regions of the genome. Xeroderma pigmentosum (XP) complementation group C (XPC) and HR23B heterodimerize, recognize distortions within the DNA double helix [114, 115], and recruit the TFIIH complex. TFIIH is a multiprotein complex composed of nine proteins including the helicases XPB and XPD. XPB and XPD unwind 20-30 nucleotides surrounding the damaged base in the 3′-5′ and 5′-3′ direction respectively [116]. The opened DNA structure is stabilized by recruitment of XPA and RPA [117, 118]. After the structure is stabilized, XPF and XPG endonucleases remove the damaged base [119, 120] and the gap is repaired by polymerase δ and ε [121].

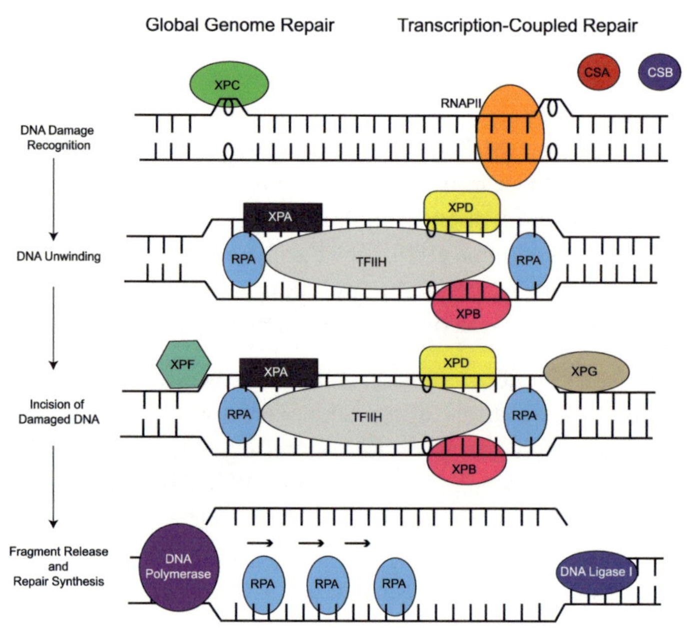

Figure 6. The nucleotide excision repair (NER) pathway is the major way cells rid themselves of bulky DNA lesions such as UV photoproducts. NER is accomplished through the cooperative action of a variety of proteins, working in concert to (1) recognize DNA damage, (2) access and unwind the DNA in the region of the lesion, (3) incise and remove the damage, and (4) repair the gap with a high degree of fidelity using the undamaged strand as a template. Without effective NER, UV mutations accumulate and skin cancers of all kinds occur with high incidence. (Adapted from [3]).

http://dx.doi.org/10.5772/58994

TCR recognizes damage in transcribed regions of the genome after transcription by RNA polymerase II has stalled [122, 123]. Following exposure to UV radiation, Cockayne syndrome B (CSB), Cockayne syndrome A (CSA), and the core NER factors (excluding XPC) are recruited to the sites of stalled RNA polymerase II [124-126]. After damage recognition, either by GGR or TCR, many NER factors work in concert to unwind the double helix in the area of photodamage, excise the damaged strand, and repair the gap using the undamaged sister strand as a template. In this way, NER corrects UV photodamage with a high degree of fidelity and minimizes the chances for UV-induced mutagenesis..

The importance of DNA repair in preventing melanoma is evident in individuals diagnosed with xeroderma pigmentosum (XP) [127, 128]. They are highly sensitive to UV radiation and develop epidermal thinning, telangiectasias, and altered pigmentation in addition to increased prevalence of skin malignancies [129], with a large number of UV-induced mutations in oncogenes and tumor suppressors [130]. These patients have defective DNA repair due to mutations in one of 8 factors associated with NER [131]. Since DNA repair is not possible, patients with XP are encouraged to limit exposure to UV radiation in order to prevent cellular damage. Individuals diagnosed with XP have a 1000 fold increase in skin cancer risk compared to the average population and are often diagnosed with melanoma in the second decade (on average over 40 years before the general public) [132].

3.2.5. Skin complexion

The amount of melanin pigment present in the skin determines skin complexion, and low basal pigmentation (having a fair-skinned phenotype) constitutes a major risk factor for the development of melanoma. Melanin pigments, all derived from the amino acid tyrosine, are synthesized by melanocytes, transported to the keratinocytes where they absorb UV radiation, and prevent damage to the sensitive layers of the skin. In fact, melanocytes produce two distinct forms of melanin. Eumelanin is a dark brown/black chemically inert pigment that potently blocks penetration of UV energy into the skin. Pheomelanin, in contrast, is a lighter-colored pigment that is much less effective at blocking UV penetration and that may even potentiate oxidative UV damage [133] (Figure 7).

The amount of eumelanin in the epidermis largely determines skin complexion. The Fitzpatrick skin phototype was developed by a Harvard University Medical School dermatologist to classify an individual's UV susceptibility based on basal pigment levels, tendency to burn, and ability to tan [134]. Individuals with a lower Fitzpatrick score have fair skin (less pigment), red or blonde hair, burn easily and are unable to tan, while individuals with a higher Fitzpatrick score have a darker complexion (more pigment), do not burn, and tan easily (Table 2). Compared to individuals with a Fitzpatrick score of IV, individuals with a Fitzpatrick score of I have a relative risk of 2.09 developing melanoma [71]. A recent study demonstrated that pigment and race were not sufficient to predict an individual's Fitzpatrick score and sun sensitivity; this finding highlights the importance of physician-based counseling to all patients regarding sun safety and prevention of sun-induced malignancies [135].

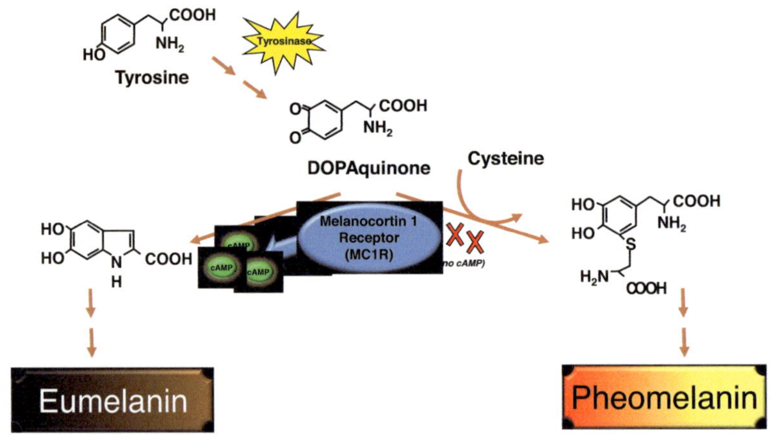

Figure 7. Synthesis of eumelanin and pheomelanin is regulated by the melanocortin 1 receptor (MC1R). Eumelanin, a dark brown/black pigment with excellent UV protective properties, is produced when melanocytes are stimulated through MC1R signaling and cytoplasmic cAMP levels are increased. In contrast, pheomelanin, a sulfated pigment with poorer UV-blocking properties is made when MC1R is inactive.

Phototype	Skin color	MED (mJ/cm^2 UV)	UV Response	Melanoma Risk
I	Ivory/pale white	15-30	Burns easily and strongly, never tans	++++
II	Very white	25-40	Burns easily, tans minimally with difficulty	+++/++++
III	White	30-50	Burns moderately, tans somewhat	+++/++
IV	Light brown, beige, olive	40-60	Burns minimally, tans moderately	++
V	Moderate brown	60-90	Rarely burns, tans well	+
VI	Dark brown/black	90-150	Never burns, tans profusely	+/-

Table 2. The Fitzpatrick scale of skin complexion. MED represents the minimal erythematous dose (the least amount of UV required to cause a sunburn).

4. Pigmentation and MC1R

The melanocortin 1 receptor (MC1R) is a major determinant of skin pigmentation and UV sensitivity. UV exposure activates the MC1R, which directly controls not only the adaptive tanning response (UV-induced pigmentation) but regulates melanocyte DNA repair and, thus, the mutagenic risk as well.

4.1. Eumelanin versus pheomelanin

Melanocytes, derived from neural crest cells, produce pigment in the skin. As described above, lack of basal skin pigmentation is a major risk factor for the development of melanoma. The two major types of pigment produced by the melanocyte are eumelanin and pheomelanin. Pigmentation depends on the type and amount of melanin produced in addition to its cellular distribution rather than number of melanocytes present in the skin [136-138]. Eumelanin is a dark insoluble polymer that absorbs UV light [139, 140] and oxidants [141], protecting DNA from the damaging effects of these factors. Pheomelanin is a soluble red/yellow polymer containing cysteine, which provides little protection from UV light and reports demonstrate that pheomelanin can promote oxidative damage [133, 142]. Synthesis of both eumelanin and pheomelanin begins with the conversion of tyrosine to DOPA and then to DOPAquinone via the enzyme tyrosinase [143]. Incorporation of a cysteine into DOPAquinone molecule eventually leads to the production of pheomelanin rather than eumelanin. Individuals without a functional tyrosinase are unable to produce any pigment and have a condition known as albinism [140]. Control of the ratio of pheomelanin to eumelanin in a cell is determined by multiple factors including pH of the cellular milieu and levels of the tyrosinase enzyme [133, 144]. Higher levels of tyrosinase and neutral pH favor eumelanin production and darker pigmentation [144, 145]. In addition to pH and tyrosinase, the melanocortin 1 receptor is one of the major factors controlling the pigment ratio.

4.2. MC1R and pigment switch

The melanocortin 1 receptor (MC1R) is one of the major proteins controlling the switch between the production of eumelanin and pheomelanin, and therefore is a one of the major control points of pigment production. Increased activation of MC1R by melanotropic hormones leads to an increase in tyrosinase expression and eumelanin production [146]. MC1R is a G-coupled protein receptor that is activated by alpha-melanocyte stimulating hormone (α-MSH) leading to the activation of adenylate cyclase and an accumulation of cAMP. cAMP promotes two pathways: 1) it activates protein kinase A (PKA) and 2) it up-regulates cAMP responsible binding element (CREB) and microphthalmia transcription factor (MITF); these factors ultimately cause an increased expression of enzymes involved in pigment production [136, 140, 147-149]. MC1R is a highly polymorphic protein with over 100 variants reported [150-152]. Five specific variants, D84E, R142H, R151C, R160W, and D294H, are associated with a decrease in pigment production and the red hair/fair skin phenotype [153-155]. These individuals are more susceptible to melanoma due to a decrease in eumelanin production coupled with inefficient DNA repair; this latter point suggests that MC1R plays a role not only in pigment production, but also in nucleotide excision repair [156, 157].

Studies using agouti signaling protein (ASIP) confirm the role of MC1R in the production of eumelanin. ASIP is a competitive antagonist of MSH and binds to MC1R causing an increase in the production of pheomelanin [158]. The effects of ASIP on melanocyte pigment production require a functional MC1R [158, 159]. The reduction in eumelanogenesis and increase in pheomelanogensis accompanied by ASIP signaling is only partially due to inhibition of MSH binding to MC1R. Binding of ASIP to MC1R causes a decrease in tyrosinase activity as well as tyrosinase related protein 1 and 2 protein levels, thus promoting pheomelanin synthesis [158-161]. ASIP also signals through a cAMP independent pathway via attractin and mahoguin to influence MC1R signaling and increase pheomelanin levels [162].

4.3. MC1R and adaptive pigmentation

The inability to have an adequate adaptive tanning response is a major risk factor for the development of melanoma. As explained above, the tanning response increases the production of pigment in the skin and serves as a protective barrier from the damaging effects of UV radiation. Adaptive pigmentation is dependent upon MC1R signaling [163]. UV radiation promotes cellular damage in keratinocytes, activating the damage response protein p53. p53 activation increases the transcription of proopiomelanocortin, which is processed and cleaved to MSH [164]. MSH is secreted from the keratinocytes and diffuses to the melanocyte membrane where it binds to and activates MC1R promoting the synthesis of eumelanin [146, 165]. Individuals with defective MC1R signaling, whether from inability of MC1R to bind to its ligands or from an inert response upon binding, cannot increase their pigment production following exposure to UV radiation and instead are highly susceptible to burning [163] (Figure 8).

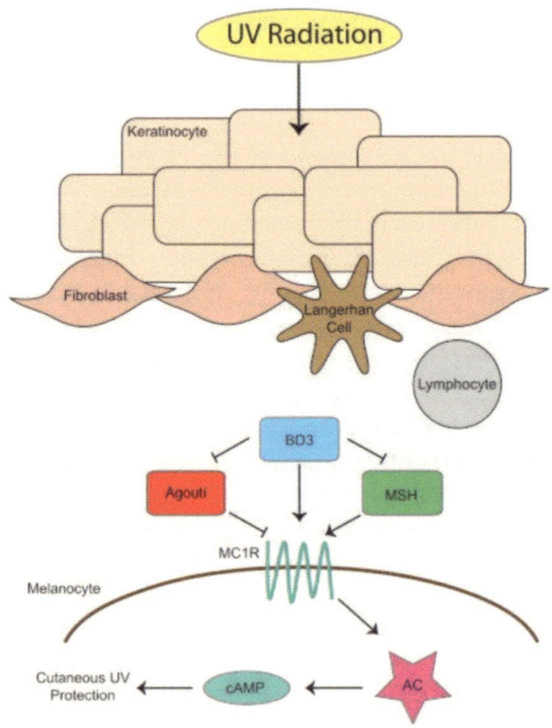

Figure 8. Cutaneous response to UV radiation. UV radiation induces the secretion of MSH and agouti signaling protein. MSH binds to MC1R and activates adenylyl cyclase (AC) which leads to the accumulation of cAMP. cAMP signaling to promote pathways responsible for cutaneous UV protection. Agouti signaling protein binds to MC1R and prevents activation of adenylyl cyclase inhibiting the adaptive tanning pathways.

Current research is investigating pharmacological methods to increase the tanning response in order to prevent damage, particularly in those individuals who have defective MC1R signaling. Forskolin is an activator of adenylyl cyclase and functions downstream of MC1R leading to an increase in the production of cAMP. Forskolin applied to a transgenic mouse model with humanized skin promoted the synthesis of eumelanin and adaptive pigmentation [166]. Phosphodiesterase inhibitors including rolipram prevent cAMP degradation and is hypothesized to have similar effects to forskolin. Rolipram is currently an FDA-approved drug and may have clinical applications for this condition.

5. Conclusion

The incidence of melanoma has dramatically increased throughout the past century. Although the cause for the increase is unknown, it is clear there are a number of environmental and genetic factors responsible for melanoma risk. The major environmental risk factor is exposure to UV radiation via ambient sunlight or artificial tanning beds. The intensity of the ambient sunlight varies with geography throughout the world. Countries located on latitudes closer to the equator have a higher incidence rate compared to countries located further away from the equator. Exposure to UV radiation, however, does not entirely explain the increase in melanoma diagnoses. Other environmental factors also play a role including certain medications (PUVA, NBLP) and exposure to heavy metals. Genetic factors also play a major role in melanoma risk. As melanoma often originates from pre-existing nevi, the presence of a large number of nevi, nevi with large diameters, or the presence of dysplastic nevi increase the risk. A past medical history of cutaneous or non-cutaneous cancer also increases the risk of subsequently developing melanoma. Although there are many intrinsic factors which play a role in determining one's risk of developing melanoma, the most important is the ability to produce pigment. Eumelanin protects the skin from UV induced damage. Individuals with fair skin and a low Fitzpatrick phototype are highly susceptible to melanoma. A subset of individuals with fair skin also has defective MC1R signaling and is unable to promote the adaptive tanning pathway. Clearly, much is known about the risk factors for developing melanoma, and hopefully as we better understand the pathogenesis of the disease, we will develop therapeutics and strategies to prevent melanoma from occurring.

Acknowledgements

We are indebted to Dr. Catherine Anthony of the Markey Cancer Center Research Communications Office for useful edits. This work was supported by the following NIH grants: R01 CA131075, UL1TR000117, ES07266, T32 ES007266, and T32CA165990. We also thank the Drury Pediatric Research Endowed Chair Fund, Wendy Will Case Cancer Research Fund, Markey Cancer Foundation, Children's Miracle Network, and Jennifer and David Dickens Melanoma Research Foundation.

Author details

Erin M. Wolf Horrell, Kalin Wilson and John A. D'Orazio*

*Address all correspondence to: jdorazio@uky.edu.

University of Kentucky College of Medicine, Markey Cancer Center, Department of Pediatrics, the Graduate Center for Toxicology and the Department of Physiology, Lexington, USA

References

[1] Surveillance, E., and End Results (SEER) Program (http://www.seer.cancer.gov) Research Data (1973-2011)National Cancer Institute, DCCPS, Surveillance Research Program, Surveillance Systems Branch, *SEER Stat Fact Sheets: Melanoma of the Skin*, April 2014.

[2] J, F., et al., *GLOBOCAN 2010 v1.0 Cancer Incidence and Mortality Worldwide: IARC CancerBase No. 11*, I.A.f.R.O. Cancer, Editor 2013: Lyon, France.

[3] Berquist, B.R. and D.M. Wilson, 3rd, *Pathways for repairing and tolerating the spectrum of oxidative DNA lesions.* Cancer Lett, 2012. 327(1-2): p. 61-72.

[4] Lens, M.B. and M. Dawes, *Global perspectives of contemporary epidemiological trends of cutaneous malignant melanoma.* Br J Dermatol, 2004. 150(2): p. 179-85.

[5] Rigel, D.S. and J.A. Carucci, *Malignant melanoma: prevention, early detection, and treatment in the 21st century.* CA Cancer J Clin, 2000. 50(4): p. 215-36; quiz 237-40.

[6] Linos, E., et al., *Increasing burden of melanoma in the United States.* J Invest Dermatol, 2009. 129(7): p. 1666-74.

[7] Mariotto, A.B., et al., *Projections of the cost of cancer care in the United States: 2010-2020.* J Natl Cancer Inst, 2011. 103(2): p. 117-28.

[8] Rigel, D.S., *The effect of sunscreen on melanoma risk.* Dermatol Clin, 2002. 20(4): p. 601-6.

[9] Balducci, L. and C. Beghe, *Cancer and age in the USA.* Crit Rev Oncol Hematol, 2001. 37(2): p. 137-45.

[10] Balk, S.J., D.E. Fisher, and A.C. Geller, *Teens and indoor tanning: a cancer prevention opportunity for pediatricians.* Pediatrics, 2013. 131(4): p. 772-85.

[11] Howlander N, N.A., Krapcho M et al., *SEER Cancer Statistics Review, 1975-2009.* Bethesda, MD: National Cancer Institute, 2002.

[12] Society, A.C., *Cancer Facts and Figures 2013*, 2013, American Cancer Society: Atlanta.

[13] Jemal, A., et al., *Cancer statistics, 2010.* CA Cancer J Clin, 2010. 60(5): p. 277-300.

[14] Fisher, D.E. and A.C. Geller, *Disproportionate burden of melanoma mortality in young U.S. men: the possible role of biology and behavior.* JAMA Dermatol, 2013. 149(8): p. 903-4.

[15] Purdue, M.P., et al., *Recent trends in incidence of cutaneous melanoma among US Caucasian young adults.* J Invest Dermatol, 2008. 128(12): p. 2905-8.

[16] Siegel, R., et al., *Cancer treatment and survivorship statistics, 2012.* CA Cancer J Clin, 2012. 62(4): p. 220-41.

[17] Mashiah, J. and S. Brenner, *Malignant melanoma: it pays to be a woman.* Skinmed, 2003. 2(3): p. 183-7.

[18] Hu S, S.-V.R., Parker DF, Kirsner RS, *Comparison of stage at diagnosis of melanoma among Hispanic, black, and white patients in Miami-Date County, Florida.* Arch Dermatol, 2006. 142(6): p. 704-708.

[19] Kumar, V., et al., *Robbins and Cotran Pathologic Basis of Disease.* Eighth ed, ed. W. Schmitt2010, Philadelphia, PA: Saunders.

[20] Gloster, H.M., Jr. and K. Neal, *Skin cancer in skin of color.* J Am Acad Dermatol, 2006. 55(5): p. 741-60; quiz 761-4.

[21] Rigel, D.S., *Epidemiology of melanoma.* Semin Cutan Med Surg, 2010. 29(4): p. 204-9.

[22] Parkin, D.M., D. Mesher, and P. Sasieni, *13. Cancers attributable to solar (ultraviolet) radiation exposure in the UK in 2010.* Br J Cancer, 2011. 105 Suppl 2: p. S66-9.

[23] Gilchrest, B.A., et al., *The pathogenesis of melanoma induced by ultraviolet radiation.* N Engl J Med, 1999. 340(17): p. 1341-8.

[24] Baier, J., et al., *Singlet oxygen generation by UVA light exposure of endogenous photosensitizers.* Biophys J, 2006. 91(4): p. 1452-9.

[25] Babu, V. and P.C. Joshi, *Tryptophan as an endogenous photosensitizer to elicit harmful effects of ultraviolet B.* Indian J Biochem Biophys, 1992. 29(3): p. 296-8.

[26] Davies, H., et al., *Mutations of the BRAF gene in human cancer.* Nature, 2002. 417(6892): p. 949-54.

[27] Sage, E., *Distribution and repair of photolesions in DNA: genetic consequences and the role of sequence context.* Photochem Photobiol, 1993. 57(1): p. 163-74.

[28] Tadokoro, T., et al., *UV-induced DNA damage and melanin content in human skin differing in racial/ethnic origin.* FASEB J, 2003. 17(9): p. 1177-9.

[29] Markovitsi, D., T. Gustavsson, and A. Banyasz, *Absorption of UV radiation by DNA: spatial and temporal features.* Mutat Res, 2009. 704(1-3): p. 21-8.

[30] Dumaz, N., et al., *The role of UV-B light in skin carcinogenesis through the analysis of p53 mutations in squamous cell carcinomas of hairless mice.* Carcinogenesis, 1997. 18(5): p. 897-904.

[31] Hodis, E., et al., *A landscape of driver mutations in melanoma.* Cell, 2012. 150(2): p. 251-63.

[32] Bulliard, J.L., *Site-specific risk of cutaneous malignant melanoma and pattern of sun exposure in New Zealand.* Int J Cancer, 2000. 85(5): p. 627-32.

[33] Armstrong, B.K. and A. Kricker, *The epidemiology of UV induced skin cancer.* J Photochem Photobiol B, 2001. 63(1-3): p. 8-18.

[34] Boniol, M., et al., *Seasonal variation in the occurrence of cutaneous melanoma in Europe: influence of latitude. An analysis using the EUROCARE group of registries.* Eur J Cancer, 2005. 41(1): p. 126-32.

[35] Moan, J., A. Dahlback, and R.B. Setlow, *Epidemiological support for an hypothesis for melanoma induction indicating a role for UVA radiation.* Photochem Photobiol, 1999. 70(2): p. 243-7.

[36] Lee, J.A. and J. Scotto, *Melanoma: linked temporal and latitude changes in the United States.* Cancer Causes Control, 1993. 4(5): p. 413-8.

[37] AIHW and AACR, *Cancer in Australia: an overview 2012.* Cancer series no. 742012, Canberra: AIHW. 216.

[38] Moan, J., et al., *Solar radiation, vitamin D and cancer incidence and mortality in Norway.* Anticancer Res, 2009. 29(9): p. 3501-9.

[39] Rigel, D.S., E.G. Rigel, and A.C. Rigel, *Effects of altitude and latitude on ambient UVB radiation.* J Am Acad Dermatol, 1999. 40(1): p. 114-6.

[40] Atkinson, S.K., et al., *Environmental factors affecting ultraviolet photodegradation rates and estrogenicity of estrone and ethinylestradiol in natural waters.* Arch Environ Contam Toxicol, 2011. 60(1): p. 1-7.

[41] Walter, S.D., W.D. King, and L.D. Marrett, *Association of cutaneous malignant melanoma with intermittent exposure to ultraviolet radiation: results of a case-control study in Ontario, Canada.* Int J Epidemiol, 1999. 28(3): p. 418-27.

[42] MacKie, R.M. and T. Aitchison, *Severe sunburn and subsequent risk of primary cutaneous malignant melanoma in scotland.* Br J Cancer, 1982. 46(6): p. 955-60.

[43] Lew, R.A., et al., *Sun exposure habits in patients with cutaneous melanoma: a case control study.* J Dermatol Surg Oncol, 1983. 9(12): p. 981-6.

[44] Holman, C.D. and B.K. Armstrong, *Cutaneous malignant melanoma and indicators of total accumulated exposure to the sun: an analysis separating histogenetic types.* J Natl Cancer Inst, 1984. 73(1): p. 75-82.

[45] Pfahlberg, A., K.F. Kolmel, and O. Gefeller, *Timing of excessive ultraviolet radiation and melanoma: epidemiology does not support the existence of a critical period of high susceptibility to solar ultraviolet radiation-induced melanoma.* Br J Dermatol, 2001. 144(3): p. 471-5.

[46] Robinson, J.K., *Sun exposure, sun protection, and vitamin D.* JAMA, 2005. 294(12): p. 1541-3.

[47] Hanson, K.M., E. Gratton, and C.J. Bardeen, *Sunscreen enhancement of UV-induced reactive oxygen species in the skin.* Free Radic Biol Med, 2006. 41(8): p. 1205-12.

[48] Xu, C., et al., *Photosensitization of the sunscreen octyl p-dimethylaminobenzoate by UVA in human melanocytes but not in keratinocytes.* Photochem Photobiol, 2001. 73(6): p. 600-4.

[49] Green, A.C., et al., *Reduced melanoma after regular sunscreen use: randomized trial follow-up.* J Clin Oncol, 2011. 29(3): p. 257-63.

[50] Kwon HT, M.J., Walker KK, Yu H, Lewis EC, Belch GE, *Promotion of frequent tanning sessions by indoor tanning facilities: two studies.* J Am Acad Dermatol, 2003. 46: p. 700-705.

[51] Swerdlow, A.J. and M.A. Weinstock, *Do tanning lamps cause melanoma? An epidemiologic assessment.* J Am Acad Dermatol, 1998. 38(1): p. 89-98.

[52] Demierre, M.F., *Time for the national legislation of indoor tanning to protect minors.* Arch Dermatol, 2003. 139(4): p. 520-4.

[53] Geller, A.C., et al., *Use of sunscreen, sunburning rates, and tanning bed use among more than 10 000 US children and adolescents.* Pediatrics, 2002. 109(6): p. 1009-14.

[54] Boniol, M., et al., *Cutaneous melanoma attributable to sunbed use: systematic review and meta-analysis.* BMJ, 2012. 345: p. e4757.

[55] Ting, W., et al., *Tanning bed exposure increases the risk of malignant melanoma.* Int J Dermatol, 2007. 46(12): p. 1253-7.

[56] Cancer, I.A.f.R.o.C.W.G.o.A.U.L.a.S., *The association of use of sunbeds with cutaneous malignant melanoma and other skin cancers: A systematic review.* Int J Cancer, 2007. 120(5): p. 1116-22.

[57] El Ghissassi, F., et al., *A review of human carcinogens--part D: radiation.* Lancet Oncol, 2009. 10(8): p. 751-2.

[58] Stern, R.S., *The risk of melanoma in association with long-term exposure to PUVA.* J Am Acad Dermatol, 2001. 44(5): p. 755-61.

[59] Csoma, Z., L. Kemeny, and J. Olah, *Phototherapy for neonatal jaundice.* N Engl J Med, 2008. 358(23): p. 2523-4; author reply 2524-5.

[60] Liebel, F., et al., *Irradiation of skin with visible light induces reactive oxygen species and matrix-degrading enzymes.* J Invest Dermatol, 2012. 132(7): p. 1901-7.

[61] Bauer, J., et al., *Blue light phototherapy of neonatal jaundice does not increase the risk for melanocytic nevus development.* Arch Dermatol, 2004. 140(4): p. 493-4.

[62] Matichard E, L.H.A., Sanders A, Leguyadec J, Crickx B, Descamps V, *Effect of neonatal phototherapy on melanocytic nevus count in children.* Arch Dermatol, 2006. 142(12): p. 1599-1604.

[63] Csoma, Z., et al., *Neonatal blue-light phototherapy could increase the risk of dysplastic nevus development.* Pediatrics, 2007. 119(6): p. 1269.

[64] Csoma, Z., et al., *Neonatal blue light phototherapy and melanocytic nevi: a twin study.* Pediatrics, 2011. 128(4): p. e856-64.

[65] Fortes, C. and E. de Vries, *Nonsolar occupational risk factors for cutaneous melanoma.* Int J Dermatol, 2008. 47(4): p. 319-28.

[66] Dong, S., et al., *UVA light-induced DNA cleavage by isomeric methylbenz[a]anthracenes.* Chem Res Toxicol, 2002. 15(3): p. 400-7.

[67] Imlay, J.A., S.M. Chin, and S. Linn, *Toxic DNA damage by hydrogen peroxide through the Fenton reaction in vivo and in vitro.* Science, 1988. 240(4852): p. 640-2.

[68] Marghoob, A.A., et al., *Basal cell and squamous cell carcinomas are important risk factors for cutaneous malignant melanoma. Screening implications.* Cancer, 1995. 75(2 Suppl): p. 707-14.

[69] Gandini, S., et al., *Meta-analysis of risk factors for cutaneous melanoma: III. Family history, actinic damage and phenotypic factors.* Eur J Cancer, 2005. 41(14): p. 2040-59.

[70] Pielop, J.A., I. Brownell, and M. Duvic, *Mycosis fungoides associated with malignant melanoma and dysplastic nevus syndrome.* Int J Dermatol, 2003. 42(2): p. 116-22.

[71] Gandini, S., et al., *Meta-analysis of risk factors for cutaneous melanoma: II. Sun exposure.* Eur J Cancer, 2005. 41(1): p. 45-60.

[72] Hemminki, K., H. Zhang, and K. Czene, *Familial and attributable risks in cutaneous melanoma: effects of proband and age.* J Invest Dermatol, 2003. 120(2): p. 217-23.

[73] Ferrone, C.R., et al., *Clinicopathological features of and risk factors for multiple primary melanomas.* JAMA, 2005. 294(13): p. 1647-54.

[74] Bradford PT, F.D., Goldstein AM, Tucker MA, *Increased risk of second primary cancers after a diagnosis of melanoma.* Arch Dermatol, 2010. 146(6): p. 265-72.

[75] Begg, C.B., et al., *Lifetime risk of melanoma in CDKN2A mutation carriers in a population-based sample.* J Natl Cancer Inst, 2005. 97(20): p. 1507-15.

[76] Tucker, M.A., et al., *Familial and cutaneous features of dysplastic nevi: a case-control study.* J Am Acad Dermatol, 1993. 28(4): p. 558-64.

[77] Clark, W.H., Jr., et al., *A study of tumor progression: the precursor lesions of superficial spreading and nodular melanoma.* Hum Pathol, 1984. 15(12): p. 1147-65.

[78] Kruger, S., et al., *Epidemiologic evidence for the role of melanocytic nevi as risk markers and direct precursors of cutaneous malignant melanoma. Results of a case control study in melanoma patients and nonmelanoma control subjects.* J Am Acad Dermatol, 1992. 26(6): p. 920-6.

[79] Bataille, V., et al., *Risk of cutaneous melanoma in relation to the numbers, types and sites of naevi: a case-control study.* Br J Cancer, 1996. 73(12): p. 1605-11.

[80] Reimer, R.R., et al., *Precursor lesions in familial melanoma. A new genetic preneoplastic syndrome.* JAMA, 1978. 239(8): p. 744-6.

[81] Lynch, H.T., B.C. Frichot, 3rd, and J.F. Lynch, *Familial atypical multiple mole-melanoma syndrome.* J Med Genet, 1978. 15(5): p. 352-6.

[82] Brose, M.S., et al., *BRAF and RAS mutations in human lung cancer and melanoma.* Cancer Res, 2002. 62(23): p. 6997-7000.

[83] Pollock, P.M., et al., *High frequency of BRAF mutations in nevi.* Nat Genet, 2003. 33(1): p. 19-20.

[84] Yazdi, A.S., et al., *Mutations of the BRAF gene in benign and malignant melanocytic lesions.* J Invest Dermatol, 2003. 121(5): p. 1160-2.

[85] Snels, D.G., et al., *Risk of cutaneous malignant melanoma in patients with nonfamilial atypical nevi from a pigmented lesions clinic.* J Am Acad Dermatol, 1999. 40(5 Pt 1): p. 686-93.

[86] Chang, Y.M., et al., *A pooled analysis of melanocytic nevus phenotype and the risk of cutaneous melanoma at different latitudes.* Int J Cancer, 2009. 124(2): p. 420-8.

[87] Garbe, C., et al., *Associated factors in the prevalence of more than 50 common melanocytic nevi, atypical melanocytic nevi, and actinic lentigines: multicenter case-control study of the Central Malignant Melanoma Registry of the German Dermatological Society.* J Invest Dermatol, 1994. 102(5): p. 700-5.

[88] Abadir, M.C., et al., *Case-control study of melanocytic nevi on the buttocks in atypical mole syndrome: role of solar radiation in the pathogenesis of atypical moles.* J Am Acad Dermatol, 1995. 33(1): p. 31-6.

[89] Kelly, J.W., et al., *Sunlight: a major factor associated with the development of melanocytic nevi in Australian schoolchildren.* J Am Acad Dermatol, 1994. 30(1): p. 40-8.

[90] Barnhill, R.L. and G.C. Roush, *Histopathologic spectrum of clinically atypical melanocytic nevi. II. Studies of nonfamilial melanoma.* Arch Dermatol, 1990. 126(10): p. 1315-8.

[91] Tsao, H., et al., *The transformation rate of moles (melanocytic nevi) into cutaneous melanoma: a population-based estimate.* Arch Dermatol, 2003. 139(3): p. 282-8.

[92] Tucker, M.A., et al., *Clinically recognized dysplastic nevi. A central risk factor for cutaneous melanoma.* JAMA, 1997. 277(18): p. 1439-44.

[93] Gandini, S., et al., *Meta-analysis of risk factors for cutaneous melanoma: I. Common and atypical naevi.* Eur J Cancer, 2005. 41(1): p. 28-44.

[94] Tucker, M.A., *Melanoma epidemiology.* Hematol Oncol Clin North Am, 2009. 23(3): p. 383-95, vii.

[95] Swerdlow, A.J., J.S. English, and Z. Qiao, *The risk of melanoma in patients with congenital nevi: a cohort study.* J Am Acad Dermatol, 1995. 32(4): p. 595-9.

[96] Krengel, S., A. Hauschild, and T. Schafer, *Melanoma risk in congenital melanocytic naevi: a systematic review.* Br J Dermatol, 2006. 155(1): p. 1-8.

[97] Marghoob, A.A., et al., *Large congenital melanocytic nevi, risk of cutaneous melanoma, and prophylactic surgery.* J Am Acad Dermatol, 2006. 54(5): p. 868-70; discussion 871-3.

[98] Lanoy, E., et al., *Epidemiology of nonkeratinocytic skin cancers among persons with AIDS in the United States.* AIDS, 2009. 23(3): p. 385-93.

[99] Olsen, C.M., L.L. Knight, and A.C. Green, *Risk of melanoma in people with HIV/AIDS in the pre-and post-HAART eras: a systematic review and meta-analysis of cohort studies.* PLoS One, 2014. 9(4): p. e95096.

[100] Dahlke, E., et al., *Systematic review of melanoma incidence and prognosis in solid organ transplant recipients.* Transplant Res, 2014. 3: p. 10.

[101] Frankenthaler, A., et al., *Impact of concomitant immunosuppression on the presentation and prognosis of patients with melanoma.* Melanoma Res, 2010. 20(6): p. 496-500.

[102] Brewer JD, C.L., Weaver AL, Dapprich DC, Weenig RH, Lim KK, Walsh JS, Otley CC, Cherikh W, Buell JF, Woodle ES, Arpey C, Patton PR, *Malignant melanoma in solid transplant recipients: collection of database cases and comparison with surveillance, epidemiology, and end results data for outcome analysis.* Arch Dermatol, 2011. 147(7): p. 790-6.

[103] Zwald, F.O., et al., *Melanoma in solid organ transplant recipients.* Am J Transplant, 2010. 10(5): p. 1297-304.

[104] Yang, G.B., et al., *Risk and survival of cutaneous melanoma diagnosed subsequent to a previous cancer.* Arch Dermatol, 2011. 147(12): p. 1395-402.

[105] Pappo, A.S., et al., *Melanoma as a subsequent neoplasm in adult survivors of childhood cancer: a report from the childhood cancer survivor study.* Pediatr Blood Cancer, 2013. 60(3): p. 461-6.

[106] Hayat, M.J., et al., *Cancer statistics, trends, and multiple primary cancer analyses from the Surveillance, Epidemiology, and End Results (SEER) Program.* Oncologist, 2007. 12(1): p. 20-37.

[107] Karagas, M.R., et al., *Pregnany history and incidence of melanoma in women: a pooled analysis.* Cancer Causes Control, 2006. 17(1): p. 11-9.

[108] Elling, S.V. and F.C. Powell, *Physiological changes in the skin during pregnancy.* Clin Dermatol, 1997. 15(1): p. 35-43.

[109] Thoma, B.S. and K.M. Vasquez, *Critical DNA damage recognition functions of XPC-hHR23B and XPA-RPA in nucleotide excision repair.* Mol Carcinog, 2003. 38(1): p. 1-13.

[110] Setlow, R.B. and W.L. Carrier, *The Disappearance of Thymine Dimers from DNA: An Error-Correcting Mechanism.* Proc Natl Acad Sci U S A, 1964. 51: p. 226-31.

[111] Boyce, R.P. and P. Howard-Flanders, *Release of Ultraviolet Light-Induced Thymine Dimers from DNA in E. Coli K-12.* Proc Natl Acad Sci U S A, 1964. 51: p. 293-300.

[112] Setlow, R.B., P.A. Swenson, and W.L. Carrier, *Thymine Dimers and Inhibition of DNA Synthesis by Ultraviolet Irradiation of Cells.* Science, 1963. 142(3598): p. 1464-6.

[113] Setlow, R.B. and J.K. Setlow, *Evidence that ultraviolet-induced thymine dimers in DNA cause biological damage.* Proc Natl Acad Sci U S A, 1962. 48: p. 1250-7.

[114] Sugasawa, K., et al., *Xeroderma pigmentosum group C protein complex is the initiator of global genome nucleotide excision repair.* Mol Cell, 1998. 2(2): p. 223-32.

[115] Sugasawa, K., et al., *A multistep damage recognition mechanism for global genomic nucleotide excision repair.* Genes Dev, 2001. 15(5): p. 507-21.

[116] Gerard, M., et al., *Purification and interaction properties of the human RNA polymerase B(II) general transcription factor BTF2.* J Biol Chem, 1991. 266(31): p. 20940-5.

[117] Park, C.J. and B.S. Choi, *The protein shuffle. Sequential interactions among components of the human nucleotide excision repair pathway.* FEBS J, 2006. 273(8): p. 1600-8.

[118] Tapias, A., et al., *Ordered conformational changes in damaged DNA induced by nucleotide excision repair factors.* J Biol Chem, 2004. 279(18): p. 19074-83.

[119] Mu, D., D.S. Hsu, and A. Sancar, *Reaction mechanism of human DNA repair excision nuclease.* J Biol Chem, 1996. 271(14): p. 8285-94.

[120] Houtsmuller, A.B., et al., *Action of DNA repair endonuclease ERCC1/XPF in living cells.* Science, 1999. 284(5416): p. 958-61.

[121] Shivji, M.K., et al., *Nucleotide excision repair DNA synthesis by DNA polymerase epsilon in the presence of PCNA, RFC, and RPA.* Biochemistry, 1995. 34(15): p. 5011-7.

[122] Mellon, I., G. Spivak, and P.C. Hanawalt, *Selective removal of transcription-blocking DNA damage from the transcribed strand of the mammalian DHFR gene.* Cell, 1987. 51(2): p. 241-9.

[123] Mu, D. and A. Sancar, *Model for XPC-independent transcription-coupled repair of pyrimidine dimers in humans.* J Biol Chem, 1997. 272(12): p. 7570-3.

[124] Kamiuchi, S., et al., *Translocation of Cockayne syndrome group A protein to the nuclear matrix: possible relevance to transcription-coupled DNA repair.* Proc Natl Acad Sci U S A, 2002. 99(1): p. 201-6.

[125] Donahue, B.A., et al., *Transcript cleavage by RNA polymerase II arrested by a cyclobutane pyrimidine dimer in the DNA template.* Proc Natl Acad Sci U S A, 1994. 91(18): p. 8502-6.

[126] Venema, J., et al., *Xeroderma pigmentosum complementation group C cells remove pyrimidine dimers selectively from the transcribed strand of active genes.* Mol Cell Biol, 1991. 11(8): p. 4128-34.

[127] Li, C., et al., *Polymorphisms in the DNA repair genes XPC, XPD, and XPG and risk of cutaneous melanoma: a case-control analysis.* Cancer Epidemiol Biomarkers Prev, 2006. 15(12): p. 2526-32.

[128] Paszkowska-Szczur, K., et al., *Xeroderma pigmentosum genes and melanoma risk.* Int J Cancer, 2013. 133(5): p. 1094-100.

[129] Eugene, D.W. and K.D. Joshi, *Xeroderma pigmentosa--a disfiguring disease.* Kathmandu Univ Med J (KUMJ), 2006. 4(1): p. 78-81.

[130] D'Errico, M., et al., *UV mutation signature in tumor suppressor genes involved in skin carcinogenesis in xeroderma pigmentosum patients.* Oncogene, 2000. 19(3): p. 463-7.

[131] Cleaver, J.E., *Defective repair replication of DNA in xeroderma pigmentosum.* Nature, 1968. 218(5142): p. 652-6.

[132] Bradford, P.T., et al., *Cancer and neurologic degeneration in xeroderma pigmentosum: long term follow-up characterises the role of DNA repair.* J Med Genet, 2011. 48(3): p. 168-76.

[133] Mitra, D., et al., *An ultraviolet-radiation-independent pathway to melanoma carcinogenesis in the red hair/fair skin background.* Nature, 2012. 491(7424): p. 449-53.

[134] Fitzpatrick, T.B., *Soleil et peau.* J Med Esthet, 1975. 2: p. 33-4.

[135] He, S.Y., et al., *Self-reported pigmentary phenotypes and race are significant but incomplete predictors of Fitzpatrick skin phototype in an ethnically diverse population.* J Am Acad Dermatol, 2014.

[136] D'Orazio, J., et al., *UV Radiation and the Skin.* Int J Mol Sci, 2013. 14(6): p. 12222-48.

[137] Rees, J.L., *Genetics of hair and skin color.* Annu Rev Genet, 2003. 37: p. 67-90.

[138] Dessinioti, C., et al., *Melanocortin 1 receptor variants: functional role and pigmentary associations.* Photochem Photobiol, 2011. 87(5): p. 978-87.

[139] Kaidbey, K.H., K.H. Grove, and A.M. Kligman, *The influence of longwave ultraviolet radiation on sunburn cell production by UVB.* J Invest Dermatol, 1979. 73(3): p. 743-5.

[140] Scherer, D. and R. Kumar, *Genetics of pigmentation in skin cancer--a review.* Mutat Res, 2010. 705(2): p. 141-53.

[141] Hoogduijn, M.J., et al., *Melanin protects melanocytes and keratinocytes against H2O2-induced DNA strand breaks through its ability to bind Ca2+.* Exp Cell Res, 2004. 294(1): p. 60-7.

[142] Thody, A.J., et al., *Pheomelanin as well as eumelanin is present in human epidermis.* J Invest Dermatol, 1991. 97(2): p. 340-4.

[143] Riley, P.A., *Melanin.* Int J Biochem Cell Biol, 1997. 29(11): p. 1235-9.

[144] Ancans, J., et al., *Melanosomal pH controls rate of melanogenesis, eumelanin/phaeomelanin ratio and melanosome maturation in melanocytes and melanoma cells.* Exp Cell Res, 2001. 268(1): p. 26-35.

[145] Burchill, S.A., A.J. Thody, and S. Ito, *Melanocyte-stimulating hormone, tyrosinase activity and the regulation of eumelanogenesis and phaeomelanogenesis in the hair follicular melanocytes of the mouse.* J Endocrinol, 1986. 109(1): p. 15-21.

[146] Suzuki, I., et al., *Binding of melanotropic hormones to the melanocortin receptor MC1R on human melanocytes stimulates proliferation and melanogenesis.* Endocrinology, 1996. 137(5): p. 1627-33.

[147] Yasumoto, K., et al., *Microphthalmia-associated transcription factor as a regulator for melanocyte-specific transcription of the human tyrosinase gene.* Mol Cell Biol, 1994. 14(12): p. 8058-70.

[148] Bertolotto, C., et al., *A SUMOylation-defective MITF germline mutation predisposes to melanoma and renal carcinoma.* Nature, 2011. 480(7375): p. 94-8.

[149] Bertolotto, C., et al., *Regulation of tyrosinase gene expression by cAMP in B16 melanoma cells involves two CATGTG motifs surrounding the TATA box: implication of the microphthalmia gene product.* J Cell Biol, 1996. 134(3): p. 747-55.

[150] Seabrook, T.J., et al., *A novel mechanism of immune regulation: interferon-gamma regulates retention of CD4 T cells during delayed type hypersensitivity.* Immunology, 2005. 116(2): p. 184-92.

[151] Perez Oliva, A.B., et al., *Identification and functional analysis of novel variants of the human melanocortin 1 receptor found in melanoma patients.* Hum Mutat, 2009. 30(5): p. 811-22.

[152] Gerstenblith, M.R., et al., *Comprehensive evaluation of allele frequency differences of MC1R variants across populations.* Hum Mutat, 2007. 28(5): p. 495-505.

[153] Valverde, P., et al., *Variants of the melanocyte-stimulating hormone receptor gene are associated with red hair and fair skin in humans.* Nat Genet, 1995. 11(3): p. 328-30.

[154] Flanagan, N., et al., *The relation between melanocortin 1 receptor genotype and experimentally assessed ultraviolet radiation sensitivity.* J Invest Dermatol, 2001. 117(5): p. 1314-7.

[155] Box, N.F., et al., *Characterization of melanocyte stimulating hormone receptor variant alleles in twins with red hair.* Hum Mol Genet, 1997. 6(11): p. 1891-7.

[156] Bohm, M., et al., *alpha-Melanocyte-stimulating hormone protects from ultraviolet radiation-induced apoptosis and DNA damage.* J Biol Chem, 2005. 280(7): p. 5795-802.

[157] Hauser, J.E., et al., *Melanin content and MC1R function independently affect UVR-induced DNA damage in cultured human melanocytes.* Pigment Cell Res, 2006. 19(4): p. 303-14.

[158] Suzuki, I., et al., *Agouti signaling protein inhibits melanogenesis and the response of human melanocytes to alpha-melanotropin.* J Invest Dermatol, 1997. 108(6): p. 838-42.

[159] Abdel-Malek, Z.A., et al., *The melanocortin 1 receptor is the principal mediator of the effects of agouti signaling protein on mammalian melanocytes.* J Cell Sci, 2001. 114(Pt 5): p. 1019-24.

[160] Sakai, C., et al., *Modulation of murine melanocyte function in vitro by agouti signal protein.* EMBO J, 1997. 16(12): p. 3544-52.

[161] Hunt, G. and A.J. Thody, *Agouti protein can act independently of melanocyte-stimulating hormone to inhibit melanogenesis.* J Endocrinol, 1995. 147(2): p. R1-4.

[162] Hida, T., et al., *Agouti protein, mahogunin, and attractin in pheomelanogenesis and melanoblast-like alteration of melanocytes: a cAMP-independent pathway.* Pigment Cell Melanoma Res, 2009. 22(5): p. 623-34.

[163] D'Orazio, J.A., et al., *Topical drug rescue strategy and skin protection based on the role of Mc1r in UV-induced tanning.* Nature, 2006. 443(7109): p. 340-4.

[164] Cui, R., et al., *Central role of p53 in the suntan response and pathologic hyperpigmentation.* Cell, 2007. 128(5): p. 853-64.

[165] Hunt, G., et al., Nle4DPhe7 alpha-melanocyte-stimulating hormone increases the eumelanin:phaeomelanin ratio in cultured human melanocytes. J Invest Dermatol, 1995. 104(1): p. 83-5.

[166] Amaro-Ortiz, A., et al., Pharmacologic induction of epidermal melanin and protection against sunburn in a humanized mouse model. J Vis Exp, 2013(79).

Chapter 2

Acral Melanoma — A Distinct Molecular and Clinical Subtype

R. Barra-Martínez, N.E. Herrera-González,
F. Fernández –Ramírez and L.A. Torres

Additional information is available at the end of the chapter

http://dx.doi.org/10.5772/59093

1. Introduction

Skin cancer represents one-third of all cancers that are diagnosed every year worldwide. From all types of skin cancer, cutaneous melanoma is the least frequent among this group of malignant tumors, it is however, the most highly invasive and metastatic tumor. It has also shown an important growth of around 150% in its appearance since 1971, having an estimation of 76,250 new cases diagnosed in the USA in 2012. In 1971 there was only 1 case in 600 white people. In the period of 1992 to 2004, its annual growth was of 3.1%. This led to an estimated incidence of 1 in every 90 white people by 2000. By 2010 it was 1 in every 50, for people above 50 years old in the USA. Its epidemiological importance lies in its high mortality rate, since it is the cause of 90% of deaths for skin cancer and it is potentially the most dangerous form of skin tumor [1]. The outlook for patients with advanced melanoma is often fatal due to a lack of effective treatments.

In Mexico, melanoma incidence is around 1.7 per 100 000 people, and the Histopathologic Record of Malignancies in 2001 reported that it is the second most frequent. Women are the gender most affected by Melanoma (1.6/1). The median age of presentation in this country is 54 years and in 77% of the cases there is no relation to sun exposure. On the other hand, it is important to point out that there is a lack of formal registration of neoplasias in health institutions of our nation [1, 2, 3].

There are four clinicopathological subtypes that Melanoma presents, which usually are correlated to ethnic differences and to exposition to UV radiation: Superficial spreading melanoma (SSM), Lentigo maligna melanoma (LMM), Nodular melanoma (NM) and Acral lentiginous melanoma (ALM) [1, 4]. SSM and LMM, are the most common among Caucasians and their presence has been directly related to sun exposure. Nodular melanoma is less frequent (10%) than SSM (70%), but both melanomas share pigmentary characteristics in patients. It is probable, however, that these two types of melanoma have a direct relation with sun exposure. However, this risk factor has not been proven in NM, given that this type can be found in any place on the body, not just in skin areas frequently exposed to sun light.

The most frequent subtypes of Melanoma in our population are, NM and ALM [4, 5] (Figure 1). Studies supporting the hypothesis that ALM may be a biological and genetically different subtype, will be mentioned in the following sections. Its distinct development pattern suggests that it may possess molecular and cellular uniqueness.

This may be because of different genetic alterations that control the transformation of melanocytes to acral melanoma, leading to the need for a specific-therapeutic target towards this subtype of melanoma with a high rate among Mexicans and Latin-Americans.

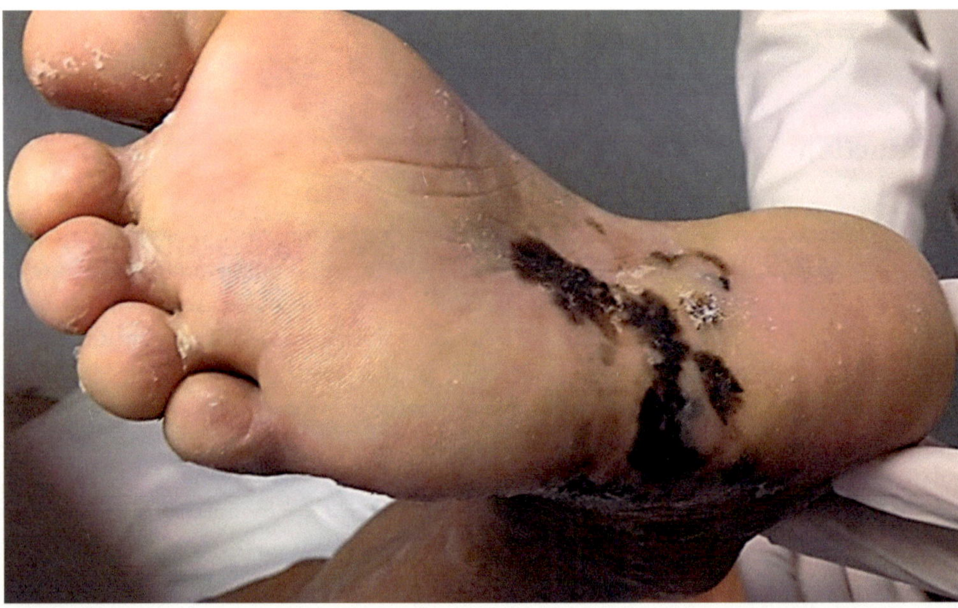

Figure 1. An indolent ALM subtype on the foot of a 58-year-old male patient, with 8 months of evolution. Nodular melanoma (NM) and Acral Lentiginous Melanoma (ALM) are the most frequent subtypes of Melanoma in our population. The lower extremities (mainly on the feet) are the most common anatomic locations reported for ALM.

2. Risk factors

Several studies have identified certain variables associated with an increased risk of developing melanoma: European ancestry, phenotype, UV radiation exposure, personal or family history of malignant melanoma, and molecular alterations are some of the most relevant [6]. Genetic alterations, will receive particularly emphasis later in this review. It is important to mention, that the risk factors traditionally associated with melanoma are related principally to Caucasians, where most clinical and basic studies are carried out. However, there are not enough studies supporting the predisposition of such factors for the subtypes of melanoma occuring in Mexican or Latin-American population.

Yamaguchi et al, reported that the risk factors traditionally described such as UV exposure, have a small influence in the pathogenesis of dark skin population. It has been postulated that UV radiation plays a smaller role in the pathogenesis of melanoma in the darker-skinned population. This is due to the fact that with an increase in melanin content, the larger melanosomes (in darker skin), absorb and scatter more energy than the smaller ones in lighter skin [7].

3. Sun exposure

Although various phenotypic characteristics enhance or reduce the risk of developing melanoma, sun exposure has been reported as the main cause of SSM, LMM and NM subtypes. The incidence of this disease is much higher in people who tend to burn rather than tan. (8)

UVA rays constitute 90% of solar radiation. However, UVB rays are greater risks for those who traditionally work or have recreational and daily activities outside. Among those with SSM and LMM, 75% of the affected individuals are sunburned by UVB rays. However, ALM has not been related to this risk factor. In addition, it is known that excessive sun exposure at early ages (childhood and adolescence) has a negative outcome in DNA reparation. The most important exogenous factor for melanoma is UV radiation exposure, particularly intermittent exposition, and it is known as the only etiological agent that can be modified. The increase in sun exposure and the damage to higher levels of the atmosphere because of contamination has resulted in an increase of the amount of radiation [9,10,11].

Sun exposure increases the expression of α-melanocyte stimulating hormone (α-MSH) and of the peptides of pro-opiomelanocortin in the skin. Melanocyte- stimulating hormone belongs to a group called the melanocortins. α-MSH is the most important melanocortin for pigmentation and shows a high affinity for melanocyte stimulating hormone receptor (MSHR). Once α-MSH binds to MSHR, cellular cAMP is activated, as well as other signal transduction pathways. The final result is the production of eumelanin.

Eumelanin, the primary pigment that colors the skin, hair and eyes in humans, also protects the body from UV and other hazardous radiations that can damage skin cells. When eumelanin has been crystalized, it forms both a geometric and a chemical disorder at the same time. It turns out that both kinds of disorders, may play a complementary role in producing eumelanin's broadband absorption. The tiny crystals of eumelanin have a chemically ordered state with intrinsic randomness: the orientations of the stacked molecules are arbitrary and the sizes of the crystals are different. That combination of order and disorder contributes to eumelanin's broadband absorption (12). Recently, it was reported that eumelanin is a naturally existing nanocomposite that has very critical macroscopic properties as a result of its nanostructure properties. All eumelanin molecules share very similar chemistry, although there are more than 100 variations. It has been proposed that the small variations from one molecule to another may contribute to the disorder that broadens the ability to absorb UV light (13).

Additionally, different alleles for melanocortin 1 receptor (MC1R) gene have been identified. The subtypes related to loss of function reduce the production of cAMP after stimulation of α-MSH, and thus increase the expression of pheomelanin. This is observed in individuals of light skin, increasing the risk of developing melanoma by the formation of free radicals after UV ray exposure.

Recently, a study was performed in 789 patients with diagnosis of melanoma. In order to characterize these patients according to their levels of sun exposure, three groups were established in the study: intermittent, chronic, and absence of exposure [14]. The vast majority of patients were in the first group. These melanomas were present in skin locations exposed to sun radiation in an intermittent manner. SSM and NM belong to this group. Multiple common and atypical nevi may constitute a marker of risk of these melanomas. The second group was formed by patients with melanomas in skin areas with chronic sun exposure, showing all the damage and premise typical of this location. LMM belongs to this group. Finally, the third group corresponds to melanomas present in skin areas with no sun exposure, usually diagnosed in late stages. This group includes ALM and mucosa melanoma, which usually are thicker at diagnosis and have worse prognosis [15, 16, 17]

4. Acral lentiginous melanoma

Acral lentiginous melanoma (ALM) distinguishes itself from the other subtypes for many characteristics, mainly histological and clinical-prognostic. A huge controversy regarding the cause of its worse prognosis, has been going on since its description.

ALM usually occurs on palmoplantar or subungual areas (Fig 2), lacking hair. Similar to NM, it is very aggressive when its proliferative vertical phase develops. It is more commonly found in individuals with dark skin (35-60%), oriental population and Afro-Caribbean. Considering its localization, it is thought to be UV-protected by the thickened stratum corneum and the nail matrix. ALM is rare in Caucasian populations (1-5%), but has a higher incidence among our population and Latin-Americans with dark skin(8, 9, 18). However, for individuals with lighter skin in our population, SSM is the most frequent.

According to the data of The National Cancer Institute Surveillance, Epidemiology and End Results, ALM is the least frequent histological subtype in the USA, with a 2-3% frequency. However, it shows a higher percentage among afroamerican people and Asians.

Reed described for the first time ALM as pigmented lesions of the extremities, mainly of the plantar and palmar regions, that were characterized by a phase of lentiginous (radial) growth, which evolved in months or years to the invasive vertical phase.(19)

Arrington was the first to notice that this type of melanoma was more prevalent among the African American population and that their prognosis was less favorable due to being diagnosed at an advanced stage. Yet, it was not documented by the SEER as a different histological subtype until 1986 [20]. Usually, ALM is not associated with nevi, family history or gene susceptibility known to melanoma. In its great majority, ALM are diagnosed as thick melanomas which in most cases are usually presented in their late phase, with a worse prognosis and a lower survival rate than the most common subtypes of melanoma associated with chronic sun exposure [20].

Pereda et al, reported the Clinical presentation of ALM in patients from Spain. In seventeen of them, ALM was found on a foot and in six on a hand. Four ALMs of the hand were subungueal. Most of the foot ALMs were located on the sole (twelve cases) [22].

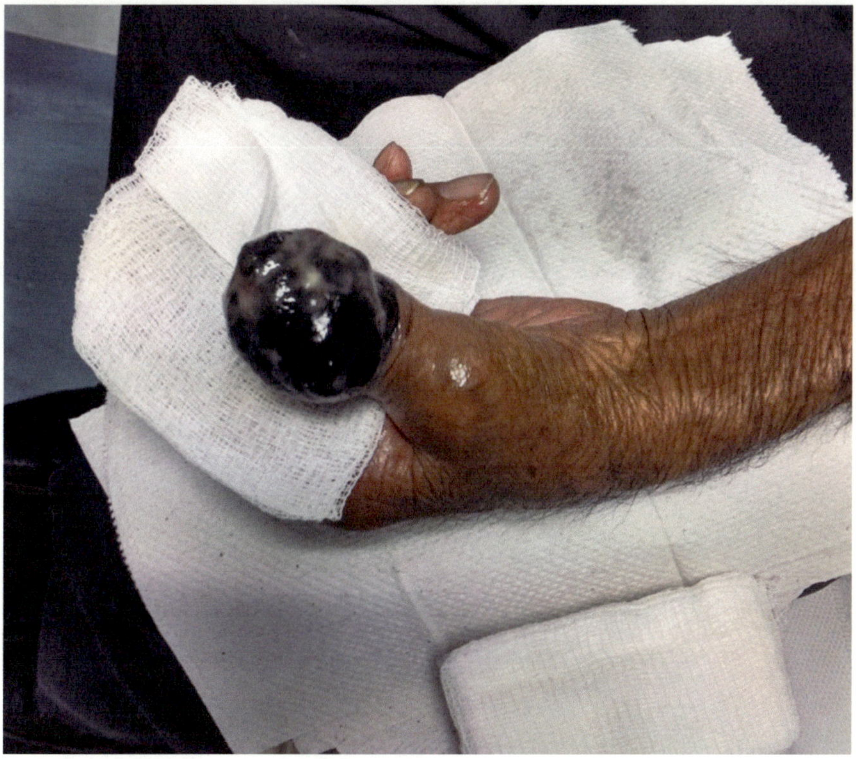

Figure 2. A subungueal tumor of a 71-year-old male patient with an advanced ALM (thick Breslow), on the thumb of the left hand. ALM is the most prevalent subtype in Mexicans and LatinAmericans. It is usually found on hands and feet: palms and soles, wrists and heels, and under the nails. ALM and NM are usually diagnosed in later stages, unlike SSM and LMM. The most affected sites are by far the feet and nails. Initially, they may be misdiagnosed as a mole, an ulcer, an abscess, a wart, a nail bed dystrophy or as the result of a trauma.

The most frequent location of ALM is in the feet (Figure 1), mainly the plantar region and the first finger, as in subungual areas in the majority of non caucasians racial groups. This has led to the conclusion that trauma may be an important factor of ALM, and not sun exposure [22]. Even when the superficial region of the palms and plantar region are similar, in the plantar region there is a continuous exposure to pressure, friction, maceration and irritation. Nevertheless, there are counterarguments towards this theory, including that the hands are more exposed to UV radiation and acute trauma. In addition, it has not been possible to prove changes in the incidence of plantar melanoma when some African tribes began urbanization and the use of shoes.

Another important factor in the predominance of plantar ALM, is the fact that there is a 50% greater amount of melanocytes there than in the palms [23, 24]. The research of Ghadially proposed that trauma during less than 12 months, did not increase the risk of melanoma in the Xiphophorus fish model [25]. Troyanova [26] described mechanical trauma on previous pigmented skin lesions as a risk factor for the formation of melanoma and remarks that trauma has to be carefully checked. Recently, an amelanotic subungueal melanoma arising after trauma was reported by Rangwala [27]. Melanomas formed on burns scars and tattoos have also been frequently publishedin recent years.Of 687 Chinese melanoma patients, 15.2% showed a strong association between trauma in the extremities and melanoma [28].

Clinical experience coming from medical attention given to patients of melanoma treated in two of the major oncological centers of our nation, shows that AM occurs in no photo exposed areas [5], mainly in lower extremities (more than 80% of the cases) and in subungual regions (Figure 3). This information has been reported by the Mixed Tumor Unit from the Oncologic Service (General Hospital of Mexico) and the Dermatologic Center "Ladislao de La Pascua", Mexico City [18]

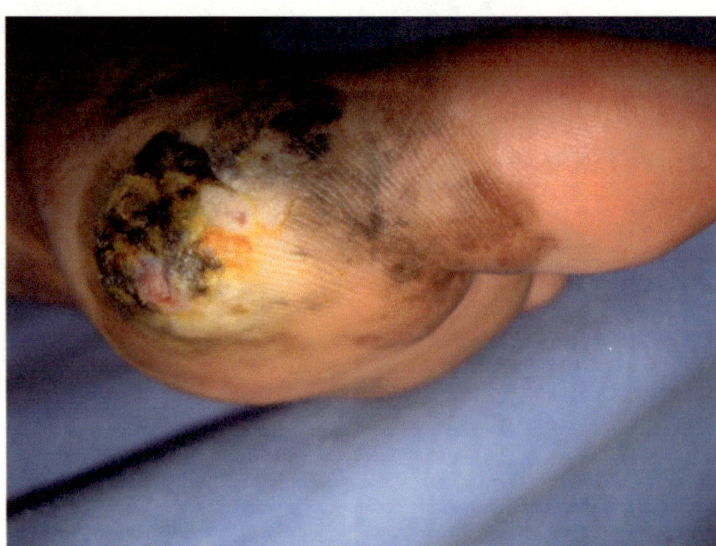

Figure 3. ALM on the foot of a 61-year-old male patient, with indolent growth. The Oncology Unit of the General Hospital of Mexico reports that more than 50% of ALMs are presented on the lower extremities (mainly on the soles and subungueal areas. Being the toe by far, the most affected).

http://dx.doi.org/10.5772/59093

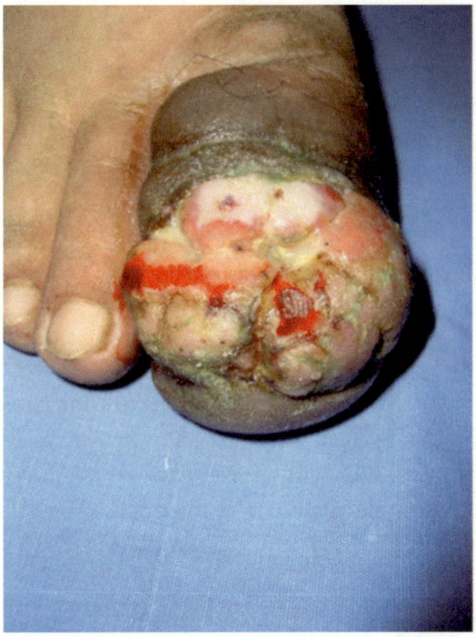

Figure 4. A subungueal tumor of a 54-year-old male patient with an advanced amelanic melanoma. ALMs are usually diagnosed in the later stages unlike SSM and LMM. It was misdiagnosed as a bleeding ulcer of progressive growth.

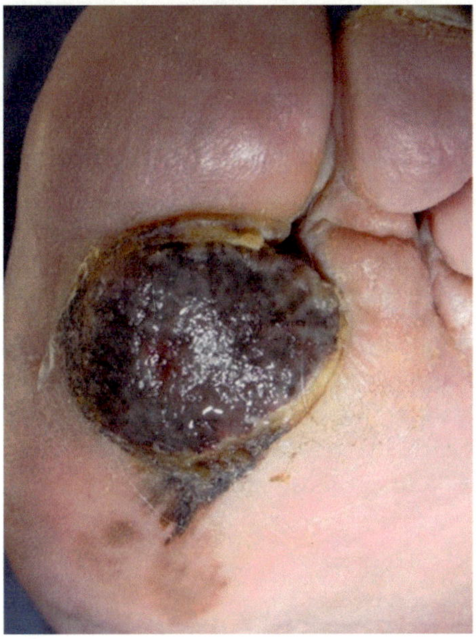

Figure 5. A plantar tumor of a 65-year-old male patient. The lower extremity is the most common anatomic location reported for mexicans. Initially this case was diagnosed as a pigmented lesion of a fast vertical phase progression.

5. Molecular alterations in melanoma

Melanoma arises through a complex process of cellular mutations and a loss of keratinocyte control over growth and differentiation. As malignant melanoma progresses, it develops through interaction between dysfunctional melanocytes and the tumor microenvironment. This in turn, allows the formation of nevocyte nests at the demal-epidermal junction and is accompanied with changes in both, keratinocytes and local adhesion molecules (29). The progression from healthy melanocyte to melanoma occurs through mutations within the tumor and through alterations of the cellular environment.

In the skin, tissue homeostasis is critical in cellular regulation and melanoma breaks this regulation through multiple processes. Defining intercellular molecular dialogues in human skin promises to provide key information about the transformation of melanocyte to melanoma. A great number of genes and proteins have been reported to play an essential role in this transformation. The most important are: B-RAF, c-KIT, PTEN, p16, p53, cyclin1, ARF, K-RAS (30).

6. Familial melanoma

It has been reported by a meta-analysis that the presence of at least one-first degree relative with melanoma increases to double or more, the risk of developing this disease.

Many genetic studies in melanoma-prone families lead to the identification of *CDKN2A* as the main familial melanoma gene. This gene is located at the chromosome 9p21 region. *CDKN2A* encodes two different proteins: INK4A (p16) and ARF (p14). In order to produce these two proteins, the use of alternative promoters and different first exons is necessary. Exon 1α is used for INK4A and 1β for ARF. The second exons of the two transcripts are translated in distinct reading frames, encoding two completely different proteins (with no amino acid homology). Nevertheless, both proteins share potent anticancer activities. *INK4A* inhibits the G1 cyclin-dependent kinases (CDKs) 4/6, which phosphorylate and inactivates the retinoblastoma protein (RB). After that, the S-phase is allowed to occur. Loss of INK4A function promotes RB inactivation resulting in cell cycle progression. *ARF* (Alternative Reading Frame) inhibits MDM2 mediated ubiquitination and degradation of p53. Loss of ARF, inactivates p53. Alterations of p16 are associated to familial melanoma in 20% and in 40% to sporadic melanoma [31].

7. Melanomas with intermitent sun exposure

As it was mentioned earlier, more than 90% of melanomas are diagnosed in white and light skinned populations. The majority of the international studies have addressed these populations, since they are at higher risk of developing melanoma. Thus, most reports are drawn from data of white and light skinned populations. The main alterations reported in SSM and NM, are B-RAF and N-RAS mutations.

7.1. BRAF

It is a tyrosine and threonine kinase that participates in the signal transduction known as Ras/Raf/MEK/ERK/MAP kinase. *BRAF* functions to regulate the MAPK/ERK pathway, which is conserved in all eukaryotes. This pathway acts as a signal transducer between the extracellular environment and the nucleus, activating downstream transcription factors to induce a range of biochemical processes including growth and differentiation, proliferation and migration associated to the ability of tissue invading [32, 33, 34]. Through direct secuentiation of PCR products, three substitutions of simple bases have been demonstrated. The most prevalent (95% of the cases) is constituted by the transversion of T1799A, occurring on exon 15 of *BRAF*, and causes the substitution of the amino acid valine for glutamic acid in position 599 (V599E). Such position has recently been modified to V600E.

Other *BRAF* mutations that cause carcinogenesis exist, such as K601E or those affecting exon 11, but they rarely occur in melanoma. A fusion of *BRAF* to *AKAP9*, by a paracentromeric inversion of the long arm of chromosome 7 has been observed in cases associated to ionized radiation exposure. This produces an oncogene, *AKAP9-BRAF*, which also results in a constitutive activation of the MAP kinase pathway [35, 36, 37].

Exon 15 BRAF mutations in melanoma were first reported in 2002. The number of reports of BRAF mutations in primary melanoma tissue increases continually. Varying prevalences in primary melanoma tissue have been detected, from 41% to 88% in SSM. These BRAF alterations alone, are not capable of demonstrating neither the immortalization of malignant cells, nor the progression of the disease further more than a nevus [37].

A pilot BRAF mutation study in ALM patients was carried out by collaboration between the Genetic Service of the General Hospital of Mexico and the Molecular Oncology Laboratory of the School of Medicine at the National Polytechnic Institute. DNA sequencing of seven ALM samples of Mexican patients (General Hospital of Mexico) showed no T1799A mutation in any of the studied samples (M. Sc. Thesis, 2012) [38].

7.2. NRAS

RAS are among the most frequently mutated oncogenes in human cancers. They show different mutation patterns and spectrums in all members: *NRAS*, *HRAS* and *KRAS*. The isoforms share a high degree of similarity, although each one displays preferential coupling to particular cancer types.

RAS play a fundamental role in the signaling pathway of MAP kinase. Extracellular signals such as hormones, cytokines, and various growth factors interact with their receptors to activate the small G-proteins of the RAS family. This pathway includes *BRAF* and it contributes to the control of cellular proliferation, particularly malignant cell proliferation. *RAS* also controls apoptosis through the PI3K-PTEN-Akt pathway.

SSM shows mutations almost exclusively in *NRAS*. A prevalence of 5% to 10% *NRAS* mutation has been reported. However for hereditary melanomas, the prevalence increases to 80%. Most cases of *NRAS* mutation are in codon 61. *NRAF* and *BRAF* mutations are mutually exclusive [39].

8. Melanoma with chronic sun exposure

There are similarities between this type of melanoma and those without sun exposure. However, there are differences with ALM since they show much lower mutational characteristics.

KIT (CD117) encodes a tyrosine kinase receptor for stem cells factor and plays a key role in melanocyte development, migration and proliferation. *KIT* is found on chromosome 4 and may be altered in a variety of different types of cancers. It is mutated in 28% of LMM, 36% in ALM, and is absent in melanomas with intermittent sun exposure. KIT over expression during the vertical growth phase of melanoma development supports the hypothesis of its participation in late stages of the disease. It is the target of several small molecules inhibitors such as imatinib, being a therapeutic target for this type of melanoma. Different roles of KIT among different types of melanoma, give additional evidence that each subtype can be considered different biologically and genetically [40].

9. Melanoma without sun exposure

ALM and mucosal melanomas have an inverse correlation among mutations of *BRAF* and *NRAS*. The increase in the copy number of Cyclin D1, CDK4, KIT and ABCB5 has also been reported.

9.1. CYCLIN D1

It is an important regulator of transition of the cell cycle for phases G1/S. It also participates in the phosphorylation of RB protein by binding kinase 4, cyclin dependent. Many studies have revealed a highly organized sequence of events indispensable for promotion of continued proliferation. The decision to continue cell cycle progression occurs when cellular RAS induces the elevation of cyclin D1. These levels are maintained through G1 phase and are necessary for the initiation of S phase, thus resulting in immediately reduced cyclin D1 levels. One requirement for DNA synthesis, is the reduction of cyclin D1 to low levels during the S phase. This forces the cell when it enters G2 phase, to induce high cyclin D1 levels once more. Thus, cyclin D1 is proposed to be a switch activator in the regulation of continued cell cycle progression [41, 42].

Cyclin D1 frequent amplification was reported in 44.4% of ALM by Sauter et al, Cyclin D1 was overexpressed in all cases with amplifications and in 20% of cases without amplification.

Cyclin D1 may be an oncogene in melanoma and that targeting its expression can be therapeutically useful in the future for ALM [42].

9.2. CDK4

It is a union protein of cyclin D1, found in chromosome 12q14. During early stages of phase G1 of the cell cycle, Cyclin D binds to kinase dependent cyclin 4 or 6 (CDK4 or CDK6) and the resulting complex "frees the brake" that limits the progression towards late G1, going into phase S. The cyclin D-CDK4/6 complex releases a potent inhibitor of the cell cycle progression: the one formed by protein pRB and inactive transcription factors. The types of melanoma having an increase in the number of copies of CyclinD1 and CDK4 have less possibilities of responding to the therapeutic target used in BRAF, such as Vemurafenib.

9.3. ABCB5

Human ATP-binding cassette transporter, also known as P-glycoprotein, is related to the subfamily of multidrug resistant genes (MDR). The ABCB subfamily includes eleven members that have different expression patterns. Whereas the functions of several transporters of the ABCB family are not known, there is some information about ABCB5 in relation to its pattern of expression or its associated function [43]. It has been described by Frank et al [44, 45] described it and it was implicated in the regulation of progenitor cell fusion (located in chromosome 7p21-15). Their study used an enriched culture of human epidermal melanocytes isolated from the foreskins of healthy donors and melanoma cell lines. They showed a higher and more intense ABCB5 expression in ALM than in SSM. Herrera-Gonzalez and her team [46], reported a 90% overexpression of ABCB5 in ALM samples of Mexican patients by using RT-PCR. A direct relationship between mRNA expression and the aggressiveness of ALM was also shown.

10. Conclusion

In regard to the progression of human cancer, it is universally thought, that it develops from a single mutated cell, followed by malignant clonal expansion secondary to additional genomic and genetic alterations. As the malignant cells continue to acquire these alterations, tumor subclones with distinct phenotypic advantages (47) for its progression may be produced: for example invasion, proliferation, ability to colonize different organs, etc. In many cancers, regulation of specific signaling molecules also goes awry, affecting a host of other proteins and cellular processes.

In recent years, the histological and phenotypic characteristics of ALM combined with its high proportion among melanomas in Afro-Americans, Asian and Latin Americans, has confirmed the thought that this histological type of melanoma may differ biological and molecularly from its most common counterparts, recognized by its sun exposure and its greater frequency among Caucasians. While ALM is characterized by a high frequency of focal amplifications (mainly involving CCND1, CDK4) and deletions, the most common cutaneous melanomas exhibit few changes in the number of genetic copies. In a similar way, while *BRAF* and *NRAS* are mutated in 50% and 20% of the cases respectively, mutation in *KIT* (which codifies the tyrosine kinase receptor) seems to be absent in the most common cutaneous melanoma. However, BRAF mutations in ALM constitute approximately 16% of the cases reported by Curtin et al. [40, 41]

A systematic sequencing was used for the human genome sequence. New technologies allow sequencing of randomly generated DNA fragments from cancer genomes and thus detect alterations and copy number variation as well as base substitutions, to identify most somatic mutations in an individual cancer genome. Pleasance et al, sequenced the complete genome of the COLO-829 cell line, an immortal and cancer derived from a metastasis of a melanoma from a 43 year-old-male. In their study they identified 33,345 somatic base substitutions [48, 49]

The study of Turajlic et al. [50] is the first to characterize the mutational spectra in ALM. They used a whole genome sequencing to characterize punctual somatic mutations and structural variation in a primary acral melanoma and its lymph node metastasis. Evidence of transcription-coupled repair was suggested by the lower mutational rate in the transcribed regions and expressed genes. Primary melanoma and metastasis, at the level of global gene copy number alterations, loss of heterozygosity and single expressed genes are very similar[50].

These results may be controversial since their sequenced results were on the genome of only one patient. They cite that despite the perception that acral skin is sun protected, the dominant mutational signature reveals sun damage. We judge that there is no solid data regarding the presence of solar exposure on sites where ALM is developed.

Studies suggest that ungual matrix does not provide a complete protection against UV radiation and it has previously been suggested that UVB can penetrate the human nail [51]. There are substantial variations in the number and pattern of mutations in individual cancers reflecting different exposures, DNA repair defects and cellular origins [52, 53]. It is also possible that characteristics of different mutations are induced by the inefficiency of pyrimidine dimers repaired by excision of nucleotide due to the presence of a mutation in ERCC5 [54, 55].

Several studies support the hypothesis that ALM is a different genetic subtype and its inherent heterogeneity represents a challenge in the era of directed therapy [56].

Author details

R. Barra-Martínez[1], N.E. Herrera-González[2], F. Fernández –Ramírez[3] and L.A. Torres[1]

1 Oncology Unit of General Hospital of Mexico, Mexico

2 Molecular Oncology Laboratory. Postgraduate Section. Superior School of Medicine, IPN, Mexico

3 Genetic Unit of General Hospital of Mexico, Mexico

References

[1] Alfeirán RA, Escobar AG Epidemiologia del melanoma de piel en México. Rev INCAN I (1999) 44(4): 168-174.

[2] Fernández CSB, León AG, Herrera TMC, Salazar SE, Sánchez DMR, Alcalá ORB et al. Perfil epidemiológico de los tumores malignos en México. Dir. Gral. Epidem. Secretaría de Salud México, D.F. (SINAIS / SINAVE / DGE / SALUD). (2011). p. 46 - 138.

[3] Vásquez MI, Villanueva LCG, Meraz R MA, Magaña M, Herrera GN. Biología molecular del melanoma. Actas Dermatol & Dermatopatol Méx. (2005); 5:5 - 15.

[4] Garbe C., Peris K, Hauschild A, Saiag P. Middleton M, Spatz A. Diagnosis and treatment of melanoma: European consensus-based interdisciplinary guideline Eur J of cancer (2010); 46: 270-283.

[5] Vázquez MI, Meraz RM, Magaña M, Sánchez GD, Herrera-González NE. Quimiorresistencia en el melanoma. Informe preliminar. Act Dermat y Dermapat (2006);6: 8-10

[6] Lascano AR, Kuznitzky R, Cuestas E, Mainard C et al. Factores de riesgo para melanoma cutáneo. Estudio de casos y controles en Córdoba, Argentina. Medicina (Buenos Aires). (2004); 64 (6) : 504-508

[7] Yuji Yamaguchi, Vicent J. Hearing. Melanocytes and their diseases. Cold spring harb perspect med. (2014); 4 : a017046

[8] De la Fuente GA, Ocampo CJ. Melanoma Cutáneo. Gac Méd Méx. (2010); 146: 126 – 135.

[9] Martínez SH, Vega GM, Toussaint CS, Gutiérrez VR, Orozco TR, León E, et al. El primer Consenso Nacional de Expertos en Melanoma. GAMO. (2005); 4: 11 – 13.

[10] Hayat MJ, Howlader N, Reichman ME y Edwards KB. Cancer statistics, trends, and multiple primary cancer analyses from the Surveillance, Epidemiology, and End Results (SEER) Program. The Oncologist (2007);12: 20 – 37.

[11] Geller CA y Swetter S. Screening and early detection of melanoma. CA Cancer J Clin (2011); 61:69-77.

[12] Massachusetts Institute of Technology (2014). Eumelanin's secrets: Discovery of melanin structure may lead to better sun protection. *Sciencedaily*. Retrieved January, 2015 from www.sciencedaily.com/releases/2014/05/140522115754.htm

[13] Chen, C.T., Chuang, J. Cao, V. Ball, D. Ruch, and M. J. Buehler. "Excitonic effecs from geometric order and disorder explain broadband optical absorption in eumelanin" Nature communications 5 (2014): 3859

[14] Nagore E, Botella ER, Requena C, Serra G, Martorell A, Hueso L, et al. Perfil clínico y epidemiológico de los pacientes con melanoma cutáneo según el grado de exposición solar de la localización del melanoma. Act Dermosifil (2009); 100: 205-211

[15] Rouhani P, Hu S, Kirsner RS. Melanoma in Hispanics and Black Americans. Cancer Control (2008); 15: 248-253

[16] Boriani, F O'Learly, Tohill M, Orlando A. EUR REB MED PHARMACOL SCI (2014); 08:1990-1996

[17] Schmerling R, Loria D, Cinat G, Ramos W, Cardona F, Sánchez J, Martínez-Said H, Buzaid A. Cutaneus melanoma in Latin America: the need for more data..Rev Panam Salud Publica. (2011);30(5):431-8

[18] Hernández ZS, Medina BA, López-Tello SA, Alcalá PD. Epidemiología del cáncer de piel en pacientes de la Clínica de Dermato-oncología del Centro Dermatológico Dr. Ladislao de la Pascua. Rev Mex Dermatol. (2012); 56: 30-37.

[19] Reed WB, Becker S, SR., Becker S, JR., Nickel WR. Giant Pigmented Nevi, Melanoma, and Leptomeningeal Melanocytosis: A Clinical and Histopathological Study. Arch Dermatol. (1965); 91(2):100-119.

[20] Arrington JH III, Reed RJ, Ichinose H, Krementz ET. Plantar lentiginous melanoma: a distinctive variant of human cutaneous malignant melanoma. Am J Surg Pathol. (1977); 1:131-143.

[21] Bradford PT, Goldstein AM, McMaster ML, Tucker MA. Acral Lentiginous Melanoma Incidence and Survival Patterns in the United States, 1986-2005. Arch Dermatol. (2009); 145: 427-434.

[22] C. Pereda, V. Traves, C. Requena, C. Serra-Guillén. B. Llombart, O. Sanmartín, C. Guillén, E. Nagore. Clinical presentation of acral lentiginusos melanoma: a descriptive study. Actas dermo-sifiliograficas (2012) 104: 220-226

[23] Feibleman CE, Stoll H, Maize JC. Melanomas of the palm, sole, and nailbed: a clinicopathologic study. Cancer. (1980); 46: 2492-2504.

[24] Phan A, Touzet S, Dalle S, Ronger-Salve S, Balme B, Thomas L. Acral lentiginous melanoma: a clinicoprognostic study of 126 cases. Br J Dermatol. (2006); 155: 561-569.

[25] Ghadially FN, trauma and melanoma production. Nature (1966); 211: 1199

[26] Troyanova P. The role of trauma in the melanoma formation. J Boun (2002); 7: 347-350

[27] Ranwala S, Hunt C, Modi G, Krishnan B, Orengo I. Amelanotic subungual melanoma after trauma: an unusual clinical presentation. Dermatol online j (2011); 17:8

[28] Zanhg N., Wang. L, Zhu.G., Sun. D., He. H., Luang. Q., Liu. L., Hao. F., Lee. C., Gao. P. The associatiom between trauma and melanoma in the Chinese population: a ret-

rospective study. J of the European Academy of Dermatology and Venereology. (2013).

[29] Hsu M, Meier F, Herlyn M. Melanoma development and progression: a conspiracy between tumor and host. Differentiation (2002) 70: 522-536

[30] Herrera-González Norma Estela. "Interaction between the Immune System and Melanoma", Recent Advances in the Biology Therapy and Management of Melanoma" (2013)

[31] Young, R. J., Waldeck, K., Martin, C., Foo, J. H., Cameron, D. P., Kirby, L., Do, H., Mitchell, C., Cullinane, C., Liu, W., Fox, S. B., Dutton-Regester, K., Hayward, N. K., Jene, N., Dobrovic, A., Pearson, R. B., Christensen, J. G., Randolph, S., McArthur, G. A. and Sheppard, K. E. Loss of CDKN2A expression is a frequent event in primary invasive melanoma and correlates with sensitivity to the CDK4/6 inhibitor PD0332991 in melanoma cell lines. Pigment Cell & Melanoma Research, (2014), 27: 590–600.

[32] Sullivan RJ, Flaherty KT. BRAF in Melanoma: Pathogenesis, Diagnosis, Inhibition, and Resistance. J of Skin Cancer 2011; (2011): 1 – 8.

[33] Avruch J. MAP kinase pathways: the first twenty years. Biochim Biophys Acta. (2007); 1773:1150-1160.

[34] Vidwans SJ, Flaherty KT, Fisher DE, Tenenbaum JM, Travers MD, Shrager J. A Melanoma Molecular Disease Model. PLoS One (2011); 6: 1 – 10.

[35] Ciampi R, Nikiforov YE. Alterations of BRAF gene in human tumors. Endocr Pathol. (2005);16: 163-172.

[36] Zafon C y Obiols G. Vía de señalización dependiente de la proteincinasa de activación mitogénica. De las bases moleculares a la práctica clínica. Endocrinol Nutr. (2009); 56(4):176-186

[37] Cantwell-Dorris ER, O'Leary JJ, and Sheils OM. BRAFV600E: Implications for Carcinogenesis and Molecular Therapy. Mol Cancer Ther. (2011); 10: 385 – 394.

[38] Barra-Martínez R. Estudio de la mutación de T-1799A BRAF en melanoma acral lentiginoso y nodular de pacientes del Hospital General de México 2010. Maestría en Ciencias de la Salud. Sección de Posgrado. Escuela Superior de Medicina, IPN.

[39] Jakob, J. A., Bassett, R. L., Ng, C. S., Curry, J. L., Joseph, R. W., Alvarado, G. C., Rohlfs, M. L., Richard, J., Gershenwald, J. E., Kim, K. B., Lazar, A. J., Hwu, P. and Davies, M. A. (2012), *NRAS*mutation status is an independent prognostic factor in metastatic melanoma. Cancer, 118: 4014–4023.

[40] Curtin JA, Busam K, Pinkel D, Bastian BC. Somatic activation of KIT in distinct subtypes of melanoma. J Clin Oncol. (2006); 24:4340- 4346.

[41] Curtin JA, Fridlyand J, Kageshita T, Patel HN, Busam KJ, Kutzner H, et al. Distinct sets of genetic alterations in melanoma. N Engl J Med. (2005); 353:2135-2147

[42] Sauter. E., Yeo Un-Cheol., Streem. A., Zhu. W., Litwin. S., Tichansky. E., Pistritto. G., Nesbit. M., Pinkel. D., Herlyn. M., Bastian. B. Cyclin D1 Is a Candidate Oncogene in Cutaneus Melanoma. The American Journal of Cancer. (2002):62;3200-3206.

[43] Ambudkart. S., Dey. S., Ihrycyna. C., Ramachandra. M., Pastan. I., Gottesman. M. Biochemical cellular and pharmacological aspects of the multidrug transported. Pharmacol Toxicol. (1999); 39:361-98.

[44] Frank N, Pendse S, Lapchak P, Margaryan A., Schlain D., Doeing C, et al. Regulation of progenitor cell fusion by ABCB P-glycoprotein, a novel human ATP- binding cassette transporter. J Biol Chem. (2003); 278:47156–47165.

[45] Frank N, Margaryan A, Huang Y, Schatton T, Waaga-Gasser AM, Gasser M et al. ABCB5-mediated doxorubicin transport and chemoresistance in human malignant melanoma. Cancer Res. (2005); 65: 4320–4333.

[46] Vásquez-Moctezuma I, Meraz-Ríos MA, Villanueva-López CG, Magaña M, Martínez-Macias R, Herrera-González NE. ATP-binding cassette transporter ABCB5 gene is expressed with variability in malignant melanoma. IPN. Actas Dermosifil. (2010); 101: 341-348.

[47] Yancovitz Molly, Adam Litterman, Joane Yoo, Elise Ng, Richard L. Shapiro et al. Intra- and Inter-Tumor heterogeneity of $BRAF^{V600E}$ mutations in primary and metastic melanoma. PLoS ONE (2012); 07(1); e29336

[48] Pleasance, E.D., Cheetham, R.K., Stephens, P.J., McBride DJ, Humphray SJ, Greenman CD et al. A comprehensive catalogue of somatic mutations from a human cancer genome. Nature. (2010); 463: 191–196.

[49] Lee JT, Li L, Brafford PA,Van Den Eijnden M, Halloran MB. PLX4032, a potent inhibitor of the B-Raf V600E oncogene, selectively inhibits V600E-positive Melanomas. Pigment Cell & Melanoma Res.(2010); 23: 820–827.

[50] Turajlic S, Furney SJ, Lambros MB, Mitsopoulos C, Kozarewa I, Geyer FC, et al. Whole genome sequencing of matched primary and metastatic acral melanomas. Genome Res (2012) 22:196–207.

[51] Parker SG, Diffey BL. The transmission of optical radiation through human nails. Br. J. Dermat (1983); 108:11-16.

[52] Greenman C, Stephens P, Smith R, Dalgliesh GL, Hunter C, Bignell G, et al. Patterns of somatic mutation in human cancer genomes. Nature. (2007); 446: 153–158.

[53] Stratton MR, Campbell PJ, Futreal PA. The cancer genome. Nature. (2009); 458:719–724.

[54] Pfeifer GP, You YH, Besaratinia A. Mutations induced by ultraviolet light. Mutat. Res. (2005); 571:19–31.

[55] Gaddameedhi S, Kemp MG, Reardon JT, Shields JM, Smith-Roe SL, Kaufmann WK et al. Similar Nucleotide Excision Repair Capacity in Melanocytes and Melanoma Cell. Cancer Res. (2010); 70: 4922- 4930

[56] Furney SJ, Turajlic S, Fenwick K, Lambros MB, MacKay A, Ricken G, et al. Genomic characterisation of acral melanoma cell lines. Pigment Cell Melanoma Res. (2012); 25; 488–492.

Chapter 3

Signaling Pathways Altered During the Metastatic Progression of Melanoma

Ana Carolina Monteiro, Mariana Toricelli and
Miriam Galvonas Jasiulionis

Additional information is available at the end of the chapter

http://dx.doi.org/10.5772/59747

1. Introduction

Metastasis is one of the most important parameters that affect cancer patient's prognosis. It is associated with resistance to treatments, high recurrence rates and poor cancer patient survival rates [1]. Although melanoma is an aggressive type of skin cancer that carries significant morbidity and mortality, the prognosis for patients with localized tumor is quite good, the aggravation being the metastatic capacity of the tumor. When the process of metastasis takes place, the prognosis is generally very poor, with the metastatic melanoma being rarely curable [2-3].

The establishment of metastatic lesions is a complex process and requires a series of sequential steps, each of which is rate limiting, and although substantial progress has been made in understanding the molecular mechanisms of metastasis, new data suggest this process is perhaps even more complicated than originally suspected [4]. Another issue in defining the factors involved in the melanoma metastasis is that melanoma is highly heterogeneous and for this its classification and staging is until today a challenge for specialists [1]. Because of that, there is still a lot unclear understanding about the progression of the disease, making it difficult to ensure which molecular pathways are involved in each step of the disease development. Therefore, for the development of new prognostic and therapeutic targets of melanoma metastasis, it is important to elucidate which pathways are involved specifically in the progression of the localized tumor to its metastasis [2]. For that, a deep review of the literature, analysing carefully which pathologic classification each study considered, may clarify the molecular alterations involved specifically in the most aggressive step in melanoma progression.

Signaling pathways, such as the canonical Wnt pathway, the c-kit receptor and the MITF transcription fator are among pathways found altered during melanoma [5]. The reactivation of melanocyte-specific programs seems to contribute, in combination with other oncogenic changes, with melanoma aggressiveness. Others pathways that are classically altered in melanoma metastasis are the MAPK and PI3K pathways, with gain-of-function mutations leading to melanoma metastasis progression [1].

Besides these pathways that are consistently involved in the metastasis of melanoma, there are some other potentially altered pathways in this process. For example, it is known that the tumor microenvironment has an important role in determining melanoma progression to metastasis [6], and in this scope the importance of metalloproteinases is being highlighted. In addition, numerous studies report modulation of the metastatic properties of melanoma cells by microRNAs, suggesting this as a common occurrence. MicroRNAs regulate tumor suppressor genes and oncogenes, each miRNA being able to regulate a great number of genes. Besides, due to its stable and lineage-specific expression nature, microRNAs are attractive candidate as biomarkers and therapeutic targets [7].

Although there are a great number of studies trying to elucidate the molecular mechanisms of melanoma progression, the process of melanoma metastasis is still unclear. Finding core mediators of different processes in metastasis is a formidable challenge, and may provide opportunities for developing new prevention and treatment strategies. This chapter will discuss basic concepts of malignant melanoma metastasis, focusing on the pathways that the literature indicate as consistently altered in this process and will describe how the host's environment influences the biological behavior of metastatic cells.

2. Melanoma metastasis

Cutaneous melanoma is the most aggressive type of skin cancer, and the high mortality rates worldwide caused by this disease is due to its great ability to form metastases and resist to current therapies [8,9,10]. Genetic and epigenetic alterations contribute to the development of cells able to invade and metastasize [11]. These changes ensure the features that allow cells to modulate the microenvironment, and change their interactions with the extracellular matrix and other cells [8]. Although our knowledgement about the molecular pathogenesis of melanoma has increased, the molecular changes occuring during the malignant transformation of melanocytes are not very well described.

3. Adhesion molecules

One of the main characteristics of metastatic melanoma is cell heterogeneity [10]. This characteristic provides the cell ability to invade and colonize different tissues [11]. Local invasion and metastasis processes are responsible for the morbidity and mortality associated with melanoma. The development of invasive cells occurs in the vertical growth phase (VGP) when melanoma cells are able to penetrate the basement membrane, grow in the dermis and metastasize [12]. Moreover, these cells have many cytogenetic abnormalities, suggesting a significant genomic instability [13]. The development of metastatic melanoma from primary VGP melanomas occurs when these cells dissociate from the primary tumor, migrate through the adjacent stroma and invade the lymphatic and/or blood vessels to form tumors at distant sites [13]. The invasion and migration of melanoma are related to changes in cell adhesion. Typically, cell adhesion controls cell migration, organization, organogenesis and tissue architecture [14]. Disturbances in adhesion contribute to tumor invasion, tumor-stroma interactions and signaling between tumor cells and normal cells [14]. There are numerous cell adhesion molecules, which are sub-grouped based on their structural similarity and are categorized as integrins, cadherins, immunoglobulin superfamily or selectins. The expression of these molecules is influenced by the environment, microenvironment and genetic/epigenetic factors [14]. Therefore, determining changes in the expression of these molecules during metastasis may help to define future therapeutic targets. Several adhesion molecules have been reported to play a role in melanoma progression.

As previously stated, the extracellular matrix (ECM) surrounding the cell provides a physical support for the cell adhesion. The anchorage of cell in the ECM is not just structural, considering that this binding stimulates signal transduction cascades that mediate signaling required for the proliferation, migration, differentiation and cell survival [15]. The type of apoptosis triggered by the loss of anchorage is called "*anoikis*". Currently, the role of anchorage in the cell survival is widely accepted and studied in numerous adherent cell types, such as fibroblasts, endothelial, bronchial epithelial, liver, intestine, prostate cells and in keratinocytes [16]. The acquisition of *anoikis*-resistant phenotype is one of the critical steps during tumor progression. In melanoma, we and others [17-19] demonstrated that malignant transformation is associated with resistance to *anoikis* [16]. One of the key molecules involved in *anoikis* are integrins. The physical connection between extracellular matrix and the cytoskeleton of actin is mainly mediated by receptors of the integrin family. Besides being involved in the interaction of the cell with the extracellular matrix, integrins are also responsible for signaling between the cell and its microenvironment. The integrin family is among the best-characterized adhesion molecules. Currently, 18 types of α subunits and 8 types of β subunits are known, which combine to form at least 24 integrins already described [20]. The expression pattern of integrins on cell surface causes the cell to fit perfectly into its microenvironment. In this regard, integrins have altered interactions with their microenvironment may give drastic consequences for cell fate as provide cell tend to lose their original adhesion, recognizing a different substrate and reconfigure it with characteristics that enable metastasize [21-22]. It is known that the increase and alteration of integrin expression is indicative of progression of melanoma [23]. Many integrins are found altered in metastatic melanoma (TABLE 1). Thus, a large number of studies have shown that expression of $\alpha v\beta 3$ and $\alpha v\beta 1$ integrins is related with malignant transformation of melanocytes or melanoma progression [24-28]. $\alpha v\beta 3$ integrin is an integrin expressed only in melanoma cells and not in benign melanocytes [24]. $\beta 3$ integrins have also been associated with angiogenesis [29]. $\alpha v\beta 3$ and $\alpha v\beta 1$ integrins are expressed in metastatic melanoma and late melanoma compared with early melanoma and nevi [28-30]. The $\alpha v\beta 3$ integrin is associated with melanoma progression, acting as a receptor for vitronectin, which self-regulates the expression of matrix metalloproteinase-2 (MMP-2] and increases invasive proteins [24-25]. Alpha-v integrin antibodies block the growth of human melanoma transplants in mice and a new inhibitor of αvβ3 integrin blocks *anoikis* and metastasis in human melanoma cell line M21[31-32].

Integrins	Reference
Alpha1 beta1	[26]
Alpha2 beta1	[26]
Alpha3 beta1	[25]
Alpha4 beta1	[26]
Alpha5 beta1	[33]
Alpha6 beta1	[14, 26]
Alpha7 beta1	[34]
alphaV beta3	[14]
alphaV beta5	[34]

Table 1. Main integrins found altered in metastatic melanomas

Immunoglobulin superfamily adhesion molecules are cell surface glycoproteins that express a variable number of loops in its extracellular domain. Most of these molecules has a transmembrane domain but is linked to the cell surface only by a glycophosphatidilinositol anchor [35]. Heterophilic interactions with members of the immunoglobulin superfamily, integrins, cadherins and extracellular matrix components may occur, as well as homophilic interactions, which are essential in Ca^{2+}-dependent cell adhesion [36-37]. The family of immunoglobulins has an important relevance in the pathophysiology of melanoma, among which we can highlight the CD54 (ICAM), CD66 (CEACAM), CD146 (MCAM or Mel-CAM) and CD166 (ALCAM). These molecules appear to be important in the melanoma progression, although many of their functions are still uncertain. Through literature review, it is possible to note their participation in advanced cases of melanoma and metastatic disease [14, 38]. Particularly, CD54 (ICAM) has been associated with melanoma progression and risk of metastasis [39]. Its expression is evident in melanoma when compared with nevi [26, 40-42]. The CD66 (CEACAM) is a glycoprotein surface molecule involved in intercellular adhesion and associated with diverse cellular functions that regulate growth and differentiation and play an important role in insulin homeostasis, vasculogenesis and immunomodulation. Furthermore, it implies in many intracellular signaling mediated processes involved in the growth and differentiation of tumor cells, performing thus a key role in the modulation of many types of cancer. A strong correlation between the expression of this molecule in primary tumors and subsequent development of metastatic disease was observed. An apparently gradual increase in CD66 expression in cutaneous melanocytic lesions in more advanced stages of neoplastic progression was observed, indicating that CD66 may play an important role in the development and progression of melanoma. Furthermore, this molecule interacts with integrins (especially with beta-3 subunit) and this interaction appears to be important in cell migration and metastasis [43]. The CD146 molecule was first identified as a cell adhesion molecule specific for melanoma and capable of providing homologous and heterologous interactions between neoplastic melanocytes and endothelial cells in a calcium-independent manner [14]. Also known as MELCAM, MCAM and MUC18 [44], CD146 plays a pro-migratory key role in the vascular system, normal development and tumor progression, displaying overexpression in many tumors, including melanoma, prostate cancer and cancer breast [45-47]. The expression of CD146 in melanocytes, nevi and melanoma cells from radial growth phase is environmentally regulated through direct contact cell-cell with keratinocytes, but the mechanisms of this regulation are not well-established [48]. Moreover, in melanoma progression, the expression of this molecule increases gradually and reaches its peak in metastatic disease [14, 20, 49]. It is reported that CD146 displays strictly correlation with cadherins and experimental situations where an increased expression of cadherins is stimulated, CD146 levels return to normal levels [50]. The CD166, also named ALCAM, was first identified on activated leukocytes, hematopoietic stem cells and myeloid progenitors. Furthermore, it is possible to observe its expression in neuronal cells, mesenchymal stem cells, stromal cells from bone marrow, but also in cultured metastatic melanoma cells [51]. Like other adhesion molecules, CD166 shows homophilic and heterophilic interactions and has represented a marker of metastatic development similarly to beta-3 integrin, since its expression reaches peak levels in metastatic melanoma cells [52].

Another major family of adhesion molecules found to be altered in metastatic melanoma is the cadherin family. Cadherins are calcium-dependent cell adhesion molecules with important functions in the formation and maintenance of normal tissue architecture [11]. Cadherins are a superfamily of at least 30 different molecules, whose expression is temporally and spatially controlled. Classic cadherins are divided into three subtypes: N (neural), E (epithelial) and P (placental) [53]. The E-cadherin molecule, which is expressed by epithelial cells, is the one most frequently altered in tumors. Different studies have shown that E-cadherin is frequently inactivated in the development of human carcinomas, including carcinomas of breast, colon, prostate, stomach, liver, esophagus, skin, kidney and lung and is associated with invasion and metastases formation in lymph nodes [53-54]. The inhibition of the E-cadherin function may occur by several mechanisms, including mutation or deletion of *CDH1* gene, chromosomal rearrangement or promoter hypermethylation [53]. In fact, deletions or hypermethylation of 16q22 region, where the E-cadherin gene is located, are common in carcinomas but, in melanoma cells, deletions, mutations and methylation of the E-cadherin gene are apparently not involved [54]. Three transcriptional factors, AP-2, Snail and SIP1, have recently been shown to be important in the transcriptional silencing of the E-cadherin gene in melanomas [55-57]. Loss of AP-2 expression in metastatic melanoma cells results in the deregulation of MCAM/MUC18, c-Kit and E-cadherin expression, all of which are involved in melanoma progression [57]. In experimental models, inhibition of E-cadherin expression in carcinoma cells facilitates tumor invasion, while the reestablishment of the expression results in proliferation inhibition and invasion and metastasis reduction [58]. E-cadherin is partially responsible for the phenomenon of contact inhibition, a characteristic of normal epithelial cells, associated with the proliferation blockade when cells come into contact with each other [53]. This feature is essential for maintaining epithelia architecture. In animal models, functional loss of E-cadherin is associated with acceleration of tumor progression. Adenocarcinomas and metastatic lesions appear earlier in animals that do not express E-cadherin function [59]. These E-cadherin properties allowed classifying it as a metastasis suppressor molecule. Loss E-cadherin expression appears to be a critical step in the melanoma progression, allowing the tumor cells to be released from the epidermis and to invade the dermis [60]. The cadherin switch from E-cadherin to N-cadherin results in disassociation of melanoma cells from keratinocytes and promotes melanoma cell invasion through the dermis. The N-cadherin expression in melanoma cells correlates with increased motility and invasion, suggesting that N-cadherin potentiates the interaction between tumor cells and stromal cells, including fibroblasts and endothelial cells [61]. Anti-N-cadherin antibodies can delay the trans-endothelial migration of melanoma cells and induce apoptosis of melanoma cells [61]. The E-cadherin cytoplasmic portion interacts with alpha-and ß-catenin. Besides the ß-catenin be part of E-cadherin adhesion complex, it plays an essential role as a mediator of the signal transduction pathway of Wnt/Wingless (glycoprotein that plays a role in embryogenesis), which activates the transcription factors LEF/Tcf [53]. The transcription factors LEF/Tcf are responsible for controlling expression of genes encoding cyclin D1, MYC and metalloproteinases [54]. In a simplified manner, the cytoplasmic pool of ß-catenin can be considered regulatory elements of epithelial cells proliferation and invasion. In tissues where there is interaction between cells and formation of adherent junctions mediated by E-cadherin, ß-catenin molecules are recruited to the sub-membrane region. The lack of degradation mechanism or the functional loss of E-cadherin leads to the ß-catenin cytoplasmic accumulation and its translocation to the nucleus. The ß-catenin also plays a role in the control of proliferation and apoptosis and is also increased in some cancers. Data show that E-cadherin suppresses the growth of metastatic melanoma cells by inhibiting beta-catenin signaling pathway/Wnt [54]. Therefore, these data suggest that E-cadherin may play an important role early in the metastatic cascade.

4. Matrix metalloproteinases

Proteolytic enzymes, by their ability to degrade ECM proteins, become important components in the process of tumor progression. With the sequencing of the human genome, more than 500 genes were identified as encoding proteases or protease-like proteins, with a large number being associated with the tumor process [62]. Among these, the matrix metalloproteinases (MMPs)-a group of 24 enzymes that degrade ECM components and the basal membrane [63]-have been the focus of much research on cancer [63-64]. This family of glycoproteins is secreted as a latent pro-enzyme, activated by proteolysis of a conserved region present in the N-terminal domain and is divided into six groups depending on the type of substrate that degrades: collagenases, gelatinases, stromelysins and extracellular matrix metalloproteinases [62]. MMPs are regulated both at transcriptional and post-transcriptional level. These regulation mechanisms operate to ensure their coordinated expression [63]. MMPs activity occurs only where proteolysis is required. Cytokines and peptide factors, such as interleukin (IL)-4 and IL-10, growth factors (transforming growth factor (TGF-α), basic fibroblast growth factor (bFGF), and TGF-beta1, induce the expression of different members of MMPs family [65]. However, malignant tumors have strategies that avoid these regulatory mechanisms and provide proteolytic activity that accompanies cancer development and metastasis [65]. Increased MMP activity is associated with the stages of tumor invasion and metastasis and is frequently overexpressed in different cancers. Upon activation, MMP activity is modulated by common endopeptidase inhibitors, such as α2-macroglobulins (present in plasma and tissue fluids) and, more specifically, by the inhibitors of matrix metalloproteases (TIMPs) [63-65]. MMPs mediate the extracellular matrix and basement membrane degradation during early stages of tumorigenesis process, contributing to the formation of a microenvironment that promotes tumor growth. MMPs also participate in later stages of cancer development, promoting the sustained growth of both primary tumors and metastases by activating growth factors, inactivating protein binding to growth factors or releasing mitogenic molecules residing on the extracellular matrix. One of the first steps in the carcinoma invasion is the disruption of the basement membrane and subsequent migration through extracellular matrix [9]. The basement membrane is composed of molecules such as laminin, type IV collagen and proteoglycans containing heparan sulfate [66]. More recently, it was shown that laminin-5 (molecule present in basement membranes of epithelium) is associated with the control of melanoma cells migratory phenotype [67]. The cleavage of laminin-5 by MMP-2 or MMP-14 shows a cryptic site of laminin that triggers cell motility [67]. This laminin-5 cleaved form is found in experimental tumors. In human cancers, MMP-14 co-localizes with laminin-5, which suggests that it is associated with microinvasive cancers [68]. E-cadherin is cleaved by MMP-3 or 7, and the release of E-cadherin promotes the invasion of tumor cells in a paracrine manner *in vitro*, possibly acting as a competitive inhibitor of other E-cadherin [69]. Cleavage of E-cadherin also triggers epithelial to mesenchymal transition associated with the invasive behavior of tumors, including metastatic melanomas [69]. Other molecules such as CD44, also regulate this process [70]. MMPs activation is also among the mechanisms that tumor cells use to escape the "surveillance" of the immune system. MMPs also activate TGF-ß, a suppressor factor of T lymphocytes in the response against tumors. Genetically modified animals that do not express some MMPs have smaller tumors than normal animals, and develop tumors later [71]. These molecules, which have been considered tumor-associated molecules, are not produced only by the tumor cells themselves. Studies using the technique of *in situ* hybridization showed that several MMPs mRNA are also produced by stromal fibroblasts and inflammatory cells present in the tumor microenvironment [72-74]. The inflammatory cells such as mast cells, macrophages and neutrophils, as well as producing MMPs also produce cytokines that may act as positive modulators of this process [65]. This creates a tissue network of transcriptional activation, synthesis, secretion and MMPs activation. The phenomenon discussed above clearly illustrates the concept that the tumor behavior depends not only on tumor cells, but also on their interactions with elements of the host. Likewise, the tumor cells invade the host tissues and endothelial cells are recruited by the tumor, forming vascular structures (blood vessels and lymphatics) that comprise an important element of the tumor microenvironment. The tumor vascularization occurs by angiogenesis. At the same time it creates vascular routes inflow nutrients necessary for the tumor mass growth. The newly formed vessels may give way to the efflux of tumor cells to the hematogenic or lymphatic circulation, thus resulting in systemic tumor dissemination [9].

5. Tissue inhibitors of metalloproteinases

Inhibitors of matrix metalloproteinases have been identified in various species, such as *C. elegans, Drosophila*, zebrafish and humans, suggesting that these genes are present from the start of the evolutionary process [75]. Recent studies have shown developmental defects in Timps-deficient organisms in both mammals and in non-mammals, revealing the importance of these proteins during embryonic development. In mammals, the family of tissue inhibitors of metalloproteases (Timps) consists of four distinct members: TIMP1, 2, 3 and 4, which share substantial sequence homology and structural identity at the protein level [75]. TIMPs have basically two structural domains: an N-terminal domain containing 6 conserved cysteine residues forming three "loops", having the inhibitory activity of MMPs; and a C-terminal, which also contains six conserved cysteine residues and form three "loops". The balance between activities of the protease inhibitor and the proteolytic potential determines the tumor progression [75]. Thus, increases in expression and activity of MMPs are found in almost all human cancers. Interestingly, the expression of their inhibitors, TIMPs, is also generally increased in several cancers. Among them, TIMP1 has been associated with poor prognosis in metastatic melanoma, suggesting promising value of TIMP1 as a prognostic marker of the tumor [76-77]. In our laboratory, a model that allows us to study different stages of melanoma progression was developed. Murine melan-a melanocytes surviving after 1, 2, 3 and 4 cycles of adhesion impediment (named respectively 1C, 2C, 3C and 4C cell lines) showed changes in morphology and growth independent of phorbol myristate acetate (PMA). Different melanoma cell lines (such as 4C3-, 4C3+, 4C11-, and 4C11+) were established after subjecting the surviving spheroids formed after blocking the adhesion of 4C cell line to a limiting dilution [17]. Previous data from our laboratory show a progressive increase in the TIMP1 expression along the melanoma genesis, and this increase is related to resistance to *anoikis* and to a more aggressive phenotype *in vivo* [76]. We also observed that soluble TIMP1 in non-tumorigenic lineage melan-a confers *anoikis* resistance and it is differentially associated with CD63 and β1-integrin along the melanoma genesis [77]. CD63, β1-integrin and TIMP1 are not interacting in the murine melan-a melanocytes. The 4C cell line, corresponding to pre-malignant melanocytes, shows interaction between CD63 and β1-integrins, and CD63 and TIMP1, which could initiate the signaling pathways for cell survival, since 4C cell line is more *anoikis*-resistant when compared with its parental melan-a cell line. In 4C11- and 4C11+ melanomacell lines, a tighter CD63/β1integrins/TIMP1 complex seem to be formed, which could result in a more efficient activation of cell survival signals, giving to these cells a higher resistance to *anoikis* (Figure 1). However, the mechanisms regulating the functions of TIMP1 and signaling pathways activated by this complex along the tumorigenesis are still unclear. Studies are in progress to further elucidate the role of TIMP1 in metastatic melanoma.

http://dx.doi.org/10.5772/59747

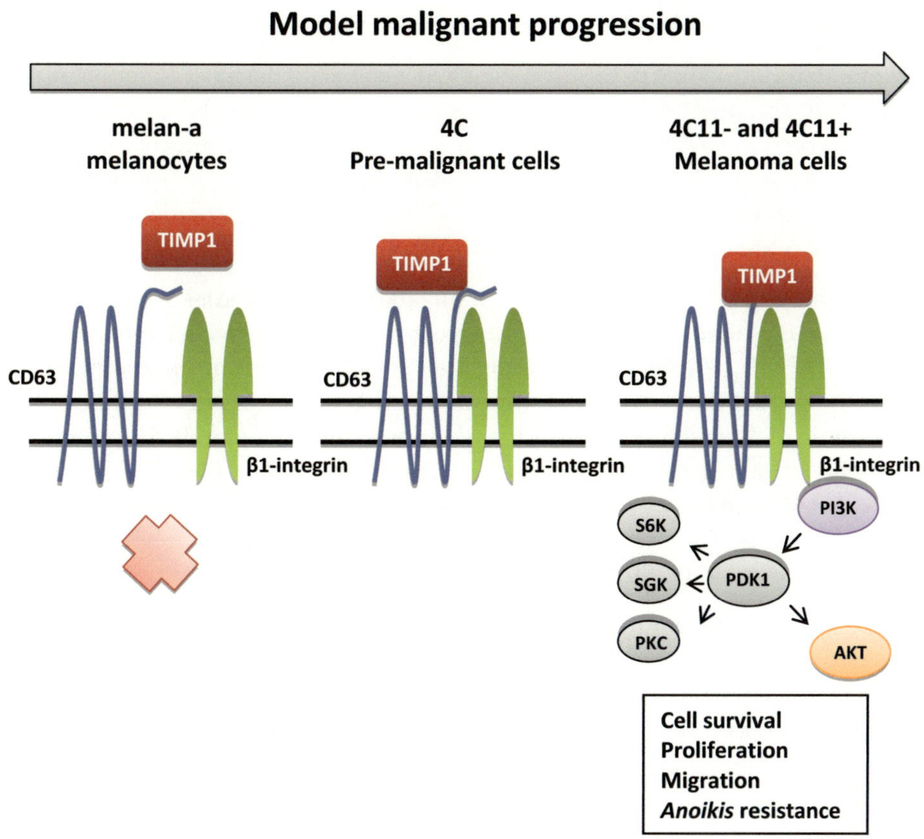

Figure 1. Schematic representation of the interaction among CD63, β1-integrin and TIMP1 along melanoma progression. A. In the melanocyte lineage melan-a, there is no interaction among CD63, β1-integrin and TIMP1. In the pre-malignant 4C cell line, TIMP1 associates with CD63, but not with β1-integrins, and CD63 interacts with β1-integrins. In 4C11- and 4C11+ melanoma cell lines, the formation of CD63/β1-integrin/TIMP1 complex occurs, which could be related to a more efficient activation of cell survival signals [77].

6. Pathways classically involved in melanoma and their involvement in melanoma metastasis

6.1. BRAF

The MAPK pathway is an important intracellular signal transduction pathway, which regulates cellular proliferation, differentiation, gene expression, cell survival and apoptosis [78]. This pathway is activated by different factors through different receptors, as tyrosine kinases and G-protein-coupled receptors. The activation of those membrane receptors promotes RAS activation, which activates several effector proteins, as the ones in RAF family.

RAF then activate the kinase cascade (MEK1/2 and ERK1/2), which can phosphorylate nuclear and cytoplasmic substrates involved in several cellular processes [1].

The most mutated gene in this pathway is the *BRAF* gene, with the most common mutation in melanoma being the $BRAF^{V600E}$ mutation. This mutation involves the change of valine to glutamic acid at codon 600 (V600E) in the exon 15, which causes a conformational change in the protein structure leading to its activation. Therefore, since the BRAF is constitutively activated, cells with $BRAF^{V600E}$ present hyperactivation of the MAPK pathway and are able to signal through it without activation by RAS [78-79].

Since the first report by Davies and colleagues in 2002, several studies have confirmed that activating BRAF mutations are present in approximately 60% of melanoma, and over 90% of them are $BRAF^{V600E}$ [80]. *BRAF* mutations are not only present in melanoma but also in nevi. Some shows that the incidence of this mutation is higher in nevi (up to 80%) than in melanoma (up to 65%) and this brought the question if mutations in BRAF can be acquired during primary tumor development or even during metastasis [78, 81]. Several results suggest that BRAF mutation occurs early in the malignant transformation of melanocytes but is not sufficient to cause melanoma and so this mutation is probably acquired during the melanoma progression [78].

It is predicted that the constitutive activation of the MAPK pathway can lead to oncogenic transformation of cells by promoting cell proliferation, invasion, metastasis, migration, survival and angiogenesis [82]. Specifically, MAPK is predicted to mediate melanoma metastasis by inducing proteolytic enzymes, as MMPs, which leads to degradation of basement membrane, and by regulating genes involved in cell migration, cell survival, and growth [83]. However, this has been poorly studied.

In 2012, Colombino and colleagues analyzed primary and metastatic melanoma samples and found that overall 43% of primary melanomas have mutated BRAF with no significant frequency increase in metastatic lesions [84]. However, Shinozaki and collaborators in 2004 analyzed the BRAF mutation in tumor specimens and showed that this mutation is more frequent in melanoma metastasis (57%) than in primary melanomas (31%), which suggests that it can be acquired during metastasis. They also analyzed 13 pairs of primary melanomas with their respective metastases. Four pairs were not mutated in the primary or the metastatic tumor, other four pairs were mutated in both stages and five pairs (38%) present the wild type gene in the primary tumors and the mutated one in the metastatic tumors. This suggests that BRAF is not a key factor for the development of metastasis, although it can be acquired during this process. However, the frequency of mutation found in the study was lower than the report in the literature [81].

Another report that analyzed metastatic tumors in an Australian cohort demonstrated that 48% of the patients had a BRAF mutation, with 74% being the $BRAF^{V600E}$. Interestingly, the presence of the BRAF mutation led to a poorer survival unless patients were treated with BRAF inhibitor [85].

Another study shows that inhibition of $BRAF^{V600E}$ expression causes a significant decrease in the metastatic ability of the metastatic cell lines Lu1205 and UACC 903M. This impaired ability to metastasize was due the reduction of cell extravasation through the endothelium, process mediated by IL-8 and ICAM [79]. Mutated BRAF can also participate of metastasis development by the generation of new blood vessels by promoting macrophage inhibitory cytokine-1 (MIC-1) and vascular endothelial growth factors (VEGF) secretion [82]. MIC-1 was shown to be upregulated in metastatic melanoma cell lines and patient biopsies in comparison with melanocytes. A trend was also observed in comparison with primary melanomas [86]. A RNA interference targeting $BRAF^{V600E}$ blocks melanoma cell invasion *in vitro* and decreases MMP-2 activity while $BRAF^{V600E}$ induces activity of MMP-1, also suggesting that this mutation can be involved in the metastatic process [82].

Mutation in BRAF can also activate ERK1/2, which was seen activated by Jorgensen and collaborators in 54% of primary melanomas and 33% of metastatic tumors [87]. However, Mirmohammadsadegh and collaborators analyzed the expression of phosphorylated ERK1/2 (pERK) in human cells and specimens and saw that it levels was low in melanocytes, upregulated in melanoma cell lines and abundant in melanoma metastasis. Yet, this study did not distinguish between non-metastatic and metastatic cell lines and did not analyze samples of primary tissue [88].

The successful treatment of metastatic melanomas with $BRAF^{V600E}$ inhibitors [89] and the events here forehead mentioned suggests that this mutation is involved somehow in the process of metastasis, but the exact mechanisms involved are still unclear [82].

6.2. MITF

Microphthalmia-associated transcription factor (MITF) is a master regulator of melanocyte development and regulates survival, growth, differentiation and pigmentation of these cells [90]. There are several isoforms of MITF described, but in melanocytes and melanoma there is a predominance of the isoform MITF-M [91].

The levels of MITF expression are very important to cell fate. High levels of MITF induce cell cycle arrest and differentiation, while low levels promote cell cycle arrest, apoptosis and even invasion and metastasis. If MITF levels are depleted for long time, melanoma can enter quiescence or senescence. Thus, only an intermediate level of MITF favors cell proliferation [1, 90]. Wherefore, levels of MITF have to be tightly regulated during melanocytic development and even during melanoma progression.

Several reports indicate that most human melanomas express MITF [1], and that MITF is expressed in high levels in benign and primary tumors [91]. MITF is genomically amplified in 10% of primary melanomas and 21% of metastatic melanoma, and the amplification in the metastatic samples correlates with a significant decrease in the 5-year survival rate of patients [92]. However, expression of MITF in metastatic lesion is variable. Beyond the specimens that present MITF amplification and therefore high levels of expression, other metastatic lesions present predominantly downregulation of MITF [93]. A report demonstrated that depletion of MITF expression in mouse and human cells is sufficient to induce experimental lung metastasis [91]. Consistently, high levels of MITF in melanoma patients are associated with low invasiveness and fewer metastases [90]. Because some metastatic lesions present low expression of MITF while others present MITF amplification, it is proposed that MITF can have paradoxical effects in different sub-groups of melanomas. For example, the decrease in MITF expression in metastatic melanomas can be beneficial for tumor growth because it reduces pigmentation, and therefore the cellular energy utilized for pigment production [93]. However, in specimens with high expression of MITF, it can regulate c-Met expression, which upregulation appears to have a functional role in metastatization of melanoma [94].

Because MITF is part of a complex pathway, alterations in factors upstream or downstream to MITF can affect melanoma development [90]. However, this has not been properly investigated in metastatic melanoma. Until now, the expression and functional role of MITF in metastatic melanoma is not determined.

6.3. TGF-β

The transforming growth factor-β (TGF-β) is a cytokine implies in several cellular processes, as cell proliferation, differentiation and survival. TGF-β interacts with its receptor, leading to the receptor phosphorylation, which then phosphorylates the cytoplasmatic proteins SMAD. The SMADs proteins accumulate in the nucleus and acts as transcription factors. TGF-β can also signal through a non-canonical pathway. In this respect, TGF-β can activate phosphatidylinositol-3-kinase (PI3K) and several mitogen activated protein kinases (MAPKs), leading to cell signaling independent of SMAD [95].

There are three isoforms of TGF-β in mammalian, TGF-β1, TGF-β2, TGF-β3. *In vitro*, normal melanocytes and malignant melanomas express TGF-β1 and TGF-β3, but TGF-β2 is only found in melanoma cells. The expression of TGF-β2 correlates with the deepness of melanoma. Thus, metastatic and highly invasive tumors present TGF-β2 expression, while a minority of primary melanomas minimally invasive express TGF-β and *in situ* tumors does not express it [95]. In addition, melanoma secretes large amounts of TGF-β, and high amounts of TGF-β in plasma are associated with advanced tumor stages [96] since it foments tumor growth, angiogenesis, invasiveness and dissemination.

The overexpression of an inhibitory SMAD, SMAD 7, is effective in reducing secretion of MMPs and impairing bone metastasis development. The blockage of TGF-β receptor has the same effect. TGF-β also promotes the epithelial to mesenchymal transition (EMT), an event associated with increase in metastasis, increase in MMP2 and MMP9 expression, and angiogenesis by modulating IL-8, MMPs, VEGF, among other important factors [95, 97].

TGF-β also promotes metastasis through expression induction of the transcription factor GLI2. High expression of GLI2 correlated with increased cell invasiveness and bone metastasis emergence. In a murine model of induced metastasis, cells with elevated expression of GLI2 caused bone metastasis, while cells with low level of this factor have reduced and heterogenic capacity to form metastasis. In addition, the GLI2 knockdown in an aggressive melanoma cell line (1205Lu) dramatically diminishes their ability to form bone metastasis [96].

6.4. Wnt (β-catenin and WNTs)

β-catenin is an adherent junction protein and a transcriptional coativator. It mediates cell adhesion, proliferation, survival and migration [1]. It participates in the WNT pathway and the interaction between WNT ligands and receptors leads to the accumulation of β-catenin in the nucleus, where it promotes transactivation of target genes [98].

The role of β-catenin in melanoma it is still unclear. Some show β-catenin is frequently constitutively activated in melanomas and that its accumulation promotes metastasis, while others show its high expression suppresses invasion and indicates a better prognosis for patients [1, 99].

A report shows that β-catenin is an important regulator of melanoma metastasis to lymph nodes and lungs. In this case, β-catenin cooperates with PTEN loss and $BRAF^{V600E}$ to promote primary tumor and metastasis, but the mechanism was not enlightened [1]. In other study, activation of β-catenin signaling increased metastatic potential in NRAS-driven melanoma in mice, although it repressed cell migration, indicating that β-catenin inhibits the initial steps of metastasis, as cell migration, but can be involved in the latest steps of this process [100].

However, another study that analyzed β-catenin expression by immunohistochemistry in melanocytic samples identified that β-catenin was strongly stained in 96% of melanocytic nevi, in 94% of radial growth phase primary melanoma, in 65% of vertical growth phase primary melanoma and in only 38% of metastatic melanomas [101]. The involvement of β-catenin decrease in melanoma metastasis was also seen indirectly by decrease in WLS, an important component to WNT ligands secretion. The reduction of WLS expression by shRNA in the melanoma cell line A375 caused spontaneous metastasis in the lung of mice. Of 36 animals injected with WLS shRNA cells, 10 developed lung metastasis while none of the 18 animals injected with control shRNA cell presented metastasis. This was due to the inhibition of the WNT/ β-catenin pathway [98].

Therefore, β-catenin effects on melanoma metastasis are still not fully understood and may depend on cellular context [100]. Some state that WNT signaling via the canonical pathway, which involves β-catenin, is associated with a less metastatic phenotype, while the non-canonical pathway, involving Wnt5A, would be related with increased malignancy [6]. The overexpression of Wnt5A appears to be consistently associated with a more aggressive disease and metastasis development [1] and this is probably due the upregulation of metastatic markers, as CD44 and Snail, and the promotion of EMT [6].

Wnt5 activity is regulated by heparan sulfate proteoglycans (HSPGs), glycoproteins that are categorized based on the structure of their glycosaminoglycan (GAG) chains and although has been poorly studied in melanomas, has been recently associated with melanoma metastasis. For example, HSPGs are important to cell signaling through the non-canonical Wnt pathway. The HSPGs syndecans 1 and 4 are necessary to the presentation of Wnt5A to its receptor ROR2 and its consequent internalization and signaling. Cleavage of the syndecans GAGs result in less Wnt5A at the cell surface and a consequent decrease in the cell metastatic potential [6].

6.5. PI3K

The phosphoinositide-3 kinase (PI3K) pathway is another key signaling cascade that controls cell survival, proliferation and motility. PI3K is activated by receptor tyrosine kinases or RAS leading to the release of second messenger PIP3, which can activate several downstream effectors, as AKT. PTEN (Phosphatase and Tensin Homolog) is an important negative regulator of this pathway [1].

PI3K pathway is commonly hyperactivated in melanomas. A report that analyzed 68 metastatic melanomas showed that 41% presented a mutation in this pathway [102]. Besides 3% of metastatic melanomas presents activating mutation of PI3K and 5-20% of late-stage melanoma present mutations that leads to PTEN loss, which is the protein most commonly mutated in this pathway [1]. Another study that analyzed PI3K protein expression demonstrated that PI3K expression was low in nevi and high in melanomas. Interestingly this expression was even higher in metastatic specimens [103].

Inactivation of PTEN by mutation leads to a constitutive activation of PI3K pathway. Because PTEN mutations are rarely found in primary melanomas, it is proposed that the activation of the PI3K pathway may be important to the late events of melanoma progression, as invasion and metastasis [103]. An interesting study demonstrated that mice with PTEN loss and $BRAF^{V600E}$ develop malignant melanoma that is able to metastasize to lymph nodes and distant organs, while mice with only $BRAF^{V600E}$ produced benign melanocytic hyperplasia, showing that PTEN loss cooperate with $BRAF^{V600E}$ to induce metastasis [104].

AKT is also able to induce tumor cell invasion and metastasis to the lung in a mouse model by inhibiting the small GTPase RhoB [105]. Moreover, a higher percentage of biopsies present strong phospho-AKT (the activated form of AKT) staining in metastatic melanoma than in primary melanomas and nevi and high levels of phospho-AKT are associated with poor patient survival rates (Dai 2005).

7. Other pathways

7.1. Telomerase

Telomerase is a ribonucleoprotein complex and its main function is to maintain the telomeric repeats that cap the ends of eukaryotic chromosomes and therefore preserve their integrity by preventing end-to-end fusions [106]. In melanocytic lesions, is seen that nevi have low or even absent telomerase activity, primary melanomas have intermediate levels of activity and metastatic melanomas present increased telomerase activity. Telomerase promoter seems to be frequently mutated in melanoma and two mutational hotspots were found in 85% of melanoma metastases [107].

The inhibition of the RNA portion of the telomerase, called TER (telomerase RNA), results in severe decrease in metastatic tumor development. In an experiment, mice that received injection of melanoma cells with TER downregulated presented 70% fewer metastases in the lung then mice injected with control cells. The inhibition of TER also led to the downregulation of several genes, including genes involved in transcriptional regulation, cell proliferation and adhesion, chromatin assembly and others. Interestingly, it was also seen a regulation of genes of the glycolytic pathway, as aldolase, suggesting that telomerase can mediate its metastatic properties through activation of glycolysis in cancer [106].

7.2. ACP5

The analysis of the expression of ACP5 (Tartrate-resistant acid phosphatase 5), a protein involved in bone development [108], in a melanoma tissue microarray comparing primary and metastatic specimens demonstrated that ACP5 is upregulated in the metastatic lesions. To confirm the role of ACP5 in metastasis, the authors overexpressed ACP5 in a human poorly metastatic melanoma cell line (1205Lu) and observed an increase in the metastatic ability of those cells *in vivo*. Animals that received injection of the parental 1205Lu cell did not develop spontaneous metastasis, while 40% of the animals that were injected with the cells overexpressing ACP5 developed metastasis to the lung and lymph nodes [109].

7.3. Chemokines

Chemokines are secreted chemotactic cytokines that were first identified as modulators of leukocytes trafficking to inflammatory sites. Chemokines realize its biological function through the binding in chemokine receptors, G-protein coupled receptors. It has been seen by several authors that melanoma cells have a high expression of chemokines and that its interaction with its receptors stimulates tumor growth, angiogenesis and metastasis [110].

The expression of CXCL8, a potent chemokine also known as IL-8, has been associated with tumor angiogenesis, progression and metastasis in some mouse models. In one case, the induction of CXCL8 expression by ultraviolet-B radiation potentiated tumor and metastasis development. In addition, metastatic melanoma cell lines express higher levels of CXCL8 than its non-metastatic variants [110]. Moreover, in an analysis of tumor specimens, it was seen that radial growth tumors do not present CXCL8 expression, while half of the vertical growth tumors present it. A significant increase in CXCL8 expression was also seen in metastatic samples in comparison with thin melanomas [111]. The CXCL8 receptor, CXCR2, was also seen to be involved in melanoma metastasis. *In vivo* murine studies using knockout models demonstrated that CXCR2 played a major role in melanoma metastasis to the lung [112].

Chemokines receptors also appear to be important to specific organ metastasis. CXCR4 was identified as the most frequent expressed chemokine receptor in liver metastasis of paraffin-embedded tissue, with 89% of the samples expressing it [113]. CCR9 was observed as expressed in a great majority of intestine metastasis of melanoma, but not in other organs [114].

7.4. NEDD9

NEDD9 (neural precursor expressed, developmentally downregulated 9) is an adaptor protein that belong to the Cas family of signal transduction molecules. NEDD9 is genomically amplified in melanomas and its high expression correlates with melanoma progression and metastasis. NEDD9 is frequently overexpressed in human metastatic tumor in comparison to primary ones and its expression enhances invasion *in vitro* and metastasis *in vivo* of both normal and transformed melanocytes. NEDD9 appears to mediate melanoma invasive behavior through interaction with focal adhesion kinase and modulation of focal contact formation [115].

7.5. MicroRNAs

MicroRNAs (miRNAs) are small non-coding RNA Molecules - 17 to 22 nucleotides - that regulate gene expression post-transcriptionally. MiRNAs are negative regulators of gene expression. These regulatory RNAs act by binding to mRNA molecules of specific gene targets and inducing their cleavage or translation repression. Because just approximately seven nucleotides of the miRNA – the so-called seed region - interact with the target mRNA, each miRNA may have a large number of targets. Therefore, a unique miRNA can influence the expression of even hundreds of proteins and, for that, miRNAs participate of several processes in the cell as development, cell proliferation, differentiation and metabolism [116-117].

Because of the critical role miRNAs have in the cell biology, changes in their expression patterns have impact in different disorders, as cancer itself [116]. After miRNAs being related with tumorigenesis, it did not take long until they were specifically related with metastasis. The first microRNA linked with metastasis was described in 2007 by Ma, Weinberg and colleagues. In this paper, the authors demonstrated that microRNA-10b is highly expressed in metastatic breast cancer cells and that its overexpression in non-metastatic breast tumors leads to metastasis [91, 118]. Two years later, in 2009, Hurst termed the miRNAs involved in the metastasis process, metastamiRs. The metastamiRs modulate key signaling pathways and can promote or suppress metastasis [117].

Recently, miRNAs have been linked with melanoma metastasis, but there is still limited information about it. Most time, there is only one study analyzing the involvement of certain miRNA with melanoma aggressiveness. Here, we will present some of miRNAs that are consistently associated with melanoma metastasis, but are not necessarily defined as metastamiRs.

A miRNA that appears to act as a metastamiR in melanoma is the miR-214. MiR-214 expression was evaluated in the poorly metastatic lineage A375 and in its highly metastatic variant cell lines, originated from several passages *in vivo*. It was seen an upregulation of miR-214 in the highly metastatic melanoma cells lines in comparison with the parental one. Beyond that, the overexpression of miR-214 in a metastatic lineage that expressed intermediate levels of this miRNA resulted in a higher number of lung metastases than the control in a metastasis formation assay *in vivo*. In addition, miR-214 silencing in a highly metastatic lineage, which expressed high levels of this miRNA, caused a significantly reduction of lung metastases formation. Furthermore, as primary tumor growth was not influenced by miR-214, these results indicate miR-214 as a metastamiR with an important role in the melanoma progression [119].

Other metastamiRs which involvement with melanoma has been recently discovered are miR-30b and miR-30d. These clustered miRNAs (miRNAs that are transcribed together) are upregulated in melanoma metastasis samples related to primary melanomas and nevi. Overexpression and underexpression assays *in vivo* proved the importance of this cluster expression to metastasis occurrence. In addition to the increased metastatic potential, the upregulation of these miRNAs correlates with shorter time to recurrence and reduced overall survival. Overexpression of miR-30b/30d promotes melanoma metastasis by modifying the glycosylation pattern of transmembrane proteins, more specifically by directly repressing GalNAc transferase GALNT7, which culminates in pro-invasive and immunosuppressive effects [120].

The miR-1908, miR-199a-5p and miR-199a-3p also promote human melanoma metastasis. These miRNAs are overexpressed in highly metastatic cell lines in comparison with their poorly metastatic parental cells. Ectopic expression of these miRNAs in the parental cell lines (MeWo) caused increased metastatic potential and individual inhibition of these miRNAs in the metastatic cells suppressed metastatic colonization. Interestingly, the expression of these miRNAs are upregulated in primary melanomas that had metastasized in comparison with those that had not, indicating that the expression of them in primary tumors is an early event that can be predictive of melanoma metastasis. Another indicator that those are metastamiRs is that they do not affect tumor growth [121].

An important genomic region involved in melanoma development is the 7q31-34 region, because it is commonly amplified in melanomas. This region includes the BRAF and c-MET oncogenes, and the miR-182. It was observed a higher expression of this miRNA in metastatic melanoma tumors compared with primary melanomas and nevi, and this is caused, at least in part, by gene amplification. It was seen that this overexpression promotes metastatic properties as cell ability to extravasate or to seed at a distant site, through the downregulation of FOX3 and MITF-M [122].

Another miRNA that is upregulated in metastatic melanoma in comparison with primary melanoma and dysplastic nevi is the miR-21. MiR-21 expression also correlates positively with Breslow thickness, advanced clinical stage and metastatic behavior [123-124]. miR-532-5p also presents higher expression levels in metastatic melanoma tumors than in primary melanomas. An important target of miR-532-5p in metastatic tumor is the transcription factor RUNX3, which may act through β-catenin [125].

miR-221/222 are also upregulated in metastatic cells relative to primary melanomas or melanocytes. They are not expressed in compound nevus, but are progressively increased in the melanoma progression, with the higher level being in the metastases samples. Although they have increased expression in metastatic melanomas, they increase during tumorigenesis, which suggests that they are not metastamiRs *per se* [126].

In comparison with miRNAs that are overexpressed in melanoma, little is known about miRNAs that are diminished during melanoma progression [127], so even less is known about miRNAs downregulated in melanoma metastasis. Fortunately, there is some information in this area and we will present it here.

The miR-200 family (miR-200a, miR-200b, miR-200c, miR-141 and miR-429) is important in melanoma development, however its function is controversial, with some showing that miR-200 is upregulated during melanoma progression and some showing that it is downregulated. Importantly for metastasis, miR-200c was shown to be downregulated in metastatic melanoma compared with primary melanoma and melanocytic nevi [128]. In addition, miR-200c levels were different in melanoma samples located at primary versus distant metastatic sites [129]. The role in suppressing metastasis was confirmed by a miR-200c overexpression assay, which showed inhibition of melanoma growth and metastasis *in vivo*. It appears that one pathway that this miRNA act is through Bmi-1 (a Polycomb group protein) and E-cadherin, which, together, regulate proliferation and motility [128]. Interestingly, the combination of miR-200c overexpression with the tumor vaccine B16F10/GPI-IL-21 potentiated the metastasis inhibition effect of the vaccine, which has previously shown some protective anti-melanoma immunity but failed to completely inhibit tumor and metastases development [130].

One of the first discovered miRNAs, let-7b, is also related with the aggressiveness of melanoma. This miRNA has been implicated as a tumor suppressor in several tumors and its levels are diminished in metastatic melanoma cell lines compared to primary melanoma cell lines [131]. The ectopic expression of let-7b in the highly metastatic cells B16-F10 originated a great decrease in the number of tumor nodules formed in the lung. The authors also suggested that the low expression of miR-7b facilitates metastasis through the upregulation of its target Basigin (an extracellular matrix metalloproteinase inducer), that consequently increases MMPs production [132].

MiR-9 is also frequently lost in metastatic melanoma tissues related to primary melanoma tissues. In addition, the same expression was observed in metastatic melanoma cell lines compared with cells from radial growth phase melanomas and vertical growth phase melanomas. The low expression of miR-9 correlates with high cell proliferation, migration, and metastasis development *in vivo*. The low levels of this miRNA stimulate the metastatic phenotype through the upregulation of NF-kB (a direct target of miR-9) and consequent high levels of Snail and downregulation of E-cadherin [133].

Others miRNAs that are downregulated in metastatic melanoma in comparison with primary melanoma are the miR-20b and miR-145, however to confirm their role in metastasis it would be important to do other experiments beyond its expression analysis. The mechanism of action of miR-145 is still unknown [134], however miR-20b seems to act through the regulation of the proteinase-activated receptor 1 (PAR-1), a thrombin receptor that it is involved in thrombosis and hemostasis and appears to have a key role in the progress of malignant melanoma [135].

Although there are still limited studies about the role of miRNAs in the process of melanoma metastasis, it is already a fact that the miRNA circuit is altered in this process and therefore the miRNA processing machinery may be deregulated. However, this has been poorly studied. A study shows that TARBP2 e SND1 (two RISC components) are overexpressed in cutaneous malignant melanoma metastases related to primary cutaneous malignant melanoma. This study also shows that Dicer, Drosha and other molecules of the miRNA machinery are not altered in the metastasis process [136]. In another study with tissue samples, it was observed Dicer upregulation in metastatic melanoma in comparison with *in situ* melanoma. Furthermore, high expression of Dicer correlated with aggressive cancer features as increased tumor mitotic index, Breslow's depth of invasion and nodal metastasis and with metastasis to the non-sentinel lymph node. High levels of Dicer expression also appears to be related with elevate rates of metastasis to organs and to the sentinel lymph node, but this relation was not statistically significant [131]. Both studies were performed with a restrict number of samples, so further studies are important to confirm which enzymes of the miRNA machinery are altered in the melanoma metastasis process.

8. Conclusion

Cutaneous melanoma is a melanocytic tumor whose incidence and mortality are on the rise worldwide. Prognosis of patients with melanoma depends on the stage of the tumor and is usually based on microstaging and radiological evaluation of metastases. Among the numerous prognostic parameters, tumor thickness is the most sensitive in predicting the risk of metastasis. However, it is still difficult to determine the prognosis for melanoma patients individually. More specific prognostic indicators for metastatic melanoma are needed.

The homeostasis of skin melanocytes is controlled by the keratinocytes of the epidermis and the balance between these cells is maintained by regulating the division of melanocytes. Mutations in genes regulating growth, changes in the production of paracrine growth factors and loss of adhesion molecules (integrins, cadherins, selectins and family of immunoglobulins) contribute to the disruption of cell signaling. Thus, the melanocytes may escape regulation, spread and proliferate and thereby form melanoma.

Several genes are involved in the pathogenesis of malignant melanoma. The best known in metastatic melanoma are the mutations in BRAF, MITF and changes in WNT and PI3K pathways. Due to the heterogeneity of metastatic lesions many changes have been described for metastatic melanoma, thus leading to greater difficulty of classifying major pathways altered in melanoma. Therefore, studies on the molecular biology of melanoma seeking to identify molecular markers for prognosis are interesting. Immunohistochemical (Mel-CAM), enzyme (Tyrosinase), protein (integrins, ICAM-1, cyclin D1), microRNAs and genetic (CDKN2A, p53) markers could be used for this purpose.

In this way, although there are several molecular alterations described in melanoma metastasis, there are some inconsistent data, probably due driver factors, as the heterogeneity of metastatic lesions, difficulty of correctly classifying the different stages of the tumor and difficulty in obtaining appropriate samples. Moreover, there is complicacy in the classification of cell lines and use of inappropriate technique. For example, today it is well established that metastatic characteristics can only be analyzed *in vivo*, but there are cases that only *in vitro* assays, as migration and invasion assays, are performed and the authors quote an involvement with metastasis. In addition, the same cell line is considered as highly aggressive in some studies and as poorly metastatic in others. These issues complicate a proper understanding of the melanoma metastasis biology.

Acknowledgements

This work was supported by FAPESP (2012/08776-5 to MGJ, 2013/04829-0 to ACM, and 2010/18715-8 to MT) and CNPq (470681/2012-8 to MGJ).

Author details

Ana Carolina Monteiro, Mariana Toricelli and Miriam Galvonas Jasiulionis*

*Address all correspondence to: mjasiulionis@gmail.com

Pharmacology Department, Universidade Federal de São Paulo, São Paulo, SP, Brazil

Ana Carolina Monteiro and Mariana Toricelli share the first authorship

References

[1] Orgaz JL, Sanz-Moreno V. Emerging molecular targets in melanoma invasion and metastasis. Pigment Cell Melanoma Res. 2013 Jan;26(1):39-57.

[2] Hoon DS, Ferris R, Tanaka R, Chong KK, Alix-Panabieres C, Pantel K. Molecular mechanisms of metastasis. J Surg Oncol. 2011 May 1;103(6):508-17.

[3] Leibowitz-Amit R, Sidi Y, Avni D. Aberrations in the micro-RNA biogenesis machinery and the emerging roles of micro-RNAs in the pathogenesis of cutaneous malignant melanoma. Pigment Cell Melanoma Res. 2012 Nov;25(6):740-57.

[4] Gupta GP, Massague J. Cancer metastasis: building a framework. Cell. 2006 Nov 17;127(4):679-95.

[5] Chin L, Garraway LA, Fisher DE. Malignant melanoma: genetics and therapeutics in the genomic era. Genes Dev. 2006 Aug 15;20(16):2149-82.

[6] O'Connell MP, Weeraratna AT. A spoonful of sugar makes the melanoma go: the role of heparan sulfate proteoglycans in melanoma metastasis. Pigment Cell Melanoma Res. 2011 Dec;24(6):1133-47.

[7] Segura MF, Greenwald HS, Hanniford D, Osman I, Hernando E. MicroRNA and cutaneous melanoma: from discovery to prognosis and therapy. Carcinogenesis. 2012 Oct;33(10):1823-32.

[8] Zbytek B, Carlson JA, Granese J, Ross J, Mihm MC, Jr., Slominski A. Current concepts of metastasis in melanoma. Expert Rev Dermatol. 2008 Oct;3(5):569-85.

[9] Hanahan D, Weinberg RA. Hallmarks of cancer: the next generation. Cell. 2011 Mar 4;144(5):646-74.

[10] Bennett DC. How to make a melanoma: what do we know of the primary clonal events? Pigment Cell Melanoma Res. 2008 Feb;21(1):27-38.

[11] Charames GS, Bapat B. Genomic instability and cancer. Curr Mol Med. 2003 Nov; 3(7):589-96.

[12] Mazzocca A, Carloni V. The metastatic process: methodological advances and pharmacological challenges. Curr Med Chem. 2009;16(14):1704-17.

[13] Edelman GM. Cell adhesion molecules in the regulation of animal form and tissue pattern. Annu Rev Cell Biol. 1986;2:81-116.

[14] Johnson JP. Cell adhesion molecules in the development and progression of malignant melanoma. Cancer Metastasis Rev. 1999;18(3):345-57.

[15] Valentijn AJ, Zouq N, Gilmore AP. Anoikis. Biochem Soc Trans. 2004 Jun;32(Pt3): 421-5.

[16] Grossmann J. Molecular mechanisms of "detachment-induced apoptosis--Anoikis". Apoptosis. 2002 Jun;7(3):247-60.

[17] Oba-Shinjo SM, Correa M, Ricca TI, Molognoni F, Pinhal MA, Neves IA, et al. Melanocyte transformation associated with substrate adhesion impediment. Neoplasia. 2006 Mar;8(3):231-41.

[18] Cai Q, Yan L, Xu Y. Anoikis resistance is a critical feature of highly aggressive ovarian cancer cells. Oncogene. 2014 Aug 18;0.

[19] Yao X, Jennings S, Ireland SK, Pham T, Temple B, Davis M, et al. The anoikis effector Bit1 displays tumor suppressive function in lung cancer cells. PLoS One. 2014;9(7):e101564.

[20] Haass NK, Smalley KS, Herlyn M. The role of altered cell-cell communication in melanoma progression. J Mol Histol. 2004 Mar;35(3):309-18.

[21] Kuphal S, Bauer R, Bosserhoff AK. Integrin signaling in malignant melanoma. Cancer Metastasis Rev. 2005 Jun;24(2):195-222.

[22] Clark EA, Brugge JS. Integrins and signal transduction pathways: the road taken. Science. 1995 Apr 14;268(5208):233-9.

[23] Gahmberg CG, Fagerholm SC, Nurmi SM, Chavakis T, Marchesan S, Gronholm M. Regulation of integrin activity and signalling. Biochim Biophys Acta. 2009 Jun; 1790(6):431-44.

[24] Albelda SM, Mette SA, Elder DE, Stewart R, Damjanovich L, Herlyn M, et al. Integrin distribution in malignant melanoma: association of the beta 3 subunit with tumor progression. Cancer Res. 1990 Oct 15;50(20):6757-64.

[25] Natali PG, Nicotra MR, Bartolazzi A, Cavaliere R, Bigotti A. Integrin expression in cutaneous malignant melanoma: association of the alpha 3/beta 1 heterodimer with tumor progression. Int J Cancer. 1993 Apr 22;54(1):68-72.

[26] Schadendorf D, Gawlik C, Haney U, Ostmeier H, Suter L, Czarnetzki BM. Tumour progression and metastatic behaviour in vivo correlates with integrin expression on melanocytic tumours. J Pathol. 1993 Aug;170(4):429-34.

[27] Moretti S, Martini L, Berti E, Pinzi C, Giannotti B. Adhesion molecule profile and malignancy of melanocytic lesions. Melanoma Res. 1993 Aug;3(4):235-9.

[28] Li X, Chen B, Blystone SD, McHugh KP, Ross FP, Ramos DM. Differential expression of alphav integrins in K1735 melanoma cells. Invasion Metastasis. 1998;18(1):1-14.

[29] Brooks PC, Montgomery AM, Rosenfeld M, Reisfeld RA, Hu T, Klier G, et al. Integrin alpha v beta 3 antagonists promote tumor regression by inducing apoptosis of angiogenic blood vessels. Cell. 1994 Dec 30;79(7):1157-64.

[30] Trikha M, Timar J, Lundy SK, Szekeres K, Cai Y, Porter AT, et al. The high affinity alphaIIb beta3 integrin is involved in invasion of human melanoma cells. Cancer Res. 1997 Jun 15;57(12):2522-8.

[31] Mitjans F, Sander D, Adan J, Sutter A, Martinez JM, Jaggle CS, et al. An anti-alpha v-integrin antibody that blocks integrin function inhibits the development of a human melanoma in nude mice. J Cell Sci. 1995 Aug;108 (Pt 8):2825-38.

[32] Zhang Y, Yang M, Ji Q, Fan D, Peng H, Yang C, et al. Anoikis induction and metastasis suppression by a new integrin alphavbeta3 inhibitor in human melanoma cell line M21. Invest New Drugs. 2011 Aug;29(4):666-73.

[33] Friedl P, Zanker KS, Brocker EB. Cell migration strategies in 3-D extracellular matrix: differences in morphology, cell matrix interactions, and integrin function. Microsc Res Tech. 1998 Dec 1;43(5):369-78.

[34] Hartstein ME, Grove AS, Jr., Woog JJ. The role of the integrin family of adhesion molecules in the development of tumors metastatic to the orbit. Ophthal Plast Reconstr Surg. 1997 Dec;13(4):227-38.

[35] Cavallaro U, Dejana E. Adhesion molecule signalling: not always a sticky business. Nat Rev Mol Cell Biol. 2011 Mar;12(3):189-97.

[36] Aricescu AR, Jones EY. Immunoglobulin superfamily cell adhesion molecules: zippers and signals. Curr Opin Cell Biol. 2007 Oct;19(5):543-50.

[37] Maness PF, Schachner M. Neural recognition molecules of the immunoglobulin superfamily: signaling transducers of axon guidance and neuronal migration. Nat Neurosci. 2007 Jan;10(1):19-26.

[38] Thies A, Moll I, Berger J, Wagener C, Brummer J, Schulze HJ, et al. CEACAM1 expression in cutaneous malignant melanoma predicts the development of metastatic disease. J Clin Oncol. 2002 May 15;20(10):2530-6.

[39] Johnson JP, Stade BG, Holzmann B, Schwable W, Riethmuller G. De novo expression of intercellular-adhesion molecule 1 in melanoma correlates with increased risk of metastasis. Proc Natl Acad Sci U S A. 1989 Jan;86(2):641-4.

[40] Natali P, Nicotra MR, Cavaliere R, Bigotti A, Romano G, Temponi M, et al. Differential expression of intercellular adhesion molecule 1 in primary and metastatic melanoma lesions. Cancer Res. 1990 Feb 15;50(4):1271-8.

[41] Natali PG, Hamby CV, Felding-Habermann B, Liang B, Nicotra MR, Di Filippo F, et al. Clinical significance of alpha(v)beta3 integrin and intercellular adhesion molecule-1 expression in cutaneous malignant melanoma lesions. Cancer Res. 1997 Apr 15;57(8):1554-60.

[42] Schadendorf D, Heidel J, Gawlik C, Suter L, Czarnetzki BM. Association with clinical outcome of expression of VLA-4 in primary cutaneous malignant melanoma as well as P-selectin and E-selectin on intratumoral vessels. J Natl Cancer Inst. 1995 Mar 1;87(5):366-71.

[43] Brummer J, Ebrahimnejad A, Flayeh R, Schumacher U, Loning T, Bamberger AM, et al. cis Interaction of the cell adhesion molecule CEACAM1 with integrin beta(3). Am J Pathol. 2001 Aug;159(2):537-46.

[44] Liu WF, Ji SR, Sun JJ, Zhang Y, Liu ZY, Liang AB, et al. CD146 Expression Correlates with Epithelial-Mesenchymal Transition Markers and a Poor Prognosis in Gastric Cancer. Int J Mol Sci. 2012;13(5):6399-406.

[45] Kristiansen G, Yu Y, Schluns K, Sers C, Dietel M, Petersen I. Expression of the cell adhesion molecule CD146/MCAM in non-small cell lung cancer. Anal Cell Pathol. 2003;25(2):77-81.

[46] Aldovini D, Demichelis F, Doglioni C, Di Vizio D, Galligioni E, Brugnara S, et al. M-CAM expression as marker of poor prognosis in epithelial ovarian cancer. Int J Cancer. 2006 Oct 15;119(8):1920-6.

[47] Zabouo G, Imbert AM, Jacquemier J, Finetti P, Moreau T, Esterni B, et al. CD146 expression is associated with a poor prognosis in human breast tumors and with enhanced motility in breast cancer cell lines. Breast Cancer Res. 2009;11(1):R1.

[48] Li G, Herlyn M. Dynamics of intercellular communication during melanoma development. Mol Med Today. 2000 Apr;6(4):163-9.

[49] Shih LM, Hsu MY, Palazzo JP, Herlyn M. The cell-cell adhesion receptor Mel-CAM acts as a tumor suppressor in breast carcinoma. Am J Pathol. 1997 Sep;151(3):745-51.

[50] Hsu M, Andl T, Li G, Meinkoth JL, Herlyn M. Cadherin repertoire determines partner-specific gap junctional communication during melanoma progression. J Cell Sci. 2000 May;113 (Pt 9):1535-42.

[51] Weidle UH, Eggle D, Klostermann S, Swart GW. ALCAM/CD166: cancer-related issues. Cancer Genomics Proteomics. 2010 Sep-Oct;7(5):231-43.

[52] van Kempen LC, Meier F, Egeblad M, Kersten-Niessen MJ, Garbe C, Weidle UH, et al. Truncation of activated leukocyte cell adhesion molecule: a gateway to melanoma metastasis. J Invest Dermatol. 2004 May;122(5):1293-301.

[53] Vleminckx K, Kemler R. Cadherins and tissue formation: integrating adhesion and signaling. Bioessays. 1999 Mar;21(3):211-20.

[54] Gruss C, Herlyn M. Role of cadherins and matrixins in melanoma. Curr Opin Oncol. 2001 Mar;13(2):117-23.

[55] Poser I, Dominguez D, de Herreros AG, Varnai A, Buettner R, Bosserhoff AK. Loss of E-cadherin expression in melanoma cells involves up-regulation of the transcriptional repressor Snail. J Biol Chem. 2001 Jul 6;276(27):24661-6.

[56] Comijn J, Berx G, Vermassen P, Verschueren K, van Grunsven L, Bruyneel E, et al. The two-handed E box binding zinc finger protein SIP1 downregulates E-cadherin and induces invasion. Mol Cell. 2001 Jun;7(6):1267-78.

[57] Jean D, Gershenwald JE, Huang S, Luca M, Hudson MJ, Tainsky MA, et al. Loss of AP-2 results in up-regulation of MCAM/MUC18 and an increase in tumor growth and metastasis of human melanoma cells. J Biol Chem. 1998 Jun 26;273(26):16501-8.

[58] Valyi-Nagy IT, Hirka G, Jensen PJ, Shih IM, Juhasz I, Herlyn M. Undifferentiated keratinocytes control growth, morphology, and antigen expression of normal melanocytes through cell-cell contact. Lab Invest. 1993 Aug;69(2):152-9.

[59] Tang A, Eller MS, Hara M, Yaar M, Hirohashi S, Gilchrest BA. E-cadherin is the major mediator of human melanocyte adhesion to keratinocytes in vitro. J Cell Sci. 1994 Apr;107 (Pt 4):983-92.

[60] Danen EH, de Vries TJ, Morandini R, Ghanem GG, Ruiter DJ, van Muijen GN. E-cadherin expression in human melanoma. Melanoma Res. 1996 Apr;6(2):127-31.

[61] Li G, Satyamoorthy K, Herlyn M. N-cadherin-mediated intercellular interactions promote survival and migration of melanoma cells. Cancer Res. 2001 May 1;61(9): 3819-25.

[62] Chang C, Werb Z. The many faces of metalloproteases: cell growth, invasion, angiogenesis and metastasis. Trends Cell Biol. 2001 Nov;11(11):S37-43.

[63] Coussens LM, Fingleton B, Matrisian LM. Matrix metalloproteinase inhibitors and cancer: trials and tribulations. Science. 2002 Mar 29;295(5564):2387-92.

[64] Egeblad M, Werb Z. New functions for the matrix metalloproteinases in cancer progression. Nat Rev Cancer. 2002 Mar;2(3):161-74.

[65] Westermarck J, Kahari VM. Regulation of matrix metalloproteinase expression in tumor invasion. FASEB J. 1999 May;13(8):781-92.

[66] Welgus HG, Campbell EJ, Bar-Shavit Z, Senior RM, Teitelbaum SL. Human alveolar macrophages produce a fibroblast-like collagenase and collagenase inhibitor. J Clin Invest. 1985 Jul;76(1):219-24.

[67] Zhang R, Premi S, Kilic SS, Bacchiocchi A, Halaban R, Brash DE. Clonal growth of human melanocytes using cell-free extracellular matrix. Pigment Cell Melanoma Res. 2013 Nov;26(6):925-7.

[68] Veitch DP, Nokelainen P, McGowan KA, Nguyen TT, Nguyen NE, Stephenson R, et al. Mammalian tolloid metalloproteinase, and not matrix metalloprotease 2 or membrane type 1 metalloprotease, processes laminin-5 in keratinocytes and skin. J Biol Chem. 2003 May 2;278(18):15661-8.

[69] Grieve AG, Rabouille C. Extracellular cleavage of E-cadherin promotes epithelial cell extrusion. J Cell Sci. 2014 Aug 1;127(Pt 15):3331-46.

[70] Mashita N, Yamada S, Nakayama G, Tanaka C, Iwata N, Kanda M, et al. Epithelial to mesenchymal transition might be induced via CD44 isoform switching in colorectal cancer. J Surg Oncol. 2014 Jun 29.

[71] Overall CM, Lopez-Otin C. Strategies for MMP inhibition in cancer: innovations for the post-trial era. Nat Rev Cancer. 2002 Sep;2(9):657-72.

[72] Depner S, Lederle W, Gutschalk C, Linde N, Zajonz A, Mueller MM. Cell type specific interleukin-6 induced responses in tumor keratinocytes and stromal fibroblasts are essential for invasive growth. Int J Cancer. 2014 Aug 1;135(3):551-62.

[73] Sekiuchi M, Kudo A, Nakabayashi K, Kanai-Azuma M, Akimoto Y, Kawakami H, et al. Expression of matrix metalloproteinases 2 and 9 and tissue inhibitors of matrix metalloproteinases 2 and 1 in the glomeruli of human glomerular diseases: the results of studies using immunofluorescence, in situ hybridization, and immunoelectron microscopy. Clin Exp Nephrol. 2012 Dec;16(6):863-74.

[74] Rosewell KL, Curry TE, Jr. Detection of ovarian matrix metalloproteinase mRNAs by in situ hybridization. Methods Mol Biol. 2009;590:115-29.

[75] Stetler-Stevenson WG. Tissue inhibitors of metalloproteinases in cell signaling: metalloproteinase-independent biological activities. Sci Signal. 2008;1(27):re6.

[76] Ricca TI, Liang G, Suenaga AP, Han SW, Jones PA, Jasiulionis MG. Tissue inhibitor of metalloproteinase 1 expression associated with gene demethylation confers anoikis resistance in early phases of melanocyte malignant transformation. Transl Oncol. 2009 Dec;2(4):329-40.

[77] Toricelli M, Melo FH, Peres GB, Silva DC, Jasiulionis MG. Timp1 interacts with beta-1 integrin and CD63 along melanoma genesis and confers anoikis resistance by activating PI3-K signaling pathway independently of Akt phosphorylation. Mol Cancer. 2013;12:22.

[78] Menzies AM, Long GV, Murali R. Dabrafenib and its potential for the treatment of metastatic melanoma. Drug Des Devel Ther. 2012;6:391-405.

[79] Liang S, Sharma A, Peng HH, Robertson G, Dong C. Targeting mutant (V600E) B-Raf in melanoma interrupts immunoediting of leukocyte functions and melanoma extravasation. Cancer Res. 2007 Jun 15;67(12):5814-20.

[80] Davies H, Bignell GR, Cox C, Stephens P, Edkins S, Clegg S, et al. Mutations of the BRAF gene in human cancer. Nature. 2002 Jun 27;417(6892):949-54.

[81] Shinozaki M, Fujimoto A, Morton DL, Hoon DS. Incidence of BRAF oncogene mutation and clinical relevance for primary cutaneous melanomas. Clin Cancer Res. 2004 Mar 1;10(5):1753-7.

[82] Evans MS, Madhunapantula SV, Robertson GP, Drabick JJ. Current and future trials of targeted therapies in cutaneous melanoma. Adv Exp Med Biol. 2013;779:223-55.

[83] Tang YQ, Jaganath IB, Manikam R, Sekaran SD. Inhibition of MAPKs, Myc/Max, NFkappaB, and hypoxia pathways by Phyllanthus prevents proliferation, metastasis and angiogenesis in human melanoma (MeWo) cancer cell line. Int J Med Sci. 2014;11(6):564-77.

[84] Colombino M, Capone M, Lissia A, Cossu A, Rubino C, De Giorgi V, et al. BRAF/NRAS mutation frequencies among primary tumors and metastases in patients with melanoma. J Clin Oncol. 2012 Jul 10;30(20):2522-9.

[85] Long GV, Menzies AM, Nagrial AM, Haydu LE, Hamilton AL, Mann GJ, et al. Prognostic and clinicopathologic associations of oncogenic BRAF in metastatic melanoma. J Clin Oncol. 2011 Apr 1;29(10):1239-46.

[86] Boyle GM, Pedley J, Martyn AC, Banducci KJ, Strutton GM, Brown DA, et al. Macrophage inhibitory cytokine-1 is overexpressed in malignant melanoma and is associated with tumorigenicity. J Invest Dermatol. 2009 Feb;129(2):383-91.

[87] Jorgensen K, Holm R, Maelandsmo GM, Florenes VA. Expression of activated extracellular signal-regulated kinases 1/2 in malignant melanomas: relationship with clinical outcome. Clin Cancer Res. 2003 Nov 1;9(14):5325-31.

[88] Mirmohammadsadegh A, Mota R, Gustrau A, Hassan M, Nambiar S, Marini A, et al. ERK1/2 is highly phosphorylated in melanoma metastases and protects melanoma cells from cisplatin-mediated apoptosis. J Invest Dermatol. 2007 Sep;127(9):2207-15.

[89] Flaherty KT, Puzanov I, Kim KB, Ribas A, McArthur GA, Sosman JA, et al. Inhibition of mutated, activated BRAF in metastatic melanoma. N Engl J Med. 2010 Aug 26;363(9):809-19.

[90] Bell RE, Levy C. The three M's: melanoma, microphthalmia-associated transcription factor and microRNA. Pigment Cell Melanoma Res. 2011 Dec;24(6):1088-106.

[91] Mobley AK, Braeuer RR, Kamiya T, Shoshan E, Bar-Eli M. Driving transcriptional regulators in melanoma metastasis. Cancer Metastasis Rev. 2012 Dec;31(3-4):621-32.

[92] Garraway LA, Widlund HR, Rubin MA, Getz G, Berger AJ, Ramaswamy S, et al. Integrative genomic analyses identify MITF as a lineage survival oncogene amplified in malignant melanoma. Nature. 2005 Jul 7;436(7047):117-22.

[93] Levy C, Khaled M, Fisher DE. MITF: master regulator of melanocyte development and melanoma oncogene. Trends Mol Med. 2006 Sep;12(9):406-14.

[94] McGill GG, Haq R, Nishimura EK, Fisher DE. c-Met expression is regulated by Mitf in the melanocyte lineage. J Biol Chem. 2006 Apr 14;281(15):10365-73.

[95] Busse A, Keilholz U. Role of TGF-beta in melanoma. Curr Pharm Biotechnol. 2011 Dec;12(12):2165-75.

[96] Alexaki VI, Javelaud D, Van Kempen LC, Mohammad KS, Dennler S, Luciani F, et al. GLI2-mediated melanoma invasion and metastasis. J Natl Cancer Inst. 2010 Aug 4;102(15):1148-59.

[97] Javelaud D, Mohammad KS, McKenna CR, Fournier P, Luciani F, Niewolna M, et al. Stable overexpression of Smad7 in human melanoma cells impairs bone metastasis. Cancer Res. 2007 Mar 1;67(5):2317-24.

[98] Yang PT, Anastas JN, Toroni RA, Shinohara MM, Goodson JM, Bosserhoff AK, et al. WLS inhibits melanoma cell proliferation through the beta-catenin signalling pathway and induces spontaneous metastasis. EMBO Mol Med. 2012 Dec;4(12):1294-307.

[99] Webster MR, Weeraratna AT. A Wnt-er migration: the confusing role of beta-catenin in melanoma metastasis. Sci Signal. 2013 Mar 26;6(268):pe11.

[100] Gallagher SJ, Rambow F, Kumasaka M, Champeval D, Bellacosa A, Delmas V, et al. Beta-catenin inhibits melanocyte migration but induces melanoma metastasis. Oncogene. 2013 Apr 25;32(17):2230-8.

[101] Kageshita T, Hamby CV, Ishihara T, Matsumoto K, Saida T, Ono T. Loss of beta-catenin expression associated with disease progression in malignant melanoma. Br J Dermatol. 2001 Aug;145(2):210-6.

[102] Shull AY, Latham-Schwark A, Ramasamy P, Leskoske K, Oroian D, Birtwistle MR, et al. Novel somatic mutations to PI3K pathway genes in metastatic melanoma. PLoS One. 2012;7(8):e43369.

[103] Kyrgidis A, Tzellos TG, Triaridis S. Melanoma: Stem cells, sun exposure and hallmarks for carcinogenesis, molecular concepts and future clinical implications. J Carcinog. 2010;9:3.

[104] Dankort D, Curley DP, Cartlidge RA, Nelson B, Karnezis AN, Damsky WE, Jr., et al. Braf(V600E) cooperates with Pten loss to induce metastatic melanoma. Nat Genet. 2009 May;41(5):544-52.

[105] Jiang K, Sun J, Cheng J, Djeu JY, Wei S, Sebti S. Akt mediates Ras downregulation of RhoB, a suppressor of transformation, invasion, and metastasis. Mol Cell Biol. 2004 Jun;24(12):5565-76.

[106] Bagheri S, Nosrati M, Li S, Fong S, Torabian S, Rangel J, et al. Genes and pathways downstream of telomerase in melanoma metastasis. Proc Natl Acad Sci U S A. 2006 Jul 25;103(30):11306-11.

[107] Bastian BC. The molecular pathology of melanoma: an integrated taxonomy of melanocytic neoplasia. Annu Rev Pathol. 2014;9:239-71.

[108] Xia L, Huang W, Tian D, Chen Z, Zhang L, Li Y, et al. ACP5, a direct transcriptional target of FoxM1, promotes tumor metastasis and indicates poor prognosis in hepatocellular carcinoma. Oncogene. 2014 Mar 13;33(11):1395-406.

[109] Scott KL, Nogueira C, Heffernan TP, van Doorn R, Dhakal S, Hanna JA, et al. Proinvasion metastasis drivers in early-stage melanoma are oncogenes. Cancer Cell. 2011 Jul 12;20(1):92-103.

[110] Singh S, Singh AP, Sharma B, Owen LB, Singh RK. CXCL8 and its cognate receptors in melanoma progression and metastasis. Future Oncol. 2010 Jan;6(1):111-6.

[111] Varney ML, Johansson SL, Singh RK. Distinct expression of CXCL8 and its receptors CXCR1 and CXCR2 and their association with vessel density and aggressiveness in malignant melanoma. Am J Clin Pathol. 2006 Feb;125(2):209-16.

[112] Singh S, Varney M, Singh RK. Host CXCR2-dependent regulation of melanoma growth, angiogenesis, and experimental lung metastasis. Cancer Res. 2009 Jan 15;69(2):411-5.

[113] Kim J, Mori T, Chen SL, Amersi FF, Martinez SR, Kuo C, et al. Chemokine receptor CXCR4 expression in patients with melanoma and colorectal cancer liver metastases and the association with disease outcome. Ann Surg. 2006 Jul;244(1):113-20.

[114] Amersi FF, Terando AM, Goto Y, Scolyer RA, Thompson JF, Tran AN, et al. Activation of CCR9/CCL25 in cutaneous melanoma mediates preferential metastasis to the small intestine. Clin Cancer Res. 2008 Feb 1;14(3):638-45.

[115] Kim M, Gans JD, Nogueira C, Wang A, Paik JH, Feng B, et al. Comparative oncogenomics identifies NEDD9 as a melanoma metastasis gene. Cell. 2006 Jun 30;125(7): 1269-81.

[116] Dykxhoorn DM. MicroRNAs and metastasis: little RNAs go a long way. Cancer Res. 2010 Aug 15;70(16):6401-6.

[117] Hurst DR, Edmonds MD, Welch DR. Metastamir: the field of metastasis-regulatory microRNA is spreading. Cancer Res. 2009 Oct 1;69(19):7495-8.

[118] Ma L, Teruya-Feldstein J, Weinberg RA. Tumour invasion and metastasis initiated by microRNA-10b in breast cancer. Nature. 2007 Oct 11;449(7163):682-8.

[119] Penna E, Orso F, Cimino D, Tenaglia E, Lembo A, Quaglino E, et al. microRNA-214 contributes to melanoma tumour progression through suppression of TFAP2C. EMBO J. 2011 May 18;30(10):1990-2007.

[120] Gaziel-Sovran A, Segura MF, Di Micco R, Collins MK, Hanniford D, Vega-Saenz de Miera E, et al. miR-30b/30d regulation of GalNAc transferases enhances invasion and immunosuppression during metastasis. Cancer Cell. 2011 Jul 12;20(1):104-18.

[121] Pencheva N, Tran H, Buss C, Huh D, Drobnjak M, Busam K, et al. Convergent multi-miRNA targeting of ApoE drives LRP1/LRP8-dependent melanoma metastasis and angiogenesis. Cell. 2012 Nov 21;151(5):1068-82.

[122] Segura MF, Hanniford D, Menendez S, Reavie L, Zou X, Alvarez-Diaz S, et al. Aberrant miR-182 expression promotes melanoma metastasis by repressing FOXO3 and microphthalmia-associated transcription factor. Proc Natl Acad Sci U S A. 2009 Feb 10;106(6):1814-9.

[123] Jiang L, Lv X, Li J, Li X, Li W, Li Y. The status of microRNA-21 expression and its clinical significance in human cutaneous malignant melanoma. Acta Histochem. 2012 Oct;114(6):582-8.

[124] Yang CH, Yue J, Pfeffer SR, Handorf CR, Pfeffer LM. MicroRNA miR-21 regulates the metastatic behavior of B16 melanoma cells. J Biol Chem. 2011 Nov 11;286(45): 39172-8.

[125] Kitago M, Martinez SR, Nakamura T, Sim MS, Hoon DS. Regulation of RUNX3 tumor suppressor gene expression in cutaneous melanoma. Clin Cancer Res. 2009 May 1;15(9):2988-94.

[126] Felicetti F, Errico MC, Bottero L, Segnalini P, Stoppacciaro A, Biffoni M, et al. The promyelocytic leukemia zinc finger-microRNA-221/-222 pathway controls melanoma progression through multiple oncogenic mechanisms. Cancer Res. 2008 Apr 15;68(8): 2745-54.

[127] Mazar J, DeYoung K, Khaitan D, Meister E, Almodovar A, Goydos J, et al. The regulation of miRNA-211 expression and its role in melanoma cell invasiveness. PLoS One. 2010;5(11):e13779.

[128] Liu S, Tetzlaff MT, Cui R, Xu X. miR-200c inhibits melanoma progression and drug resistance through down-regulation of BMI-1. Am J Pathol. 2012 Nov;181(5):1823-35.

[129] Elson-Schwab I, Lorentzen A, Marshall CJ. MicroRNA-200 family members differentially regulate morphological plasticity and mode of melanoma cell invasion. PLoS One. 2010;5(10).

[130] Wang X, He X, Zhao F, Wang J, Zhang H, Shi F, et al. Regulation gene expression of miR200c and ZEB1 positively enhances effect of tumor vaccine B16F10/GPI-IL-21 on inhibition of melanoma growth and metastasis. J Transl Med. 2014;12:68.

[131] Ma Z, Swede H, Cassarino D, Fleming E, Fire A, Dadras SS. Up-regulated Dicer expression in patients with cutaneous melanoma. PLoS One. 2011;6(6):e20494.

[132] Fu TY, Chang CC, Lin CT, Lai CH, Peng SY, Ko YJ, et al. Let-7b-mediated suppression of basigin expression and metastasis in mouse melanoma cells. Exp Cell Res. 2011 Feb 15;317(4):445-51.

[133] Liu N, Sun Q, Chen J, Li J, Zeng Y, Zhai S, et al. MicroRNA-9 suppresses uveal melanoma cell migration and invasion through the NF-kappaB1 pathway. Oncol Rep. 2012 Sep;28(3):961-8.

[134] Dynoodt P, Speeckaert R, De Wever O, Chevolet I, Brochez L, Lambert J, et al. miR-145 overexpression suppresses the migration and invasion of metastatic melanoma cells. Int J Oncol. 2013 Apr;42(4):1443-51.

[135] Saleiban A, Faxalv L, Claesson K, Jonsson JI, Osman A. miR-20b regulates expression of proteinase-activated receptor-1 (PAR-1) thrombin receptor in melanoma cells. Pigment Cell Melanoma Res. 2014 May;27(3):431-41.

[136] Sand M, Skrygan M, Georgas D, Sand D, Gambichler T, Altmeyer P, et al. The miRNA machinery in primary cutaneous malignant melanoma, cutaneous malignant melanoma metastases and benign melanocytic nevi. Cell Tissue Res. 2012 Oct;350(1): 119-26.

Section 2

Clinical Disease Management

Chapter 4

Surgery and Staging of Melanoma

Rolland Gyulai, Zsolt Kádár and Zsuzsanna Lengyel

Additional information is available at the end of the chapter

http://dx.doi.org/10.5772/59471

1. Introduction

Surgical management of melanoma encompasses primary biopsy and complete wide local excision (WLE) of the tumor, as well as the surgical treatment of metastatic melanoma, including both cutaneous and internal metastases. The management of a melanoma suspect lesion starts with the initial biopsy of the lesion. A great variety of techniques can be used for the biopsy of melanomas, and the choice of the technique is dependent on multiple factors (patient's age, strength of clinical suspicion of melanoma, thickness of the tumor, localization, etc.). Once the clinical diagnosis of melanoma is confirmed histologically, local tumor control is established by wide local excision. The margins for WLE are determined by the T stage of the tumor, and are between 0.5-2.0 cm. Certain clinical melanoma types (e.g. lentigo maligna) require special attention, as the recommended margins can differ from those generally advised for other melanoma types.

Important surgical procedures include wide local excision with safety margins, sentinel lymph node biopsy, regional lymph node dissection and reconstruction of defects after melanoma excision. A plastic surgeon of the appropriate specialty should perform the excision and reconstruction.

Performing surgery of locoregional and distant metastases depends on various factors. However, in highly selected patients, complete surgical resection of the metastases may result in prolonged survival. In addition, combination of surgery with novel immuno-, and targeted therapies, may result in an even better outcome in the future for patientswith stage IV disease.

2. Primary treatment of suspicious pigmented lesion/melanoma

Early diagnosis and complete removal of the malignant cells are of paramount importance in the treatment of malignant melanoma. This usually requires a two-step approach. First, pigmented or amelanotic lesions suspicious for melanoma should be promptly biopsied and submitted to pathological evaluation, and second, the tumor should be subsequently excised with adequate surgical margins. The margins of the final excision are determined with the tumor characteristics in mind, as determined by the histopathological analysis of the biopsy specimen. Thus, removal of appropriate biopsy sample containing the fragment with the worst prognostic characteristics, is of substantial importance. As extensive loss of tissues may potentially influence the feasibility of further surgical interventions, such as the sentinel lymph node biopsy, the use of proper biopsy techniques is essential during the primary treatment of melanoma.

Recommendations regarding the width of the surgical margin of excision are nowadays clearly defined for primary melanoma, and are based on the histopathological features of the melanoma. These recommendations, however, are sometimes difficult or impossible to follow, like in the case of specially localized melanomas, or certain melanoma subtypes. This chapter summarizes the available evidence regarding different biopsy techniques and the surgical management of primary melanoma.

2.1. Biopsy of melanoma suspect lesions

The primary aim of performing biopsy in the case of a melanoma suspect lesion is to establish or exclude the diagnosis of melanoma. An additional goal is to ensure accurate pathological staging of the tumor in order to enable adequate surgical management by performing wide local excision (WLE). Excisional, incisional and shave biopsy techniques are used in the surgical treatment of melanoma.

2.1.1. Excisional biopsy

The preferred biopsy technique for most melanomas is excisional biopsy.[1,2] This means that the entire lesion is removed with an additional 1-3 mm margin of normal-appearing skin. Wider excisions, however, should be avoided, to permit subsequent lymphatic mapping for sentinel lymph node biopsy. Generally, the excised tissue sample should contain part of the subcutaneous fat as well, and should be oriented to aid subsequent histopathological evaluation. The positioning of the excision also should possibly allow for subsequent wider excisions. The excisional biopsy technique can be used in most melanomas, when primary closure of the wound is feasible. Although the lowest frequency of positive margins is reported when excisional biopsy is used, positive margins and even residual melanoma on WLE do occur.[3]

2.1.2. Incisional biopsy

The reported frequency of excisional biopsy technique used for diagnosing melanoma varies significantly with centers, countries, and individuals, and ranges between 10 and 86 percent.

[1,3-6] Thus, in a significant portion of melanoma suspect lesions, a biopsy technique other than excisional biopsy are used. Even guidelines that emphasize the importance of excisional biopsy in melanoma management state that incisional biopsy may be appropriate in certain clinical circumstances. Such clinical scenarios may include cases when excisional biopsy is not feasible due to the large size or the location (nose, ear, face, palm, and sole) of the lesion, concerns about cosmesis or low clinical suspicion of melanoma.

In the case of incisional biopsy only a portion of the lesion is removed, either by a punch biopsy or using a scalpel (Figure 1.a-c). As incisional biopsy specimens contain only part of the lesion, concerns regarding misdiagnosis, staging inaccuracy or diagnostic uncertainty may arise. Careful selection of the biopsy site is therefore crucial to ensure that the biopsy best represents the entire lesion, both in terms of the type and the T stage of the tumor. This is usually achieved by sampling the thickest, most raised area of the tumor, or the darkest part of flat lesions. Complex lesions containing multiple suspicious foci may require more than one simultaneous biopsy sampling. Both in case of punch biopsy and incisional biopsy adequate depth (reaching to the subcutaneous fat) of the sampling should be guaranteed.

The theory that incisional biopsy, by cutting through the neoplastic tissue, represents an increased risk for lymphatic or hematologous metastatisation, and thus it should be regarded as a harmful procedure, has been refuted by several earlier studies.[3,7] Moreover, Molenkamp et al. reported slightly better survival in patients with residual tumor cells in their re-excision samples, compared to patients without residual cells in their re-excision specimen.[3] The authors speculated that immunity against residual tumor cells, triggered by biopsy induced wound healing, might be responsible for this finding.

2.1.3. Shave biopsy

In the case of shave biopsy a superficial, a few mm deep flat section of the skin is removed (Figure 1.d). Shave biopsy is ideally performed at the level of the deep dermis, however, the depth of excision is often compromised with the desire to provide a cosmetically good result. Shave biopsy of primary melanoma, as it often results in incomplete removal of the tumor and thus compromises pathological staging of the tumor, is not recommended in most of the cases for melanoma biopsy. However, if the index of melanoma suspicion is low, shave biopsy may be performed. When performing shave biopsy in pigmented lesions, deep scoop shave biopsy is the preferred technique.

2.1.4. The effect of biopsy techniques on staging, prognosis and treatment of melanoma

The biopsy of the pigmented lesion should not only establish or exclude the diagnosis of melanoma, but also provide information on the T stage of the tumor. Ideally, this initial T stage will be the same as the one achieved after the wide local excision of the tumor. This will ensure that the original treatment plan regarding the width of the surgical margin and the requirement for sentinel lymph node biopsy, does not need subsequent adjustment. As these treatment parameters are primarily determined by Breslow's depth of the tumor, achieving appropriate deep margin sampling is of paramount importance during melanoma biopsy.

Theoretically, sampling errors may stem from several scenarios (Figure 1.a-d). Tumor depth determination may be compromised by not representative tissue sampling (Figure 1a), positive deep biopsy margin (Figure 1b) or not representative tumor depth (Figure 1c). Diagnostic inaccuracy, as a consequence of inappropriate tumor depth measurement, may (Figure 1b) or may not (Figure 1c) lead to upstaging after wide local excision. In a recent study, positive deep margins were found in 12%, 32%, 17% and 24% of cases undergoing excisional, shave, punch and incisional biopsies, respectively.[4] After wide local excision, tumor depth was more than the biopsy depth in 44% of the cases with residual tumors in WLE, and resulted in T-stage reclassification in 22% of cases. Reclassification was necessary in 2%, 7%, 24% and 24% of cases when the initial diagnosis was established by excisional, shave, punch or incisional biopsy, respectively. Diagnostic inaccuracy led to subsequent treatment change in 2%, 5%, 18% and 18% of cases when excisional, shave, punch or incisional biopsy, respectively, was used for initial sampling. Although there is no data regarding the tumor thickness in the individual biopsy groups, it is likely that shave biopsy was more frequently used for thinner and incisional techniques for thicker melanomas. This may explain why initial punch and incisional biopsy so frequently required later reclassification in this study.

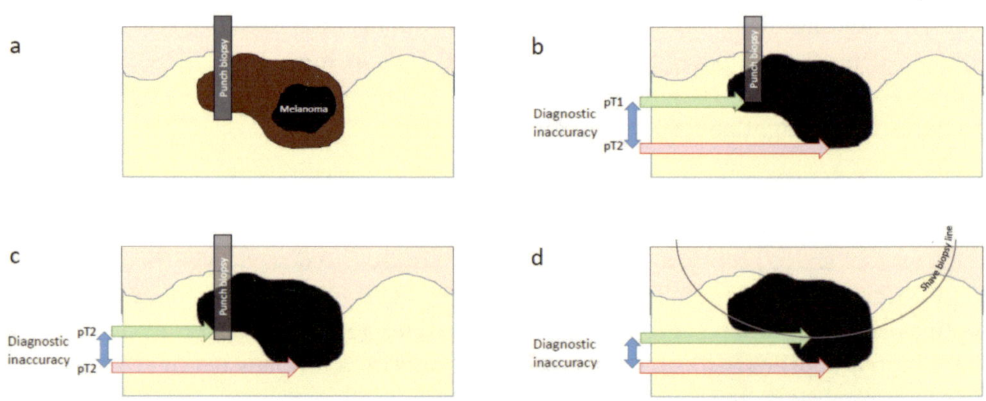

Figure 1. Diagnostic inaccuracy arising from different forms of sampling error using incisional (punch) biopsy or shave biopsy techniques. Inadequate punch biopsy sampling of pigmented lesion (a) may result in non-representative tissue sampling. Tissue sample is removed from the benign part of the pigmented lesion, while missing the malignant part leading to false negative diagnosis. Inadequate depth of punch biopsy sampling (b) results in positive deep margin on histology. Accurate T stage cannot be established, and histological reevaluation after WLE will result in the upstaging of the tumor from T1 to T2. Inadequate assessment of melanoma depth due to failure in sampling the deepest part of the tumor (c). Accurate T stage cannot be established, however, reevaluation will not result in upstaging. Positive deep margin after shave biopsy sampling of melanoma (d). Proper T stage cannot be established, and diagnostic inaccuracy may result in upstaging after WLE.

It must also be emphasized that a rather substantial part of excised melanomas are clinically not suspected to be melanoma, and vice versa, in a smaller, but significant portion of pigmented lesions, the clinical diagnosis of melanoma is not confirmed by the histopathological examination. The mean number of pigmented lesions to be excised to detect one melanoma

http://dx.doi.org/10.5772/59471

was 29 (range 11-83) in a study among general practitioners in Perth, Australia.[8] Thus, in cases of clinical uncertainty, shave or incisional biopsies may help to establish early melanoma diagnosis, and biopsies may also help to avoid unnecessary wide excisions in case of benign lesions.

Several studies have compared the effect of biopsy techniques on the prognosis of melanoma. [9-13] While in some studies a decreased survival rate was associated with incisional, shave or needle aspiration biopsy compared to those who had excisional biopsy, these studies included either low number of patients or significant age differences among patient groups. [12,13] Other, more recent studies, involving significantly higher numbers of patients, found no negative effect of non-radical diagnostic techniques on the survival of melanoma patients. [10,11] Moreover, Molenkamp et al. reported slightly better survival in patients with residual tumor cells in their re-excision samples,[3] and speculated that biopsy induced wound healing may theoretically trigger immunity against residual tumor cells. In summary, incisional (punch or scalpel) and shave biopsies may be used for the initial diagnosis of melanoma, although, excisional biopsy, when feasible, is recommended as the first choice.

2.1.5. Biopsy techniques in different melanoma types and special locations

Although, when feasible, excisional biopsy is the recommended technique for initial diagnosis of melanoma, there are certainly significant differences among melanoma subtypes, which, consequently, require different surgical approaches. The most critical factors when choosing the appropriate biopsy technique are clinical estimate of depth and size and localization of the lesion. Although there are no general rules regarding biopsy techniques for different clinical types of melanoma, some practical recommendations can be formulated. It must be emphasized as well that in case of lesions requiring amputation of the anatomical unit (e.g. digit or ear), histological confirmation of the diagnosis of melanoma is necessary before performing the final procedure.

- *Superficial spreading melanomas,* when primary closure of the wound is feasible, should be removed by excisional biopsy. However, these melanomas usually invade only the upper dermis, which makes them ideal candidates for shave biopsy. In case of large lesions, when complete excision of the lesion is not feasible, incisional biopsy is the preferred choice.

- *Nodular melanomas,* on the other hand, are deeply infiltrating lesions with usually smaller diameter. In most instances, therefore, nodular melanomas may and should be managed by excisional biopsy.

- *Lentigo maligna* usually presents clinically as an extensive, several centimeter large lesion on the head of elderly patients. Due to its size, location, and the frequent uncertainty in the diagnosis, as well as the advanced age of the patients, lentigo maligna often requires one or more initial incisional biopsy sampling to establish the diagnosis of melanoma, and to select subsequent management strategies.

- *Acral-lentiginous melanomas* frequently pose a diagnostic challenge on first presentation. Moreover, their size and location commonly makes them impossible to be treated by excisional biopsy. Therefore, especially when surgical management involves amputation, an initial incisional biopsy is essential to confirm the clinical diagnosis of melanoma.

- *Ulcerated and/or regressive melanomas* should be managed with special attention, as these clinical features are usually associated with poorer outcome. Furthermore, both ulceration and regression can interfere with histopathological evaluation, and can obscure the establishment of proper diagnosis. Therefore, excisional biopsy sampling is highly recommended in these cases to avoid false negative diagnosis or understaging.

- *Melanomas in special anatomical regions* (eyelid, ear, nose, genitoanal) usually require individual approach, as excisional biopsy sampling is often not feasible with primary wound closure. For that reason, it is recommended that an incisional biopsy is taken before final management of pigmented lesions in these locations.

2.2. Wide Local Excision (WLE) of malignant melanoma

Once the histopathological examination of the biopsy sample established the diagnosis of melanoma, the entire tumor should be surgically removed with adequate safety margins from the surrounding healthy-appearing skin. The wide local excision is intended to provide adequate surgical control of the tumor spread by removing all tumor cells from the primary tumor bed and the potential satellite lesions from the immediate vicinity of the tumor. Additionally, WLE provides tissue samples for the final T staging of melanoma.

2.2.1. General recommendations for surgical margins for wide local excision of melanoma

Current recommendations for surgical management of melanoma are based on randomized clinical trials completed several years ago.[14-20] The margin of wide local excision depends on the T stage of the melanoma, which is primarily determined by the depth of tumor invasion (see Table 1. for staging). While there has been considerable debate regarding the radicality of surgery, current guidelines recommend 0.5 – 2.0 cm surgical margins (see Table 1. for recommended surgical margins).[1]

2.2.2. Surgical margins for wide local excision in clinical types and special anatomical regions

Most melanomas on the trunk and the proximal part of the extremities may be surgically managed according to the generally recommended margins for re-excision. Certain melanoma types, however, owing to their unique localization (face, acral region of the extremities) or type (lentigo maligna), require special approach, and allow only compromised excisional margins.

2.2.2.1. Melanoma in situ (lentigo maligna and non lentigo maligna type)

In general, the NCCN guideline recommends 0.5-1.0 mm margins for in situ melanomas.[1] These recommendations, however, are based on expert consensus, as there are no randomized prospective studies that have examined the surgical margins for melanoma in situ. Recently it has been shown that almost all (99%) melanoma in situ lesions are completely removed with a 0.9 mm margin, and a margin of 0.6 mm provides negative resection margins in 86% of cases.

T classification	Thickness (mm)	Ulceration status/ mitoses	Recommended surgical margin (cm)	Remarks
Tis	in situ	NA	0.5-1.0	0.5 cm on face, neck, hands, feet 1.0 cm if significant residual pigment near the biopsy site
T1	≤1.0	a: w/o ulceration and mitosis <1/mm^2 b: with ulceration or mitoses ≥1/mm^2	1.0	
T2	1.01-2.00	a: w/o ulceration b: with ulceration	1.0-2.0	
T3	2.01-4.00	a: w/o ulceration b: with ulceration	2.0	
T4	≥4.00	a: w/o ulceration b: with ulceration	2.0	

Table 1. Summary of T staging and current National Comprehensive Cancer Network (NCCN) recommended wide local excision margins for melanoma.

[21] Another recent study found that in situ melanoma lesions that were not lentigo maligna type, were unlikely to recur if completely removed, even with narrow margins (Figure 2.a).[22] On the other hand, a significantly higher incomplete excision rate was found in the lentigo maligna group (Figure 2.b), compared with the non-lentigo maligna type in situ melanomas (29.3% vs. 5.9%, respectively). Thus, the authors propose more aggressive treatment, if possible, for in situ melanomas of lentigo maligna type.

2.2.2.2. *Eyelid melanoma*

There is no generally accepted consensus regarding the appropriate surgical margins for eyelid melanomas. In this melanoma group, guidelines for WLE are impractical, and cannot be used in the majority of cases. In a recent retrospective study, local, nodal and distant metastases occurred in 21%, 11% and 4% of 56 cases with eyelid melanomas, respectively.[23] Pathological margins of >2 mm were associated with increased disease-free survival, compared with margins ≤2 mm. Lower eyelid melanomas were found to have significantly higher recurrence rate than upper eyelid tumors.

2.2.2.3. *External ear melanoma*

Although external ear melanoma had been considered to be a more aggressive type of melanoma, this hypothesis is not supported by more recent evidence. Histologically, melanomas arising on the external ear are most frequently superficial spreading melanomas (33-46%), followed almost equally by lentigo maligna (19.6%-26%) and nodular (16-22%) types. While narrower excisional margins and Mohs surgery are gaining acceptance in the treatment of ear melanoma as well, the use of these techniques are associated with significant (30%) recurrence rates.[24] Therefore, management should follow standard melanoma treatment recommendations in external ear melanoma cases, if feasible (Figure 2.c).

2.2.2.4. Mucosal melanoma of the head and neck

Achieving melanoma-free resection margins is often difficult in this melanoma type (Figure 2.d). This may be attributed to the close proximity of critical anatomic structures, the presence of satellite formation, multifocality, angiolymphatic invasion, and submucosal spread, which are common features in oral cavity and sinonasal melanoma. The 2-year and 5-year survival rates for mucosal melanoma of the head and neck are 54% and 32%, respectively. Taking into account the high recurrence rate in this melanoma subtype, even apparently localized lesions may require radical surgery with planned reconstruction.[25,26]

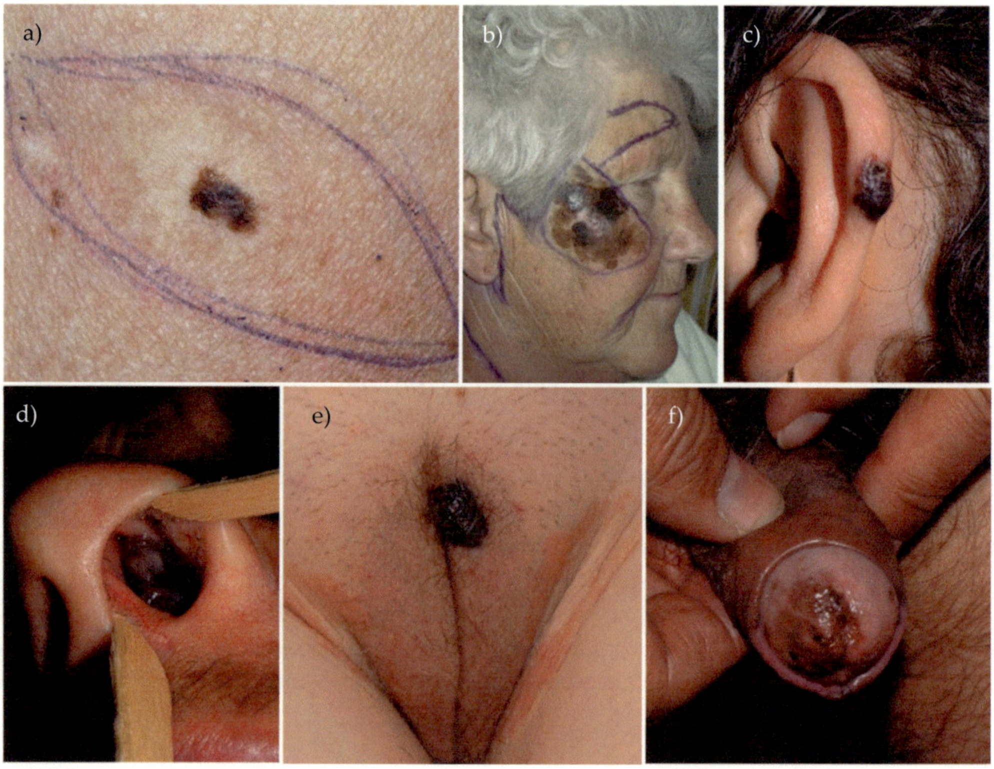

Figure 2. Melanomas in special anatomical regions require individual surgical approach. In case of in situ melanoma not lentigo maligna type (a), a 5-6 mm surgical margin is sufficient to ensure clear resection margins. In case of lentigo maligna type in situ melanomas (b), a wider, 10 mm margin is recommended, if feasible. Management of external ear melanomas (c) should follow standard melanoma treatment recommendations, if feasible. Mucosal melanomas of the head and neck region (d) require radical surgery with planned reconstruction in most cases. For mucosal melanoma of the female genitalia (e) wide excision with a 1-2 cm margin is recommended. Melanoma of the glans, preputium or urethra (f) wide local excision or penectomy provides effective local control.

2.2.2.5. Mucosal melanoma of the female genitalia

Although 70% of patients present with clinically localized disease, the overall prognosis of this melanoma type is poor. Surgical management of vulvar melanoma (Figure 2.e) consist of wide excision with a 1-cm margin for melanomas with a thickness of <1 mm, and a 2-cm margin for thicker lesions.[27,28]

2.2.2.6. Mucosal melanoma of the male genitalia

Melanoma of the glans, preputium or urethra is certainly an uncommon entity. Therefore, standard recommendations are not available for the management of this subtype of melanoma. Partial penectomy or WLE provided effective local control for low stage penile (Figure 2.f) or urethral melanomas and all scrotal lesions.[29]

2.2.2.7. Anorectal melanoma

Because of the rarity and the advanced stage at which most patients present, a standard surgical intervention has not been established to date for anorectal melanoma. Usually, wide local excision (with negative margin) is the preferred surgical management in most patients. Extensive disease that is not amenable to local excision, may require abdominoperineal resection.[30]

2.3. Surgical techniques

2.3.1. Neck and face

The face is an important area because it encompasses the eyes, nose, mouth and it is in proximity to the ears. The surgical radicality of extension must often be compromised to avoid injury to these structures. These structures limit the excision margins for surgical treatment of melanomas occurring on the face. In the management of cutaneous melanoma the first step is the wide local excision.

The first goal is to treat the cancer with maximal protection of function and aesthetics. We need take notice of the size and the localization of the defect, what kind of tissues are missing (bone, muscle, fat, skin, cartilage, etc.), the base of the wound, the acceptable functional impairment, the morbidity of the donor area, the moveable area around the defect, the history of the patient (previous operation or irradiation) and the expectations of the patient too. Ideally incisions should be within the relaxed skin tension lines (RSTL) or parallel to them, so the scars will be functionally and aesthetically superior. The RSTL is a complex interaction of the external and internal factors, which contains the skin as well.

If there is a melanoma on the neck, middle or lower area of the face, we can perform an elliptical excision parallel to the RSTL with a 3 to 5 mm safety border, undermining the surrounding area and closing the wound primarily.[17] If the tumor size is bigger we need to prepare local flaps to cover the defect. Local flaps' blood supply are very reliable, random pattern from the surrounding tissues or axial pattern from a named source artery. The laxity, quality and texture of the surrounding skin is the best to prepare local flaps and it is the nearest approach to the defect's skin.

If the size of the defect is too big and there is no possibility for local flaps,skin grafting can be performed. There are split-thickness and full-thickness skin grafting. The split-thickness skin is0.25-0.75 mm thick, the procedure is simple, fast, and not demanding. The donor area heals spontaneously and is fit to be used again as a donor area, although the graft may contract and become hypo-or hyperpigmented. The full-thickness skin is 0.8-1.1 mm thick, it rarely contracts and/or gets pigmented, it is more resistant against external cues compared to split-thickness grafts, and the subcutaneous layer may regenerate. On the other hand, this surgical technique ismore demanding for the patient, and it requires a good blood supply of therecipient area, which limits the size of the graft. Lastly, the donor area need to be sutured /closed primarily.

Recommended flaps are: rotational facial flaps, bilobed flaps, transpositonal flaps, V-Y advancement flaps (Figure 3.). It is uncommon to use distant flaps on the face except for some cases, when there is not enough skin in the surrounding areas, due to irradiation or previous operations.

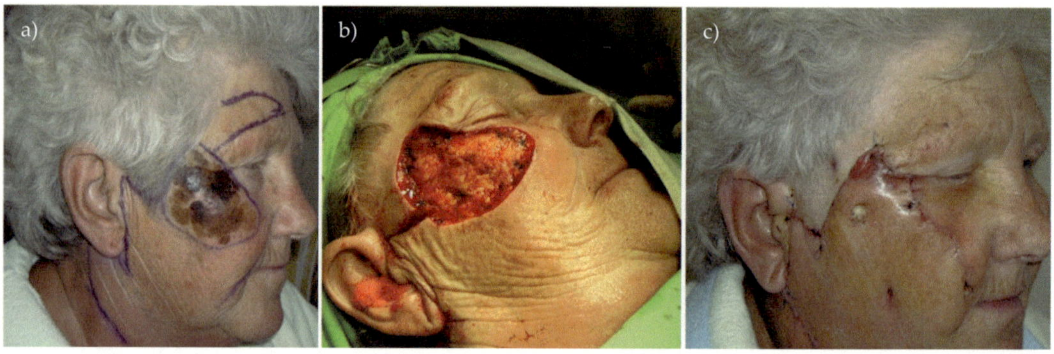

Figure 3. Removal of extensive melanoma from the face and reconstruction with combined local flaps. Melanoma (lentigo maligna type) on the face. Note markings of planned flaps (a). Extensive tissue defect after excision of melanoma with surgical margins. Reconstruction with combined local flaps (b). Good cosmetical result on 10th postoperative day (c).

2.3.2. *Eye*

After primary melanoma excision the choice of repair depends on the size and location of the defect, surrounding tissue mobility, degree of vascular compromise, extent of lamella loss, skin texture and color match. It is not common to excise and primarily close the wounds around the eyes.[31] In general it is done, if the size of the melanoma is very small, the melanoma is in situ, there is a sufficient skin laxity, or the patient's general health status does not permit more intensive surgical intervention. In the periocular region a 5 mm margin of excision for thin eyelid melanomas is recommended.[32,33] Care must be taken to avoid placing too much tension on the eyelid. If the defect involves one third of the eyelid margins, we can perform pentagonal wedge closure after the excision.

We have to pay attention to the canthal regions and the lower eyelid to avoid their injuries, leading to dryness and ectropium. We should also pay attention to the eyebrows and try to reconstruct them.

In this region primarily we perform local flaps and skin grafting or cartilage grafting to cover the defects after melanoma excision. The local flaps can be skin, skin-subcutaneous and skin-muscles flaps from the surrounding area, where the laxity, quality and texture are the best suited to cover these defects. Their blood supply can show random pattern from the subcutaneous layer or axial pattern from a named source artery. In these cases it is advisable to do cantopexy to prevent ectropium evolution.

Recommended flaps are: V-Y advancement flap, Tenzel and Mustarde rotation flaps, Romboid-Limberg transpositional flaps, Median and Paramedian forehead flaps and Glabellar flap.[31,33]

Full-thickness skin graft is used in this region to minimize scaring and pigmentation. It protects against extrinsic factors and the subcutaneous layer may regenerate. Disadvantages of full-thickness skin grafting include demanding surgery, the need for good blood supply in the recipient area and the need for suturing in the donor area. The size of this graft is also limited (Figure 4.).

If the tumor involves the tarsal plates and after the excision of the melanoma a tarsal defect develops, auricular or nasal free cartilage graft can be used to cover the defect. Generally, the cartilage graft can be covered with a local flap to reconstruct the total eyelid layers. In these cases composite grafts may be used as well, which contain skin, cartilage and, if necessary, conjunctiva.

Occasionally, if the patient's general health status is poor, it is acceptable in the medial canthal area to leave the defect open, and let it heal by second-intention. Adequate wound management and dressing should be applied to help the granulation and epithelisation. Another use of second-intention healing is to delay skin grafting. After granulation the skin graft procedure can be performed.[31,33]

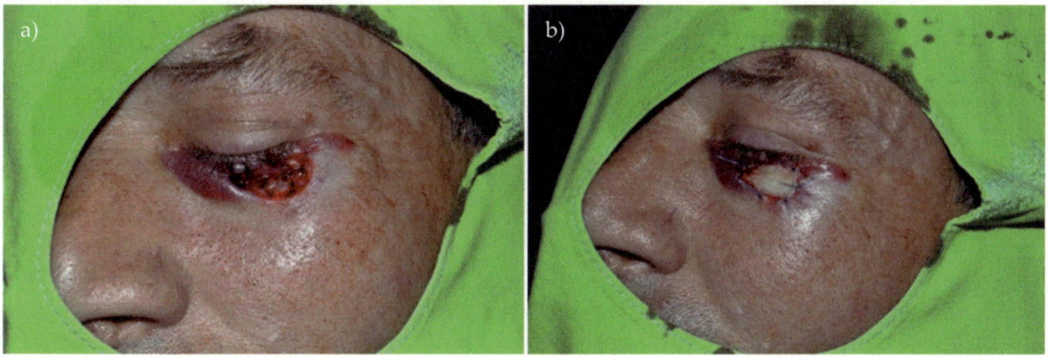

Figure 4. Full-thickness skin grafting for the reconstruction of lower eyelid defect after excision of melanoma. Lower eyelid defect (a) and full-thickness skin graft covering of the defect (b).

2.3.3. Nose

The nose is a three-layered structure of a skin and fibrofatty covering, a bony and cartilaginous framework and an inner lining of vestibular skin and nasal mucosa. Nasal defect may involve these layers alone or in combination.[34,35] The nose is divided into topographic subunits, as tip, dorsum, sidewalls, alar lobules, soft triangles and columella.[34,35] A wide range of techniques including defect and subunit reconstruction – using simple as well as more complex flap and multistaged procedures – must be in the surgeon's armamentarium. When a defect involves greater than 50% of a subunit, replacement of the entire subunit should be considered. We can perform primary wound closure after elliptical excision with undermining the surrounding area only on the dorsal region if the size of the tumor is not too large and the skin is loose. Second-intention healing is good only for superficial wounds on concave surfaces.[34] If the tumor size is bigger we can use local flaps from the middle face and the frontal region. (Figure 5. and 6.) The nasal tip, columella and alar regions are more difficult, and primary closure is usually not possible. Instead we use local flaps, skin grafting and composite grafting in these regions. The advantages of local flaps over skin grafts include better contour, color and texture match and less scar contracture. The most common local flap is the nasolabial flap, while the forehead flap remains the workhorse for major nasal reconstruction with numerous modifications.[34] Some others are the dorsonasal flap, glabellar flap, advancement flap from the middle face, and flaps from the upper perioral region. These local flaps are useful for defects of about 2 cm or less. If the tumor is large enough to require a tip and alar nose amputation, we can use reconstructive surgical methods or prosthetic devices. Full-thickness skin grafting is easy to perform and it is useful in the reconstruction of superficial defects in the areas of the tip and alar lobules (Figure 7.). On the other hand, it may heal with a contrasting flattened and shiny appearance.[34,35] The term composite graft means that skin and cartilage are grafted together from the conchal region, helical rim or helical root.

2.3.4. Ear

On the ear after wide excision, which includes skin and subcutaneous tissue removing, primary closure is usually not performed. There are many options for the reconstruction of aurical defects including direct closure, second-intention healing, full thickness skin grafts and local flaps.[36,37] The defects of the posterior wall of the ear, where the skin is more abundant and loose, can often be closed primarily. If the defect is in the central and anterior region with intact cartilage, most defects will do well by second intention healing or full thickness skin grafting.[37] If the defect involves the cartilage the most common surgical procedure is wedge excision, which means excising the skin and cartilage together in a V or W form. After these excisions we should reconstruct the cartilage and then the skin. If larger excisions are necessary, we need to use local flaps, which are from the earlobe, pre-and retroauricular regions. These flaps iclude direct advancement flap, rotational flaps, transposition and subcutaneous island flaps. If more than one third of the ear is involved by the tumor, we need to perform partial amputation. If the tumor is in an advanced stage, it may be necessary to amputate the whole ear. Amputation requires more complex reconstructive surgical methods to restore the ear or prosthetic devices can be used.

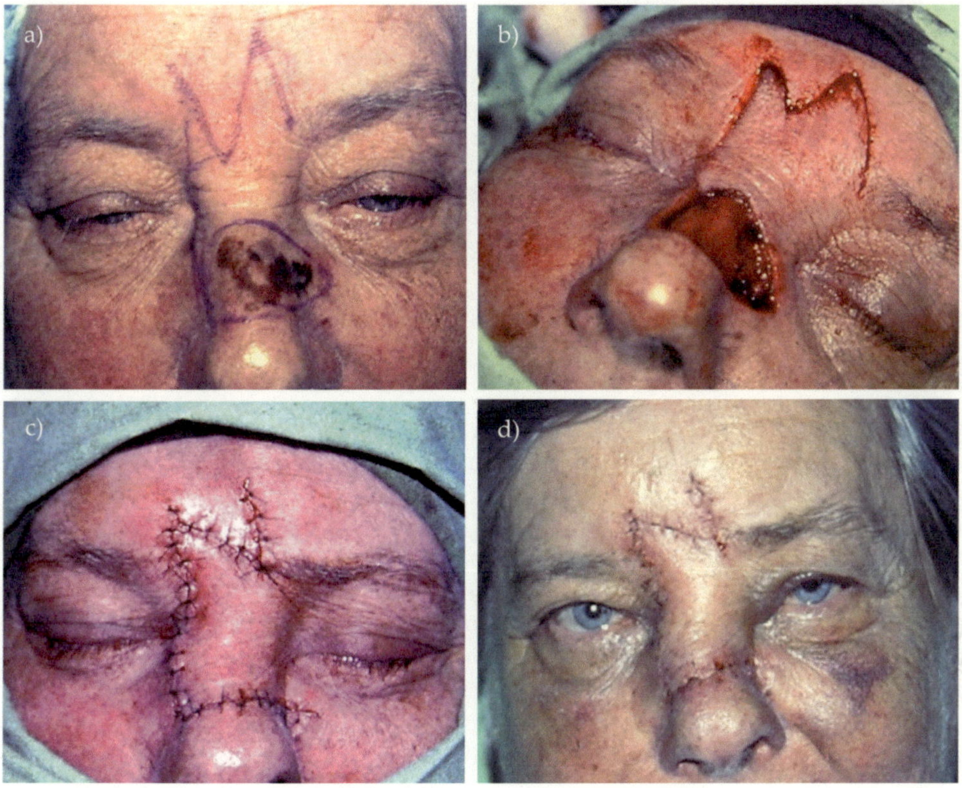

Figure 5. Glabellar flap for the reconstruction of a defect on the dorsum of the nose after wide excision of melanoma. Extensive melanoma on the dorsum of the nose (a). The defect and preparing glabellar flap (b). Suturing the flap (c) and postoperative results 3 weeks after operation (d).

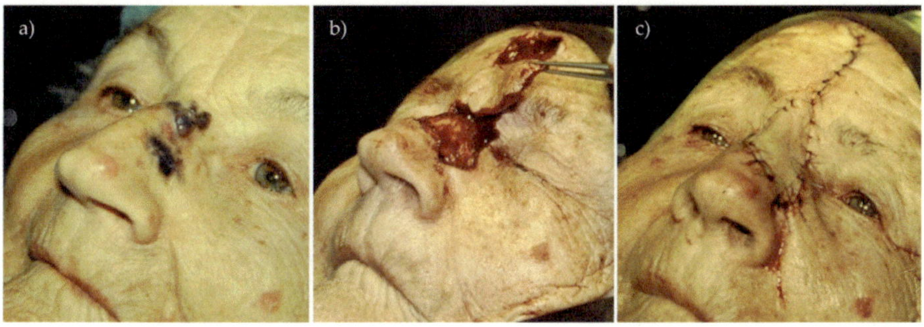

Figure 6. Forehead flap for the resonstruction of nasal and glabellar defect after melanoma excision. Melanoma on the nose and glabellar region (a). After ecxision and performing forehead flap (b) Suturing the flap. Good cosmetical result (c).

2.3.5. Mouth and perioral region

Melanomas in the perioral regions are not common. The tumor can involve the skin, the oral orbicular muscle and the mucosal layer alone or together.[37] In this region we should pay

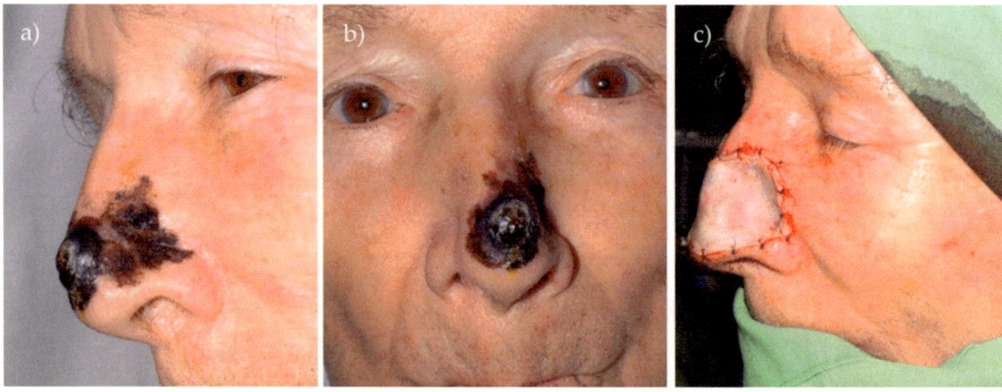

Figure 7. Split-thickness skin grafting for the reconstruction of extensive defect on the tip of the nose after excision of melanoma. Melanoma involving the tip and alar lobules of the nose (a-b) Split-thickness skin graft covering of the defect (c).

attention to protect the muscular-, sensorial-, and the closing function of the mouth, the adequate oral access for eating and to the use of dentures, to the symmetry, the upper/lower lip ratio and the quality of scars.[37] After tumor excision, if the defect is less than one half of the lip width, we can use primary wound closure after undermining the surrounding layers. Primary closure offers the best aesthetic result and should be prioritized. In the upper lip we can perform wedge excision while in the lower lip W-shape excision is used. In cases of large tumor size the defect can be covered by local skin-, and skin-mucosal flaps originating from the perioral region or from the lips and the inner surface of the mouth. The ideal donor areas for labial reconstruction are the remaining labial tissue and the opposing lip.[37] The lip is elastic and can be elongated, which is a very useful for reconstruction.

Recommended local flaps are: V-Y advancement flap, Rotational flap, Nasolabial flap, Forehead flap, Abby flap, Estlander flap, Karapandzic flap (Figure 8.).

2.3.6. Digits

The skin of the hand and toe is specialized and structurally unique, balancing the need for sensing, mobility for complex motor skills on the hand, durability to withstand wear and tear on the toe.[38] Earlier melanomas arising on the skin and/or nail bed of the digits were mostfrequently managed with amputation at the proximal joint from the tumor. Recently tissue- sparing excision is performed increasingly.[38] When excising melanomas on the toes, amputations should be limited to preserve as much length and function of the digit as possible without compromising the necessary safety border. It requires a more conservative surgery, wide excision and only partial resection of the affected phalanx.[38] The excision is done in the subcutaneous layer and on the fingertip, the entire nail complex needs to be removed. In these cases the defect can be covered with a local flap, like V-Y advancement flap, or we can use local flaps from the neighboring digits. If the bone is not directly involved it is not necessary to remove the total phalanx or metacarpus or metatarsus, since the removal of bone in these localisations does not have oncological benefit (Figure 9.).

http://dx.doi.org/10.5772/59471

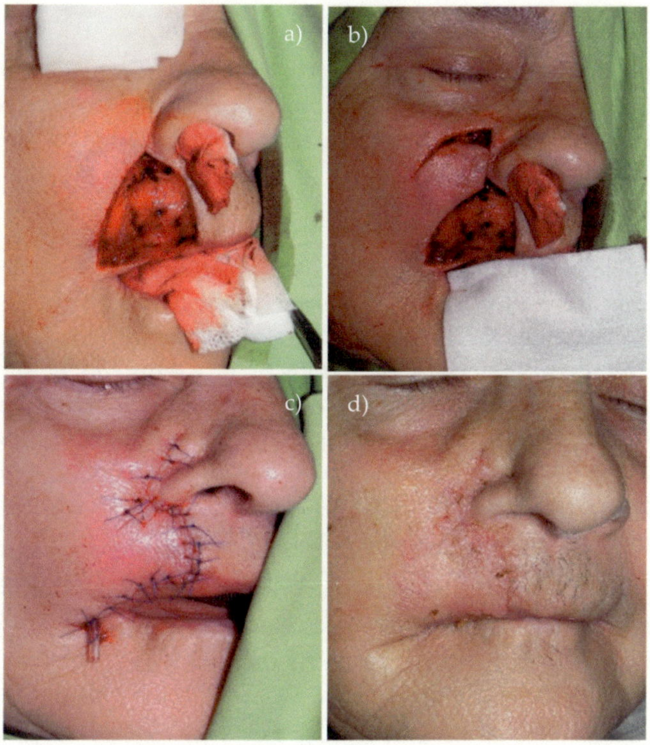

Figure 8. Reconstruction of facial defect with local flap after removal of melanoma. Large defect in the nasolabial region after melanoma excision (a). Preparing the local flap (b). Closing the wound with sutures (c). Good postoperative result 2 weeks after the operation (d).

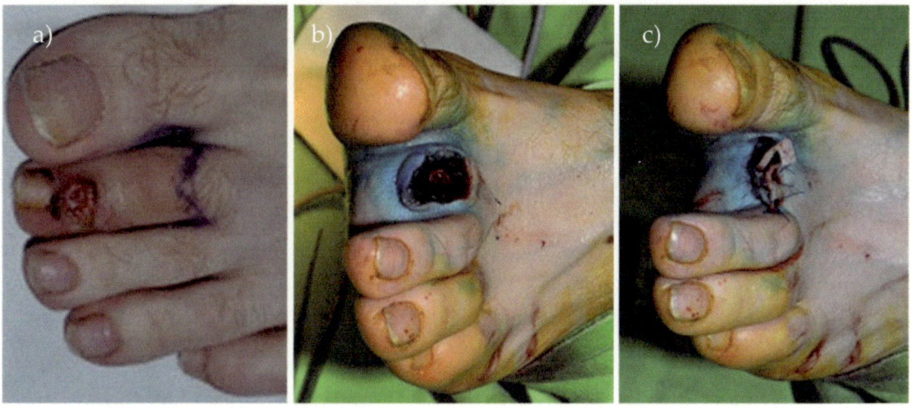

Figure 9. Surgical management of amelanotic melanoma on the toe. Melanoma present on the distal phalanx of the toe (a). Amputation at the distal phalanx (b). Suturing of the wound (c).

2.3.7. Interdigital spaces

Melanomas arising between the digits is difficult to treat. Covering to these defects can be done with full thickness skin grafts and local flaps. It may be necessary to remove the phalanx and metacarpuses and/or metatarsuses depending on the progression of the tumor.

2.3.8. Hand and foot

Acral lentiginous melanoma tends to be diagnosed at later stages due to medical diagnostic mistakes and patients' poor attention to lesions arising on extremities.[38] The reconstruction of the defects after melanoma excision on the dorsal or plantar region of the hand is challenging. Generally we can use full thickness skin grafts or local flaps and we should pay attention to retaining function. First, it is important to cover the joints, tendons and bones. If the defect is large we can perform distal flaps with microsurgical techniques. It is important to mind the weight-bearing regions of the foot, because reconstructing these defects requires a flap from the adjacent area or a free flap with microvascular anastomoses that contain adequate soft tissue to cover the defect and to supply the function too.

3. Surgery of locoregional recurrence of melanoma

Locoregional recurrence can occur as regional nodal disease or as satellite or in-transit metastases.

In-transit metastases are locoregional relapses found between the primary melanoma and the draining lymphatic basin. By definition lesions that occur more than 2 cm from the primary melanoma are termed in-transit metastases. The ones that are located closer (≤ 2 cm) are regarded as satellite lesions (Figure 10). The risk factors for the development of in-transit metastases include lymph node involvement and was confirmed as the most important prognostic factor by Weide et al.[39] Furthermore the risk of local recurrence increases significantly as the thickness of the primary melanoma increases and with the presence of ulceration.[15,39] Both satellite and in-transit metastases are regarded as stage IIIB (without regional nodal metastases) or stage IIIC (with regional nodal metastases) disease by the 2009 American Joint Committee on Cancer staging system and are associated with worse prognosis than local recurrence.[40] Patient with locoregional recurrences should undergo staging procedures (e.g. PET, CT scans) to rule out presence of distant metastatic disease. If there is no evidence of extraregional disease, the treatment strategies for in-transit metastatic disease depend on the size, number and location of the lesions.

In case of solitar lesion or limited disease surgical excision of the metastases with histologically negative margins is the adequate treatment. The precise width of surgical margin is not determined. The resection should be with generous margin depending on the anatomic site involved. Multifocal metastases within a circumscribed area may be resected en-bloc. Primary closure is prefered if possible, however skin grafting or flaps may be done for skin coverege. In patients, who have surgical resectable in-tranist metastases and have not had a lymphane-

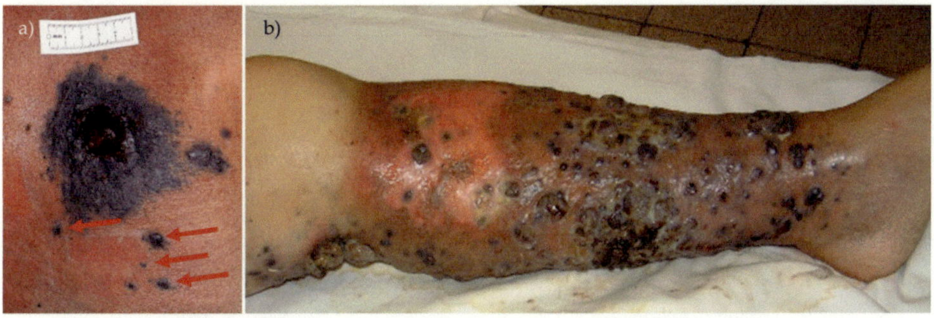

Figure 10. Satelitte metastases (red arrows) around primary melanoma (a) and multiple cutaneous and subcutaneous in transit metastases on the lower leg (b).

dectomy previously a sentinel lymph node biopsy (SLNB) may be considered.[41,42] Some authors recommend performing SLNB even for patients who had undergone SLN biopsy earlier or lymph node dissection suggesting a potential benefit for proper staging and for administering the adequate therapy.[43,44]

In the presence of multiple, inoperable, locoregional cutaneous metastases on the extremity isolated limb perfusion (ILP) should be considered.[45,46] A systematic review of twenty two studies, including 2 018 patients[47] who had isolated limb perfusion concluded that the median complete response rate to ILP was of 58.20%, with a median overall response rate of 90.35%. Amputation for extensive regional recurrence is rarely indicated, as patients in such cases have a high risk of development of metastases in distant organs and no survival benefit can be achived.

For refractory-, recurrent and for anatomically unresectable lesions intralesional (interferon, interleukin-2) or topical (imiquimod, diphencyprone) therapy, cryosurgery, electrochemotherapy, laser-, radio-, and systemic therapy may also be an effective treatment opition.[48-51] Electrochemotherapy combines inravenous or intralesional cytotoxic drug, most commonly cisplatin or belomycin and intralesional electric pulses (Figure 11.). The electric pulse creates cell membrane poration resulting in a better penetration of the chemotherapeutic agent.[52,53] A study has reported a 72% objective response rate of the total of 54 lesions treated with electrochemotherapy.[53] However, superiority of one over the other has not been proven and the choice of the method depends on individual factors.

Patients suspicious for regional lymphnode recurrence should have a fine needle biopsy to confirm the diagnosis and a workup (PET CT or CT scans) to rule out distant metastases. Then lymphadenectomy should be performed in patients who did not have one or the lymphnode disscetion was uncompleted. For patients who have undergone previous lymphadenectomy, excision of the recurrent tumor is still indicated, if feasible. In this case the marking of the lymphnodes by ultrasound prior the surgery makes the surgeon's job easier. In patients with recurrent disease limited to the regional lymph node basin, completion lymphadenectomy offers the best potentially curative treatment option and can provide excellent long-term survival for selected patients.[54]

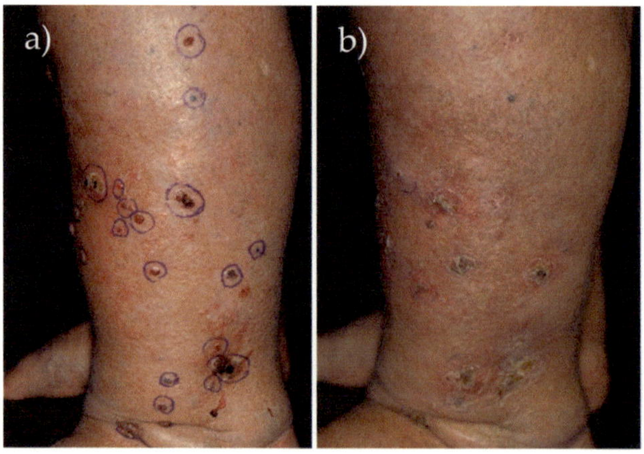

Figure 11. Electrochemoterapy (bleomycin) of multiple cutaneous and subcutaneous melanoma metastases. Before (a) and 10 days after (b) therapy. Photos courtesy of Erika Kis MD, PhD, Department of Dermatology and Allergology, University of Szeged, Hungary.

4. Surgery of stage IV disease

Metastatic melanoma has a poor prognosis and a median survival of 6-10 months depending on the site of metastasis.[40] These patients are classified as stage IV according to the American Joint Committee on Cancer (AJCC 2009) staging manual and seperated into three groups (Table 2.). Stage IV patients with M1a disease have higher survival rates than patients with lung metastases (M1b), who have a better prognosis than those with M1c disease with or without elevated lactate dehydrogenase serum levels (LDH).[55]

M classification	Site of distant metastases	LDH level
M1a	Metastases of the skin, subcutis or lymph nodes beyond regional lymph nodes	normal
M1b	Lung metastases	normal
M1c	Distant metastases at other location or	normal
	Distant metastases at any location with elevated serum levels of LDH	elevated

Table 2. M classification of distant metastases in melanoma according to AJCC 2009.

Currently there is no gold standard care for treatment of stage IV disease. The therapeutic landscape for melanoma is rapidly changing. The first novel agent showing overall survival benefit in unresectable stage III or metastatic melanoma was an anti-CTLA4 blocking monoclonal antibody (ipilimumab) approved by the FDA in 2011.[56] Since then target therapies have been approved for the treatment of metastatic melanoma (BRAF inhibitors: dabrafenib, vemurafenib, MEK inhibitor: trametinib).[57-59] Moreover new immun (e.g. PD-1 inhibitors) and target therapies are on their way. The impact of these drugs on survival rates are clear and promising, but surgery of distant metastases could increase this rate.

Numerous studies, mainly retrospective, showed that patients in whom complete surgical excision of metastases was carried out have a 5-year survival rate of 15–28 % vs. 5-10% in patients who received systemic therapy alone.[60-64] The prospective trial of the Southwest Oncology Group showed a median overall survival of 21 months (overall survival at 3 and 4 years were 36% and 31% respectively) in 64 patients whose metastases had been completely resected. The majority of the patients had one disease site (n=50) and skin and soft tissue sites were present in more than 50% of the cases. The authors concluded that aggressive surgical therapy with follow up adjuvant therapy can be an appropriate cure for these selected patients.[65] International MMAIT-IV trial further supported the role of surgery for stage IV melanoma. In this prospective trial patients who had undergone complete resection of their metatstatic disease were treated with two types of immunotherapy. The 5-year survival was 40–45%.[66] The Multicenter Selective Lymphadenectomy Trial (MSLT-I) also suggested that patients with complete resection exhibit an improved survival compared to patients receiving systemic therapy alone, regardless of site and number of metastases.[67]

Despite that these data are persuasive for surgery in patients with distant metastases, surgery is rarley used in stage IV melanoma except for palliation. Many oncologists believe that once melanoma has spread to a distant site, surgery is not helpful because patients already have occult micrometastases and circulating tumor cells. In the report of Koyanagi et al[68,69] 52% of stage IV patients had detectable circulating tumor cells. However the presence of tumor cells in the blood do not obviously generate metastatic lesions. Most of stage IV melanoma patients at first have disease progression in one organ and the number of metastases in the site can vary.

The advantage of surgical resection of metastatic melanoma is that it may delay disease progression by interrupting the metastatic cascade associated with hematogenous seeding of cells to other sites.[70,71] Surgical resection also decreases tumor burden thus reducing tumor-induced immunosuppression. Metastases greater than 2 cm are eradicated easier with surgery than with systemic treatments.[72] In addition, surgical resection has less side-effects than systemic therapeutic agents.

The recent development of imaging techniques has led to more accurate detection of metastases (size of 5-10mm), aiding surgeons in improved delineation of the extent of the disease and planing for the operation. In line with this development in surgical techniques, anesthesia and intensive supportive care have reduced operative mortality and morbidity rate even for multiple metastectomy.[71] It is evident that appropriate patient selection is essential for a good outcome.

Surgery in metastatic diseases is most effective in patients with small number of metastases and/or few metastatic organ sites.[73] Based on the MSLT-I study and Wevers et al, the percent of stage IV patients eligible for surgery can range widely from more than half to only 22%.[67, 74] In deciding about surgery, one should consider underlying co-morbidities, performance status and life expectany. If no survival benefit and/or advantage in quality of life can be achieved with surgical metastectomy, it may be disregarded. It has been shown by numerous studies that complete (R0) resection is associated with a better survial and in all cases com-

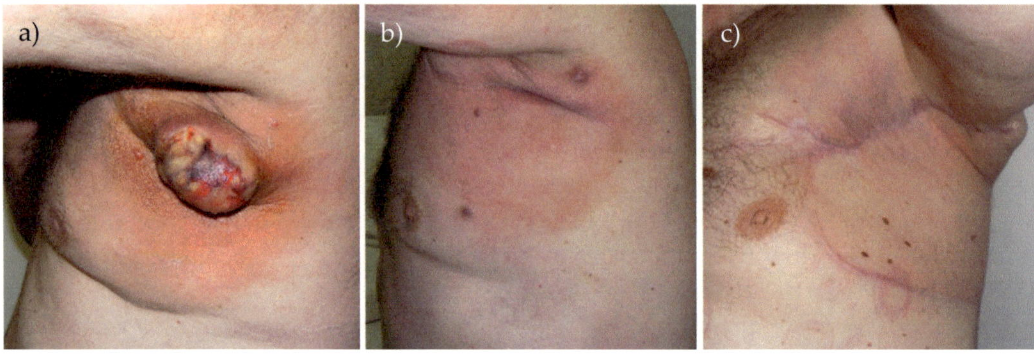

Figure 12. Neoadjuvant BRAFi in the treatment of melanoma. The 52 year-old patient with unknown primary melanoma and inoperable metastases in the left axillary region (a). BRAF inhibitor (vemurafenib) was initiated. After 3 months of BRAF inhibitor treatment the tumor almost completly regressed (b). Subsequently, the patient underwent surgery for the remnant disease (c).

pletness should be strained by the surgeon.[75-78] Further prognostic factors are prolonged disease-free survival and a tumour-volume doubling time of >60 days.[73,79,80] (Table 3.).

• Feasibility of complete surgical resection (R0)
• Number of metastases
• Site of metastases
• Tumor doubling time
• Disease free interval
• Other therapy modalities
• Acceptable functional deficit
• Co-morbidities

Table 3. Factors to consider prior to surgical resection in stage IV melanoma

Multiple disease sites are not a contraindication to surgical resection but all of the factors mentioned above should be considered before procedure. Reccurent disease can be treated with repeated metastectomy.[81-83] Ollila et al points out that prolonged disease-free interval prior to recurrence and complete surgical metastasectomy of the recurrence were the two most important prognostic factors for survival after recurrence.

In the case of large tumor masses, when surgery can not be carried out, effective systemic treatment prior to surgery is advisable in order to treat the initially unresectable disease. Neoadjuvant setting has been successfully applied in several solid tumors (e.g. breats, head and neck cancer) but it has not been used in advanced cutaneous melanoma, because no effective systemic treatments were available for this disease. The presence of new systemic therapies (biological and target) may change this. Several case reports have shown the beneficial effects of BRAF inhibitors. Patients with unresectable bulky disease regained surgical suitabilty after taking the drug for a couple of months[84-86] (Figure 12).

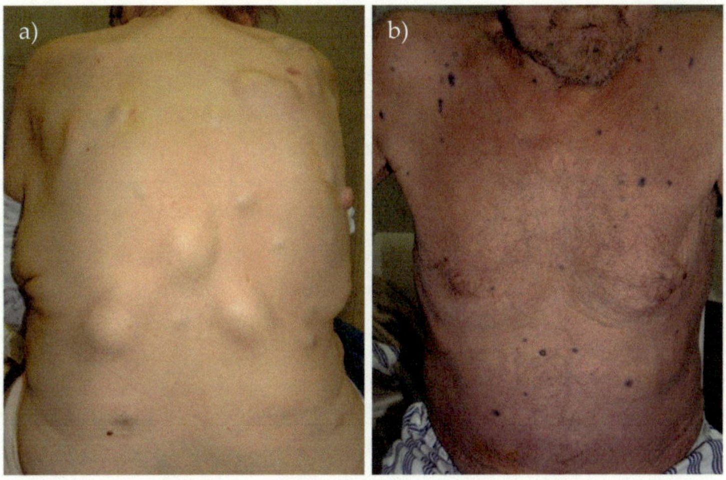

Figure 13. Multiple distant soft tissue metastases (a) and multiple distant skin metastases (b).

In contrast to BRAF inhibitors, ipilimumab seems to be a less effective agent in neoadjuvant setting because of its mechanism of action and relatively slow pattern of time response. However the surgical excision of lesions that are resistant to treatment with ipilimumab may improve outcomes for some patients. Other immuntherapies are in development (PD-1 inhibitors) which show an earlier tumor response compared to ipilimumab.[87] Overall, surgical resection of metastatic lesion in highly selected patients appears to offer a survival advantage over systemic treatment modalities alone. The decision for surgery of stage IV melanoma patients should be discussed at an interdisciplinary tumor board. After complete metastectomy, adjuvant therapy may be indicated as melanoma is likely to recur. Surgical resection should be considered more often than it is currently practiced, since the combined advances in imaging techniques and promising novel systemic agents can improve patients' quality of life and clinical outcomes.

4.1. Surgery of distant skin, soft tissue and lymphnode metastases (Stage IV M1a)

Almost 40% of patients with stage IV melanoma have M1a disease.[88] Median survival of patients in this group is 18-40 months. Skin and soft tissue metastases are usually associated with a better prognosis than distant lymph node disease (Figure 13.). Positive prognostic factors for M1a disease are fewer lesions, longer disease-free interval, and smaller size of tumors.[61] Skin and soft tissue metastases should be resected as soon as possible before the metastases becomes large and, if applicable, with wide margins (2 cm). In case of lymphnode metastases regional lymphnode dissection is performed (for details see section on lymph node dissection). Factors to consider prior to surgical resection in stage IV melanoma are summarized in Table 3. Complete surgical resection of M1a disease can promote survival up to 60 months, even after recurrence.[81] Metastases can ulcerate causing pain, bleeding, infection, and decreased quality of life. Surgical resection for palliation may be indicated in these situations.

4.2. Surgery of pulmonary metastases (Stage IV M1b)

The lung is the most typical site of visceral metastases (40%) for melanoma. Pulmonary metastases are associated with a longer survival than metastases to other visceral sites.[40] A growing number of studies have shown that pulmonary metastectomy improves survival [89-96] (Table 4). Tafra et al reported that of 984 melanoma patients with lung metastases, the 106 patients that underwent metastectomy had better 5 year survival than patients treated with non-surgical methods (27% vs. 3%, respectively).[79] Chua et al conducted a large single center study with 1737 patients.[89] 292 patients had surgery for lung metastases and the 5-year survival for this patient group was 38%.

According to the various reports, factors predictive of improved survival are: ability to achieve a complete resection, prolonged disease-free interval (>36 months), 2 or fewer pulmonary nodules,[89-91] size of the largest metastasis <2 cm, prior response to chemotherapy/immunotherapy, and male sex.[92] While the disease may recurr, most of the data demonstrate that long term survival can be achieved with repeated metastectomy (in cases of extra-thoracic lesions also) in suitable patients.[91]

The presence of multiple and even bilateral pulmonary nodules is not a contraindication to surgery.[89,97] Interestingly, hilar or mediastinal lymph node involvement did not have an effect on survival.[93] In most cases pulmonary metastectomy involves wedge resection and segmentectomy with occasional indication for lobectomy.

Author	**Number of patients undergoing surgery**	**Median OS (months)**	**5 year survival (%)**
Andrews et al[91]	86	35	33
Chua et al[89]	292	23	34
Leo et al[93]	282	19	22
Neuman et al[94]	26	40	29
Ollila et al[61]	45	23.1	15.6
Petersen et al[90]	318	19	21
Schunan et al[92]	30	18.3	35.1
Tafra et al[79]	106	23	27
Younes et al[96]	48	32	36

OS: overall survival

Table 4. Studies of pulmonary metastectomy in patients with lung metastases from melanoma

As mentioned earlier, patient selection in Stage IV disease is very important. Tumor doubling time (TDT), an index calculated on the basis of tumour growth rate as detected on the chest radiographs, is one of the major factors predictive of survival and should be used as a consideration in the decision of whether or not to operate.[80] Patients undergoing surgical managment of lung metastases should have pulmonary function and clinical condition suitable for the operation, controlled primary lesion, metastases that appeared technically resectable on diagnostic imaging, and preoperative biopsy consistent with melanoma.

The spread of advanced imaging techniques (CT, PET) contribute to the earlier detection of melanoma metastases and give a more precise preoperative image of the location, thus aiding the accurate selection of surgery candidates (Figure 14.).

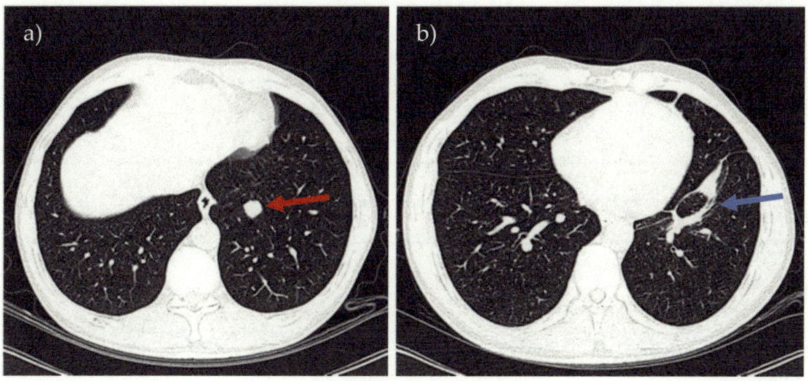

Figure 14. Solitary pulmonary metastases in a 40 year-old patient (red arrow). b. Post surgical scarring at the site of the metastases (blue arrow).

Upper aerodigestive tract metastases of melanoma are extremily rare. The patients are usually symptomatic with hemoptysis or cough. Treatments with approriate aggressive multimodal therapies are needed in such cases (metastectomy, segmental resection, laser excision, external beam radiation).[98-100]

In conclusions, findings are suggestive that pulmonary metastectomy for carefully selected patients warrant a favourable outcome.

4.3. Surgery of visceral metastases

4.3.1. Liver metastases (Stage IV M1c)

Liver metastases can occur both in cases of cutaneous and/or ocular melanoma. It is important to distinguish them, as in metastastic ocular melanoma the liver is the predominant metastatic site (89% of cases) and often the first and only site of metastases.[100,101] In contrast, cutaneous melanoma metastases can occur in the lungs, lymph nodes, brain and soft tissue. Only few patients develop liver (15%-20%) and bowel metastases.[102,103] The difference in metastatic presentation is most likely driven by the absence of lymphatics in the uveal tract, therefore melanoma spreads hematogenously.[104]

Studies evaluating the role of surgery in the treatment of hepatic metastases from melanoma are mainly retrospective case series from single institutions. Some of these studies included non-surgical (chemotherapy, best supportive care etc) comparator arm, while others did not have a control group.[76-78,105-108] (Table 5.)

The comparative studies showed a longer median overall survival in patients who underwent hepatic resection compared to non-surgical treatment in both ocular and cutaneous melanomas. Overall survival was 2-4 months for patients with unresected hepatic metastases versus 28 months for those with completly resected liver metastases.[78] A recent metaanalysis of five studies also revealed a significant improvment in overall survival after surgery compared to non-surgical procedures.[109] The majority of noncomparative studies also reported benefit from resection of metastases.[66,75,110-114]

All studies observed that R0 resection was associated with longer overall survival than R1 or R2 surgery.[75-78]

Author	Melanoma type	Number of patients	Median OS (months)	5 year survival (%)
Adam et al[110]	Cutaneous and ocular	1452	19	21
Caralt et al[117]	Cutaneous and ocular	NR	26.3	NR
Chua et al[115]	Cutaneous and ocular	23	21	NR
de Ridder et al[75]	Ocular, cutanous and unknown	32	29	3
Faries et al[107]	Cutaneous and ocular	1078	24.8	30
Frenkel et al[76]	Ocular	74	23	NR
Groeschl et al[111]	NR	NR	39	36
Herman et al[118]	Cutaneous and ocular	367	22	NR
Kim et al[119]	Cutaneous and GI tract	NR	9.5	4
Kodjikian et al[116]	Ocular	63	20.5	24
Mariani et al[77]	Ocular	798	23.0	NR
Marshall et al[105]	Ocular	188	24.0	NR
Pawlik et al[114]	Cutaneous and ocular	40	29.4	21 for ocular
Pilati et al[66]	Cutaneous and ocular	36	15	NR
Piperno-Neumann et al[108]	Ocular	470	21	NR
Ripley et al[112]	Cutaneous and ocular	539	36	53
Rivoire et al[106]	Ocular	63	25	NR
Rose et al[78]	Cutaneous	1750	28	29
Ryu et al[113]	Cutaneous and ocular	33	29	42

OS: overall survival; NR: not reported

Table 5. Studies of hepatic resection in patients with liver metastases from melanoma

The outcome of surgery is also influenced by the number of metastases, length of disease-free interval and limited disease distribution.[78,115,116] However, eligibility for surgery upon the extent of disease and the number of metastases varied in the studies. In the Kodjikian study[116], the cut-off number for resection liver metastases was 10 or less lesions.

Recurrence rates following hepatic resection in the studies ranged between 72% to 75%. [78,111] All in all the hepatic resection for malignant melanoma is a safe operation.

60-day mortality rates were recorded in some reviews at 1.9% and 2.3% and postoperative complications after metastectomy occured in 15% to 20% of cases.[78,111]

In the treatment of hepatic metastases, systemic and /or non-surgical therapies can be applied in the form of adjuvant or neoadjuvant settings that supplement surgical resection. There are no clear data yet to determine the most efficacious time for the administration of systemic therapy secondary to surgery. Pawlik et al found that patients who had received adjuvant systemic therapy prior the hepatic resection had increased survival compared to patients having resection alone.[114] Adam et al reported increased survival in patients responsive to neoadjuvant chemotherapy.[110]

The data mentioned above indicate that both ocular and cutaneous metastatic melanoma patients with liver metastases benefit from surgery. To achieve this outcome, accurate patient selection is crucial. Only patients with limited disease/metastases who can be rendered surgically free of disease should be considered as candidates for hepatic resection. For patients with unresectable metastatic melanoma, systemic and /or regional (hepatic intra-arterial chemotherapy, hepatic arterial embolization, isolated/percutaneous hepatic perfusion) therapies should be taken into consideration.

4.3.2. Gastrointestinal metastases (Stage IV M1c)

Gastrointestinal (GI) tract is an uncommon metastatic site for melanoma malignum occuring in only 2-5% of patients. However, more than a quarter of patients with melanoma at autopsy revealed GI metastases.[120,121] Patients with metastases to the GI are often symptomatic with pain (29–64%), obstruction (27%), bleeding (27%), palpable mass (12%) or weight loss (9%). [122] In addition, the high incidence of metastases of melanoma in the small intestine has been recently assigned to the presence of functionally active chemokine CCR9 on melanoma cells that facilitate metastases to the small bowel.[123] In a large number of cases palliative surgery is needed to alleviate bleeding and /or obstruction. Looking at the survival benefit of surgery, some studies found significantly improved survival in patients who underwent surgery and had a complete resection.[121,124,125] Ollila et al. reported a 5-year survival rate of 41% after complete resection.[121]

In conclusion, metastatic melanoma of the gastrointestinal tract is very rare, but should be suspected in any patient with a history of cutaneous melanoma and new gastrointestinal symptoms. Surgical interventions for symptomatic patients with melanoma of the gastrointestinal tract significantly relieve pain and improve quality of life and may confer a survival advantage.

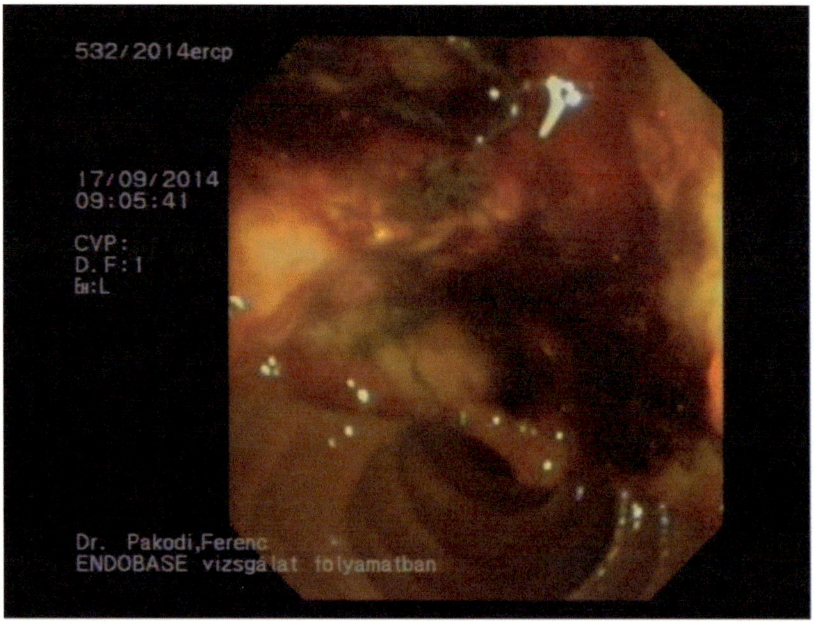

Figure 15. Duodenal melanoma metastasis.

4.3.3. Metastases to the spleen, the pancreas, or the adrenal glands (Stage IV M1c)

Isolated metastases to the spleen, pancreas or the adrenal glands are extremely rare. Few reports have demonstrated that surgical resection improves the 5-year survival.[62,126] Analysis of patients with solitary metastases to the adrenal glands yielded median survival times of 60 months.[127] In the study of Wood et al, sixty patients underwent adrenalectomy, hepatectomy, splenectomy, or pancreatectomy for melanoma metastases. The reported 5-year survival in the group after complete resection was 24%, whereas in the incomplete resection group, there were no 5-year survivors.[62,126]

4.4. Surgery of brain metastases (Stage IV M1c)

Metastatic disease to the brain is a frequent manifestation of melanoma with cerebral metastases accounting for 20-54% of deaths from melanoma.[128] It is associated with significant morbidity and mortality and poor prognosis. The median survival upon diagnosis of the cranial metastases is approximately 4 months.[129] Non-systemic treatment options are surgery, and stereotactic or palliative whole-brain radiotherapy.[130,131]

Usually patients present with symptoms such as seizures, vertigo, nausea, and vision alteration. In patients with good performance status and controlled primary disease, the surgical resection of solitary cerebral metastases is preferred. Positive prognostic factors in cases of brain metastases are younger age, good performance status, lack of neurologic symptoms, lack of extracranial disease and single focus of disease. Surgery might also be indicated for palliative reasons. If the solitary lesion is unresectable due to localization or extracranial disease, the determination of BRAF status is essential, since the efficacy of BRAF inhibitor dabrafenib in cerebral metastatic disease has been shown.[132] If no mutation is detected in BRAF, ipilimumab might be a treatment option[133] (for details see chapter 'Treatment of Brain metastases').

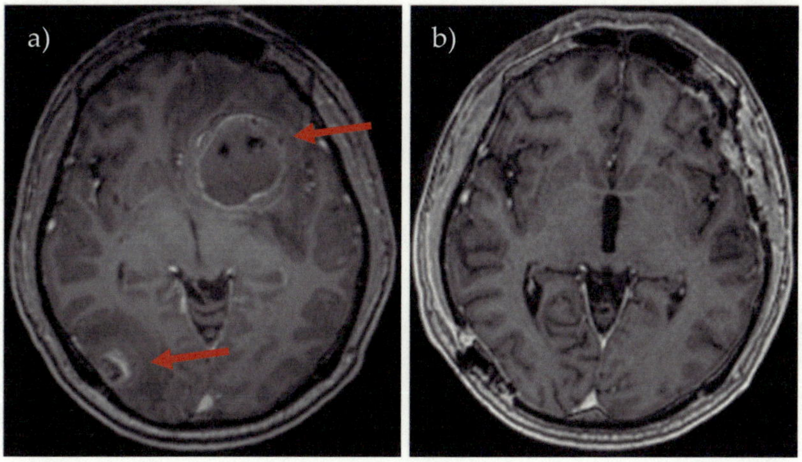

Figure 16. Pre-operative CT scan with multiple melanoma metastases. Brain metastases are indicated with red arrows (a). Post surgical CT scan (b).

4.5. Bone metastases (Stage IV M1c)

Skelatal metastases are present in 5-17% of stage IV patients and have a poor prognosis. [134] Colman et al conducted the largest retrospective analysis of melanoma patients with bone metastases.[135] The study compared the survival rate of the group of patients who underwent surgery with wide resection of metastases with the group who received other surgery or were treated without operation. The observed 1-year overall survival rate in the resection group was twice as high as that of matched historical controls (50.0 vs. 24.8%). They found that overall survival may be improved in carefully selected patients where all known macroscopic tumor can be resected.[134-137]

Author details

Rolland Gyulai*, Zsolt Kádár and Zsuzsanna Lengyel

*Address all correspondence to: gyulai.rolland@pte.hu

Department of Dermatology, Venerology and Oncodermatology, University of Pécs, Pécs, Hungary

References

[1] Coit DG, Thompson JA, Andtbacka R, Anker CJ, Bichakjian CK, Carson WE,3rd, et al. Melanoma, version 4.2014. J Natl Compr Canc Netw 2014 May;12(5):621-629.

[2] Bishop JA, Corrie PG, Evans J, Gore ME, Hall PN, Kirkham N, et al. UK guidelines for the management of cutaneous melanoma. Br J Plast Surg 2002 Jan;55(1):46-54.

[3] Molenkamp BG, Sluijter BJ, Oosterhof B, Meijer S, van Leeuwen PA. Non-radical diagnostic biopsies do not negatively influence melanoma patient survival. Ann Surg Oncol 2007 Apr;14(4):1424-1430.

[4] Hieken TJ, Hernandez-Irizarry R, Boll JM, Jones Coleman JE. Accuracy of diagnostic biopsy for cutaneous melanoma: implications for surgical oncologists. Int J Surg Oncol 2013;2013:196493.

[5] Yamashita Y, Hashimoto I, Abe Y, Seike T, Okawa K, Senzaki Y, et al. Effect of biopsy technique on the survival rate of malignant melanoma patients. Arch Plast Surg 2014 Mar;41(2):122-125.

[6] Austin JR, Byers RM, Brown WD, Wolf P. Influence of biopsy on the prognosis of cutaneous melanoma of the head and neck. Head Neck 1996 Mar-Apr;18(2):107-117.

[7] Rampen FH, van Houten WA, Jop WC. Incisional procedures and prognosis in malignant melanoma. Clin Exp Dermatol 1980 Sep;5(3):313-320.

[8] English DR, Del Mar C, Burton RC. Factors influencing the number needed to excise: excision rates of pigmented lesions by general practitioners. Med J Aust 2004 Jan 5;180(1):16-19.

[9] Santillan AA, Messina JL, Marzban SS, Crespo G, Sondak VK, Zager JS. Pathology review of thin melanoma and melanoma in situ in a multidisciplinary melanoma clinic: impact on treatment decisions. J Clin Oncol 2010 Jan 20;28(3):481-486.

[10] Macy-Roberts E, Ackerman AB. A critique of techniques for biopsy of clinically suspected malignant melanomas. Am J Dermatopathol 1982 Oct;4(5):391-398.

[11] Stell VH, Norton HJ, Smith KS, Salo JC, White RL,Jr. Method of biopsy and incidence of positive margins in primary melanoma. Ann Surg Oncol 2007 Feb;14(2):893-898.

[12] Martin RC,2nd, Scoggins CR, Ross MI, Reintgen DS, Noyes RD, Edwards MJ, et al. Is incisional biopsy of melanoma harmful? Am J Surg 2005 Dec;190(6):913-917.

[13] Bong JL, Herd RM, Hunter JA. Incisional biopsy and melanoma prognosis. J Am Acad Dermatol 2002 May;46(5):690-694.

[14] Veronesi U, Cascinelli N, Adamus J, Balch C, Bandiera D, Barchuk A, et al. Thin stage I primary cutaneous malignant melanoma. Comparison of excision with margins of 1 or 3 cm. N Engl J Med 1988 May 5;318(18):1159-1162.

[15] Balch CM, Soong SJ, Smith T, Ross MI, Urist MM, Karakousis CP, et al. Long-term results of a prospective surgical trial comparing 2 cm vs. 4 cm excision margins for 740 patients with 1-4 mm melanomas. Ann Surg Oncol 2001 Mar;8(2):101-108.

[16] Cohn-Cedermark G, Rutqvist LE, Andersson R, Breivald M, Ingvar C, Johansson H, et al. Long term results of a randomized study by the Swedish Melanoma Study Group on 2-cm versus 5-cm resection margins for patients with cutaneous melanoma with a tumor thickness of 0.8-2.0 mm. Cancer 2000 Oct 1;89(7):1495-1501.

[17] Khayat D, Rixe O, Martin G, Soubrane C, Banzet M, Bazex JA, et al. Surgical margins in cutaneous melanoma (2 cm versus 5 cm for lesions measuring less than 2.1-mm thick). Cancer 2003 Apr 15;97(8):1941-1946.

[18] Thomas JM, Newton-Bishop J, A'Hern R, Coombes G, Timmons M, Evans J, et al. Excision margins in high-risk malignant melanoma. N Engl J Med 2004 Feb 19;350(8): 757-766.

[19] Gillgren P, Drzewiecki KT, Niin M, Gullestad HP, Hellborg H, Mansson-Brahme E, et al. 2-Cm Versus 4-Cm Surgical Excision Margins for Primary Cutaneous Melanoma Thicker than 2 Mm: a Randomised, Multicentre Trial. Lancet 2011 Nov 5;378(9803):1635-1642.

[20] Haigh PI, DiFronzo LA, McCready DR. Optimal excision margins for primary cutaneous melanoma: a systematic review and meta-analysis. Can J Surg 2003 Dec;46(6): 419-426.

[21] Kunishige JH, Brodland DG, Zitelli JA. Surgical margins for melanoma in situ. J Am Acad Dermatol 2012 Mar;66(3):438-444.

[22] Akhtar S, Bhat W, Magdum A, Stanley PR. Surgical excision margins for melanoma in situ. J Plast Reconstr Aesthet Surg 2014 Mar;67(3):320-323.

[23] Harish V, Bond JS, Scolyer RA, Haydu LE, Saw RP, Quinn MJ, et al. Margins of excision and prognostic factors for cutaneous eyelid melanomas. J Plast Reconstr Aesthet Surg 2013 Aug;66(8):1066-1073.

[24] Jones TS, Jones EL, Gao D, Pearlman NW, Robinson WA, McCarter M. Management of external ear melanoma: the same or something different? Am J Surg 2013 Sep; 206(3):307-313.

[25] Patel SG, Prasad ML, Escrig M, Singh B, Shaha AR, Kraus DH, et al. Primary mucosal malignant melanoma of the head and neck. Head Neck 2002 Mar;24(3):247-257.

[26] Prasad ML, Patel SG, Huvos AG, Shah JP, Busam KJ. Primary mucosal melanoma of the head and neck: a proposal for microstaging localized, Stage I (lymph node-negative) tumors. Cancer 2004 Apr 15;100(8):1657-1664.

[27] Rogo KO, Andersson R, Edbom G, Stendahl U. Conservative surgery for vulvovaginal melanoma. Eur J Gynaecol Oncol 1991;12(2):113-119.

[28] Ragnarsson-Olding BK, Nilsson BR, Kanter-Lewensohn LR, Lagerlof B, Ringborg UK. Malignant melanoma of the vulva in a nationwide, 25-year study of 219 Swedish females: predictors of survival. Cancer 1999 Oct 1;86(7):1285-1293.

[29] Sanchez-Ortiz R, Huang SF, Tamboli P, Prieto VG, Hester G, Pettaway CA. Melanoma of the penis, scrotum and male urethra: a 40-year single institution experience. J Urol 2005 Jun;173(6):1958-1965.

[30] Ballo MT, Gershenwald JE, Zagars GK, Lee JE, Mansfield PF, Strom EA, et al. Sphincter-sparing local excision and adjuvant radiation for anal-rectal melanoma. J Clin Oncol 2002 Dec 1;20(23):4555-4558.

[31] Mathijssen IM, van der Meulen JC. Guidelines for reconstruction of the eyelids and canthal regions. J Plast Reconstr Aesthet Surg 2010 Sep;63(9):1420-1433.

[32] Yin VT, Warneke CL, Merritt HA, Esmaeli B. Number of excisions required to obtain clear surgical margins and prognostic value of AJCC T category for patients with eyelid melanoma. Br J Ophthalmol 2014 Jul 22.

[33] Harvey DT, Taylor RS, Itani KM, Loewinger RJ. Mohs micrographic surgery of the eyelid: an overview of anatomy, pathophysiology, and reconstruction options. Dermatol Surg 2013 May;39(5):673-697.

[34] Thornton JF, Griffin JR, Constantine FC. Nasal reconstruction: an overview and nuances. Semin Plast Surg 2008 Nov;22(4):257-268.

[35] Park SS. Nasal reconstruction in the 21st century--a contemporary review. Clin Exp Otorhinolaryngol 2008 Mar;1(1):1-9.

[36] Reddy LV, Zide MF. Reconstruction of skin cancer defects of the auricle. J Oral Maxillofac Surg 2004 Dec;62(12):1457-1471.

[37] Olbricht S, Liegeois NJ. Closing surgical defects of the external ear. Semin Cutan Med Surg 2003 Dec;22(4):273-280.

[38] Yun MJ, Park JU, Kwon ST. Surgical options for malignant skin tumors of the hand. Arch Plast Surg 2013 May;40(3):238-243.

[39] Weide B, Faller C, Buttner P, Pflugfelder A, Leiter U, Eigentler TK, et al. Prognostic factors of melanoma patients with satellite or in-transit metastasis at the time of stage III diagnosis. PLoS One 2013 Apr 29;8(4):e63137.

[40] Balch CM, Gershenwald JE, Soong SJ, Thompson JF, Atkins MB, Byrd DR, et al. Final version of 2009 AJCC melanoma staging and classification. J Clin Oncol 2009 Dec 20;27(36):6199-6206.

[41] Yao KA, Hsueh EC, Essner R, Foshag LJ, Wanek LA, Morton DL. Is sentinel lymph node mapping indicated for isolated local and in-transit recurrent melanoma? Ann Surg 2003 Nov;238(5):743-747.

[42] Gipponi M, Solari N, Giovinazzo D, Queirolo P, Bertoglio S, Villa G, et al. The role of sentinel lymph node biopsy in patients with local recurrence or in-transit metastasis of melanoma. Anticancer Res 2014 Jun;34(6):3197-3203.

[43] Beasley GM, Tyler DS. Treatment of in-transit melanoma: an opportunity to discover critical knowledge. Oncology (Williston Park) 2011 Dec;25(14):1351-2, 1355.

[44] Squires MH,3rd, Delman KA. Current treatment of locoregional recurrence of melanoma. Curr Oncol Rep 2013 Oct;15(5):465-472.

[45] Turley RS, Raymond AK, Tyler DS. Regional treatment strategies for in-transit melanoma metastasis. Surg Oncol Clin N Am 2011 Jan;20(1):79-103.

[46] Deroose JP, Grunhagen DJ, van Geel AN, de Wilt JH, Eggermont AM, Verhoef C. Long-term outcome of isolated limb perfusion with tumour necrosis factor-alpha for patients with melanoma in-transit metastases. Br J Surg 2011 Nov;98(11):1573-1580.

[47] Moreno-Ramirez D, de la Cruz-Merino L, Ferrandiz L, Villegas-Portero R, Nieto-Garcia A. Isolated limb perfusion for malignant melanoma: systematic review on effectiveness and safety. Oncologist 2010;15(4):416-427.

[48] Stevens G, Thompson JF, Firth I, O'Brien CJ, McCarthy WH, Quinn MJ. Locally advanced melanoma: results of postoperative hypofractionated radiation therapy. Cancer 2000 Jan 1;88(1):88-94.

[49] Damian DL, Thompson JF. Treatment of extensive cutaneous metastatic melanoma with topical diphencyprone. J Am Acad Dermatol 2007 May;56(5):869-871.

[50] Berman B, Poochareon VN, Villa AM. Novel dermatologic uses of the immune response modifier imiquimod 5% cream. Skin Therapy Lett 2002 Nov;7(9):1-6.

[51] Gibson SC, Byrne DS, McKay AJ. Ten-year experience of carbon dioxide laser ablation as treatment for cutaneous recurrence of malignant melanoma. Br J Surg 2004 Jul;91(7):893-895.

[52] Testori A, Intelisano A, Verrecchia F, Menicanti C, Tosti G, Grassi E, et al. Alternatives for the treatment of local advanced disease: electrochemotherapy, limb perfusion, limb infusion, intralesional IL2. What is the role? Dermatol Ther 2012 Sep-Oct; 25(5):443-451.

[53] Byrne CM, Thompson JF, Johnston H, Hersey P, Quinn MJ, Michael Hughes T, et al. Treatment of metastatic melanoma using electroporation therapy with bleomycin (electrochemotherapy). Melanoma Res 2005 Feb;15(1):45-51.

[54] Young SE, Martinez SR, Faries MB, Essner R, Wanek LA, Morton DL. Can surgical therapy alone achieve long-term cure of melanoma metastatic to regional nodes? Cancer J 2006 May-Jun;12(3):207-211.

[55] Manola J, Atkins M, Ibrahim J, Kirkwood J. Prognostic factors in metastatic melanoma: a pooled analysis of Eastern Cooperative Oncology Group trials. J Clin Oncol 2000 Nov 15;18(22):3782-3793.

[56] Hodi FS, O'Day SJ, McDermott DF, Weber RW, Sosman JA, Haanen JB, et al. Improved survival with ipilimumab in patients with metastatic melanoma. N Engl J Med 2010 Aug 19;363(8):711-723.

[57] Chapman PB, Hauschild A, Robert C, Haanen JB, Ascierto P, Larkin J, et al. Improved survival with vemurafenib in melanoma with BRAF V600E mutation. N Engl J Med 2011 Jun 30;364(26):2507-2516.

[58] Hauschild A, Grob JJ, Demidov LV, Jouary T, Gutzmer R, Millward M, et al. Dabrafenib in BRAF-mutated metastatic melanoma: a multicentre, open-label, phase 3 randomised controlled trial. Lancet 2012 Jul 28;380(9839):358-365.

[59] Kim KB, Kefford R, Pavlick AC, Infante JR, Ribas A, Sosman JA, et al. Phase II study of the MEK1/MEK2 inhibitor Trametinib in patients with metastatic BRAF-mutant cutaneous melanoma previously treated with or without a BRAF inhibitor. J Clin Oncol 2013 Feb 1;31(4):482-489.

[60] Martinez SR, Young SE. A rational surgical approach to the treatment of distant melanoma metastases. Cancer Treat Rev 2008 Nov;34(7):614-620.

[61] Ollila DW. Complete metastasectomy in patients with stage IV metastatic melanoma. Lancet Oncol 2006 Nov;7(11):919-924.

[62] Wood TF, DiFronzo LA, Rose DM, Haigh PI, Stern SL, Wanek L, et al. Does complete resection of melanoma metastatic to solid intra-abdominal organs improve survival? Ann Surg Oncol 2001 Sep;8(8):658-662.

[63] Bajetta E, Del Vecchio M, Bernard-Marty C, Vitali M, Buzzoni R, Rixe O, et al. Metastatic melanoma: chemotherapy. Semin Oncol 2002 Oct;29(5):427-445.

[64] Young SE, Martinez SR, Essner R. The role of surgery in treatment of stage IV melanoma. J Surg Oncol 2006 Sep 15;94(4):344-351.

[65] Sosman JA, Moon J, Tuthill RJ, Warneke JA, Vetto JT, Redman BG, et al. A phase 2 trial of complete resection for stage IV melanoma: results of Southwest Oncology Group Clinical Trial S9430. Cancer 2011 Oct 15;117(20):4740-4706.

[66] Morton D, Mozzillo N, Thompson J, Kelley M, Faries M, Wagner J, et al. MMAIT Clinical Trials Group. An international, randomized, phase III trial of bacillus Calmette-Guerin (BCG) plus allogeneic melanoma vaccine (MCV) or placebo after complete resection of melanoma metastatic to regional or distant sites. Journal of Clinical Oncology 2007;25(Suppl: 8508).

[67] Howard JH, Thompson JF, Mozzillo N, Nieweg OE, Hoekstra HJ, Roses DF, et al. Metastasectomy for distant metastatic melanoma: analysis of data from the first Mul-

ticenter Selective Lymphadenectomy Trial (MSLT-I). Ann Surg Oncol 2012 Aug;19(8): 2547-2555.

[68] Koyanagi K, Kuo C, Nakagawa T, Mori T, Ueno H, Lorico AR,Jr, et al. Multimarker quantitative real-time PCR detection of circulating melanoma cells in peripheral blood: relation to disease stage in melanoma patients. Clin Chem 2005 Jun;51(6): 981-988.

[69] Koyanagi K, Mori T, O'Day SJ, Martinez SR, Wang HJ, Hoon DS. Association of circulating tumor cells with serum tumor-related methylated DNA in peripheral blood of melanoma patients. Cancer Res 2006 Jun 15;66(12):6111-6117.

[70] Roth JA, Silverstein MJ, Morton DL. Metastatic potential of metastases. Surgery 1976 Jun;79(6):669-673.

[71] Leung AM, Hari DM, Morton DL. Surgery for distant melanoma metastasis. Cancer J 2012 Mar-Apr;18(2):176-184.

[72] Morton DL, Ollila DW, Hsueh EC, Essner R, Gupta RK. Cytoreductive surgery and adjuvant immunotherapy: a new management paradigm for metastatic melanoma. CA Cancer J Clin 1999 Mar-Apr;49(2):101-16, 65.

[73] Meyer T, Merkel S, Goehl J, Hohenberger W. Surgical therapy for distant metastases of malignant melanoma. Cancer 2000 Nov 1;89(9):1983-1991.

[74] Wevers KP, Hoekstra HJ. Stage IV melanoma: completely resectable patients are scarce. Ann Surg Oncol 2013 Jul;20(7):2352-2356.

[75] de Ridder J, van Walsum M, Verhoef C, Nagtegaal I, de Wilt J, Dutch Liver Working Group. Hepatic resection for metastatic melanoma in The Netherlands: survival and prognostic factors. Melanoma Res 2013 Feb;23(1):27-32.

[76] Frenkel S, Nir I, Hendler K, Lotem M, Eid A, Jurim O, et al. Long-term survival of uveal melanoma patients after surgery for liver metastases. Br J Ophthalmol 2009 Aug;93(8):1042-1046.

[77] Mariani P, Piperno-Neumann S, Servois V, Berry MG, Dorval T, Plancher C, et al. Surgical management of liver metastases from uveal melanoma: 16 years' experience at the Institut Curie. Eur J Surg Oncol 2009 Nov;35(11):1192-1197.

[78] Rose DM, Essner R, Hughes TM, Tang PC, Bilchik A, Wanek LA, et al. Surgical resection for metastatic melanoma to the liver: the John Wayne Cancer Institute and Sydney Melanoma Unit experience. Arch Surg 2001 Aug;136(8):950-955.

[79] Tafra L, Dale PS, Wanek LA, Ramming KP, Morton DL. Resection and adjuvant immunotherapy for melanoma metastatic to the lung and thorax. J Thorac Cardiovasc Surg 1995 Jul;110(1):119-28; discussion 129.

[80] Ollila DW, Stern SL, Morton DL. Tumor doubling time: a selection factor for pulmonary resection of metastatic melanoma. J Surg Oncol 1998 Dec;69(4):206-211.

[81] Ollila DW, Hsueh EC, Stern SL, Morton DL. Metastasectomy for recurrent stage IV melanoma. J Surg Oncol 1999 Aug;71(4):209-213.

[82] Faries MB, Morton DL. Melanoma: is immunotherapy of benefit? Adv Surg 2003;37:139-169.

[83] Pflugfelder A, Kochs C, Blum A, Capellaro M, Czeschik C, Dettenborn T, et al. Malignant melanoma S3-guideline "diagnosis, therapy and follow-up of melanoma". J Dtsch Dermatol Ges 2013 Aug;11 Suppl 6:1-116, 1-126.

[84] Koers K, Francken AB, Haanen JB, Woerdeman LA, van der Hage JA. Vemurafenib as neoadjuvant treatment for unresectable regional metastatic melanoma. J Clin Oncol 2013 Jun 1;31(16):e251-3.

[85] Fadaki N, Cardona-Huerta S, Martineau L, Thummala S, Cheng ST, Bunker SR, et al. Inoperable bulky melanoma responds to neoadjuvant therapy with vemurafenib. BMJ Case Rep 2012 Oct 22;2012:10.1136/bcr-2012-007034.

[86] La Greca M, Grasso G, Antonelli G, Russo AE, Bartolotta S, D'Angelo A, et al. Neoadjuvant therapy for locally advanced melanoma: new strategies with targeted therapies. Onco Targets Ther 2014 Jun 19;7:1115-1121.

[87] Robert C, Ribas A, Wolchok JD, Hodi FS, Hamid O, Kefford R, et al. Anti-programmed-death-receptor-1 treatment with pembrolizumab in ipilimumab-refractory advanced melanoma: a randomised dose-comparison cohort of a phase 1 trial. Lancet 2014 Sep 20;384(9948):1109-1117.

[88] Wong JH, Skinner KA, Kim KA, Foshag LJ, Morton DL. The role of surgery in the treatment of nonregionally recurrent melanoma. Surgery 1993 Apr;113(4):389-394.

[89] Chua TC, Scolyer RA, Kennedy CW, Yan TD, McCaughan BC, Thompson JF. Surgical management of melanoma lung metastasis: an analysis of survival outcomes in 292 consecutive patients. Ann Surg Oncol 2012 Jun;19(6):1774-1781.

[90] Petersen RP, Hanish SI, Haney JC, Miller CC,3rd, Burfeind WR,Jr, Tyler DS, et al. Improved survival with pulmonary metastasectomy: an analysis of 1720 patients with pulmonary metastatic melanoma. J Thorac Cardiovasc Surg 2007 Jan;133(1):104-110.

[91] Andrews S, Robinson L, Cantor A, DeConti RC. Survival after surgical resection of isolated pulmonary metastases from malignant melanoma. Cancer Control 2006 Jul; 13(3):218-223.

[92] Schuhan C, Muley T, Dienemann H, Pfannschmidt J. Survival after pulmonary metastasectomy in patients with malignant melanoma. Thorac Cardiovasc Surg 2011 Apr; 59(3):158-162.

[93] Leo F, Cagini L, Rocmans P, Cappello M, Geel AN, Maggi G, et al. Lung metastases from melanoma: when is surgical treatment warranted? Br J Cancer 2000 Sep;83(5): 569-572.

[94] Neuman HB, Patel A, Hanlon C, Wolchok JD, Houghton AN, Coit DG. Stage-IV melanoma and pulmonary metastases: factors predictive of survival. Ann Surg Oncol 2007 Oct;14(10):2847-2853.

[95] Harpole DH,Jr, Johnson CM, Wolfe WG, George SL, Seigler HF. Analysis of 945 cases of pulmonary metastatic melanoma. J Thorac Cardiovasc Surg 1992 Apr;103(4):743-8; discussion 748-50.

[96] Younes R, Abrao FC, Gross J. Pulmonary metastasectomy for malignant melanoma: prognostic factors for long-term survival. Melanoma Res 2013 Aug;23(4):307-311.

[97] Pfannschmidt J, Klode J, Muley T, Dienemann H, Hoffmann H. Nodal involvement at the time of pulmonary metastasectomy: experiences in 245 patients. Ann Thorac Surg 2006 Feb;81(2):448-454.

[98] Mifsud M, Padhya TA. Metastatic melanoma to the upper aerodigestive tract: a systematic review of the literature. Laryngoscope 2014 May;124(5):1143-1149.

[99] Koyi H, Branden E. Intratracheal metastasis from malignant melanoma. J Eur Acad Dermatol Venereol 2000 Sep;14(5):407-408.

[100] Diener-West M, Reynolds SM, Agugliaro DJ, Caldwell R, Cumming K, Earle JD, et al. Development of metastatic disease after enrollment in the COMS trials for treatment of choroidal melanoma: Collaborative Ocular Melanoma Study Group Report No. 26. Arch Ophthalmol 2005 Dec;123(12):1639-1643.

[101] Kivela T, Eskelin S, Kujala E. Metastatic uveal melanoma. Int Ophthalmol Clin 2006 Winter;46(1):133-149.

[102] Leiter U, Meier F, Schittek B, Garbe C. The natural course of cutaneous melanoma. J Surg Oncol 2004 Jul 1;86(4):172-178.

[103] Mourra N, Jouret-Mourin A, Lazure T, Audard V, Albiges L, Malbois M, et al. Metastatic tumors to the colon and rectum: a multi-institutional study. Arch Pathol Lab Med 2012 Nov;136(11):1397-1401.

[104] Aoyama T, Mastrangelo MJ, Berd D, Nathan FE, Shields CL, Shields JA, et al. Protracted survival after resection of metastatic uveal melanoma. Cancer 2000 Oct 1;89(7):1561-1568.

[105] Marshall E, Romaniuk C, Ghaneh P, Wong H, McKay M, Chopra M, et al. MRI in the detection of hepatic metastases from high-risk uveal melanoma: a prospective study in 188 patients. Br J Ophthalmol 2013 Feb;97(2):159-163.

[106] Rivoire M, Kodjikian L, Baldo S, Kaemmerlen P, Negrier S, Grange JD. Treatment of liver metastases from uveal melanoma. Ann Surg Oncol 2005 Jun;12(6):422-428.

[107] Faries MB, Leung A, Morton DL, Hari D, Lee JH, Sim MS, et al. A 20-year experience of hepatic resection for melanoma: is there an expanding role? J Am Coll Surg 2014 Jul;219(1):62-68.

[108] Piperno-Neumann S, Chaaba H, Plancher C, Mariani P, Couturier J, Sastre-Garau X, et al. Retrospective analysis of 470 metastatic uveal melanoma (MUM) patients managed at Institut Curie between 2000 and 2008.. Ann Oncol 2010;211 8):(suppl 8: viii401):Abstract 3777.

[109] Aubin JM, Rekman J, Vandenbroucke-Menu F, Lapointe R, Fairfull-Smith RJ, Mimeault R, et al. Systematic review and meta-analysis of liver resection for metastatic melanoma. Br J Surg 2013 Aug;100(9):1138-1147.

[110] Adam R, Chiche L, Aloia T, Elias D, Salmon R, Rivoire M, et al. Hepatic resection for noncolorectal nonendocrine liver metastases: analysis of 1,452 patients and development of a prognostic model. Ann Surg 2006 Oct;244(4):524-535.

[111] Groeschl RT, Nachmany I, Steel JL, Reddy SK, Glazer ES, de Jong MC, et al. Hepatectomy for noncolorectal non-neuroendocrine metastatic cancer: a multi-institutional analysis. J Am Coll Surg 2012 May;214(5):769-777.

[112] Ripley RT, Davis JL, Klapper JA, Mathur A, Kammula U, Royal RE, et al. Liver resection for metastatic melanoma with postoperative tumor-infiltrating lymphocyte therapy. Ann Surg Oncol 2010 Jan;17(1):163-170.

[113] Ryu SW, Saw R, Scolyer RA, Crawford M, Thompson JF, Sandroussi C. Liver resection for metastatic melanoma: equivalent survival for cutaneous and ocular primaries. J Surg Oncol 2013 Aug;108(2):129-135.

[114] Pawlik TM, Zorzi D, Abdalla EK, Clary BM, Gershenwald JE, Ross MI, et al. Hepatic resection for metastatic melanoma: distinct patterns of recurrence and prognosis for ocular versus cutaneous disease. Ann Surg Oncol 2006 May;13(5):712-720.

[115] Chua TC, Saxena A, Morris DL. Surgical metastasectomy in AJCC stage IV M1c melanoma patients with gastrointestinal and liver metastases. Ann Acad Med Singapore 2010 Aug;39(8):634-639.

[116] Kodjikian L, Grange JD, Baldo S, Baillif S, Garweg JG, Rivoire M. Prognostic factors of liver metastases from uveal melanoma. Graefes Arch Clin Exp Ophthalmol 2005 Oct;243(10):985-993.

[117] Caralt M, Marti J, Cortes J, Fondevila C, Bilbao I, Fuster J, et al. Outcome of patients following hepatic resection for metastatic cutaneous and ocular melanoma. J Hepatobiliary Pancreat Sci 2011 Mar;18(2):268-275.

[118] Herman P, Machado MA, Montagnini AL, D'Albuquerque LA, Saad WA, Machado MC. Selected patients with metastatic melanoma may benefit from liver resection. World J Surg 2007 Jan;31(1):171-174.

[119] Kim J, Mori T, Chen SL, Amersi FF, Martinez SR, Kuo C, et al. Chemokine receptor CXCR4 expression in patients with melanoma and colorectal cancer liver metastases and the association with disease outcome. Ann Surg 2006 Jul;244(1):113-120.

[120] Wysocki WM, Komorowski AL, Darasz Z. Gastrointestinal metastases from malignant melanoma: report of a case. Surg Today 2004;34(6):542-546.

[121] Ollila DW, Essner R, Wanek LA, Morton DL. Surgical resection for melanoma metastatic to the gastrointestinal tract. Arch Surg 1996 Sep;131(9):975-9; 979-80.

[122] Tsilimparis N, Menenakos C, Rogalla P, Braumann C, Hartmann J. Malignant melanoma metastasis as a cause of small-bowel perforation. Onkologie 2009 Jun;32(6): 356-358.

[123] Patti R, Cacciatori M, Guercio G, Territo V, Di Vita G. Intestinal melanoma: A broad spectrum of clinical presentation. Int J Surg Case Rep 2012;3(8):395-398.

[124] Branum GD, Seigler HF. Role of surgical intervention in the management of intestinal metastases from malignant melanoma. Am J Surg 1991 Nov;162(5):428-431.

[125] Patel K, Ward ST, Packer T, Brown S, Marsden J, Thomson M, et al. Malignant melanoma of the gastro-intestinal tract: a case series. Int J Surg 2014;12(5):523-527.

[126] Reddy S, Edil BH, Cameron JL, Pawlik TM, Herman JM, Gilson MM, et al. Pancreatic resection of isolated metastases from nonpancreatic primary cancers. Ann Surg Oncol 2008 Nov;15(11):3199-3206.

[127] Branum GD, Epstein RE, Leight GS, Seigler HF. The role of resection in the management of melanoma metastatic to the adrenal gland. Surgery 1991 Feb;109(2):127-131.

[128] Sampson JH, Carter JH,Jr, Friedman AH, Seigler HF. Demographics, prognosis, and therapy in 702 patients with brain metastases from malignant melanoma. J Neurosurg 1998 Jan;88(1):11-20.

[129] Fife KM, Colman MH, Stevens GN, Firth IC, Moon D, Shannon KF, et al. Determinants of outcome in melanoma patients with cerebral metastases. J Clin Oncol 2004 Apr 1;22(7):1293-1300.

[130] Aoyama H, Shirato H, Tago M, Nakagawa K, Toyoda T, Hatano K, et al. Stereotactic radiosurgery plus whole-brain radiation therapy vs stereotactic radiosurgery alone for treatment of brain metastases: a randomized controlled trial. JAMA 2006 Jun 7;295(21):2483-2491.

[131] Skibber JM, Soong SJ, Austin L, Balch CM, Sawaya RE. Cranial irradiation after surgical excision of brain metastases in melanoma patients. Ann Surg Oncol 1996 Mar; 3(2):118-123.

[132] Falchook GS, Long GV, Kurzrock R, Kim KB, Arkenau TH, Brown MP, et al. Dabrafenib in patients with melanoma, untreated brain metastases, and other solid tumours: a phase 1 dose-escalation trial. Lancet 2012 May 19;379(9829):1893-1901.

[133] Margolin K, Ernstoff MS, Hamid O, Lawrence D, McDermott D, Puzanov I, et al. Ipilimumab in patients with melanoma and brain metastases: an open-label, phase 2 trial. Lancet Oncol 2012 May;13(5):459-465.

[134] Huang KY, Wang CR, Yang RS. Rare clinical experiences for surgical treatment of melanoma with osseous metastases in Taiwan. BMC Musculoskelet Disord 2007 Jul 25;8:70.

[135] Colman MW, Kirkwood JM, Schott T, Goodman MA, McGough RL,3rd. Does metastasectomy improve survival in skeletal melanoma? Melanoma Res 2014 Aug;24(4): 354-359.

[136] Stewart WR, Gelberman RH, Harrelson JM, Seigler HF. Skeletal metastases of melanoma. J Bone Joint Surg Am 1978 Jul;60(5):645-649.

[137] Donaldson WF,3rd, Peppelman WC,Jr, Yaw KM. Symptomatic metastatic malignant melanoma to the spine. J Spinal Disord 1993 Aug;6(4):360-363.

Chapter 5

Current Surgical Management of Acral Lentiginous Melanoma

Yasuhiro Nakamura, Yukiko Teramoto,
Sayuri Sato and Akifumi Yamamoto

Additional information is available at the end of the chapter

http://dx.doi.org/10.5772/59133

1. Introduction

Malignant melanoma (MM) is the most common cause of death from skin cancer in Caucasians. The incidence of MM has considerably increased in most countries in the recent decades. However, the incidence rate of melanoma demonstrates a racial difference. The incidence rates range between 20 and 40 per 100,000 people in Australia and United States each year [1, 2]. In contrast, the incidence in Asians is clearly lower, approximately one per 100,000 [3, 4]. However, the most common clinical subtype of melanoma in Asians is acral lentiginous melanoma (ALM), which occurs at a rate of approximately 40%–65% of all cutaneous melanomas [4, 5] compared with only 2%–3% in Caucasians [6]. This subtype of melanoma, first described by Reed in 1976, is characterized by its predilection for the acral regions such as the soles, palms, and nail apparatus and by a pattern of radial lentiginous growth phase that evolves over months or years without any solar elastosis to a dermal (vertical) invasive stage. This subgroup has been designated as "plantar lentiginous melanoma," which corresponds to ALM [7]. Thereafter, MM was classified into the following four subtypes by Clark et al. in 1986 according to histological features; nodular melanoma (NM), superficial spreading melanoma (SSM), lentigo maligna melanoma (LMM), and ALM [8].

The prognosis of ALM is generally considered to be poorer than other subtypes such as SMM and LMM. In particular, the lesions of the sole are often overlooked by patients. In addition, ALM has a likelihood of being misdiagnosed as a benign melanocytic nevus, which leads to the development of tumor and delay in treatment [9]. This problem has improved with the advent of dermoscopy, which enables the dermatologists to distinguish between the early stages of ALM and benign melanocytic nevus.

Acral sites such as the palms and soles are not sun-exposured areas, and therefore overexposure to ultraviolet light has not been shown to be a risk factor for the development of ALM [10]. On the other hand, ultraviolet light can play an important role in the development of LMM [11]. A recent study showed that 81% of non-chronic sun-damaged melanomas such as SSM had a high likelihood of BRAF or N-RAS mutations and the other subtypes, including ALM, had a low rate of mutation in either gene. In contrast, ALM had a frequent mutation or amplification of the KIT gene [12].

Because of the biological and unique anatomical specificity of ALM, there are some controversies in the treatment of ALM. In this chapter, we review the published articles regarding the surgical treatment of primary ALM lesions, including our paper and experiences, assess the current role of surgery, and discuss several major controversies of ALM surgical treatment.

2. Problems of excision margins in ALM

The World Health Organization Melanoma Program undertook a randomized trial and compared lateral margins of 1 and 3 cm for 612 melanoma patients with thicknesses of <2 mm [13]. Disease-free and overall survival rates did not differ between the two groups. Two subsequent trials in Europe compared the results of treating melanomas with lateral margins of 2 or 5 cm. The Scandinavian Melanoma Group Study and French Cooperative Group Trial compared lateral margins of 2 cm with 5 cm for patients with 0.8–2.0 mm-thick and <2.1 mm-thick melanomas, respectively [14, 15]. Neither study showed any evidence that lateral margins of 5 cm reduced the local recurrence rate or improved survival rates. The Intergroup Melanoma Surgical Trial also reported the results of a randomized prospective trial that compared lateral margins of 2 cm with 4 cm for 740 melanoma patients with thicknesses of 1.01–4.0 mm [16]. This trial also demonstrated that the local recurrence and survival rates were similar for the two groups. This evidence suggests that lateral margins of at least 2 cm are suitable for patients with melanoma with thicknesses of >2 mm.

Although some uncertainties remain and further trial-based evidence is required for clarification, the general consensus is that at least margins of 1 cm should be adequate for melanomas with a thickness of ≤1 mm [17]. For 1.01–2mm-thick tumors, some evidence suggests that lateral margins > 1 cm are desirable [18]. As for *in situ* lesions, a lateral margin of 5 mm is generally recommended in some national guidelines, including Japan. However, a recent prospective, comparative study demonstrated that 86% of 1120 *in situ* lesions were successfully excised with lateral margins of 6 mm and 98.9% were successful with lateral margins of 9 mm and concluded that lateral margins of 9 mm were appropriate for *in situ* lesions [19].

The appropriate depth of excision for melanoma is also still controversial. The depth of excision has been recommended to be at least to the level of muscle fascia; deeper excisions have not been shown to improve outcomes [20, 21]. On the other hand, a recent study demonstrated that there was no advantage for a resection of the deep muscular fascia but a potential for an increased risk of intralymphatic recurrences [22].

Based on the evidence described above, current major melanoma guidelines such as the National Comprehensive Cancer Network Guideline recommends adequate lateral margins alone, depending on the maximum thickness of the tumor. However, most of the available evidence has been obtained from clinical trials that included melanomas that were located mainly on the trunk or proximal extremities. Most studies and trials have not included melanomas in the head and neck region and on distal extremities, including ALMs. Acral sites are locations where more complex reconstructive procedures may be required if wider and deeper excision margins are applied. It is unclear whether the application of current recommended excision margins to the treatment of ALM that is biologically different from other subtypes is appropriate.

3. Surgical management of subungual melanoma (SUM)

SUM is a rare manifestation of MM. The incidence of SUM also has a racial difference. It represents approximately 2%–3% and 20% of all cutaneous MMs in Caucasians [23-26] and Asians [4, 27], respectively.

The anatomy of the nail apparatus is complex and is composed of the proximal nail fold, nail matrix, nail bed, and hyponychium. The proximal nail fold is continuous with the dorsal aspect of the nail matrix distally and the extensor aspect of the digital skin proximally. The cuticle separates the ventral portion of the proximal nail fold from the underlying nail plate. The nail plate is the horny end product of the nail matrix. The hyponychium is the distal portion of the nail bed, which represents the site of union between the nail bed and tip of the digits [28].

3.1. Invasive SUM

In the surgical treatment of SUM, amputation has been traditionally performed [29]. Comparative studies of various amputation levels have not shown any advantages for metacarpal amputations over metacarpophalangeal (MP), proximal interphalangeal (PIP), or distal interphalangeal (DIP) amputations [30]; this means that the prognosis of SUM does not depend on the amputation level but on the clinical stage [31]. Therefore, the recent trend of surgery is to utilize more distal amputations, without compromising recurrence or survival [25, 26]. In particular, in the thumb, a more distal amputation is preferable (Fig. 1). Although amputation at the interphalangeal joint of the thumb results in only a 10% loss of function of a useful hand, amputation at the MP joint of the thumb results in a 40% loss of function [32]. In contrast, from the viewpoint of the functional and cosmetic aspects, ray amputation may be more appropriate than MP, PIP, or DIP amputation for the treatment of the other fingers (Fig. 2).

3.2. *In situ* or minimally-invasive SUM

Recently, several authors have proposed conservative surgery, which involves a narrow surgical margin without amputation followed by skin grafting for *in situ* SUM and minimally-invasive SUM (Fig. 3), which is defined as a Breslow tumor thickness (TT) ≤0.5 mm [33-38]. There have also been a few case reports of two-step surgeries using artificial dermis tissue for the tentative coverage of the defect after local excision, followed by skin graft coverage after

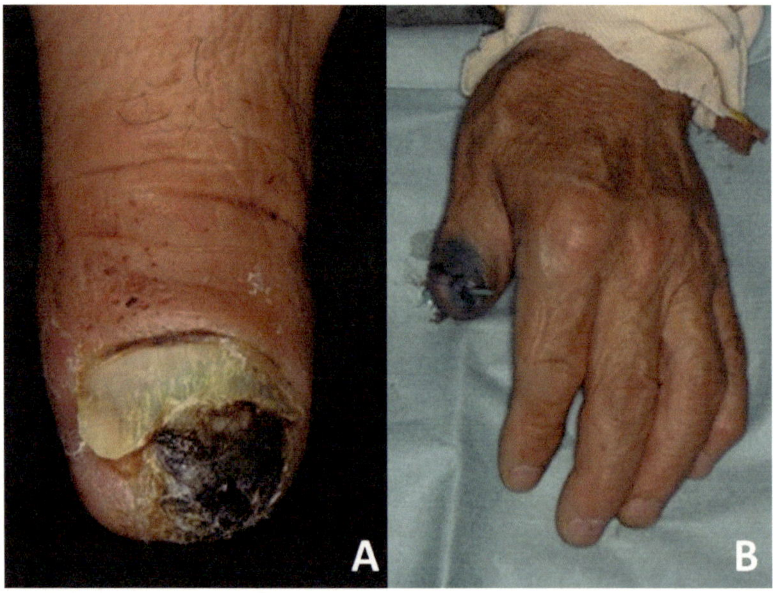

Figure 1. Minimal amputation of subungual melanoma of the thumb for avoidance of functional loss. (A) Subungual melanoma on the left thumb. (B) Amputation at the interphalangeal joint.

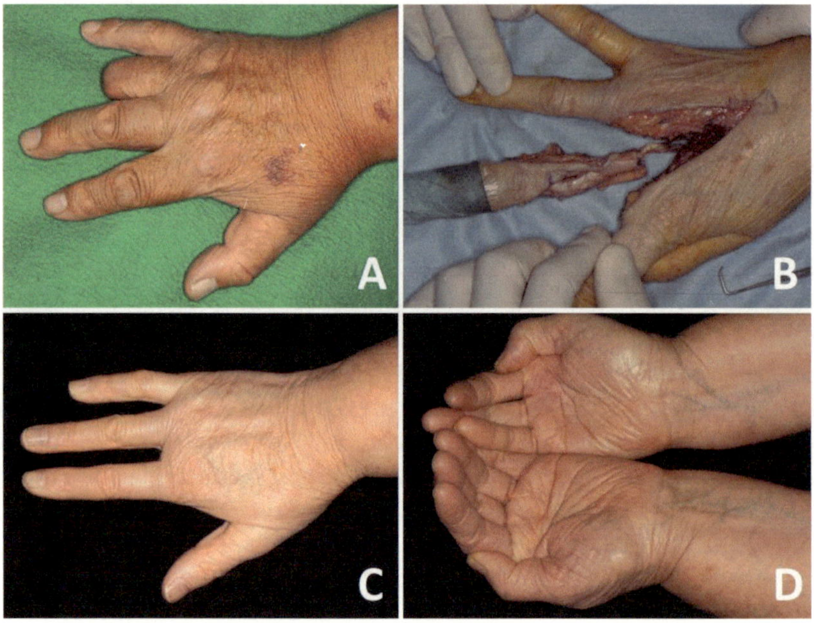

Figure 2. Cosmetic and functional advantages of ray amputation for the treatment of SUM of the finger. (A) Conspicuous amputated stump of a case of subungual melanoma on the fourth finger after proximal interphalangeal amputation. (B) A case of ray amputation for melanoma of the third fingernail. (C) Inconspicuous cosmetic result with no stump after ray amputation. (D) Hand position to "scoop up water."

the histopathological confirmation of negative surgical margins [39, 40]. These strategies are becoming more common, although the total number of such surgeries still remains small.

3.3. Possibility of conservative surgery for invasive SUM

The unique anatomy of the nail apparatus described above also demonstrates that there is scant soft tissue between the nail unit and bony surface of the distal phalanx. Haneke [41] studied the distance from the tip of the nail matrix to the extensor tendon insertion of the middle finger of a young male, and the measured distance was 0.8 mm. Kim et al. [42] also studied the shortest distances between the deepest base of the nail matrix and surface of the distal phalanx in cadavers. The mean distances were 0.90 mm for thumbs, 0.72 mm for fifth fingers, 0.87 mm for first toes, and 1.09 mm for fifth toes. The mean distance of all digits was 0.90 mm. These studies have suggested that wide local excision was insufficient for the eradication of invasive SUM with a safe, deep surgical margin and appeared to be sufficient for only *in situ* or minimally-invasive SUM.

Dermatologists sometimes encounter patients with invasive SUMs that do not invade or attach to the distal phalanx. Therefore, we measured the shortest distances of 30 surgical specimens of invasive SUM between the deepest base of the tumor and the surface of the distal phalanx [43]. There were no bone invasion cases with 4 mm-thick SUMs and the shortest tumor-to-bone distances exceeded 0.9 mm in all specimens with thicknesses of <4 mm (Fig. 4). In statistical analysis, the Pearson chi-square test showed that there was a higher likelihood of bone attachment or invasion when TT exceeded 4 mm, which was statistically significant (P=0.009). Both univariate and multivariate analyses also revealed that thick TT alone had a statistically significant effect [odds ratio 1.807 and 1.865 (95% CI 1.1085–3.008 and 1.111–3.13, P=0.023 and 0.018)]. This study only focused on the histologic evaluation of deep margins and has limitations including the lack of prognostic information; however, there have also been several reports of patients with >0.5-mm-thick SUMs who underwent non-amputative surgeries and who had no local recurrence or metastasis [36, 40, 44].

These studies indicate that the patients with invasive SUMs of intermediate thicknesses may be candidates for non-amputative surgery. However, the main problem is that it is still difficult to evaluate tumor thickness by inspection or dermoscopy preoperatively. There is a possibility of the presence of an unexpectedly thicker area in the tumor than the thickness identified from an incisional biopsy, which can consequently change the surgical strategy. High-resolution ultrasound is a noninvasive examination that can evaluate tumor thickness preoperatively, and there have been several studies that reported its accuracy for the determination of tumor thickness [45-47]. However, these studies excluded SUM; therefore, its accuracy for tumor thickness evaluation in SUM remains unclear. Furthermore, an ultrasound at 20 MHz tends to overestimate thickness because of lymphocytic infiltration around the tumor or nevus remnant [48, 49]. Reflectance confocal microscopy permits the acquisition of dynamic images of the epidermis and papillary dermis with resolution to a cellular level [50] and has been experimentally used for intraoperative imaging of the nail matrix [51]. However, its limitation is the imaging depth, which cannot be deeper than 200–300 μm [50].

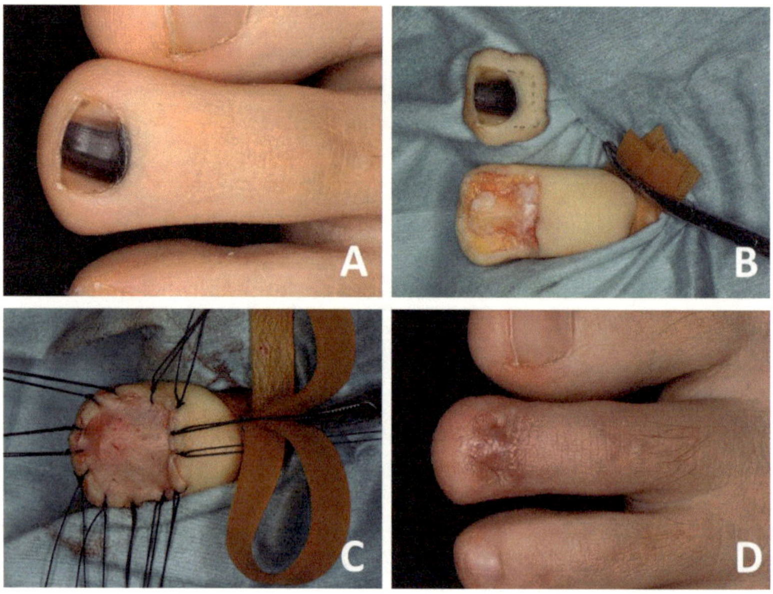

Figure 3. Non-amputative wide local excision followed by skin grafting for *in situ* subngual melanoma. (A) *In situ* subungual melanoma on the left second toe. (B) Nail apparatus excision including the periosteum of the distal phalanx. (C) Defect coverage by skin grafting. (D) Postoperative findings 8 months after surgery.

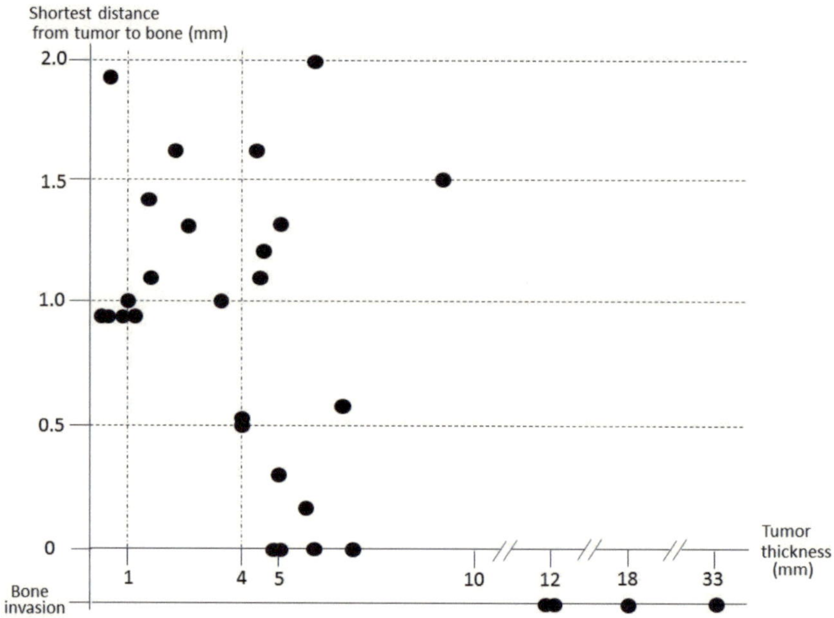

Figure 4. The relationship between shortest distance from tumor to bone and tumor thickness of invasive SUM.

http://dx.doi.org/10.5772/59133

For other surgical procedures, Chow et al. has reported on wide local excision procedures involving the removal of the nail apparatus with a layer of underlying bone of 1-mm depth running parallel to the nail bed before reconstruction with skin grafting [32]. Moehrle et al. reported on the excision of SUM with the distal part of the distal phalanx (processus unguinatus), which has led to its denotation as a "functional" surgery [52].

4. Surgical management of ALM on the volar skin

In general, ALMs start as *in situ* lesions, with brown macules that enlarge slowly and form irregularly pigmented, asymmetric macular lesions over the years, corresponding to the radial growth phase. Thereafter, indurated nodules appear within the macular lesions and sometimes the nodules ulcerate in the so-called vertical growth phase.

4.1. Problems of excision margins

Because of this very slow clinical course, ALMs on the volar skin often contain *in situ* lesions at the periphery (Fig. 5). Based on the recommended lateral margins described above, the dermatological surgeons are often confused regarding the decision for lateral margins. It is still unclear whether lateral margins of 0.5–1 cm from the peripheral border of the lesion should be suitable as the peripheral lesion is considered an *in situ* lesion, or lateral margins of 2 cm from the periphery of the lesion should be selected as the entire tumor itself is regarded as an invasive lesion.

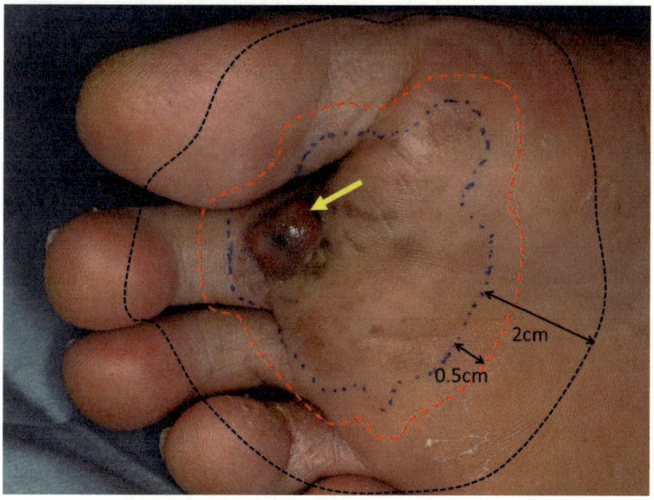

Figure 5. Confusion regarding excision margin for acral lentiginous melanoma which has *in situ* lesion. The arrow indicates the invasive lesion. Blue dotted line indicates the peripheral border of the in situ lesion. Red and black dotted lines indicate lateral margins of 0.5 cm and 2 cm from the border of the lesion, respectively.

4.2. ALM of the palm

In general, most ALMs on the palm are diagnosed at an early stage because the palm is the site where the patient easily notices the lesion at an earlier stage. Therefore, wide local excision is easily accomplished and the full-or split-thickness skin graft is adequate for the coverage of the surgical defect. The main point that the surgeon should pay attention to is avoiding intraoperative injuries of the palmar digital nerves, which are easily exposed during tumor excision because of the scant subcutaneous fatty tissue in some areas of the palm (Fig. 6). As for skin grafting, the skin obtained from non-weight-bearing areas of the foot is preferable because of the similarity to the quality of the palmar skin; however, the skin quality difference between the palmar skin and the skin obtained from other areas may be inconspicuous in elderly patients (Fig. 6).

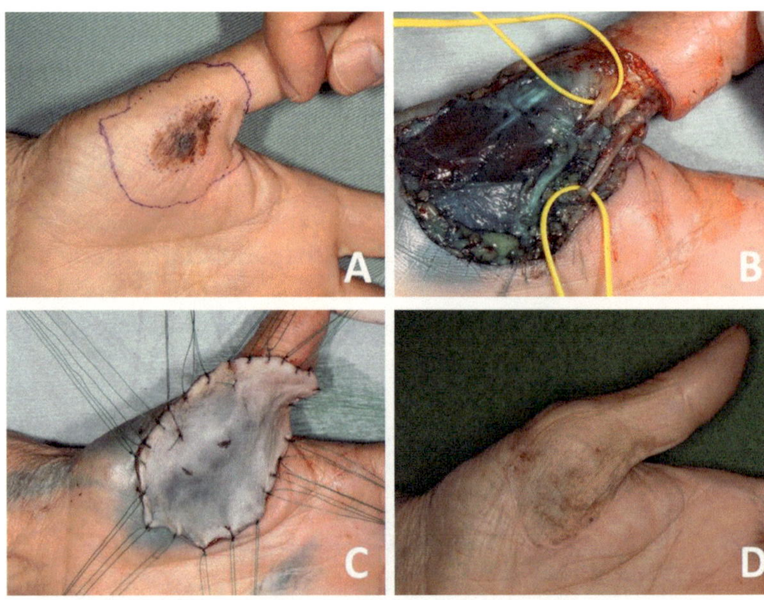

Figure 6. Surgery for the acral lentiginous melanoma on the palm. (A) The purple line indicates a lateral margin of 1 cm from the border of the lesion. (B) After wide local excision. The palmar digital nerves are safely preserved (taped by yellow vessel loops). (C) Defect coverage by full-thickness skin grafting taken from the inguinal area. (D) Postoperative findings 24 months after surgery.

4.3. ALM of the sole

ALM of the sole has been traditionally difficult to find and diagnose because of its "out-of sight" location. The lesion often precludes primary closure because of the lack of mobility of the skin on the sole and horizontal-growth of the tumor, which increases the reconstructive complexity. Therefore, after wide local excision, substantial defects have to be repaired using various methods such as skin grafting, local and distant flaps, and secondary intention healing depending on the size and site of the defect and the medical condition and lifestyle of the patient [53]. Unlike the palm of the hands, reconstruction of the sole of the foot is difficult because of its anatomy. The sole has weight-bearing areas such as the heel. In addition, a defect on the foot may result in insufficient vascular flow [54].

4.3.1. Split-thickness or full-thickness skin graft

Although split-thickness skin grafting is considered to be adequate for non-weight-bearing areas, it has been considered to be inappropriate for the heel and distal plantar area and could lead to dismal results [55]. If the surgical defect is located on the non-weight-bearing areas such as the foot and distal plantar area, or if the patient has severe medical comorbidities or is less active, the defect may be covered by split-or full-thickness skin grafting. Although skin grafting has advantages such as being much simpler than flap reconstruction, it is considered that defects of the weight-bearing areas should be repaired using local or distant flaps in ambulatory patients.

By authors' experience, the indication for skin grafting on the heel depends on the amount of the remaining subcutaneous fat pad after tumor excision. If the primary tumor is a thinner lesion and there is no need to excise the enormous subcutaneous fat pad together with the tumor, both split-or full-thickness skin grafts may be acceptable for weight-bearing reconstruction (Fig. 7A). In contrast, neither split-nor full-thickness skin grafting is appropriate when wide local excision including the subcutaneous fat beneath the tumor is required for oncologic purposes, which may lead to exposure of the calcaneum. Insufficient cushion because of the paucity of the fat pad eventually produces an erosion or ulceration of the skin graft (Fig. 7B).

As for the distal plantar area, the weight pressure on this area is not as great as on the heel. Therefore, we think that skin grafting for this area is more acceptable than that for the heel. Even through a large amount of the subcutaneous fat may be dissected with the tumor, full-thickness skin grafting may be durable for weight pressure over a long-term postoperative course (Fig. 7C). When there is remaining subcutaneous fat, reconstruction using the split-thickness skin grafting is also acceptable (Fig. 7D).

Skin grafts are generally taken from the contralateral limb because the melanoma cells were thought to primarily metastasize via lymphatic routes [56]. In contrast, a recent study has shown that there was no difference in the rates of donor site recurrence between the ipsilateral and contralateral limbs [57].

4.3.2. Local or distant flaps

A flap reconstruction is usually recommended for the closure of weight-bearing areas of the feet. The coverage of weight-bearing areas provides well-padded tissue superior to skin grafting. Among the various flaps, the medial plantar flap is the optimal reconstructive procedure. The plantar flap can provide the same quality of skin cover for weight-bearing areas and can also provide some sensation. In particular, using heel reconstruction, the donor site is located distally and away from the lymphatics of the primary site (Fig. 8).

The distally-based sural artery neurocutaneous flap is an optional procedure for heel reconstruction. Because the donor site is the posterior aspect of the lower leg, the quality of the skin is different from that of the sole. A comparative study between the medial plantar flap and distally-based sural artery flap demonstrated that the postoperative complications were higher in patients who underwent sural artery neurocutaneous flap procedures [58].

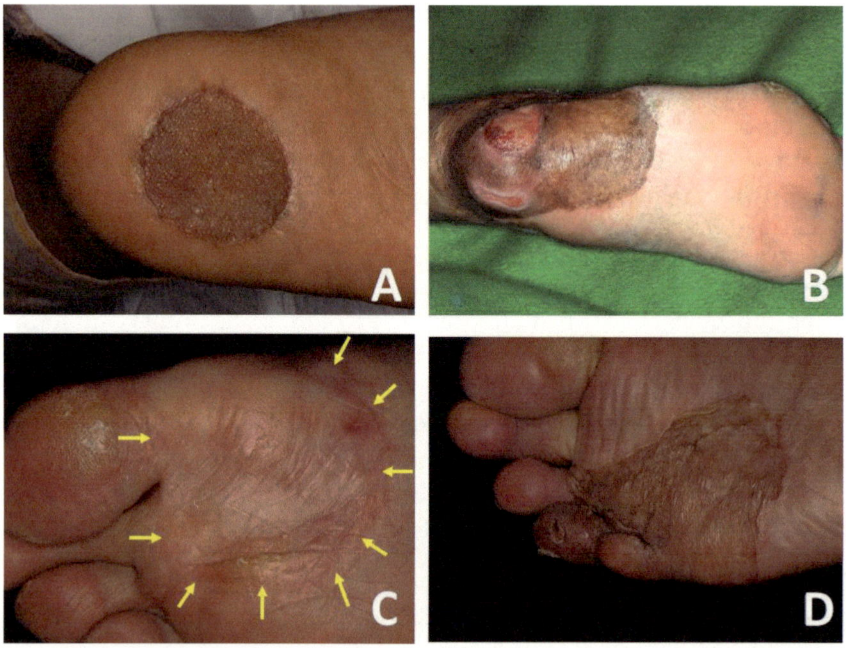

Figure 7. Skin grafting on the weight-bearing areas after excision of acral lentiginous melanoma. (A) Split-thickness skin grafting on the remaining subcutaneous fat pad of the heel. (B) Split-thickness skin grafting on the heel after excision of the tumor with a large amount of subcutaneous fat pad. The ulceration is visible on the skin graft. (C) Full-thickness skin grafting (arrows) on the plantar aponeurosis, 10 years after surgery. (D) Split-thickness skin grafting on the remaining subcutaneous fat, 2 years after surgery.

4.3.3. Secondary intention healing

Secondary intention healing requires a long-term healing period, prolonged care such as regular and frequent dressing changes, and careful observation. According to previous reports, it took approximately 12–18 weeks to close the defects (mean defect size: 32.6–36.5 cm^2) [54, 59]. Despite these drawbacks, it has the advantages of avoiding a secondary wound for tissue harvesting, a smaller scar because of the natural contraction of the wound, and granulation tissue that acts as a cushion to absorb impact while walking [54]. Recently, the effect of negative pressure wound therapy in addition to secondary intention healing has been investigated [59]. Compared with secondary intention healing alone, there was no difference in time to complete wound healing. However, the vascularity score and height of the scars was significantly better, and no wound infections during the course of treatment had occurred in the former group.

These methods clearly require a more extended period of healing time than skin grafting or flaps. Therefore, it would be appropriate to apply these methods to small-to medium-sized surgical defects.

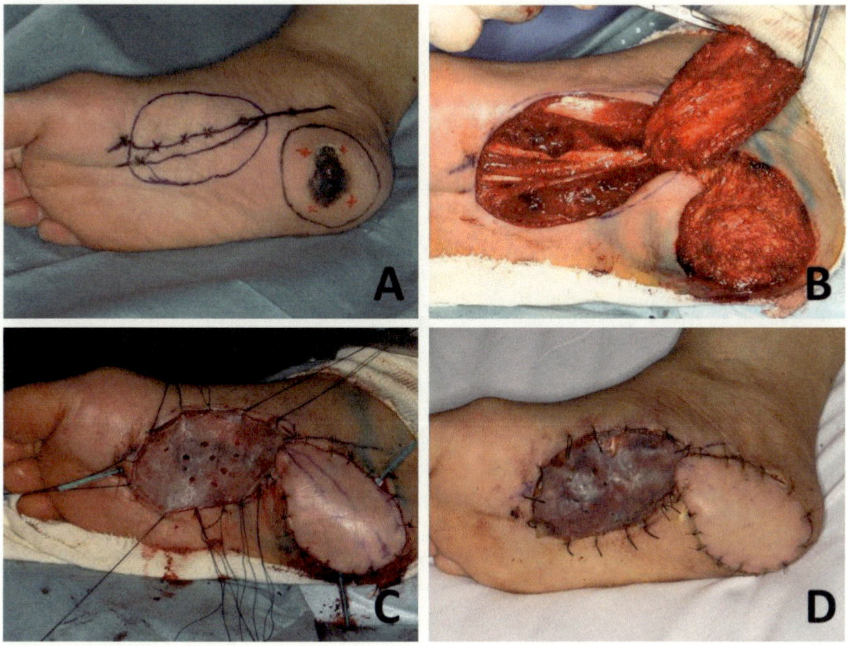

Figure 8. Reconstructive surgery of the acral lentiginous melanoma on the heel using medial plantar flap. (A) The flap design and excision margin of the tumor on the heel. (B) Elevation of the medial plantar flap. (C) Defect coverage by flap and the coverage of the donor site by skin grafting. (D) Postoperative findings 9 days after surgery.

5. Conclusions

Increased understanding of the molecular biology and pathogenesis of melanoma may lead to the development of novel therapeutic agents and treatment plans for melanoma. However, surgery is still the mainstay of treatment as there are no proven effective adjuvant systemic treatments.

Although several reliable national guidelines for melanoma have been produced using the evidence-based method, there are still some controversies in the treatment of ALM. Because of the biological and unique anatomical specificity of ALM, It is still unclear whether the thickness of ALM and recommended lateral margins are the same as that with other subtypes. Large randomized prospective studies with long-term follow up are necessary to fully evaluate surgery for ALM in the future. The accumulation of evidence produced by such studies will lead to the development of novel ALM treatments in the melanoma guidelines.

Acknowledgements

This work was partly supported by the National Cancer Center Research and Development Fund (26-A-4).

Author details

Yasuhiro Nakamura*, Yukiko Teramoto, Sayuri Sato and Akifumi Yamamoto

*Address all correspondence to: ynakamur@saitama-med.ac.jp

Department of Skin Oncology/Dermatology, Comprehensive Cancer Center, Saitama Medical University International Medical Center, Saitama, Japan

References

[1] Parkin D. M., Bray F., Ferlay J. & Pisani P. (2005). Global cancer statistics, 2002. *CA Cancer J Clin*, 55, 74-108.

[2] Sneyd M. & Cox B. (2006). The control of melanoma in New Zealand. *N Z Med J*, 119, U2169.

[3] Makredes M., Hui S. K. & Kimball A. B. (2010). Melanoma in Hong Kong between 1983 and 2002: a decreasing trend in incidence observed in a complex socio-political and economic setting. *Melanoma Res*, 20, 427-430.

[4] Ishihara K., Saida T., Otsuka F. & Yamazaki N. (2008). Statistical profiles of malignant melanoma and other skin cancers in Japan: 2007 update. *Int J Clin Oncol*, 13, 33-41.

[5] Roh M. R., Kim J. & Chung K. Y. (2010). Treatment and outcomes of melanoma in acral location in Korean patients. *Yonsei Med J*, 51, 562-568.

[6] Markovic S. N., Erickson L. A., Rao R. D., Weenig R. H., Pockaj B. A., Bardia A., Vachon C. M., Schild S. E., McWilliams R. R., Hand J. L., Laman S. D., Kottschade L. A., Maples W. J., Pittelkow M. R., Pulido J. S., Cameron J. D. & Creagan E. T. (2007). Malignant melanoma in the 21st century, part 1: epidemiology, risk factors, screening, prevention, and diagnosis. *Mayo Clin Proc*, 82, 364-380.

[7] Arrington J. H., 3rd, Reed R. J., Ichinose H. & Krementz E. T. (1977). Plantar lentiginous melanoma: a distinctive variant of human cutaneous malignant melanoma. *Am J Surg Pathol*, 1, 131-143.

[8] Clark W. H., Jr., Elder D. E. & Van Horn M. (1986). The biologic forms of malignant melanoma. *Hum Pathol*, 17, 443-450.

[9] Metzger S., Ellwanger U., Stroebel W., Schiebel U., Rassner G. & Fierlbeck G. (1998). Extent and consequences of physician delay in the diagnosis of acral melanoma. *Melanoma Res*, 8, 181-186.

[10] Phan A., Touzet S., Dalle S., Ronger-Savle S., Balme B. & Thomas L. (2006). Acral lentiginous melanoma: a clinicoprognostic study of 126 cases. *Br J Dermatol*, 155, 561-569.

[11] Newell G. R., Sider J. G., Bergfelt L. & Kripke M. L. (1988). Incidence of cutaneous melanoma in the United States by histology with special reference to the face. *Cancer Res*, 48, 5036-5041.

[12] Curtin J. A., Fridlyand J., Kageshita T., Patel H. N., Busam K. J., Kutzner H., Cho K. H., Aiba S., Brocker E. B., LeBoit P. E., Pinkel D. & Bastian B. C. (2005). Distinct sets of genetic alterations in melanoma. *N Engl J Med*, 353, 2135-2147.

[13] Veronesi U., Cascinelli N., Adamus J., Balch C., Bandiera D., Barchuk A., Bufalino R., Craig P., De Marsillac J., Durand J. C. & et al. (1988). Thin stage I primary cutaneous malignant melanoma. Comparison of excision with margins of 1 or 3 cm. *N Engl J Med*, 318, 1159-1162.

[14] Cohn-Cedermark G., Rutqvist L. E., Andersson R., Breivald M., Ingvar C., Johansson H., Jonsson P. E., Krysander L., Lindholm C. & Ringborg U. (2000). Long term results of a randomized study by the Swedish Melanoma Study Group on 2-cm versus 5-cm resection margins for patients with cutaneous melanoma with a tumor thickness of 0.8-2.0 mm. *Cancer*, 89, 1495-1501.

[15] Khayat D., Rixe O., Martin G., Soubrane C., Banzet M., Bazex J. A., Lauret P., Verola O., Auclerc G., Harper P. & Banzet P. (2003). Surgical margins in cutaneous melanoma (2 cm versus 5 cm for lesions measuring less than 2.1-mm thick). *Cancer*, 97, 1941-1946.

[16] Balch C. M., Soong S. J., Smith T., Ross M. I., Urist M. M., Karakousis C. P., Temple W. J., Mihm M. C., Barnhill R. L., Jewell W. R., Wanebo H. J. & Desmond R. (2001). Long-term results of a prospective surgical trial comparing 2 cm vs. 4 cm excision margins for 740 patients with 1-4 mm melanomas. *Ann Surg Oncol*, 8, 101-108.

[17] Karakousis C. P. (1996). Surgical treatment of malignant melanoma. *Surg Clin North Am*, 76, 1299-1312.

[18] McKinnon J. G., Starritt E. C., Scolyer R. A., McCarthy W. H. & Thompson J. F. (2005). Histopathologic excision margin affects local recurrence rate: analysis of 2681 patients with melanomas < or=2 mm thick. *Ann Surg*, 241, 326-333.

[19] Kunishige J. H., Brodland D. G. & Zitelli J. A. (2012). Surgical margins for melanoma in situ. *J Am Acad Dermatol*, 66, 438-444.

[20] Kenady D. E., Brown B. W. & McBride C. M. (1982). Excision of underlying fascia with a primary malignant melanoma: effect on recurrence and survival rates. *Surgery*, 92, 615-618.

[21] Holmstrom H. (1992). Surgical management of primary melanoma. *Semin Surg Oncol*, 8, 366-369.

[22] Grotz T. E., Glorioso J. M., Pockaj B. A., Harmsen W. S. & Jakub J. W. (2013). Preservation of the deep muscular fascia and locoregional control in melanoma. *Surgery*, 153, 535-541.

[23] Dawber R. P. & Colver G. B. (1991). The spectrum of malignant melanoma of the nail apparatus. *Semin Dermatol*, 10, 82-87.

[24] Blessing K., Kernohan N. M. & Park K. G. (1991). Subungual malignant melanoma: clinicopathological features of 100 cases. *Histopathology*, 19, 425-429.

[25] Finley R. K., 3rd, Driscoll D. L., Blumenson L. E. & Karakousis C. P. (1994). Subungual melanoma: an eighteen-year review. *Surgery*, 116, 96-100.

[26] Banfield C. C., Redburn J. C. & Dawber R. P. (1998). The incidence and prognosis of nail apparatus melanoma. A retrospective study of 105 patients in four English regions. *Br J Dermatol*, 139, 276-279.

[27] Takematsu H., Obata M., Tomita Y., Kato T., Takahashi M. & Abe R. (1985). Subungual melanoma. A clinicopathologic study of 16 Japanese cases. *Cancer*, 55, 2725-2731.

[28] Tan K. B., Moncrieff M., Thompson J. F., McCarthy S. W., Shaw H. M., Quinn M. J., Li L. X., Crotty K. A., Stretch J. R. & Scolyer R. A. (2007). Subungual melanoma: a study of 124 cases highlighting features of early lesions, potential pitfalls in diagnosis, and guidelines for histologic reporting. *Am J Surg Pathol*, 31, 1902-1912.

[29] Daly J. M., Berlin R. & Urmacher C. (1987). Subungual melanoma: a 25-year review of cases. *J Surg Oncol*, 35, 107-112.

[30] Haneke E. (2012). Ungual melanoma-controversies in diagnosis and treatment. *Dermatol Ther*, 25, 510-524.

[31] O'Leary J. A., Berend K. R., Johnson J. L., Levin L. S. & Seigler H. F. (2000). Subungual melanoma. A review of 93 cases with identification of prognostic variables. *Clin Orthop Relat Res*, 206-212.

[32] Chow W. T., Bhat W., Magdub S. & Orlando A. (2013). In situ subungual melanoma: digit salvaging clearance. *J Plast Reconstr Aesthet Surg*, 66, 274-276.

[33] Clarkson J. H., McAllister R. M., Cliff S. H. & Powell B. (2002). Subungual melanoma in situ: two independent streaks in one nail bed. *Br J Plast Surg*, 55, 165-167.

[34] Lazar A., Abimelec P. & Dumontier C. (2005). Full thickness skin graft for nail unit reconstruction. *J Hand Surg Br*, 30, 194-198.

[35] High W. A., Quirey R. A., Guillen D. R., Munoz G. & Taylor R. S. (2004). Presentation, histopathologic findings, and clinical outcomes in 7 cases of melanoma in situ of the nail unit. *Arch Dermatol*, 140, 1102-1106.

[36] Cohen T., Busam K. J., Patel A. & Brady M. S. (2008). Subungual melanoma: management considerations. *Am J Surg*, 195, 244-248.

[37] Imakado S., Sato H. & Hamada K. (2008). Two cases of subungual melanoma in situ. *J Dermatol*, 35, 754-758.

[38] Sureda N., Phan A., Poulalhon N., Balme B., Dalle S. & Thomas L. (2011). Conservative surgical management of subungual (matrix derived) melanoma: report of seven cases and literature review. *Br J Dermatol*, 165, 852-858.

[39] Hayashi K., Uhara H., Koga H., Okuyama R. & Saida T. (2012). Surgical treatment of nail apparatus melanoma in situ: the use of artificial dermis in reconstruction. *Dermatol Surg*, 38, 692-694.

[40] Smock E. D., Barabas A. G. & Geh J. L. (2010). Reconstruction of a thumb defect with Integra following wide local excision of a subungual melanoma. *J Plast Reconstr Aesthet Surg*, 63, e36-37.

[41] Haneke E. (2006). Surgical anatomy of the nail apparatus. *Dermatol Clin*, 24, 291-296.

[42] Kim J. Y., Jung H. J., Lee W. J., Kim do W., Yoon G. S., Kim D. S., Park M. J. & Lee S. J. (2011). Is the distance enough to eradicate in situ or early invasive subungual melanoma by wide local excision? from the point of view of matrix-to-bone distance for safe inferior surgical margin in Koreans. *Dermatology*, 223, 122-123.

[43] Nakamura Y., Fujisawa Y., Teramoto Y, Sato S, Yamada K, Sekine K, Fujimoto M, Otsuka F & Yamamoto A. (2014) Tumor-to-bone distance of invasive subungual melanoma: an analysis of 30 cases. *J Dermatol*, 41, 872-877.

[44] Rayatt S. S., Dancey A. L. & Davison P. M. (2007). Thumb subungual melanoma: is amputation necessary? *J Plast Reconstr Aesthet Surg*, 60, 635-638.

[45] Machet L., Belot V., Naouri M., Boka M., Mourtada Y., Giraudeau B., Laure B., Perrinaud A., Machet M. C. & Vaillant L. (2009). Preoperative measurement of thickness of cutaneous melanoma using high-resolution 20 MHz ultrasound imaging: A monocenter prospective study and systematic review of the literature. *Ultrasound Med Biol*, 35, 1411-1420.

[46] Gambichler T., Moussa G., Bahrenberg K., Vogt M., Ermert H., Weyhe D., Altmeyer P. & Hoffmann K. (2007). Preoperative ultrasonic assessment of thin melanocytic skin lesions using a 100-MHz ultrasound transducer: a comparative study. *Dermatol Surg*, 33, 818-824.

[47] Guitera P., Li L. X., Crotty K., Fitzgerald P., Mellenbergh R., Pellacani G. & Menzies S. W. (2008). Melanoma histological Breslow thickness predicted by 75-MHz ultrasonography. *Br J Dermatol*, 159, 364-369.

[48] Serrone L., Solivetti F. M., Thorel M. F., Eibenschutz L., Donati P. & Catricala C. (2002). High frequency ultrasound in the preoperative staging of primary melanoma: a statistical analysis. *Melanoma Res*, 12, 287-290.

[49] Pellacani G. & Seidenari S. (2003). Preoperative melanoma thickness determination by 20-MHz sonography and digital videomicroscopy in combination. *Arch Dermatol*, 139, 293-298.

[50] Calzavara-Pinton P., Longo C., Venturini M., Sala R. & Pellacani G. (2008). Reflectance confocal microscopy for in vivo skin imaging. *Photochem Photobiol*, 84, 1421-1430.

[51] Debarbieux S., Hospod V., Depaepe L., Balme B., Poulalhon N. & Thomas L. (2012). Perioperative confocal microscopy of the nail matrix in the management of in situ or minimally invasive subungual melanomas. *Br J Dermatol*, 167, 828-836.

[52] Moehrle M., Metzger S., Schippert W., Garbe C., Rassner G. & Breuninger H. (2003). "Functional" surgery in subungual melanoma. *Dermatol Surg*, 29, 366-374.

[53] Shapiro R. L. (2002). Surgical approaches to malignant melanoma. Practical guidelines. *Dermatol Clin*, 20, 681-699, ix.

[54] Jung J. Y., Roh H. J., Lee S. H., Nam K. & Chung K. Y. (2011). Comparison of secondary intention healing and full-thickness skin graft after excision of acral lentiginous melanoma on foot. *Dermatol Surg*, 37, 1245-1251.

[55] Evans G. R., Friedman J., Shenaq J. & Mosser S. (1997). Plantar flap reconstruction for acral lentiginous melanoma. *Ann Surg Oncol*, 4, 575-578.

[56] Roberts D. L., Anstey A. V., Barlow R. J., Cox N. H., Newton Bishop J. A., Corrie P. G., Evans J., Gore M. E., Hall P. N. & Kirkham N. (2002). U.K. guidelines for the management of cutaneous melanoma. *Br J Dermatol*, 146, 7-17.

[57] Schumacher H. H., Chia H. L. & Simcock J. W. (2010). Ipsilateral skin grafts for lower limb melanoma reconstruction are safe. *Plast Reconstr Surg*, 125, 89e-91e.

[58] Rashid M., Hussain S. S., Aslam R. & Illahi I. (2003). A comparison of two fasciocutaneous flaps in the reconstruction of defects of the weight-bearing heel. *J Coll Physicians Surg Pak*, 13, 216-218.

[59] Oh B. H., Lee S. H., Nam K. A., Lee H. B. & Chung K. Y. (2013). Comparison of negative pressure wound therapy and secondary intention healing after excision of acral lentiginous melanoma on the foot. Br J Dermatol, 168, 333-338.

Chapter 6

Changing Perceptions of Lymphadenectomy and Sentinel Lymph Node Biopsy in Melanoma

Antonio Sommariva, Camilla Cona and
Carlo Riccardo Rossi

Additional information is available at the end of the chapter

http://dx.doi.org/10.5772/59195

1. Introduction

Lymph nodes (LN) represent the most frequent site of metastases for melanoma and the main purpose of lymphadenectomy (LND) is to provide loco-regional control of disease and accurate staging as well as to eventually cure patients with AJCC stage III melanoma. Currently, lymph node involvement is mostly diagnosed after sentinel lymph node biopsy (SLNB). However, although SLNB in melanoma patients at risk for lymph node metastasis is routinely performed almost everywhere, the role of completion lymphadenectomy (CLND) after positive SLNB remains controversial, as only 15-20% of the patients operated show additional lymph node metastases in the dissected basin. The MSLT-1 trial, which evaluated the impact of SLNB and immediate LND versus simple observation and LND after clinical evidence of metastases only, did not show any survival benefit between the two randomized groups of patients [1]. Moreover, other studies have shown that some of the patients with positive sentinel nodes seem at lower risk for additional lymph node metastasis, and will probably never develop additional non sentinel lymph node metastases. On the other hand, the final analysis of the MSLT-1 trial confirmed a longer disease free survival and a gain in survival only in the patients with positive nodes in the CLND group.

Until the results of the two ongoing prospective studies (MSLT-2 and MINITUB) investigating the role of CLND after SLNB positivity are available, radical lymphadenectomy should be considered the standard of care in patients with lymph node metastases, as suggested by the NCCN guidelines, which recommend lymphadenectomy in presence of positivity of SLNB or histological/cytological confirmed clinical lymph node metastases [2].

Despite this recommendation, adherence to clinical practice guidelines remains low among melanoma surgeons. In the USA, 50% of patients with positive SLNB do not undergo completion lymphadenectomy [3]. The still evident degree of confusion on the optimal surgical treatment of AJCC stage III melanoma has been confirmed by a recent international survey on lymphadenectomy in melanoma patients with positive sentinel nodes (SN), which showed an extremely heterogeneous approach to the extent of the completion lymph node dissection (CLND), especially for SN located in the neck or groin [4]. Aside from the indication and the levels of dissection, no agreement has yet been reached on the criteria to define lymphadenectomy as adequate and, even if the minimum number of lymph nodes that should be excised achieves a reasonable consensus, other quality assurance (QA) parameters for lymphadenectomy are far from being accepted.

In this context, a consensus process on indications, technical aspects and QA parameters for SLNB and, in particular, for lymphadenectomy is desirable among melanoma surgeons and pathologists. Providing new evidence-based results in these controversial fields might help to achieve better standards of treatment. The purpose of this chapter is to critically review the most recent literature on the lymph node surgical treatment in melanoma patients providing, wherever available, new evidence and contributing to standardize the current management of this tumor.

2. State of the art on SLNB and lymphadenectomy

2.1. Rationale for indication

Cutaneous melanoma presents an increasing annual incidence worldwide and despite several advances in understanding the molecular mechanism of tumour progression and the development of more selective therapeutic strategies, a significant proportion of patients remain incurable. Lymph nodes represent the most frequent site of metastases from melanoma and the main purposes of lymphadenectomy are to provide loco-regional control of disease, accurate staging as well as to eventually cure patients with AJCC stage III melanoma. A significant number of patients with localized melanoma harbor clinical occult metastases in the regional node basin, which, if left untreated, will lead to palpable metastatic nodes (macroscopic disease). In the past, the common approach to lymph node in melanoma patients ranged between two different strategies; observation followed by therapeutic lymph node dissection (TLND) when clinical disease became evident and elective lymph node dissection (ELND) at the time of treatment of the primary in absence of macroscopic disease. However, removing lymph node metastases before they become evident is potentially a better strategy to prevent local failure and could potentially prevent systemic failure in a significant portion of patients. The drawback of ELND is that 15 to 20% of patients only have microscopic disease in the regional lymph nodes; therefore, the majority of patients will have no benefit from elective surgery and will receive surgical overtreatment. Four randomized controlled trials (RCT) [5] and one meta-analysis [6] have compared these two treatment strategies with, none demonstrating a survival advantage. The negative result in survival of ELND can be explained by the fact that more than 80% of patients in these trials will never develop lymph nodes metastases, making the studies underpowered to discover a statistical difference between the two groups. However, subgroup analysis from the WHO Melanoma Group Trial [7] showed a significant survival advantage in patients with clinically occult disease who underwent ELND compared to patients who underwent TLND for positive nodal recurrence (5-years survival 48.2 versus 26.6, P=0.04 respectively). These data suggest that there may be an improved survival in patients with occult disease, highlighting the importance of identification of early nodal disease. The difficulty in showing a survival advantage after ELND, unnecessary in 80% of patients and frequently associated with a high morbidity rate (including wound complications, lymphedema and pain), has made it, over the years, unappealing.

The controversy on performing ELND disappeared with the advent of SLNB, which determined a consistent paradigm shift in melanoma patients at risk of lymph node metastasis. After the pioneering studies of Donald Morton, who first hypothesized the role of sentinel lymph node as the first lymph node receiving lymphatic drainage from the primary tumour, SLNB emerged as a minimal invasive staging procedure for determining the nodal status in patients with melanoma [8]. The intra-operative use of a combined technique based on blue dye and radiotracer has been demonstrated to be feasible and accurate for nodal staging of patients with melanoma [9]. A recent meta-analysis of 71 studies, which includes 25240 melanoma patients who underwent SLNB in the period 1998-2009, showed that SLNB is highly accurate in melanoma with a proportion of patients successfully mapped (a least one sentinel lymph node removed) of 98.1%, a rate which tends to increase with the year of publication and quality score of the studies, female sex, ulceration and age [10]. The same study reported a false negative rate of SLNB of 12.5% (i.e. the proportion of patients with nodal recurrence in un-dissected nodal basins after a negative SLNB over the total positive patients and the false negative patients), which is inversely associated with the proportion of patients successfully mapped. The ability of SLNB to predict the negative status of the lymph node basin is expressed by the post-test probability negative (PTPN, the ratio of patients with negative SNB who recurred to all patients with negative SLNB). The PTNB in this study is 3.4%, which represents the proportion of patients with negative SLNB who recur. This risk seems inversely related to the proportion of patients successfully mapped and positively associated with the length of follow-up, younger patient age, the proportion of females, the mean Breslow thickness and the proportion of ulcerated tumours. The overall data analysis showed that, after a negative SLNB, the chances of nodal recurrence can be estimated to be equal to or lower than 5% providing reassurance that SLNB is a feasible and reliable method for accurately predicting the lymph node status of melanoma patients and is now considered a reliable staging procedure for melanoma.

SLNB status has been identified as the most important prognostic factor for overall survival in melanoma patients with no clinical evidence of metastatic disease [11] and has been included in the AJCC TNM staging system since the 6th edition in 2001 [12]. For this reason, a general consensus on performing SLNB in patients with intermediate thickness melanomas (Breslow 1-4mm)) [13] has been reached, as SLNB gives important prognostic information that can be used for planning follow-up protocols and adjuvant treatments [14]. Although the use of SLNB in thick melanomas remains uncertain, the procedure is recommended in this sub-group of patients mainly for staging purposes and local control of disease [14]. For thin melanoma (≤1mm), the role of SLNB is more controversial. It is known that the risk of node positivity in thin melanoma patients is less than 5%, but we should consider that this group accounts for the majority of patients with melanoma (about 65%) and therefore a large number of patients with microscopic disease might be left under staged and possibly undertreated. A sufficient level of evidence exists to also consider SLNB in patients with thin melanoma, particularly in presence of ulceration and/or mitotic rate ≥1 (AJCC T1b melanomas) [15]. Several studies have investigated the optimal cut-off value to consider SLNB cost-effective in thin melanomas. In patients with Breslow ≤0.50 mm, SLNB positivity is very unlikely, with a reported incidence of positive nodes of 0% [16]. Between 0.51 and 0.99 mm, the risk tends to increase and in a subgroup of patients with thin melanoma of at least 0.76 mm in depth and 1 or more mitosis, a 12.5% incidence of SN metastases has been reported [17].

It has been calculated that only 50-60% of patients with positive SLNB underwent CLND in USA [3] and Europe [18]. This proportion is probably higher among surgeons normally dealing with melanoma, as reported by a recent survey [4]. In this study, mainly involving surgeons working in melanoma or surgical oncology units, 91.8% of responders recommend CLND in patients with positive SLNB. However, the role of CLND in the presence of positive SLNB, remains uncertain. The Multicenter Selective Lymphadenectomy (MSTL-1) trial was started in 1994 and evaluated over 8 years the outcome of 2001 patients with primary cutaneous melanoma randomly assigned to undergo wide excision and nodal observation (observation group) or wide excision and SLNB, with immediate lymphadenectomy in presence of nodal metastases detected on biopsy (biopsy group). The prognostic value of SLNB was overall confirmed in patients with intermediate-thickness (1.2 to 3.5 mm) melanoma; 10-years Melanoma-Specific survival was 85.1±1.5 in negative SLNB and 62.1± 4.8 in positive SLNB [1]. Moreover, the MSLT-1 confirms that, among other established prognostic factors (Breslow thickness and ulceration), SLNB status is the most powerful indicator for disease recurrence (HR=2.64) and death from melanoma (HR=2.40). Considering survival analysis of patients with intermediate-thickness melanomas, a better 10-year disease free survival was detected in the biopsy group (71.3±1.8% versus 64.7±2.3%, HR for recurrence and metastasis=0.76, P=0.01), even though no difference was detected in the 10-year melanoma-specific survival among the two arms (81.4±1.5 and 78.3±2.0%, P=0.18). Even if no impact on overall survival has been observed in the biopsy group, at this level of evidence the present data suggest performing CLND for all patients with positive SLNB, mainly for achieving better regional control [2, 14]. Furthermore, a complete LND with therapeutical intent is recommended in presence of clinically evident, cyto/histologically proven lymph node metastasis.

2.2. Surgical techniques

SLNB involves preoperative lymphoscintigraphy, obtained through the injection of human albumin nanocolloid labelled with technetium 99mTc. The injection is in the intradermal layer, close to the scar of the removed melanoma or to the tumor if still present, and followed by scintigraphic scans (early and late) in the likely locations of lymphatic drainage [9]. Once the

http://dx.doi.org/10.5772/59195

basin and location of the sentinel node has been identified, cutaneous projection area of each single node is marked on the skin. Immediately prior to surgery, the primary site is further injected intradermally with 0.5 to 1 mL of a vital dye (patent Blu), to increase the sensitivity of the method and to facilitate the finding of the lymph node (figure 1). SLNB is performed through a small skin incision, which should take into consideration the incision necessary for a subsequent radical lymphadenectomy [14]. Under the guidance of a radioisotope probe and following the blue lymphatic channels, the sentinel lymph node(s) is identified and removed (figure 1). Care should be taken not to disrupt or cauterize the lymph node capsule. Each SLN removed is checked ex vivo for radioactivity and the nodal basin is rescanned. Drains are seldom required and most patients are operated in one day-surgery regimen. The incidence of post-operative complications is relatively low, mainly related to wound (dehiscence/ infection or lymphatic collection), although limb lymphedema occurs not so un-frequently as generally supposed [19].

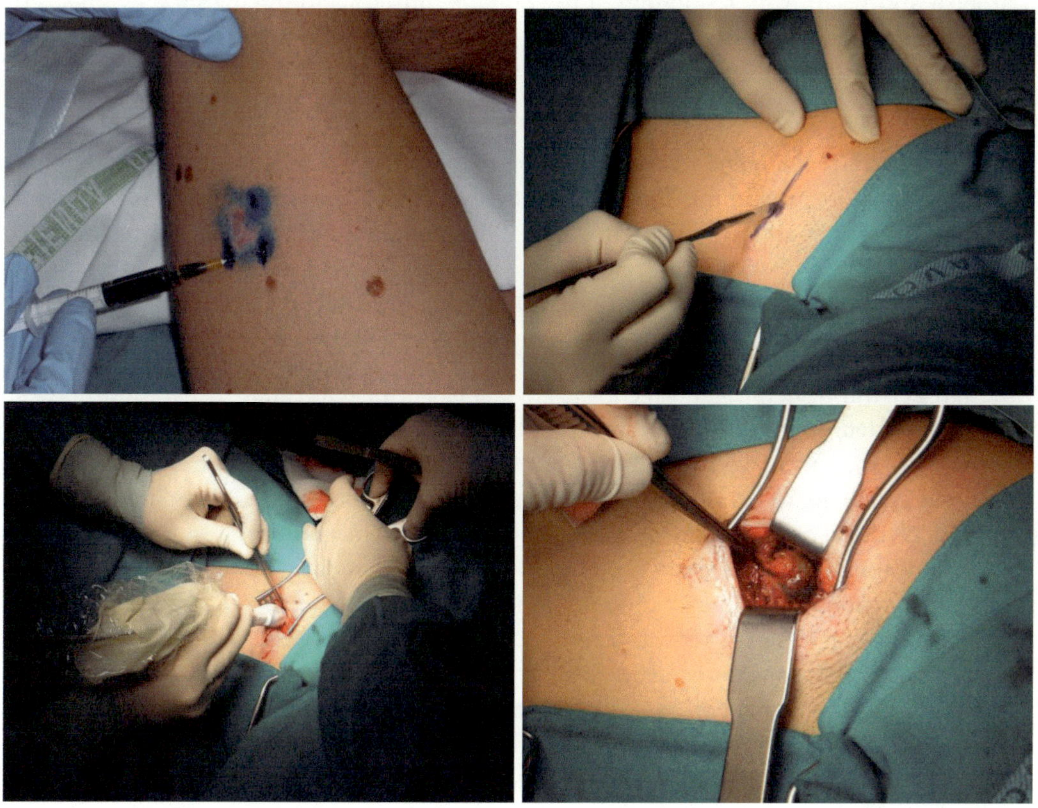

Figure 1. Surgical technique of SLNB

Radical lymphadenectomy for melanoma involves the "en bloc" excision of lymph nodes with surrounding fat tissue. In the axilla, a radical lymphadenectomy should include dissection of levels I, II and III lymph nodes around the axillary vein [20]. A section of the pectoralis minor muscle is suggested by some for a better access to level II lymph nodes or in presence of bulky level II and III nodes. Long thoracic and thoracodorsal nerves should be preserved and sectioned only if directly involved by the tumor. In case of metastasis to the inguinal lymph nodes, the standard approach involves the removal of the inguinal, external iliac and obturator lymph nodes [21]. In the classic description of inguinal dissection, a longitudinal or lazy-S-shaped skin incision is employed, extending a few centimeters cranially to the superior anterior iliac spine up to the apex of the femoral triangle (figure 2). The incision should include the SLNB scar. The cutaneous flaps are created medially and laterally, up to the pubic tubercle, the anterior margin of the gracilis and abductor muscles and up to the superior anterior iliac spine and Sartorius muscle, respectively. Deep dissection continues through the fascia lata, over the underlining muscles and femoral vessels. The saphena magna vein is generally sectioned at the apex of the femoral triangle and at the level of the saphenofemoral junction. In case of the risk of femoral vessel exposition after wound dehiscence, transposition of the sartorious muscle is warranted. Iliac and obturatory dissection is obtained through an extra-peritoneal approach. After sectioning of the oblique muscles and the inguinal ligament, the pelvic area is reached and the external iliac and obturatory lymph nodes removed, after identification of the urether and the obturator nerve.

For cervical lymph node metastastis, clear indications on the thoroughness of dissection are lacking and all the recommendations are supported by a low level of evidence and are obtained from opinions of experts in this field [22]. In case of clinically evident cervical lymph node metastasis, surgery is aimed at the removal of all five levels of lymph nodes (submandibular, jugular and supraclavicular), preserving sternocleidomastoid muscle, internal giugular vein and accessory spinal nerve (figure 3). Removal of the superficial part of the parotid is recommended only if clinically involved, because of the high risk of nerve damage observed.

Although general principles and technical details to perform adequate SLNB and LND are diffusely reported, surgeons in the clinical setting find many controversial aspects, regarding, in particular, the extent of given lymphadenectomy [22]. The question on what can be considered an adequate lymphadenectomy for metastatic melanoma is therefore largely unanswered. National guidelines are vague in defining this issue and simply suggest describing the anatomical limits of dissection [2]. This level of indeterminateness affects the attitude of melanoma surgeons in performing lymph node dissection [4]. A general agreement emerges in the presence of clinical evident lymph node metastatic disease, where a full regional lymphadenectomy is considered by most surgeons. More controversial is the thoroughness of lymphadenectomy in SLNB positive patients, in which, due to the significant risk, the approach is heterogeneous and controversial. For neck dissection, considering the risk of nerve damage as well as for the anatomic complexity, a consensus seems to emerge on performing CLND selectively and to remove the levels likely to be involved, depending on the site of the primary tumour, the site of the sentinel node and the lymphatic drainage highlighted at lymphoscintigraphy. Meanwhile, a superficial parotidectomy is associated only in presence of clinically evident metastasis [22]. For axilla, a general agreement exists on performing, in all cases, a three level dissection as the risk of lymphedema seems not affected by a more extensive lymphadenectomy. In fact, despite the risk of metastases of the third level is quite low [23],

http://dx.doi.org/10.5772/59195

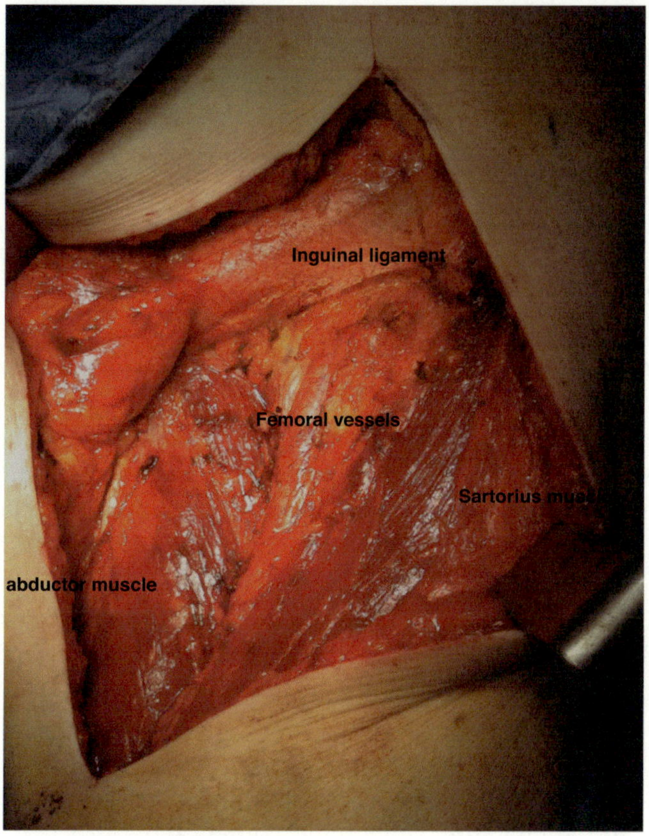

Figure 2. Intraoperative view of inguinal LND.

surgical management of recurrent disease in the apex of axilla appears more difficult. More controversial is the approach to the groin, in particular for CLND after a positive SLNB, where two distinct lymphatic basin (inguinal and pelvic) are involved. Several national guidelines suggest combining pelvic dissection out of the inguinal, only in presence of radiological evidence of pelvic metastases, >3 positive inguinal nodes and metastases to the Cloquet's lymph node (so called sentinel lymph node of the pelvis). However, the evidence is low to sustain this surgical approach and a randomized controlled trial from the Australian and New Zealand Melanoma Trial Group comparing inguinal and pelvic CLND in SLNB-positive patients with negative PET/CT pelvic scan is about to start (EAGLE FM Study, ClinicalTrials.gov Identifier, NCT02166788) [24].

3. New evidence-based results

Referring to the most recent literature on SLNB and LND in melanoma patients, new evidence-based results are now available which can contribute to answer to (and find consensus on) the three main questions still pending: 1) How can we make surgeons more confident with indications to SLNB and Lymphadenectomy (in SN positive patients)? 2) How can we get them convinced that completeness of lymphadenectomy is an important issue?, and 3) are new, more convincing, evidence-based referral values for the minimum number of lymph node to be excised now available?

3.1. Indication to lymphadenectomy in SLNB positive patients

The role of completion lymphadenectomy (CLND) after positive SLNB remains uncertain as additional non sentinel nodes (i.e. identified within lymph node dissection after SLNB) have been identified in 9 to 25% of patients. This rate is probably underestimated because, unlike the pathologic protocols normally applied for SLNB specimens, those for therapeutic lymphadenectomy are routinely limited to bisecting lymph nodes without any immunohistochemical stains. Aimed at investigating the prognostic and therapeutic impact of CLND in sentinel positive nodes two prospective trials have been undertaken: The Multicenter Selective Lymphadenectomy Trial-2 (MSTL-2) and the MiniTub trial. The MSTL-2 trial randomized patients with at least one positive SLN to observation or CLND. MSTL-2, whose patient accrual was completed in 2014, was designed to verify the incidence of nodal recurrence after removal of positive SLN(s) without CLND, the incidence and predictors of additional lymph nodes in the SLNB basin after CLND and the survival impact of CLND in SLNB positive patients. The MiniTub trial is a prospective registry investigating the outcome of patients with a T2-T3 primary melanoma and minimal SN tumour burden treated with CLND or nodal observation. While waiting for the results of these important studies, other important scientific reports have recently appeared in the literature, supporting the indication for CLND. For instance, the strength of the indication for CLND in these patients has been recently increased by the long-term results of the MSLT-1 trial [1, 25] Despite the lack of survival benefit of performing SLNB in the whole group, in a sub-group analysis, which excluded the SLNB negative patients, the node positive patients with intermediate thickness melanoma showed a 21% higher 10-year survival compared to patients who underwent lymphadenectomy for metastases discovered during follow-up. Of note is that the mean number of tumour involved nodes was significantly lower in the biopsy group with respect to the observation group (1.4 versus 3.3, P>0.001) [25]. The therapeutic effect of immediate CLND over lymphadenectomy at the time of clinically evident disease in patients with microscopic disease is confirmed by an interesting study which shows that immediate CLND is associated with a 10-year survival of 60% compared to delayed lymphadenectomy (around 45%), despite patients with early lymphadenectomy presenting worse adverse prognostic factors [26]. Moreover, a meta-analysis of non randomized studies encompassing 2633 patients, demonstrates, in patients with clinically undetectable lymph node metastasis, a 20% survival benefit after with SLNB followed by CLND [27].

Another argument in favour of the appropriateness of CLND comes from the important observation that patients with <11excised nodes were not adequately staged [28]. Furthermore, in case of sentinel node positivity, non sentinel lymph node status has an independent prognostic value in melanoma patients. The value of this observation is re-inforced by a meta-analysis suggesting the use of this new and easily reproducible prognostic factor as risk stratification criteria for clinical trials investigating adjuvant therapies and its inclusion in the future edition of the AJCC staging system [29]. Thus, not performing CLND in a SL positive patient today means lack of knowledge about his staging work-up, depriving him of important clinical information.

Taken together, all this information strongly supports that an early diagnosis of lymph node metastases (SLNB) and the removal of the affected lymphatic basin (CLND) can more effectively cure melanoma patients. Likely, some immunological events within the SL environment precede melanoma sentinel spread, suggesting that melanoma is preparing the sentinel lymph nodes to receive metastatic melanoma cells [30]. Removing SLNs and non sentinel LNs at an early stage, when probably the loco-regional immunosuppressive changes are not fully active, could explain in part the different prognostic impact of sentinel and non sentinel metastatic lymph node and opens the door to future investigations on the mechanisms of tumor response and on the immunological role of sentinel lymph nodes in melanoma.

3.2. Adequacy of lymphadenectomy and quality control

Although the extent of each LND is still argued, it has recently been demonstrated in melanoma patients that the so-called lymph node ratio (i.e. the number of positive lymph nodes over the total number of excised lymph nodes) is associated with survival [31-33]. Patients with low ratio present better prognosis independently of the number of the positive nodes, indirectly confirming the prognostic value of the number of lymph node removed during surgery. Moreover, a recent multicentric Italian study showed, in the largest caseload so far available, that patients who had a higher number of excised lymph nodes after lymphadenectomy have a better prognosis, independently of AJCC T stage, ulceration, LN tumor burden and N stage [28] (figure 3). A clear and univocal explanation of this data is not available. The association between the number of lymph nodes and prognosis can find different explanations; 1) more lymph nodes means a better immunological control of melanoma, 2) a more accurate patient staging of patients 3) a therapeutic role of more extensive surgery. The latter lends support to the hypothesis that a thorough lymphadenectomy might have a therapeutic effect in melanoma patients with lymph node metastases, in particular in those who underwent CLND for a positive SLNB with intermediate thickness primary tumour.

Once the need of a CLND in melanoma patients with lymph node metastases is accepted and the anatomical extent of a given procedure is established, how can we provide surgeons with parameters and referral values for QA? Unfortunately, shared parameters for QA of lymph node dissections for melanoma are still lacking, with the exception of the minimum number of retrieved lymph nodes, for which a general consensus seems to exist for its simplicity, reproducibility and comparability [4]. However, the benchmark values of this quality parameter (minimum number of lymph nodes for each dissected field) and the method to obtain these benchmark values are still matter of study. The minimum number values proposed in the literature are quite heterogeneous, reflecting the different method adopted for proposing it (table 1).

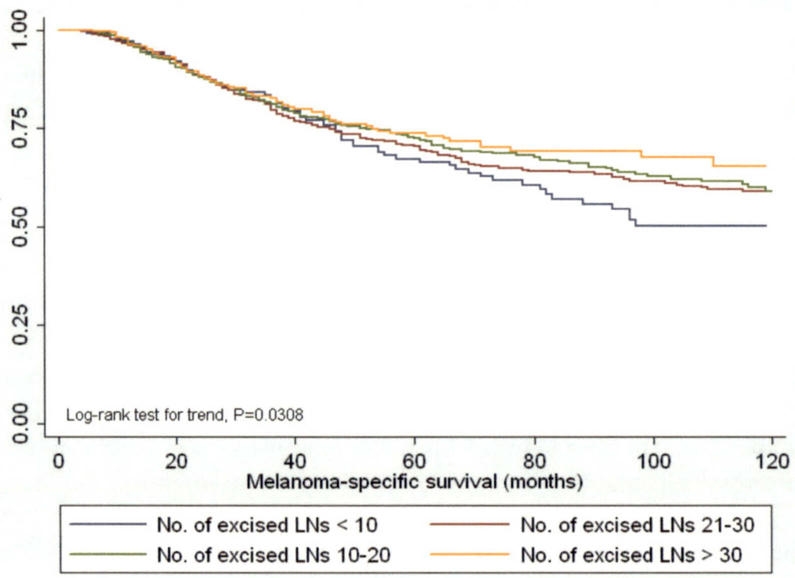

Figure 3. Patient survival according to the number of excised lymph nodes categorized as follow: ≤ 10 LNs, 11-20 LNs, 21-30 LNs and > 30 LNs. From IMI (Italian Melanoma Intergroup) caseload.

Reference	Method	Axilla	Neck ≤3 levels	Neck ≥4 levels	Groin Inguinal	Groin Inguinal and pelvic
			Minimum number of excised lymph nodes			
Balch et al. [34]	Expert opinion	10	20	20	5	5
MSLT-2 [1]	Expert opinion	15	30		6	6
Eggermont et al [35]	Expert opinion	10	15	15	5	5
Galliot-Repkat et al. [36]	Survival analysis	10	10	10	10	10
Xing et al. [33]	Survival analysis	8	15		6	6
Billimoira et al. [37]	Expert opinion	10	15	15	5	5
Spillane et al. [38, 39]	10th percentile	10	6	20	7	14
Rossi et al. [40]	10th percentile	12	7	14	6	13
Rossi et al. [28]	Survival analysis	11	14		9	12

Table 1. Minimum number values of excised lymph node for single lymphatic basin.

The most recently proposed cut-offs to deem a lymph-node dissection adequate are evidence-based (obtained by the 10th percentile/survival method) and come from two independent

http://dx.doi.org/10.5772/59195

caseloads: one from Australia [38, 39] and the other from Italy [28, 40]. As reported in table 1, the results are similar and should prompt surgeons (and pathologists) to adopt them as referral standards to measure their own performance, making a through revision of the procedure necessary when the reported numbers are below these thresholds. Another interesting evidence-based observation in this field comes from an already cited study which, besides a correlation between the absolute number of excised lymph nodes and survival, shows that, an adequate sub-staging of AJCC stage III melanoma patients is not possible below the cut-offs reported in the table [28] (figure 4).

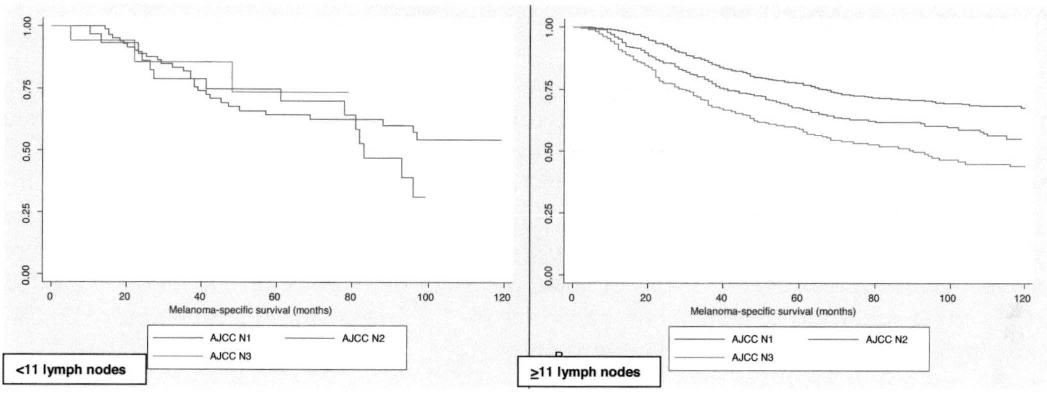

Figure 4. Loss of prognostic significance of AJCC TNM N substages according to the number of lymph nodes (< or > 11). From IMI (Italian Melanoma Intergroup) caseload.

The implementation of QA programs at institutional/multi-institutional levels needs to define other parameters for monitoring quality and the relative benchmark values. Beyond the minimum number of lymph nodes, complication rates and local recurrence rates have been suggested as QA parameters for lymphadenectomy in a recent national consensus [22]. In the near future, standardization and implementation of effective QA programs for major surgical procedures in melanoma should increase patients' standard of care as well as the likelihood of reliable results from clinical trials testing new treatments in the adjuvant setting.

4. Perspectives

4.1. Improving patient selection for SLNB and CLND

Almost 80% of patients who undergo SLNB do not harbor node metastases. Having no benefit from the procedure, they are considered to receive a surgical over-treatment. Moreover, SLNB represents a surgical procedure associated with a defined morbidity rate (10%) [41] and significant cost for the health care system [42]. For these reasons, a series of clinical pathological variables associated with SLN status has been widely studied in the literature, but the statistical predictive power of each single factor on SLNB positivity remains poorly defined (table 2).

Breslow thickness
Ulceration
Mitotic rate
Lymphovascular invasion
Clarke level IV
Young age

Table 2. Factors associated with risk of metastases in sentinel nodes

The development of statistical predictive models which analyse independent variables seems able to spare an unnecessary SLNB in between 18 to 30% of cases with an estimated error rate (i.e. patient with sentinel negative prediction even if they are sentinel positive at pathological examination) of 0.5-2.1% [43]. However, these tools need to be tested and validated in prospective studies and eventually implemented in the clinical setting. On the other hand, new markers of biologic behaviour can overcome and define the metastatic phenotype in primary melanoma and quantify the true risk of nodal metastases, but additional studies are needed to identify a subgroup of patients (in particular for thin melanomas) with defined clinical-pathological parameters at risk of SL positivity.

Identification of clinical and pathological parameters predictive of non sentinel nodes positivity represents a crucial point to improve selection of patient candidates for CLND, as it is possible to spare un-necessary CLND in a defined quota of patients [44]. Several predictors of additional non-sentinel positive LNs have been identified, including those associated with primary tumor (i.e., melanoma thickness) or sentinel nodes (i.e. metastatic burden) [45, 46]. For instance, in patients with thin melanoma, the risk of additional lymph nodes in CLND is calculated 0.1% suggesting that the potential benefit of lymph node dissection after SLNB in this group should be balanced with the morbidity of CLND [47]. Histo-pathological parameters reflecting the pattern and amount of melanoma involvement in the SNs and the related risk-assessment systems able to predict the risk of additional non sentinel lymph node metastases in CLND are reported (table 3).

As well as for predictors of SL positivity, these parameters need to be validated prospectively, and the ongoing research on new biological markers might predict the pathological status of the additional nodes, even more precisely in the near future.

4.2. Lowering the false negative rate of SLNB

The false negative rate (FNR) of SLNB probably represents the most important drawback for this procedure. The values reported in literature are wide ranging between 8.6 and 21% [10]. The main reason for this variability resides in the different methods to calculate this proportion after SLNB. In the past, many authors have erroneously considered the FNR as the ratio between the FN cases and the truly negative plus the truly positive instead the of truly positive

http://dx.doi.org/10.5772/59195

Systems	Parameters
Rotterdam system [48]	dimension of tumour deposit
Starz classification [49]	tumor penetrative depth
Hannover Scoring System (Hannover-II) [50]	dimension of the greatest deposit, tumor penetrative depth involvement of the capsula
Non-Sentinel Node Risk Score (N-SNORE) [51]	sex regression, proportion of harvested SNs maximum size perinodal lymphatic invasion
Rotterdam-Dewar Combined criteria (RDC) [52]	dimension of tumour deposit microanatomic location

Table 3. Risk assessment systems of Non-SLN involvement

plus false negative and, only recently, a standard definition has been adopted [53]. However, a recent meta-analysis shows a FNR of 12.5% [10]. This means that considering melanoma patients harbouring node metastases, approximately one out of ten of these patients has a negative SLNB. Furthermore, FNR tends to increase with the duration of follow-up and the quality of the study and is inversely correlated with the identification rate. Reasons for FNR after SLNB can involve different specialists at different steps of the SLNB procedure; lymphoschintigraphy evaluation (nuclear medicine physician), lymph node detection during surgery (surgeon) and node's pathological examination (pathologist) [54]. The number of peri-tumoral injection seems to influence the outcome of lymphoscintigraphy but controlled studies are needed to confirm the real impact on FNR [9]. Failure in lymphoscintigraphy interpretation has been demonstrated to lead to in one third of false negative results after SLNB [54]. One third of cases, a FN result is explained by the failure of surgery to remove all the nodes identified at pre-operative lymphoscintigraphy, especially in neck and groin lymphatic basin. It should be noted that the ratio of marked on lymphoscintigraphy and excised sentinel lymph nodes is equal in only 38% of patients who underwent SLNB and that 20% of patients have fewer lymph nodes removed then those marked during lymphoscintigraphy [55]. FNR after SLNB seems higher in head and neck melanomas, confirming a greater complexity of SLNB in this body district, mainly for the proximity of primary tumor and lymphatic basin, the complexity of lymphatic drainage of neck and the higher risk of complications [56]. Moreover, a lack of standardization exists between centres on the threshold beyond which radioactivity of residual lymph nodes should indicate their excision. The 10 % rule (i.e., SN defined as all the lymph nodes with >10% radioactivity of the hottest SN removed) was proposed as standardization criteria and it was demonstrated to be able to reduce the rate of missing positive nodes, but a clear consensus on this is still lacking and further research is needed in this field [57, 58].

Pathologists can also contribute to FNR. In fact, the most appropriate pathologic protocol for SN examinations is still a matter of discussion. The number of sections to be stained and the optimal distance between them can significantly influence the metastases detection in SNs.

Two main protocols have been popularized which seems to reach an acceptable compromise between diagnostic accuracy and costs [59, 60]. Although some evidence suggests that ultra-staging with polymerase chain reaction (PCR) of SNs represents an appealing prognostic tool and seems to improve melanoma cell detection in SNs, the clinical and prognostic value of molecular biology-based detection of melanoma cells in SNs needs to be further verified and supported by additional investigation in this field [61]

4.3. Videoscopic approach to lymphadenectomy

Fear of complication often influences surgeons' and patients' decision on whether or not to perform a lymphadenectomy in melanoma patients. Thus, to reduce morbidity is an important issue for surgical oncologists and for this purpose video-assisted surgery has recently been proposed for lymph node dissection. Considering the principal lymphatic basins, groin is indubitably associated with the greater incidence of wound complications. Wound infection, dehiscence/necrosis and seroma/lymphocele after traditional lymphadenectomy ranges between 15-55, 7-53 and 2-46%, respectively [62]. Videoscopic lymphadenectomy (VL) of the groin appears to be a promising tool in lowering the incidence of wound complication. Inguinal and iliac-obturator VL consists of two different surgical times. The inguinal part is performed using three trocars, placed at a variable distance from the apex of the femoral triangle (figure 5).

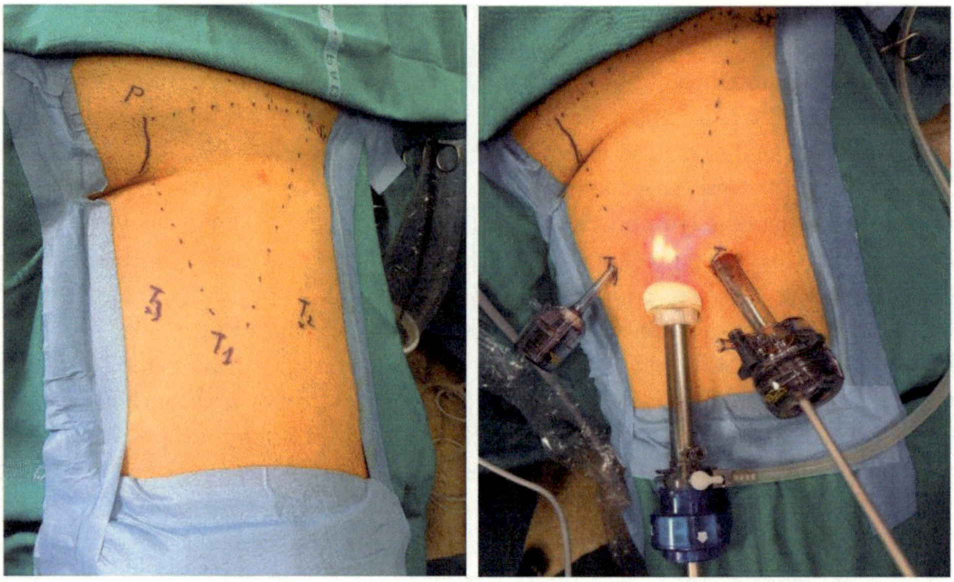

Figure 5. Trocar position for inguinal lymphadenectomy VL.

The working space is obtained after a skin incision and blunt dissection of the area under the Camper fascia. The creation of a working space using high pressure CO_2 levels (25 mm/Hg) at the beginning of the procedure make dissection easier. The saphenous vein is generally sectioned with endostaplers or endoclips. Removal of the surgical specimen is performed using endobag.

For iliac and obturator VL (figure 6), the access is extraperitoneal with the first trocar being placed infraumbilical and two trocars between the umbilicus and the pubic symphysis.

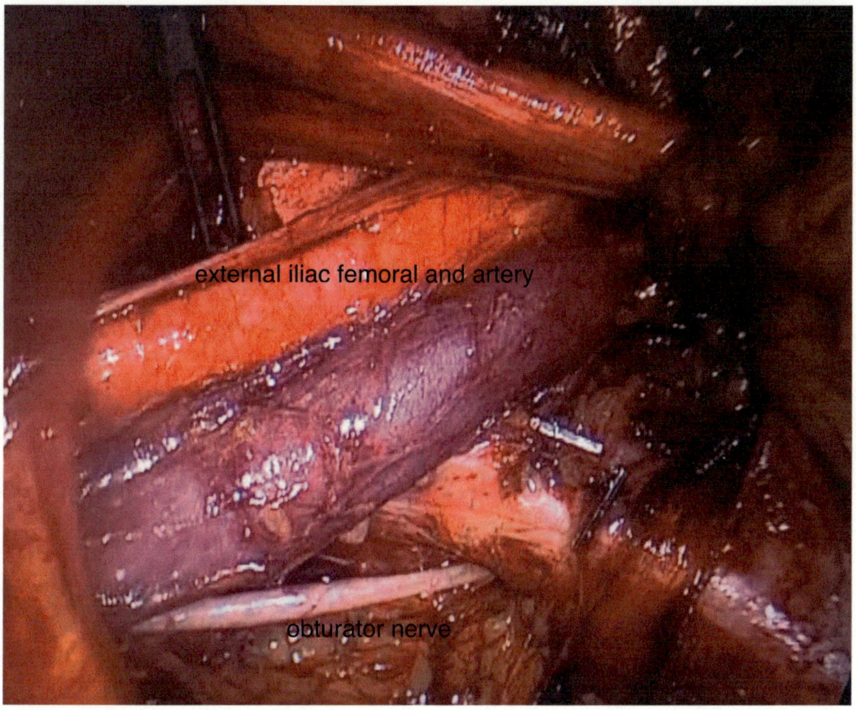

Figure 6. Intraoperative view of iliac and obturator VL

The greatest advantage of VL is probably the virtual elimination of inguinal incision and (in case of iliac lymphadenectomy) the avoidance of the parietal abdominal muscles section. This potentially leads to a significant reduction of the post-operative wound related morbidity and pain. In one uncontrolled comparative study, the incidence of complications (infection and wound dehiscence) was significantly lower after VL (47.5% versus 80%, P=0.002) [63]. In another comparative study, although the incidence of infection and wound dehiscence was not statistically different after VL compared to open lymphadenectomy, in the open group wound infections appear more serious, requiring hospital readmission and intravenous antibiotics in five of the eight patients (62 %) [64]. Although the experiences are limited and the level of evidence is low, VL for melanoma is technically feasible, seems associated with a lower post-operative morbidity profile with comparable oncological outcomes (i.e. number of excised lymph nodes, loco-regional recurrence) (table 4). Before VL becomes suitable for routine clinical practice, the lower post-operative morbidity and safe oncological profile shown in retrospective and prospective series needs to be investigated within prospective RCTs.

	Videoscopic Lymphadenectomy	Procedures (N)	Conversion rate (%)	Wound complication rate (%)	Lymph node excised (N)	Local recurrence rate (%)
Trias M, et al [65]	Iliac	12	0	16.7	10.2	Not reported
Schneider C, et al [66]	Iliac	31	0	9.7	4.6	9.7
Abbott AM, et al [64]	Inguinal	13	7.7	1.8	13	Not reported
Martin BM, et al [63]	Inguinal	40	10	15	12.6	2.5
Sommariva, et al. [unpublished data]	Inguinal and Iliac	24	16.5	4	20.4	0

Table 4. Summary of results on videoscopic groin lymphadenectomy for melanoma

5. Conclusion

Even in the present exciting era of discovering new drugs to cure patients with advanced melanoma, surgery still represents the most performed and effective treatment for this potentially lethal disease. Nevertheless, the effort to solve many controversies related to this important subject has been so far insufficient and the ongoing clinical practice guidelines often lack clear indications for an adequate clinical approach, in particular dealing with patients at high risk for or with lymph node metastasis. While waiting for the conclusion of the ongoing controlled clinical trials (MLST-2 and MiniTub), surgeons should look for new evidence based results strengthening support for indication of SLNB and lymph node dissection, completeness of the latter and QA parameters on which the surgical performance should be measured.

Indication to SLNB is accepted almost everywhere as a staging procedure. Moreover, a recent meta-analysis of retrospective studies and the last report on the long-term results of the MLST-1 controlled trial reinforce its curative value in patients with positive nodes who undergo immediate CLND. In perspective, a more precise patient selection, based on validation new statistical tools and/or identification of new molecular markers, and lowering its false negative rate might improve its efficiency and make this procedure even more appealing.

At present, LND represents the most controversial subject in the surgical treatment of melanoma, particularly in SN positive patients. Its indication can be further warranted by, besides the long-term results of the MLST-1, the demonstration of its essential role as staging procedure. A recent study shows that below the threshold of 11 excised lymph nodes an accurate sub-staging is impossible, and another one demonstrates that the status of the additional lymph nodes is an independent prognostic factor in stage III melanoma patients. These evidence-based results also prompt for their inclusion in the surgical QA process (the former), and in the forthcoming melanoma staging system (the latter). Even if the extension of each lymphadenectomy is still a matter of discussion, further evidence has been recently added to the need of its completeness, such as the demonstration that the lymph node ratio and the absolute number of excised lymph nodes are independently associated with survival. As for other solid tumours in which LND has an impact on staging and survival, melanoma surgeons are in search of simple and reproducible parameters to deem the procedure adequate. The minimum number of lymph nodes to be excised seems to meet this requirement, and the reproducible numbers provided as benchmark values by the 10th percentile method, for each type of LND, are likely to make this parameter the most reliable. Looking at the future, statistical tools and molecular markers for a better patient selection, randomized trials for devising the LND extent, and the mini-invasive surgical approach to reduce the fear of complication and improve patients' quality of life, will probably fulfil the present lack of knowledge and make surgical treatment of melanoma more standardized and cost-effective. Nevertheless, since now surgeons can be helped by the new evidence-based results in the difficult process of building consensus on some important issues in melanoma surgery.

Author details

Antonio Sommariva[1], Camilla Cona[1,2] and Carlo Riccardo Rossi[1,2]

1 Melanoma and Sarcoma Unit, Veneto Institute of Oncology IOV-IRCCS, Padova, Italy

2 Department of Surgery, Oncology and Gastroenterology, University of Padova, Padova, Italy

References

[1] Morton DL, Thompson JF, Cochran AJ, Mozzillo N, Nieweg OE, Roses DF, et al. Final trial report of sentinel-node biopsy versus nodal observation in melanoma. N Engl J Med. 2014 Feb 13;370(7):599-609.

[2] Coit DG, Andtbacka R, Anker CJ, Bichakjian CK, Carson WE, 3rd, Daud A, et al. Melanoma, version 2.2013: featured updates to the NCCN guidelines. J Natl Compr Canc Netw. 2013 Apr 1;11(4):395-407.

[3] Bilimoria KY, Balch CM, Bentrem DJ, Talamonti MS, Ko CY, Lange JR, et al. Complete lymph node dissection for sentinel node-positive melanoma: assessment of practice patterns in the United States. Ann Surg Oncol. 2008 Jun;15(6):1566-76.

[4] Pasquali S, Spillane AJ, de Wilt JH, McCaffery K, Rossi CR, Quinn MJ, et al. Surgeons' opinions on lymphadenectomy in melanoma patients with positive sentinel nodes: a worldwide web-based survey. Ann Surg Oncol. 2012 Dec;19(13):4322-9.

[5] Bedrosian I, Gershenwald JE. Surgical clinical trials in melanoma. Surg Clin North Am. 2003 Apr;83(2):385-403.

[6] Hein DW, Moy RL. Elective lymph node dissection in stage I malignant melanoma: a meta-analysis. Melanoma Res. 1992 Nov;2(4):273-7.

[7] Cascinelli N, Morabito A, Santinami M, MacKie RM, Belli F. Immediate or delayed dissection of regional nodes in patients with melanoma of the trunk: a randomised trial. WHO Melanoma Programme. Lancet. 1998 Mar 14;351(9105):793-6.

[8] Morton DL, Wen DR, Wong JH, Economou JS, Cagle LA, Storm FK, et al. Technical details of intraoperative lymphatic mapping for early stage melanoma. Arch Surg. 1992 Apr;127(4):392-9.

[9] Rossi CR, De Salvo GL, Trifiro G, Mocellin S, Landi G, Macripo G, et al. The impact of lymphoscintigraphy technique on the outcome of sentinel node biopsy in 1,313 patients with cutaneous melanoma: an Italian Multicentric Study (SOLISM-IMI). J Nucl Med. 2006 Feb;47(2):234-41.

[10] Valsecchi ME, Silbermins D, de Rosa N, Wong SL, Lyman GH. Lymphatic mapping and sentinel lymph node biopsy in patients with melanoma: a meta-analysis. J Clin Oncol. 2011 Apr 10;29(11):1479-87.

[11] Gershenwald JE, Thompson W, Mansfield PF, Lee JE, Colome MI, Tseng CH, et al. Multi-institutional melanoma lymphatic mapping experience: the prognostic value of sentinel lymph node status in 612 stage I or II melanoma patients. J Clin Oncol. 1999 Mar;17(3):976-83.

[12] Balch CM, Buzaid AC, Soong SJ, Atkins MB, Cascinelli N, Coit DG, et al. Final version of the American Joint Committee on Cancer staging system for cutaneous melanoma. J Clin Oncol. 2001 Aug 15;19(16):3635-48.

[13] Rousseau DL, Jr., Ross MI, Johnson MM, Prieto VG, Lee JE, Mansfield PF, et al. Revised American Joint Committee on Cancer staging criteria accurately predict sentinel lymph node positivity in clinically node-negative melanoma patients. Ann Surg Oncol. 2003 Jun;10(5):569-74.

[14] Wong SL, Balch CM, Hurley P, Agarwala SS, Akhurst TJ, Cochran A, et al. Sentinel lymph node biopsy for melanoma: american society of clinical oncology and society of surgical oncology joint clinical practice guideline. J Clin Oncol. 2012 Aug 10;30(23): 2912-8.

[15] Andtbacka RH, Gershenwald JE. Role of sentinel lymph node biopsy in patients with thin melanoma. J Natl Compr Canc Netw. 2009 Mar;7(3):308-17.

[16] Murali R, Haydu LE, Quinn MJ, Saw RP, Shannon K, Spillane AJ, et al. Sentinel lymph node biopsy in patients with thin primary cutaneous melanoma. Ann Surg. 2012 Jan;255(1):128-33.

[17] Kesmodel SB, Karakousis GC, Botbyl JD, Canter RJ, Lewis RT, Wahl PM, et al. Mitotic rate as a predictor of sentinel lymph node positivity in patients with thin melanomas. Ann Surg Oncol. 2005 Jun;12(6):449-58.

[18] Livingstone E, Windemuth-Kieselbach C, Eigentler TK, Rompel R, Trefzer U, Nashan D, et al. A first prospective population-based analysis investigating the actual practice of melanoma diagnosis, treatment and follow-up. Eur J Cancer. 2011 Sep;47(13): 1977-89.

[19] Hyngstrom JR, Chiang YJ, Cromwell KD, Ross MI, Xing Y, Mungovan KS, et al. Prospective assessment of lymphedema incidence and lymphedema-associated symptoms following lymph node surgery for melanoma. Melanoma Res. 2013 Aug;23(4): 290-7.

[20] Balch C. Cutaneous Melanoma. Quality Medical Pub; 2009.

[21] Spratt J. Groin dissection. J Surg Oncol. 2000 Apr;73(4):243-62.

[22] Sommariva A, Clemente C, Rossi CR. Standardization and quality control of surgical treatment of cutaneous melanoma: Looking for consensus of the Italian Melanoma Intergroup. Eur J Surg Oncol. 2014 Jul 26.

[23] Nessim C, Law C, McConnell Y, Shachar S, McKinnon G, Wright F. How often do level III nodes bear melanoma metastases and does it affect patient outcomes? Ann Surg Oncol. 2013 Jun;20(6):2056-64.

[24] Evaluation of Groin Lymphadenectomy Extent For Metastatic Melanoma (EAGLE FM); http://clinicaltrials.gov/show/NCT02166788.

[25] Morton DL, Thompson JF, Cochran AJ, Mozzillo N, Elashoff R, Essner R, et al. Sentinel-node biopsy or nodal observation in melanoma. N Engl J Med. 2006 Sep 28;355(13):1307-17.

[26] Spillane AJ, Pasquali S, Haydu LE, Thompson JF. Patterns of recurrence and survival after lymphadenectomy in melanoma patients: clarifying the effects of timing of surgery and lymph node tumor burden. Ann Surg Oncol. 2014 Jan;21(1):292-9.

[27] Pasquali S, Mocellin S, Campana LG, Bonandini E, Montesco MC, Tregnaghi A, et al. Early (sentinel lymph node biopsy-guided) versus delayed lymphadenectomy in melanoma patients with lymph node metastases : personal experience and literature meta-analysis. Cancer. 2010 Mar 1;116(5):1201-9.

[28] Rossi CR, Mozzillo N, Maurichi A, Pasquali S, Quaglino P, Borgognoni L, et al. The number of excised lymph nodes is associated with survival of melanoma patients with lymph node metastasis. Ann Oncol. 2014 Jan;25(1):240-6.

[29] Pasquali S, Mocellin S, Mozzillo N, Maurichi A, Quaglino P, Borgognoni L, et al. Nonsentinel lymph node status in patients with cutaneous melanoma: results from a multi-institution prognostic study. J Clin Oncol. 2014 Mar 20;32(9):935-41.

[30] Mansfield AS, Holtan SG, Grotz TE, Allred JB, Jakub JW, Erickson LA, et al. Regional immunity in melanoma: immunosuppressive changes precede nodal metastasis. Mod Pathol. 2011 Apr;24(4):487-94.

[31] Mocellin S, Pasquali S, Rossi CR, Nitti D. Validation of the prognostic value of lymph node ratio in patients with cutaneous melanoma: a population-based study of 8,177 cases. Surgery. 2011 Jul;150(1):83-90.

[32] Spillane AJ, Cheung BL, Winstanley J, Thompson JF. Lymph node ratio provides prognostic information in addition to american joint committee on cancer N stage in patients with melanoma, even if quality of surgery is standardized. Ann Surg. 2011 Jan;253(1):109-15.

[33] Xing Y, Badgwell BD, Ross MI, Gershenwald JE, Lee JE, Mansfield PF, et al. Lymph node ratio predicts disease-specific survival in melanoma patients. Cancer. 2009 Jun 1;115(11):2505-13.

[34] Balch CM, Durant JR, Bartolucci AA. The impact of surgical quality control in multi-institutional group trials involving adjuvant cancer treatments. Ann Surg. 1983 Aug; 198(2):164-7.

[35] Eggermont AM, Suciu S, Santinami M, Testori A, Kruit WH, Marsden J, et al. Adjuvant therapy with pegylated interferon alfa-2b versus observation alone in resected stage III melanoma: final results of EORTC 18991, a randomised phase III trial. Lancet. 2008 Jul 12;372(9633):117-26.

[36] Galliot-Repkat C, Cailliod R, Trost O, Danino A, Collet E, Lambert D, et al. The prognostic impact of the extent of lymph node dissection in patients with stage III melanoma. Eur J Surg Oncol. 2006 Sep;32(7):790-4.

[37] Bilimoria KY, Raval MV, Bentrem DJ, Wayne JD, Balch CM, Ko CY. National assessment of melanoma care using formally developed quality indicators. J Clin Oncol. 2009 Nov 10;27(32):5445-51.

[38] Spillane AJ, Cheung BL, Stretch JR, Scolyer RA, Shannon KF, Quinn MJ, et al. Proposed quality standards for regional lymph node dissections in patients with melanoma. Ann Surg. 2009 Mar;249(3):473-80.

[39] Spillane AJ, Haydu L, McMillan W, Stretch JR, Thompson JF. Quality assurance parameters and predictors of outcome for ilioinguinal and inguinal dissection in a contemporary melanoma patient population. Ann Surg Oncol. 2011 Sep;18(9):2521-8.

[40] Rossi CR, Mozzillo N, Maurichi A, Pasquali S, Macripo G, Borgognoni L, et al. Number of excised lymph nodes as a quality assurance measure for lymphadenectomy in melanoma. JAMA Surg. 2014 Jul 1;149(7):700-6.

[41] Morton DL, Cochran AJ, Thompson JF, Elashoff R, Essner R, Glass EC, et al. Sentinel node biopsy for early-stage melanoma: accuracy and morbidity in MSLT-I, an international multicenter trial. Ann Surg. 2005 Sep;242(3):302-11; discussion 11-3.

[42] Agnese DM, Abdessalam SF, Burak WE, Jr., Magro CM, Pozderac RV, Walker MJ. Cost-effectiveness of sentinel lymph node biopsy in thin melanomas. Surgery. 2003 Oct;134(4):542-7; discussion 7-8.

[43] Mocellin S, Thompson JF, Pasquali S, Montesco MC, Pilati P, Nitti D, et al. Sentinel node status prediction by four statistical models: results from a large bi-institutional series (n=1132). Ann Surg. 2009 Dec;250(6):964-9.

[44] Nagaraja V, Eslick GD. Is complete lymph node dissection after a positive sentinel lymph node biopsy for cutaneous melanoma always necessary? A meta-analysis. Eur J Surg Oncol. 2013 Jul;39(7):669-80.

[45] Gershenwald JE, Andtbacka RH, Prieto VG, Johnson MM, Diwan AH, Lee JE, et al. Microscopic tumor burden in sentinel lymph nodes predicts synchronous nonsentinel lymph node involvement in patients with melanoma. J Clin Oncol. 2008 Sep 10;26(26):4296-303.

[46] Govindarajan A, Ghazarian DM, McCready DR, Leong WL. Histological features of melanoma sentinel lymph node metastases associated with status of the completion lymphadenectomy and rate of subsequent relapse. Ann Surg Oncol. 2007 Feb;14(2): 906-12.

[47] Warycha MA, Zakrzewski J, Ni Q, Shapiro RL, Berman RS, Pavlick AC, et al. Meta-analysis of sentinel lymph node positivity in thin melanoma (<or=1 mm). Cancer. 2009 Feb 15;115(4):869-79.

[48] van Akkooi AC, de Wilt JH, Verhoef C, Schmitz PI, van Geel AN, Eggermont AM, et al. Clinical relevance of melanoma micrometastases (<0.1 mm) in sentinel nodes: are these nodes to be considered negative? Ann Oncol. 2006 Oct;17(10):1578-85.

[49] Starz H, Siedlecki K, Balda BR. Sentinel lymphonodectomy and s-classification: a successful strategy for better prediction and improvement of outcome of melanoma. Ann Surg Oncol. 2004 Mar;11(3 Suppl):162S-8S.

[50] Meier A, Satzger I, Volker B, Kapp A, Gutzmer R. Comparison of classification systems in melanoma sentinel lymph nodes--an analysis of 697 patients from a single center. Cancer. 2010 Jul 1;116(13):3178-88.

[51] Murali R, Desilva C, Thompson JF, Scolyer RA. Non-Sentinel Node Risk Score (N-SNORE): a scoring system for accurately stratifying risk of non-sentinel node positivity in patients with cutaneous melanoma with positive sentinel lymph nodes. J Clin Oncol. 2010 Oct 10;28(29):4441-9.

[52] van der Ploeg AP, van Akkooi AC, Rutkowski P, Nowecki ZI, Michej W, Mitra A, et al. Prognosis in patients with sentinel node-positive melanoma is accurately defined by the combined Rotterdam tumor load and Dewar topography criteria. J Clin Oncol. 2011 Jun 1;29(16):2206-14.

[53] Rossi CR, Pasquali S, Mocellin S. Actual false-negative rate prompts the routine use of ultrasound scan before and after sentinel node biopsy in melanoma. Ann Surg Oncol. 2008 Oct;15(10):2976-7.

[54] Karim RZ, Scolyer RA, Li W, Yee VS, McKinnon JG, Li LX, et al. False negative sentinel lymph node biopsies in melanoma may result from deficiencies in nuclear medicine, surgery, or pathology. Ann Surg. 2008 Jun;247(6):1003-10.

[55] Richtig E, Komericki P, Trapp M, Ott A, Bisail B, Egger JW, et al. Ratio of marked and excised sentinel lymph nodes and scintigraphic appearance time in melanoma patients with negative sentinel lymph node. Eur J Surg Oncol. 2010 Aug;36(8):783-8.

[56] de Rosa N, Lyman GH, Silbermins D, Valsecchi ME, Pruitt SK, Tyler DM, et al. Sentinel node biopsy for head and neck melanoma: a systematic review. Otolaryngol Head Neck Surg. 2011 Sep;145(3):375-82.

[57] McMasters KM, Reintgen DS, Ross MI, Wong SL, Gershenwald JE, Krag DN, et al. Sentinel lymph node biopsy for melanoma: how many radioactive nodes should be removed? Ann Surg Oncol. 2001 Apr;8(3):192-7.

[58] Liu LC, Parrett BM, Jenkins T, Lee W, Morita E, Treseler P, et al. Selective sentinel lymph node dissection for melanoma: importance of harvesting nodes with lower radioactive counts without the need for blue dye. Ann Surg Oncol. 2011 Oct;18(10): 2919-24.

[59] Cochran AJ. The pathologist's role in sentinel lymph node evaluation. Semin Nucl Med. 2000 Jan;30(1):11-7.

[60] Cook MG, Green MA, Anderson B, Eggermont AM, Ruiter DJ, Spatz A, et al. The development of optimal pathological assessment of sentinel lymph nodes for melanoma. J Pathol. 2003 Jul;200(3):314-9.

[61] Mocellin S, Hoon DS, Pilati P, Rossi CR, Nitti D. Sentinel lymph node molecular ultrastaging in patients with melanoma: a systematic review and meta-analysis of prognosis. J Clin Oncol. 2007 Apr 20;25(12):1588-95.

[62] Chang SB, Askew RL, Xing Y, Weaver S, Gershenwald JE, Lee JE, et al. Prospective assessment of postoperative complications and associated costs following inguinal lymph node dissection (ILND) in melanoma patients. Ann Surg Oncol. 2010 Oct; 17(10):2764-72.

[63] Martin BM, Etra JW, Russell MC, Rizzo M, Kooby DA, Staley CA, et al. Oncologic outcomes of patients undergoing videoscopic inguinal lymphadenectomy for metastatic melanoma. J Am Coll Surg. 2014 Apr;218(4):620-6.

[64] Abbott AM, Grotz TE, Rueth NM, Hernandez Irizarry RC, Tuttle TM, Jakub JW. Minimally invasive inguinal lymph node dissection (MILND) for melanoma: experience from two academic centers. Ann Surg Oncol. 2013 Jan;20(1):340-5.

[65] Trias M, Targarona EM, Piulachs J, Balague C, Bombuy E, Espert JJ, et al. Extraperitoneal laparoscopically assisted ilioinguinal lymphadenectomy for treatment of malignant melanoma. Arch Surg. 1998 Mar;133(3):272-4; discussion 5.

[66] Schneider C, Brodersen JP, Scheuerlein H, Tamme C, Lippert H, Kockerling F. Combined endoscopic and open inguinal dissection for malignant melanoma. Langenbecks Arch Surg. 2003 Mar;388(1):42-7.

Chapter 7

Current Insights Into Canine Cutaneous Melanocytic Tumours Diagnosis

Luis Resende, Joana Moreira, Justina Prada,
Felisbina Luisa Queiroga and Isabel Pires

Additional information is available at the end of the chapter

http://dx.doi.org/10.5772/59480

1. Introduction

Skin melanoma is a devastating disease, frequently diagnosed in human and dogs, accounting for 0,8% - 2% of all skin tumors in latter species [1].

Melanocytic tumours are common neoplasms in dogs, accounting for 4 to 7% of neoplastic lesions in general, and up to 7% of all malignant tumours [2,3]. They generally arise on the oral cavity (Figure 1), lip, skin (Figure 2) and digit, amongst other locations (Figure 3) [4].

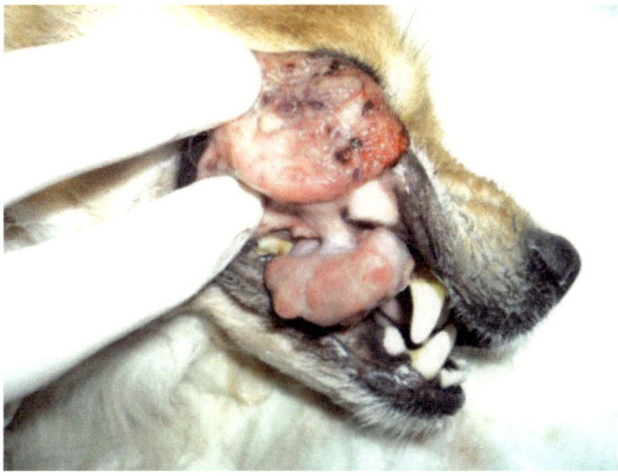

Figure 1. Canine oral melanoma (courtesy of Dr. Abel Fernandes).

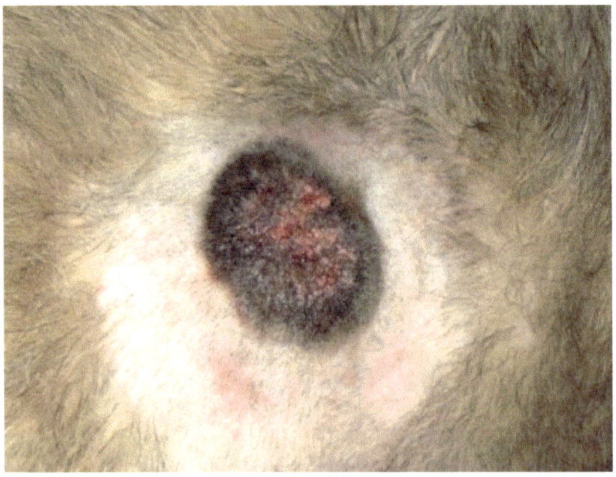

Figure 2. Canine cutaneous melanoma.

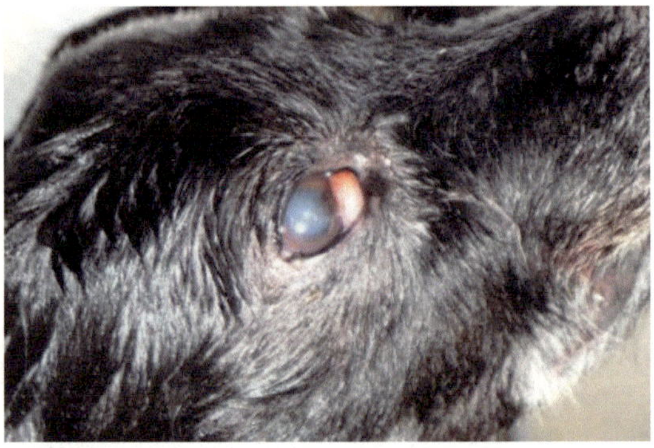

Figure 3. Canine ocular melanoma.

Biologic behaviour of these tumours is often related to its location. Over 85% of melanocytic lesions located on haired skin are described as of benign behaviour. The majority of oral and mucocutaneous junction melanomas, with the exception of the eyelid, and 50% of digital melanomas originated from the nail bed are reported as malignant [5,6].

Cutaneous canine melanocytic lesions are usually benign [7,8]. They are generally detected at a late stage, when excision is rarely curative and metastasis is often detectable in regional lymph nodes [7]. Malignant tumors are found most frequently on the head, ventral abdomen, and scrotum [7]; in the last one, they represent 3,1% of all cutaneous malignant melanomas and 4,7% of scrotal tumours [9]. Amelanotic lesions can occur as cutaneous neoplasms, but are more frequent in the oral cavity, and tend to be behaviorally malignant [10].

Metastasis are often found on regional lymph nodes and lungs, but organs as brain, heart and spleen are also commonly affected [11].

Veterinary nomenclature of canine melanocytic tumours has been subjected to many controversies and changes over time. Through this article, in accordance with the revised World

Health Organization classification system, and in order to simplify and avoid confusion, the authors describe benign lesions as melanocytoma, whereas malignant lesions are referred to as melanoma [12].

Etiology of this neoplasms is still uncertain, and several factors may be related, such as consanguinity, trauma, chemical exposure, hormones and genetic susceptibility [10]. Unlike humans, ionizing solar radiation exposure doesn't seem to be related to canine melanoma initiation [4].

Canine melanocytic tumour diagnosis often represents a challenge for the pathologist, since a high number of neoplastic lesions are quite similar in terms of its clinical and histologic appearance, including carcinoma, sarcoma, lymphoma and plasmocitoma, amongst others [10]. Indeed, cutaneous neoplasms with malignant behavior are more difficult to distinguish histologically from benign neoplasms than oral or lip neoplasms [13].

Diagnosis is usually based on fine-needle aspiration citology, but biopsy for histopathological examination is essential to determine its malignant potential [4,14]. The most reliable histologic criteria is the mitotic index, defined as the total number of mitotic figures observed per ten high-power light microscopic fields, which is known to be 90% accurate [5,6,15].

Immunochemistry has arised as an extremely useful tool, for both diagnostic and prognostic purposes. A positive diagnostic for melanocytic neoplasms is obtained with a positive labelling of S100 protein, vimentine, Neuron Specific Enolase (*NSE*) and a simoultaneous negative labelling with cytokeratine [16].

The treatment of choice for local cutaneous melanomas is surgical excision; tumours with benign histopathology criteria have an excellent prognostic after this surgery. However, for malignant tumors, the prognostic is guarded, since metastatic rates of 30-75% have been reported [5,6].

Alternative therapy methods described in the literature include systemic chemotherapy, radiotherapy [17], photodynamic therapy [18], local hyperthermia [19,20] and intralesional injection of cisplatin or carboplatin.

The poor responses to the conventional therapy are leading to a development of new immunotherapy procedures – including intralesional adenoviral vector-mediated transfer of CD40L, a tumor necrosis factor gene [21], therapy with a plasmid DNA encoding staphylococcal enterotoxin B [22], and systemic tratment with liposome-encapsulated muramyl tripeptide [23].

At last, the most promising therapy appears to be a xenogenetic human tyrosinase DNA vaccine, with minimal local reaction and no systemic toxicity signs, and a great clinical responde with significant increasing of the survival time [24].

In this paper, the authors aim to contribute to the understanding of melanocytic tumours in the dog, making a critical review of the literature and discussing the parameters currently considered valid for diagnosis use in canine melanocytic neoplams.

2. Signalment

Cutaneous melanocytic tumours are most common in older dogs (mean age of 9 years old) [25], with a higher mean age for dogs with malignant melanocytic tumours (12 years). However, age has not been related with the patient clinical outcome and survival time [26].

Although all breeds of dog (and crossbred animals) may be affected, some breeds are reported as predisposed, including Schnauzer, Doberman, Scottish Terrier, Irish Setter, Golden Retriever, Chow Chow, Cocker Spaniel, German Shepherd and Rottweiler [4,27]. Breed predisposition is thought to be related to an underlying genetic risk and/or increased pigmentation in the described above breeds [4].

One study [6] has also established a relationship between patient breed and tumour behavior, likely due to genetic susceptibility, as prior described. In the referred work, melanocytic lesions tended to be behaviorally benign in Doberman pinschers and miniature schnauzers, while miniature poodles were the mostly affected breed with malignant melanoma. However, it must be noted that oral neoplasms were also included in that study.

An early report described a higher frequency of these lesions in male dogs [28], but recent literature denies gender predisposition [6,27,29-31].

3. Pathogenesis

Melanin is a dark-brown pigment synthetized by melanocytes, dendritic cells found within the basal layer of the epidermis. These cells are dispersed from each other, located between basal keratinocytes, forming adherent and regulatory junctions mediated by epithelial cadherin (E-cadherin) molecules. After its synthesis, melanin is retained in melanosomas and transferred to the adjacent keratinocytes [32].

Conversion of normal melanocytes to clusters of neoplastic melanocytes is a process composed by a series of events: initiation, promotion, transformation and metastasis [4].

Little is known about initiation on most animal melanomas, but ionizing solar radiation exposure – the main initiator factor in Human melanomas [33] - doesn't seem to be related to canine melanomas [4]. A higher incidence of spontaneously mutated cells due to familiar clustering through inbreeding may be a critical initiation factor in domestic animals.

Malignant transformation of canine cutaneous melanocytomas is very uncommon. Regarding cutaneous melanomas, there are a few published case reports, including one by Valentine and team [34], which have described a single case of malignant transformation of a congenital melanocytic nevus is a Golden retriever. Conroy [35] described two cases of melanoma originated from junctional or dermal hamartomas and a single case of a primary melanomas originated from a subcutaneous melanocytoma have also been reported [36]. In summary, canine cutaneous melanomas are thought to arise *de novo* from epidermal and dermal melanocytes.

Promotion phase is related to mutated cells proliferation, with subsequent amplification of cell population and origin of additional mutations [4]. Melanoma promoters include chronic trauma, chemical exposure, drugs and hormones [10], and its action results in reactive hyperplasia of the epithelium, with disruption of regular keratinocyte-melanocyte interactions and proliferation of initiated cells.

The next step in carcinogenesis involves a series of transformation events. Recent developments in genetic and molecular study techniques have identified the role of a few tumour suppressors in melanoma cell lines, giving new insights on the importance of these molecules in canine melanoma development. A reduction or loss of *p16* expression was one of the most commonly found changes, in both benign and malignant tumours, suggesting that inactivation of this pathway is a critical step in the pathogenesis of melanoma [37]. Altered expression of *PTEN, TP53, Rb* and *p21* have also been related to its progression [38], as well as the presence of various oncogenes (as a result of proto-oncogenes mutation), such as *c-myc, c-erb-B-2, c-yes, c-kit* and *ras* [4].

After local proliferation phase, neoplastic cells may acquire a malignant behavior, and disseminate through hematic or lymphatic vessels to various other organs, originating secondary neoplasms known as metastasis. This complex process has it start with loss of adhesion and detachment of neoplastic cells from the primary mass, hematic and lymphatic vessels intravasion and attachment and proliferation within a secondary location [4].

Metastasis process is dependent of various adhesion molecules regulation by neoplastic cells. Several studies have shown an association between decreased and altered expression of E-cadherin, a calcium-dependent adhesion molecule responsible for melanocyte-keratinocyte interaction, and canine cutaneous melanoma progression [39,40]. CD44, a second transmembrane glycoprotein which facilitates metastasis, is required for several processes, including hyaluronate degradation, cell aggregation and migration, angiogenesis and hematopoiesis [4]. Down-regulation of regular CD44 plus up-regulation of CD44v5 has also been associated with melanoma metastasis, particularly with lymph node metastasis [41].

Autonomous growth is a key requirement for both primary and secondary neoplastic development. The most important autocrine growth factors in animal melanoma include basic fibroblast growth factor (*bFGF*), melanoma growth stimulatory activity or growth regulated proteins, platelet-derive growth factor-A, α-melanocyte stimulating hormone, and a series of interleukins (*IL-8, IL-10* and *IL-18*) [4].

4. Gross morphologic features

Macroscopically, canine malignant melanoma cannot be differentiated from melanocytoma [42]. Melanomas in dogs tend to be dermal in location, unlike Human melanomas – which are intraepidermal with some degree of dermal invasion. Prognostic schemes, such as Clark's level or Breslow thickness, built nased on depht of dermal invasion, are not applicable on canine lesions [43].

Canine melanocytomas share some aspects with Human benign melanocytic lesions, in terms of clinical evolution most common metastatic locations [42], and genetic alterations [44].

Cutaneous melanocytomas are usually symmetrical, circumscribed, but encapsulated [43], solitary, black, brown, or gray cutaneous alopecic nodules [43,45] with a variable size with range of 1-4 cm in diameter (Figure 4 and Figure 5) [43]. Epidermis is usually intact, and alopecia is frequent. Epidermal cells may be hyperpigmented, and the majority of dermal cells are replaced by the tumoral ones, which in larger masses might also extends into the subcutaneous tissue. The tumors may have a varieated appearance, with areas of pigmentation intermingled with no pigmented regions [42].

Canine cutaneous malignant melanomas can vary considerably in appearance, regardless of the location. Melanomas tend to be asymmetrical. The asymmetry may be most readily recognizable in the epidermal component of junctional tumors [43]. Melanomas size vary from some milimiteres to as large as 10 centimeters in diameter (mean range being 1 to 3 cm in diameter) [43], but this is not a reliable indicator of malignancy [13,42]. The color is variable, ranging from gray or brown to black, red, or even dark blue [7]. Cutaneous melanoma presentation includes smooth domes, sessile nodules, polypoid, plaquelike [7,43], or even lobulated masses [7]. The larger ones are often ulcerated [7,43]. The tumors may invade deeply into the subcutaneous tissue and along fascial planes [42].

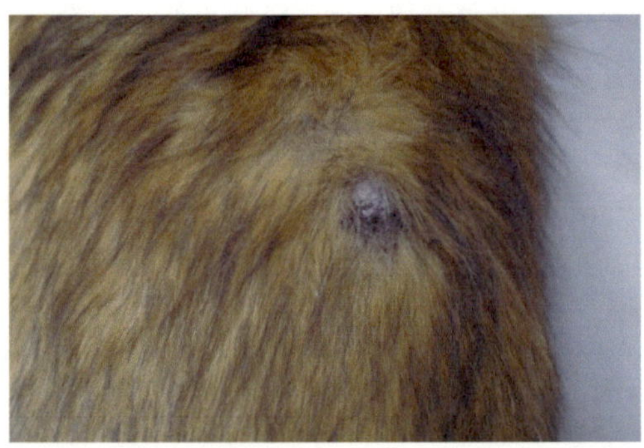

Figure 4. Canine cutaneous melanoma.

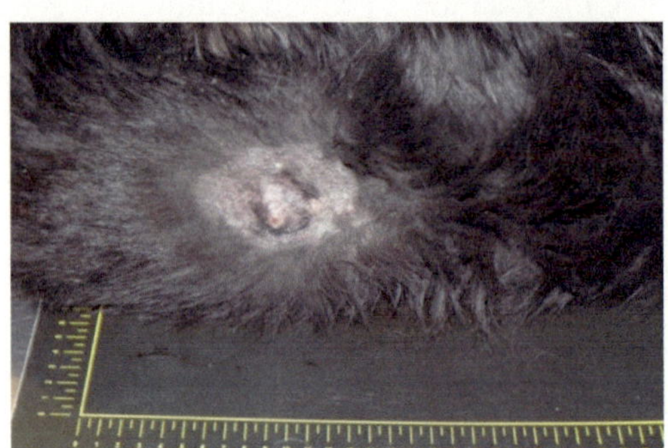

Figure 5. Canine cutaneous melanoma.

http://dx.doi.org/10.5772/59480

5. Cytological diagnosis

Microscopic examination of a cytological specimen obtained through fine needle aspiration has become a valuable technique to obtain a preliminary, and often definitive, diagnosis [46]. Being a quick, non-evasive and inexpensive procedure, it can also provide information on the stage, prognosis and metastasis evidence. Its main limitation reside on the fact that non-pigmented melanomas may strongly resemble other neoplastic lesions, and the amount of cytological sample might be very small and not fully representative of the lesion [4,46].

Several studies in Human cancer have described a strong accuracy in cytological examination in comparison with histopathological findings [47,48], but there are only few studies on the subject in Veterinary Medicine [49]. For instance, Ghisleni and others [50] evaluated a series of cutaneous and subcutaneous masses from dogs and cats through histopathology and cytology, describing an agreement between both techniques in 90.9% of the samples.

Melanocytic tumours are characterized by the presence of cells with abundant cytoplasmatic melanin granules. Neoplastic cells may appear with an epithelial (cohesive cells), mesenchymal (single oval or spindle-shaped cells) or round cell morphology. Nuclei may present a central or eccentric location, and is often solitary, though multinucleated forms are occasionally found. Nucleoli tends to be very prominent, with variable shapes such as round, oval or angular. These cells have a light basophilic cytoplasm, with a moderate to high nuclear-cytoplasmatic ratio. Varying degrees of pigmentation might be found within the same tumour smear [4,46], (Figure 6 and Figure 7).

Malignant criteria consist, most importantly, of marked anisokaryosis and nuclear pleomorphism, but also of the presence of large and atypical nucleoli [46]. Mitotic index, the most reliable criteria in histopathological evaluation, has no use in cytology. Regional lymph nodes are the most commonly evaluated site while monitoring for metastasis [4].

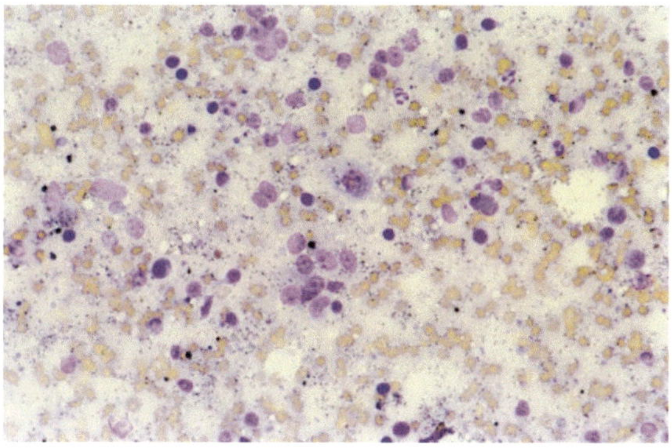

Figure 6. Canine cutaneous melanoma (Wright, 100x).

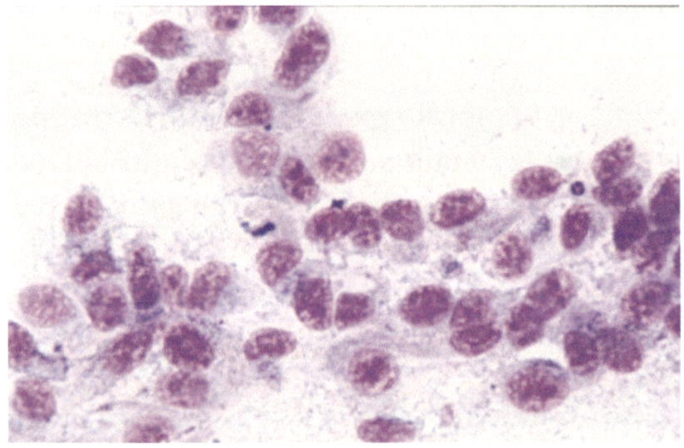

Figure 7. Canine cutaneous melanoma (Wright, 400x).

6. Histological diagnosis

Histological characteristics of canine melanocytic neoplasms were defined by World Health Organization, in *International Histological Classification of Tumours of Domestic Animals*, back in 1974 (Figure 8 and Figure 9) [13].

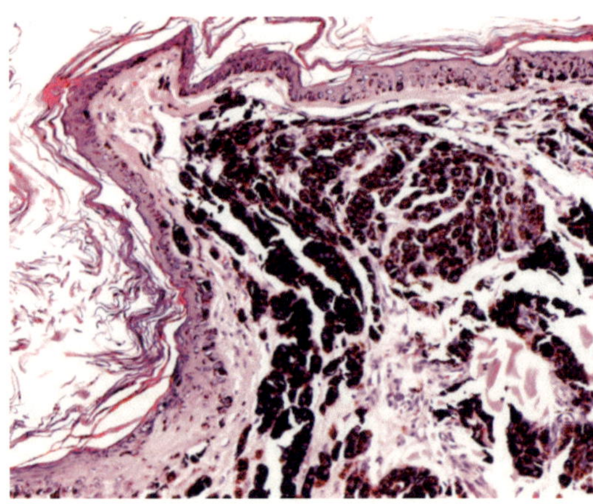

Figure 8. Canine cutaneous melanocytoma (H&E, 200x).

Histological appearance does not always correlate well with biological behavior [8]. More recent studies have provided a numerical ''tumor score'' taking into consideration mitotic index, nuclear atypia, inflammation, necrosis and volume which appears to have improved correlation between histology and behavior [8].

The term nevus, commonly used in describing pigmented melanocytic lesions of the epidermis and dermis in humans, is not used in veterinary dermatopathology [7].

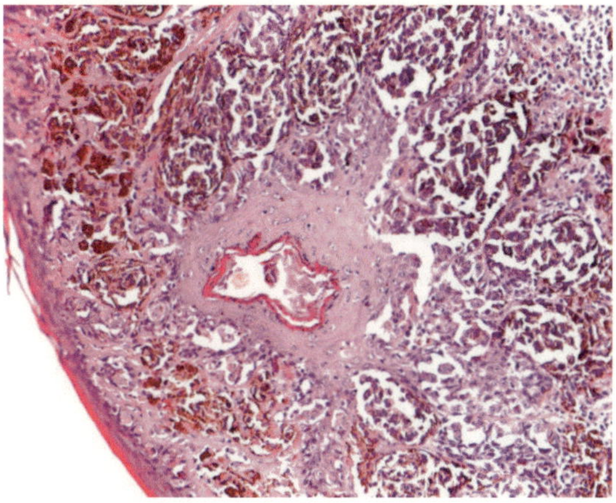

Figure 9. Canine cutaneous melanoma (H&E, 200x).

In this chapter we review several histological parameters on their ability to diagnose and predict prognosis (i.e., prediction of mortality) of canine melanocytic neoplasms. Malignancy celular features include a characteristic large nucleous, nuclear atypia, hyperchromasia, abnormal chromatin clumping and anomalous mitotic figures [51].

6.1. Predominant cell type

Melanocytic neoplasms are generally composed of one of the following cell types: epithelioid (Figure 10), spindle, mixed (Figure 11), dendritic [51,52], and round cells [43]. Other less commonly described cell types include signet ring and ballon cells [51]. All these cell types may occur either alone or in combination [43]. In melanomas, ganglion cell and multinucleated giant cell forms also may be observed [43]. The epithelioid cell type is the most common type in all locations, whereas a mixture of cell types is seen with less frequency [51].

The epithelioid cells are round, with discrete cell borders, abundant glassy cytoplasm, appearing arranged in sheets and larger nests [43]. Similar to their spindle-shaped counterparts melanomas may exhibit large ovoid nuclei and prominent nucleoli [7,43], marked anisokaryosis and variable chromatin patterns [43].

The spindle cell tumors are arranged in streams and interweaving bundles, resembling fibrosarcoma or neurofibrosarcoma presentation. In malignant lesions, the nuclei are large and fusiform with prominent nucleoli [7,43], and moderate to marked nuclear pleomorphism is seen [43]. Spindle cell predominant morphology was statistically associated with benignity in one study (in 71% melanocytomas in contrast to 29% melanomas) [43]. The mixed type consists of both cell morphologies and patterns [7].

Dendritic melanocytes have a highly angular shape, sometimes with long cytoplasmic processes, and are usually arranged in small nests [43] or organized in tightly swirling streams, often with a fingerprint pattern [7]. The dendritic or whorled forms occurs only in the skin [53].

Round cells tumors have round to polygonal cells arranged in sheets as dense packets of cells, the packets being separated by a scant stroma. The nuclei is large and round in melanomas [43].

The signet-ring cell tumors consist of compact neoplastic clusters, with round to ovoid cells presenting a faintly-eosinophilic cytoplasm and an intensely-stained periphery. A vesicular nuclei, crescent-shaped, and with a peripheral location, gives the cell a signet-ring appearance [52].

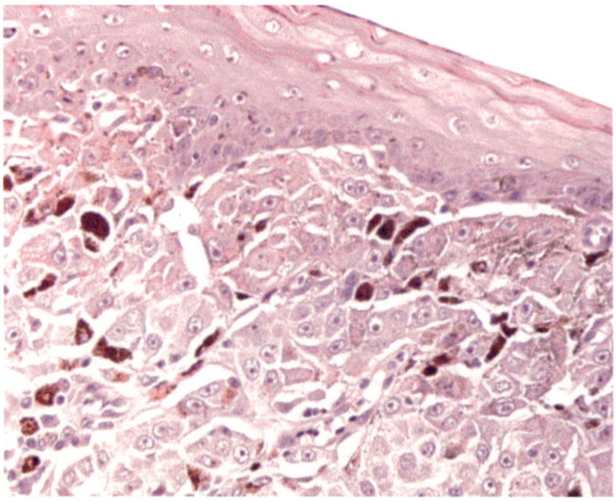

Figure 10. Epithelioid cell canine cutaneous melanoma (H&E, 400x).

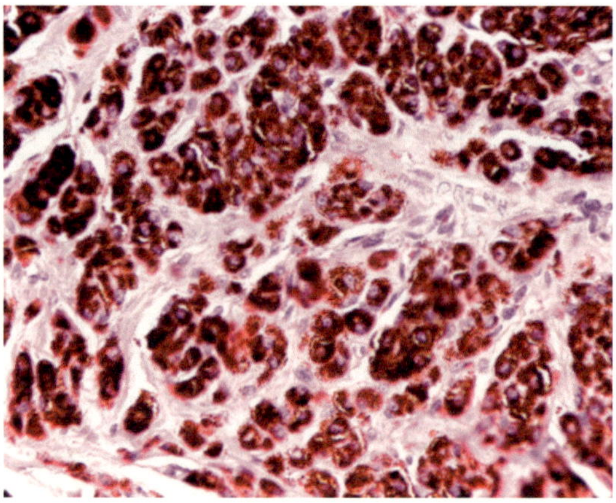

Figure 11. Mixed cell canine cutaneous melanoma (H&E, 400x).

http://dx.doi.org/10.5772/59480

Balloon cells are found organized in groups, separated by collagenous septa [52]. The cells are round to polyhedral and have clear or faintly eosinophilic cytoplasm [43,52]. In melanomas, the nuclei are round situated mainly at the periphery of the tumor cells [52]. Usually contains one central prominent nucleolus [7], which sometimes is difficult to detect. Heterochromatin, which is sparse, is dispersed throughout the nuclei [52].

Benign melanocytic cells present an enlarged vesicular nuclei with small nucleoli. Nuclear shape vary on according to the predominant tumour cell type. Mitotic figures are rare, and mitotic atypia is rarely observed. [43].

Although cell type appears to play some role in the prognosis of ocular melanocytic neoplasms, this feature lacked significance in prognosis of melanocytic tumors occurring in the mouth, feet, buccal mucosa and skin of dogs in several studies [8]. On the contrary, the epithelioid shape was associated with an unfavorable course, for 8/15 cases. The difference seems to be significant ($p = 0{,}03$) [12].

6.2. Nuclear atypia

One of the major criteria of malignancy in melanocytic neoplasms arising at any pigmented anatomic site is nuclear atypia. This feature is more valuable in epithelioid tumours than in spindle, whorled type or signet-ring cells, due to the insufficient nuclear detail associated with the later neoplasms [8,44,54]. However, not all studies are consensual [12].

Well-differentiated tumoral melanocytes have a small nucleus with one central nucleolus [8]. In contrary, undifferentiated tumours generally present cells with multiple, large, irregular and eccentrically nucleoli [8].

Several criteria are used to estimate nuclear atypia, including the percentage of nuclei involved [8]. Figures 12 and 13 (below) present moderate and severe nuclear atypia, respectively.

6.3. Mitotic index

In animal cutaneous and eye melanocytic neoplasms, mitotic index (MI) is the most reliable histological feature for distinguishing malignant from benign tumors [44,51], and also in predicting the clinical course of the disease [8]. In cutaneous melanoma, an MI of ≥3/10 hpf is significantly correlated with decreased survival [55].

The number of mitoses is usually lower in melanocytomas [<3 mitotic figures per 10 high power fields (hpf)] than melanomas [42,44,53].

In one study, the mitotic index was strongly correlated with the clinical outcome of tumors. For tumors with a favorable outcome, the mean value of the number of mitosis (on 10 randomly selected high power fields) was 1,98 (from 0 to 27). For tumors with a malignant behavior, it was 18,53 (from 0 to 75) [12].

The evaluation of the MI in conjunction with nuclear atypia classification (Figure 13) offers a more precise value the histological diagnosis [8].

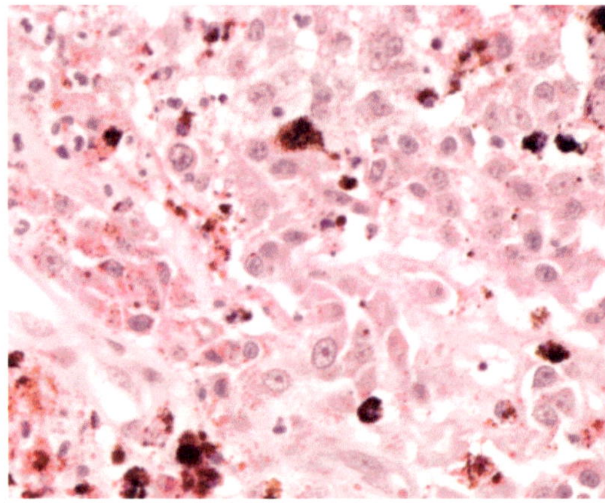

Figure 12. Canine cutaneous melanoma with moderate diferenciation (H&E, 400x).

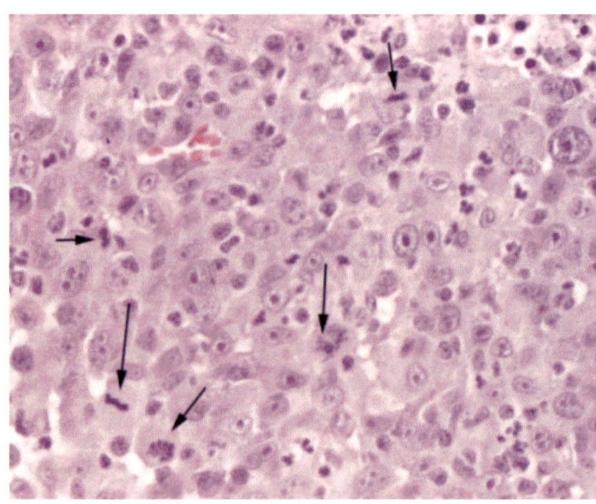

Figure 13. Canine cutaneous melanoma with evident nuclear atypia and numerous mitosis (arrow), (H&E, 400x).

6.4. Cellular pleomorphism

Cellular pleomorphism criteria include several features, such as cell size and shape, pigmentation degree and nuclear features (including prominence of nucleoli and chromatin pattern). The usefulness of these parameters as individual prognostic factors is doubtful; however, it increases when these are used together [8,27].

6.5. Degree of pigmentation

Degree of pigmentation is highly variable, even within a single smear (Figures 14, 15 and 16). Even on histological evaluation of amelanotic-classified tumours is common to detect a few very fine pigment granules in some cells. These are generally punctuate, spherical or elongated, as observed in pigmented keratinocytes. Cells with a very fine pigment may present a dusty gray appearance, instead of the typical granulation image [7]. In summary, it can be difficult to accurately diagnose an amelanotic melanocytic neoplasm and to define the degree of pigmentation [13].

Individual tumoral cells possess a different amount of melanin, which granules are generally small and uniform in size within the same cell. Splindle, round to polygonal, and balloon cells have sparsely-distributed melanin granules, while large epithelioid and dendritic cells are known to have a higher degree of pigmentation [43].

The majority of canine melanocytomas (except for ballon cell ones) have marked to moderate melanin pigmentation overall, especially in the superficial aspect of the tumors [43]. Similarly to cellular morphology, the degree of pigmentation of neoplastic cells was not an indicator of prognosis [12].

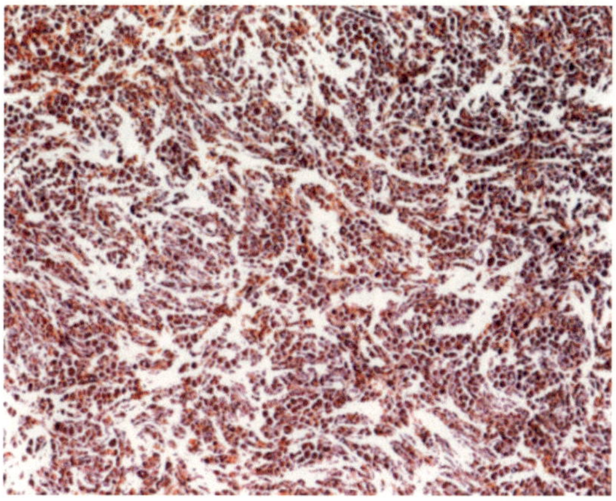

Figure 14. Canine cutaneous melanoma with marked pigmentation (H&E, 400x).

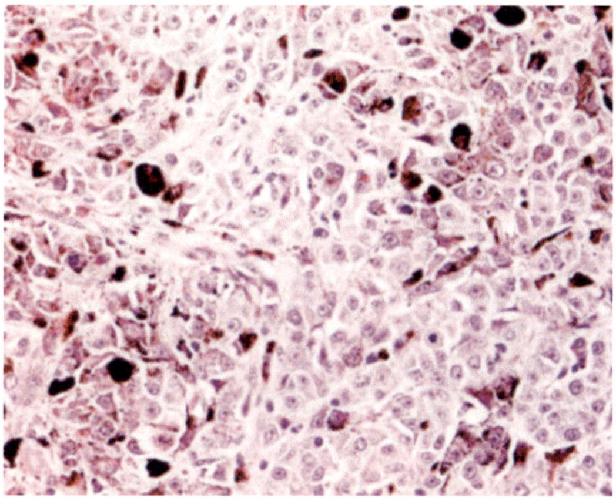

Figure 15. Canine cutaneous melanoma with moderate pigmentation (H&E, 400x).

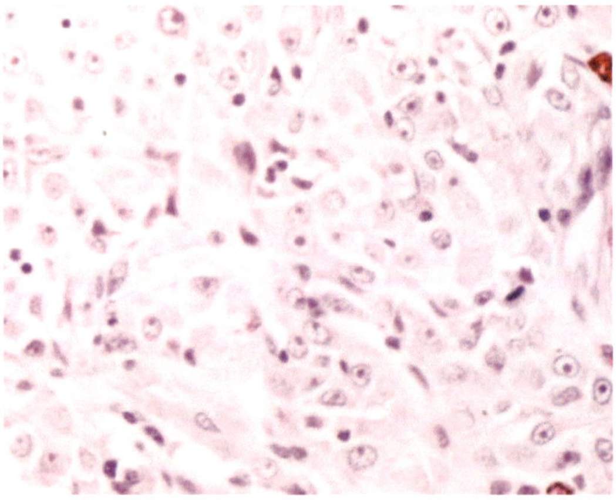

Figure 16. Amelanotic melanoma (H&E, 400x).

6.6. Junctional activity

Junctional activity refers to the proliferation of neoplastic melanocytes at the interface between the epidermis and dermis or epithelium and submucosa [53].

The presence or absence of junctional activity is not specific to melanoma and often occurs in melanocytomas [7], however, malignant melanomas arising in the skin often show marked junctional activity, (Figure 17 and Figure 18) [42].

Junctional activity was not statistically associated with survival for skin neoplasms in one study [8]. In contrast, another work considered junctional activity as an independent prognostic factor (p =0,0239) for cutaneous melanocytic neoplasms, and found that its occurrence was associated with a longer survival time (p = 0,0046) [55].

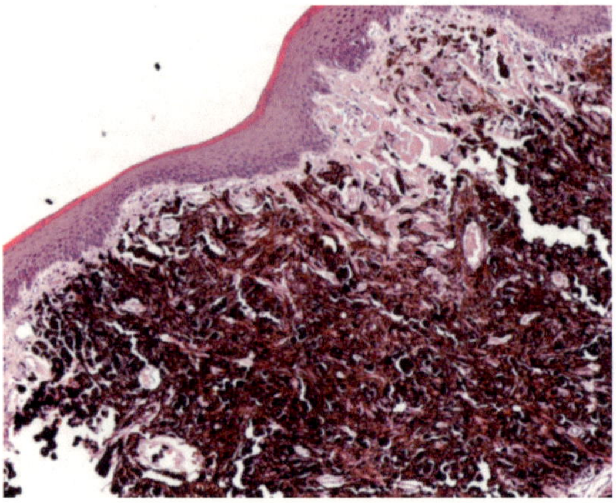

Figure 17. Canine cutaneous melanoma without junctional activity (H&E, 200x).

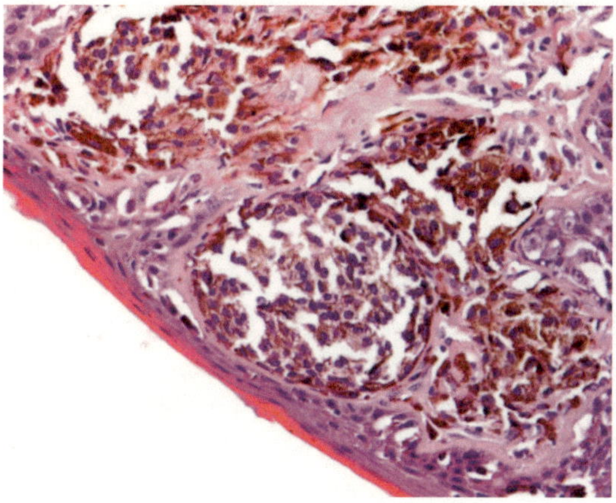

Figure 18. Canine cutaneous melanoma with junctional activity (H&E, 400x).

6.7. Intraepithelial neoplastic cells

The presence of intraepidermal tumoural cells can be graded as absent, slight (25% of neoplastic melanocytes in epidermis), moderate or prominent (more than 50% of tumour cells are present in the epidermis) [44]. However, this feature appears not to be of prognostic significance [8].

In a recent study was found that the samples of canine melanomas presented medium to prominent scatter of intraepidermal melanocytes, lower pigmentation, and higher nesting of intraepidermal melanocytes, in comparison with melanocytomas [44].

In most melanocytomas, the overlying epidermis is hyperpigmented, regardless of the presence or absence of intraepidermal clusters of neoplastic melanocytes [43].

6.8. Ulceration

Canine melanomas are most frequently ulcerated [44] and particularly larger masses [43] than melanocytomas.

According to Laprie and team [55], ulceration might be taken as a prognostic marker for this neoplasms. In the referred work, the presence of an ulcerated epidermis was associated with a shorter survival time ($p = 0,0023$) and shown to be an independent prognostic factor ($p = 0,0065$) [55]. However, two other studies found no correlation between ulceration and clinical evolution of lip, nail bed [27] or cutaneous melanocytic neoplasms [12,27].

6.9. Level of infiltration/invasion

Melanocytic tumours strictly limited to the dermis, with a shallow depth, are associated with a greater survival time ($p < 0,0001$), and deep level of infiltration has been shown to be a significant prognostic factor ($p = 0,0012$) [55]. One other study that evaluated the level of invasion (in cutaneous and subcutaneous tissues) concluded that tumors confined to the superficial dermis were associated with a benign course in 94% of cases. On the other hand, tumors reaching the deep dermis and the subcutis showed a malignant behavior; however, the sample number were too low to allow for a conclusion [12].

6.10. Necrosis

Necrosis is a common feature, particularly in larger masses [43]. The presence of necrosis was correlated with malignancy and with a short survival time in a study set of 389 melanocytic neoplasms containing both benign and malignant lesions from various locations (mouth, feet and lip, skin) [8]. In other report with a set of 38 malignant melanomas from various locations, no correlation was found with survival time [54]. In summary, necrosis is considered of limited prognostic value in animals [7].

6.11. Morphologic classification

Melanocytomas include dermal, compound, and balloon cell tumors, as well as multiple dysplastic melanocytoma syndrome in dogs [43].

Dermal melanocytoma are strictly intradermal in location and larger tumours may extend into the subcutis [43]. Melanocytomas are generally composed by spindle cells disposed in bundles, nests and whorles, with a moderate cellular concentration and a lack of stromal collagen [43,45]. Melanophages might be dispersed throughout the tumoral nodule or in aggregates [43]. Mitotic figures are ocasionally seen (inferior to 1 per 10 high power fields), and mitotic atypia is not observed [43].

Some dermal melanocytomas are composed of epithelioid or dendritic cells that are heavily pigmented [43]. Nuclear morphology may be obscured by the large amount of pigment [43]. Although nuclei may be large, there is minimal nuclear pleomorphism [43].

A compound melanocytoma has a wedge-shaped configuration, and its description refers to the fact of including both junctional and dermal components. A numerous and densely packed tumor cell population is present in the dermis, while a variable amount of tumor cells accumulate in clusters and nests within the epidermis, along the dermal–epidermal junction and in the outer follicular wall – this pattern is referred to as 'junctional activity' [43].g

Balloon cell melanocytoma have a dermal location, and are predominantly composed of large round cells [43,45], although some fusiform or polygonal melanocytes might be present [42], with an abundant, pale eosinophilic and finely granular cytoplasm [42,43,45]. These lesions often lack readily visible pigmentation; however, dust-like melanin granules may be detected in small numbers [42,43]. Nuclei are small, uniform, and ovoid [43,45] and mitotic figures are rarely observed [42,43].

Multiple dysplastic melanocytoma syndrome mostly resemble compound melanocytomas on low magnification. However, their incidence increases in larger lesions. Also, cytologic atypia and mitotic figures are present and some of the proliferating melanocytes have irregularly shaped and enlarged hyperchromatic nuclei [43].

http://dx.doi.org/10.5772/59480

Canine melanocytoma–acanthomas are mixed tumors that are composed of a benign melanocytic proliferation, resembling compound melanocytoma, and a benign epithelial proliferation [43,45]. The epithelial component usually appears follicular and resembles an isthmus-type tricholemmoma or infundibular keratinizing acanthoma [43]. The epithelial population forms a mass in the dermis composed of cords and nests with occasional small cystic structures containing keratin [45]. Melanocytic cells form nests in the epidermis and sometimes in the cords of epithelial cells within the dermal mass; melanocytic spindle cells can form whorls and bundles between the epithelial cords and nests [45]. A dermal melanocytoma– acanthoma has been immunophenotyped in a German Shepherd dog identifying the presence of keratinocytes and melanocytes [56].

Dermal melanomas have no junctional activity, but in some cases the tumour might extend deeply into the subcutaneous tissue. There might be a predominance of a certain cell type, but most tumors reveal a mixture of spindle cells, round to polygonal cells, and/or epithelioid cells. While spindle cells are poorly pigmented, more round and epithelioid cells tend to have a moderate to abundant amont of melanin granule [43]. Other important features in this kind of neoplastic lesions include a marked nuclear pleomorphism, nucleolar prominence, a moderate mitotic rate (3 or greater per 10 high power fields), atypical mitotic figures, asymmetry of the tumor nodule and a lymphoplasmacytic cell population [43].

Melanomas have an obvious 'junctional activity' pattern, with tumor cells distributed through the dermal–epidermal junction, as well as at higher levels of the epidermis, particularly in those of the nail bed and lip [43]. The intraepidermal element is mainly composed of epithelioid melanocytes, disposed individually or arranged in nests and clusters [43]. Tumours with numerous melanocytes distributed through all levels of the epidermis are referred to as lesions with a 'pagetoid' pattern [43]. Other melanomas present numerous individual neoplastic melanocytes present within the basal cell layer only, which is also referred to as an 'atypical lentiginous infiltrate' [43].

Spindle cell and desmoplastic melanomas, a subgroup of dermal melanomas, is composed predominantly of spindled melanocytes densely packed, or arranged loosely within abundant pale stroma [43]. Occasionally, there is a prominent fibroblastic component associated with the spindle shaped melanocytes, and collagen may become more abundant than the tumor cells [43]. The vast majority are amelanotic, thus a Fontana–Masson stain usually is necessary to detect the presence of melanin granules; cells are usually arranged in bundles or palisades, mimicking tumors of neural origin [43].

Balloon cell melanoma (clear cell melanoma), possess large cells with a clear eosinophilic cytoplasm [43]. The majority of balloon cell melanomas are amelanotic [43]. Some dust-like melanin granules may be present in a few tumor cells, and Fontana–Masson staining may be required for their demonstration [43,45]. These cells have a large vesicular nuclei with a prominent nucleoli [7,43]. Mitotic activity is generally low [43,45] and these dermal masses exhibit no junctional activity [45].

Signet-ring melanomas are composed of round to polygonal cells [45,52], with a pale eosinophilic cytoplasm and a darker periphery [52]. The nuclei are vesicular, crescent shaped and located at the periphery, giving the cells the appearance of signet-rings [52]. Nucleoli are prominent and occasional multinucleated cells may be present [45].

7. Histochemical diagnosis

The histological diagnosis of melanoma can be a challenge for the pathologist, especially in amelanotic tumours. On the other hand, in tumours heavily pigmented the observation of cellular features could be very difficult, requiring the use of bleaching, a histochemical method where melanin is extracted [7].

In cases where the diagnosis of a melanocytic tumor is not evident, histochemical methods specific for the cells producing melanin, such as DOPA (dihydroxyphenylalanine) reaction can be used [7,43].

8. Molecular diagnostic methods

A diagnosis of melanocytic tumors in dogs is not always easy to obtain only by conventional histological methods. Melanoma is often similar to other tumours types and has a highly variable histologic pattern which implies an accurate differential diagnosis. Furthermore, the distinction between benign and malignant tumors is not always easy [7]. Thus, it is essential the research of additional tools that can be used in melanocytic tumours diagnosis and to achieve a more accurate prognosis [57].

8.1. Classical diagnostic markers

Several markers are used to evaluate the presence of proteins normally found in melanocytes or in cells of neuroectoderm origin. The most common antibodies used are S-100 protein, *melanoma-associated antigen* (Melan-A)/MART-1, HMB-45, MEL-1, vimentin, *Neuron Specific Enolase* (NSE), microphthalmia transcription factor (MiTF), PNL2, tyrosinase, and tyrosinase-related proteins 1 and 2 (TRP-1 and TRP-2). Tumor cells are usually positive for vimentin, S100, neuron-specific enolase, and Melan-A, and negative for cytokeratin [7]. However, there is a heterogeneneity of antigen expression. The majority of melanomas are S100 positive, but other tumour types are also positive to this protein. NSE is also positive in smooth muscle and neuroendocrine tumours. Melan-A and HMB-45 expression is not a constant in every canine melanocytic tumours. Vimentin is expressed in other tumours as sarcomas [7,58-61]. HMB-45, tyrosinase, and tyrosine hydroxylase showed 100% specific but low sensitivities. One study refers that PNL2, TRP-1, and TRP-2 seems to be highly sensitive and specific for the diagnosis of canine amelanotic tumours, but it was only performed in oral melanomas [62].

In the absence of an ideal marker that excludes definitively other tumour types, confirms a diagnosis of canine melanoma and positively reacts with tumour cells in all melanomas, a diagnostic panel must be performed, including different antibodies [58-61].

8.2. Growth fraction

The proliferative activity has provided valuable information on cell growth kinetics and consequently tumour behavior in melanocytic tumours [63]. There are some markers that estimate tumor proliferation, by identifying steps associated with cell cycle [64].

MIB-1 is the monoclonal antibody which is reactive against Ki-67 nuclear antigen, a protein present in all active phases of the cell cycle (G1, S, G2 and M) while being absent in resting phase (G0) [65,66].

In canine melanocytic tumours, Ki-67 may be useful in distinction between benign and malignant tumors: melanocytomas seem to have a significant lower growth fraction than malignant melanomas [67]. Furthermore, KI-67 could be an important prognosis factor in canine cutaneous melanocytic tumours [64,68].

8.3. DNA ploidy

Changes in DNA content may reflect chromosomal alterations and represent tumour genetic instability [69-72]. Changes in the DNA ploidy constitute an early event in carcinogenesis [73,74] and detection of aneuploid cell population of pre-neoplastic lesions can be considered a factor risk of the emergence of malignant tumours [75]. Althoügh usually benign tumors were diploid [76] and aneuploidy were malignant [77], diploidy is not synonymous of a benign behavior [78]. Moreover, not all malignant tumors are aneuploid [79,80].

There are few studies about the ploidy assessment in canine melanocytic tumors [81,82] and its usefulness is still discussed. DNA index and ploidy balance seem to provide an additional tool to evaluate melanocytic tumors, being useful in the distinction of benign and malignant melanocytic tumours, mainly in amelanotic lesions [82]. Flow cytometry apparently has a limited utility for predicting the biological behavior of pigmented canine melanomas. DNA content and nuclear morphometric variables have little value in predicting survival time [83].

8.4. c-kit expression

The c-Kit protein (CD117), a transmembrane receptor that belongs to RTK III family, is a growth factor for melanocyte migration and proliferation. A loss-of-function KIT mutation are usually related with human melanocytic tumors [84,85].

In canine cutaneous melanocytic tumours, c-kit immunolabeling (both extension and intensity) were generally higher in melanocytomas than in malignant melanomas. The lack of c-kit expression in canine cutaneous malignant melanomas might be used as a criteria of tumor aggressiveness, helping to achieve a proper diagnosis [86].

8.5. Matrix metalloproteinase 2 and 9 expression

MMPs are zinc- and calcium-dependent proteases that promove not only the disruption and remodeling of structural barriers [87-89] but also a response to signaling molecules, acting as ligand for cellular adhesion receptors [90-92].

MMP-2 is widely distributed and constitutively expressed by most cells [93,94]. This protease has major roles reducing cell adhesion, stimulating cell migration and differentiation, and acting as an anti-inflammatory factor [95]. MMP-9 expression is normally induced, while almost MMPs are constitutively secreted after their translation [93,96], and may act as anti- or pro-inflammatory factors [95].

MMPs play a pivotal role in cancer development and progression [92,94,96-98] contributing to tumour proliferation, invasion, intravasation into circulation, extravasation, migration to metastatic sites and angiogenesis [90,94,99-101], deregulate the balance between growth and antigrowth signals in the tumour microenvironment [97,102,103], orchestrate inflammation [94,102,104], and evade apoptosis [89,91,102].

In canine cutaneous melanocytic tumours, MMP-2 and MMP-9 may be taken as a complement to histology in tumour diagnosis, especially in borderline lesions. Both MMP-2 and MMP-9 were expressed in the majority of canine cutaneous melanocytic tumours. MMP-2 is most commonly expressed in melanocytomas than in melanomas [105]. MMP-9 was overexpressed in malignant melanomas, compared with its expression in melanocytomas [106].

Additionally, in canine malignant melanomas a switch may occur in the MMP expression profile during tumour progression; meaning that the aggressiveness, evaluated by nuclear grade, seems to be associated with a decrease of MMP-9 and an increase of MMP-2 expression [105].

8.6. Inflammatory cells associated to tumour

The tumour associated inflammatory infiltrate may be modulate and determine tumor behavior [107]. The most studied cells in CCMT are macrophages and T-lymphocyte, however, studies on the matter are scarce.

8.6.1. Tumour Associated Macrophages (TAMs)

Macrophages constitute the most abundant leukocytes in the tumor environment, recruited by a number of chemoattractants that are produced by the tumor cells and tumor-associated stroma [108,109]. TAMs play a critical role in tumour progression and invasion by inducing neovascularization, suppressing immunocompetent cells and supporting cancer stem cells [110-113].

One study published by our group found that canine cutaneous melanocytomas present a lower number of TAMs than malignant melanomas. TAMs could constitute an important marker of canine melanocytic aggressiveness, being implicated in the progression of melanocytic precursor lesions to malignant melanoma [114].

8.6.2. T-Lymphocytic Infiltrate (TLI)

In spite of the fact that the role of the T-lymphocytic infiltrate in cancer tumourigenesis remains controversial, several studies showed that the presence of TILs are related to tumoural behavior in different tumour types [115,116].

http://dx.doi.org/10.5772/59480

Preliminary studies of our group showed that there is a difference between TILs in benign and malignant melanocytic neoplasms, whereas all melanocytomas presented little or even absence of TILs and melanomas had a more intense TILs, (Figure 19), [117].

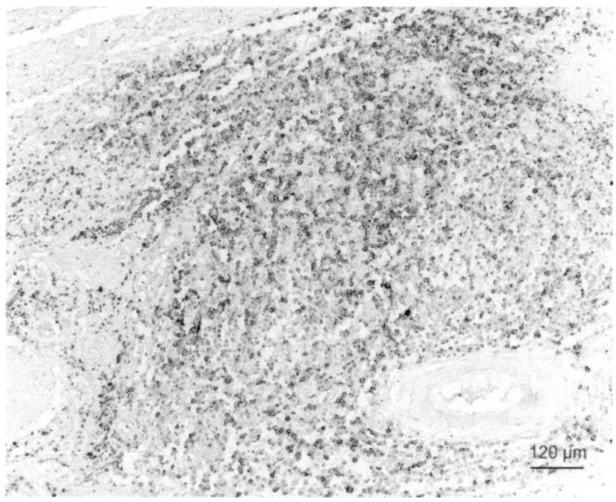

Figure 19. Abundant CD3+TILs in canine cutaneous melanoma (IHC, 100x), courtesy of Dr. Patricia Monteiro.

8.7. E-cadherin/β-catenin

Epithelial cadherin (E-cadherin) is a transmembranar glycoprotein which belongs to a family of cell to cell adhesion molecules dependent of the present of calcium molecules to bind cytoskeleton proteins through catenins. A decreased or altered expression of E-cadherin molecules often represents an increased invasiveness of tumour cells and ultimately malignancy in animal and human epithelial tumours [118,119].

In canine melanocytic tumours, the benign lesions present a membranous labelling (Figure 20) and the malignant ones an erroneous labelling, with a cytoplasmatic predominant immunostaining. Additionally, a loss of E-cadherin expression is noted in melanoma [120]. A loss of membrane E-cadherin/β-catenin complex is also detected in canine melanoma showing that a disruption of E-cadherin/β-catenin complexes and a increase of β-catenin may be associated with canine melanocytic tumours progression and aggressiveness [121].

8.8. Cox-1 and Cox-2 expression

Cyclooxygenase (COX), also known as the prostaglandin H-synthase, is an enzyme envolved on prostanoids biosynthesis. Cox-1 and Cox-2 are the two cyclooxigenase isoforms identified to date, similar in its structure but produced by different genes. The biological functions are also different: Cox-1, constitutively expressed in many tissues, plays an important role in the regulation of normal physiological, while Cox-2 is usually absent from normal cells but induced by growth factors, inflammatory reactions, tumour promoters and oncogenes [122-125].

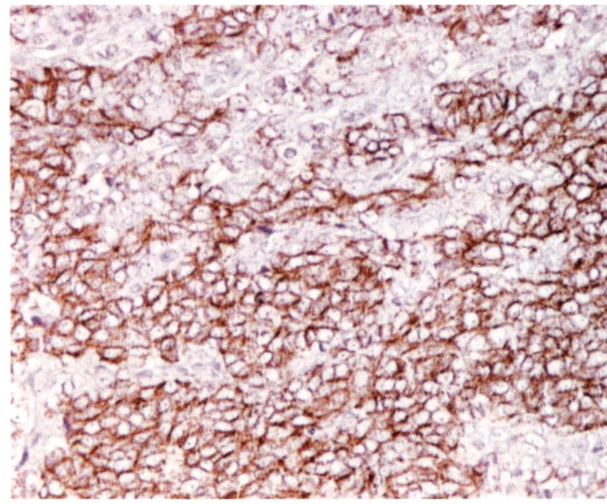

Figure 20. Strong membranar E-cadherin expression (IHC, 200x), courtesy of Dr. Mariana Santos.

Cox-1 and Cox-2 expression was recently described in canine melanocytic tumours [126-128]. Cox-1 is expressed in almost every tumours, both benign and malignant melanocytic skin lesions. Regarding Cox-2, melanocytomas did not present a positive immunolabelling, but in melanomas Cox-2 expression was present in more than 50% of the tumours [114,127]. The differences observed suggest that Cox-2 expression could be a useful tool in canine melanoma diagnosis, particularly in borderline lesions.

COX-2 expression was also observed in tumours with epithelium ulceration, necrosis, high mitotic index and nuclear grade and in less pigmented neoplasms, which could represent the higher aggressiveness of Cox-2 positive melanocytic tumours. In canine malignant melanomas, Cox-2 is associated with a higher cellular proliferation [114]. Besides the relation with tumour behavior [127], Cox-2 over-expression relates with a poor overall survival [129].

8.9. Angiogenesis

Vascular system is essential in oxygen and nutrients supply, elimination of metabolism products and promoting efficient access of leukocytes [130].

Angiogenesis is a complex process by which new blood vessels develop from pre-existing vasculature [131-133]. It is a fundamental requirement for organs development. Angiogenesis is also implicated in the pathogenesis of different pathological alterations, such as cancer and inflammation [134-136].

The tumor-associated neovascularization, by establishing continuity with the systemic circulation, allows tumor cells expressing their critical advantage in growth and facilitates metastization [137-139].

8.9.1. Vascular endothelial growth factor

Angiogenesis is a delicate process, tightly regulated by the balance of pro- and anti-angiogenic factors [140]. Among the angiogenic factors, VEGF is the more powerful and ubiquitous vascular endothelial growth factor, capable of inducing proliferation, migration, specialization and survival of endothelial cells [141,142]. Functions of VEGF family members related to neoplastic pathogenesis are linked not only to its angiogenic capacity [143], but also with the lymphangiogenesis [144,145], immunosuppression [146-148], stimulation and recruitment of endothelial and hematopoietic precursors of the bone marrow [149,150] and anti-apoptotic activity [150].

In canine melanomas, the only study published on VEGF expression is in oral melanomas. High blood concentrations of VEGF were correlated to a shorter survival time in dogs receiving definitive therapy and were associated with tumour stage [151].

This is a promising area, since VEGF may be a good indicator of preneoplastic change in melanocytic lesions [137,152]. VEGF plays a role in human melanoma progression [153,154] with a strong involvment in the switch from the radial to the vertical growth phase and the metastatic phase. So, anti-angiogenic agents might even interfere with or block melanoma progression [155].

Preliminary studies performed by Gomes J and Pires I (data unpublished) show that VEGF may be useful as a discriminating factor between malignant melanoma and benign, since it is more intensely expressed in melanomas (Figure 21) than in melanocytomas.

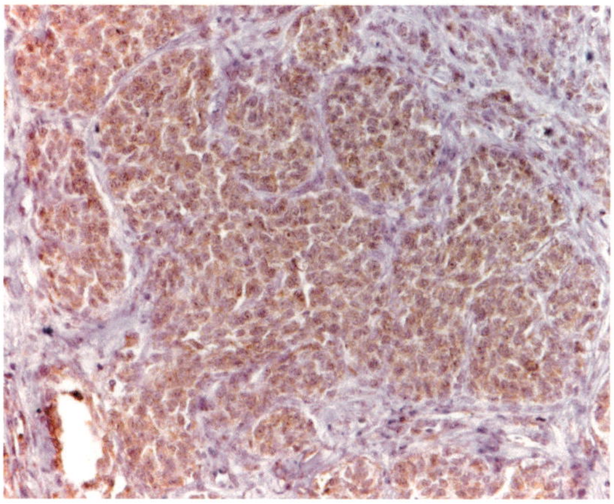

Figure 21. Canine cutaneous melanoma with a strong and diffuse VEGF expression (IHC, 200x), courtesy of Dr. Joana Gomes.

8.9.2. Microvessel Density (MVD)

Tumor angiogenesis can be estimated through a quantification of microvessel density (MVD). The most widely used method is the immunohistochemical methods, in which specific markers for endothelial cells are employed, as von Willebrand factor (Figure 22), CD34 and CD31 [156-158].

MVD seems to be important for diagnostic purposes in canine MT's. MVD is significantly higher in melanoma than in melanocytomas [159] and its expression has been associated with a high mitotic index, necrosis and ulceration (study performed by Gomes J and Pires I, data unpublished). However, its prognostic significance is still discussable [159,160].

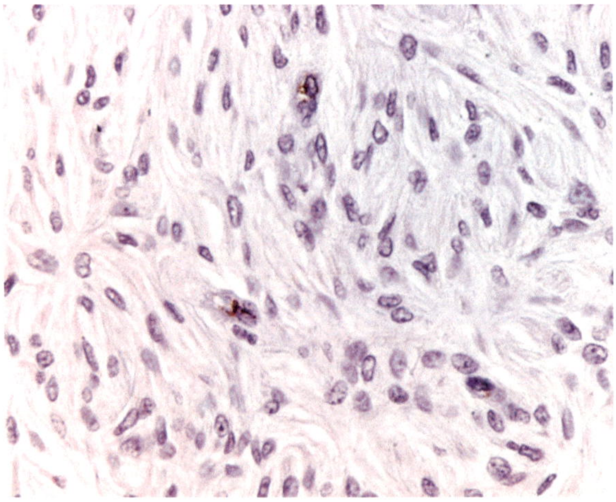

Figure 22. Tumoural neovessels positive to von Willebrand factor (IHC, 400x), courtesy of Dr. Joana Gomes.

9. Conclusions

The incidence of melanoma is increasing annually both in man and in dog. Given that dogs and humans share the same environment and similarities between human and canine melanoma it is urgent to discuss common mechanisms in melanoma development in both species.

Melanoma diagnosis in dogs can be challenging due to the variety of its histological appearances, especially when pathologists are facing amelanotic or metastatic lesions. Although the definitive diagnosis of a melanoma is often difficult by the lack of specific markers that can distinguish these lesions, immunohistochemistry plays a key role in the differential diagnosis with other neoplasms.

Additionally, the distinction between benign and malignant melanocytic tumours is not always easy, especially in borderline lesions, thus the importance of a strong knowledge of new markers of malignancy for the establishment of a definitive diagnosis and a correct therapy managment and prognosis establishment.

Author details

Luis Resende[1], Joana Moreira[2], Justina Prada[3], Felisbina Luisa Queiroga[4] and Isabel Pires[3*]

*Address all correspondence to: ipires@utad.pt

1 Veterinary Faculty, Lusófona University, Lisbon, Portugal

2 Department of Veterinary Sciences, University of Trás-os-Montes and Alto Douro, Portugal

3 Animal and Veterinary Research Centre (CECAV), Department of Veterinary Sciences, University of Trás-os-Montes and Alto Douro, Portugal

4 Center for Research and Technology of Agro-Environment and Biological Sciences (CIT-AB), Department of Veterinary Sciences, University of Trás-os-Montes and Alto Douro, Portugal

References

[1] Grandi F, Rocha RM, Miot HA, Cogliati B, Rocha NS. Immunoexpression of S100A4 in canine skin melanomas and correlation with histopathological parameters. Veterinary Quarterly 2014 1-7.

[2] Goldschmidt MH. Benign and malignant melanocytic neoplasms of domestic animals. The American Journal of Dermatopathology 1985;7 203-12.

[3] Cotchin E. Melanotic tumours of dogs. Journal of Comparative Pathology and Therapeutics 1955;65 115-IN14.

[4] Smith SH, Goldschmidt MH, McManus PM. A Comparative Review of Melanocytic Neoplasms. Veterinary Pathology 2002;39(6) 651-78.

[5] Aronsohn MG, Carpenter JL. Distal extremity melanocytic nevi and malignant melanomas in dogs. Journal of American Animal Hospital Association 1990;26 605-12.

[6] BoVeterinary Pathologylon B, Calderwood Mays MB, Hall BJ. Characteristics of canine melanomas and comparison of histology and DNA ploidy to their biologic effect. Veterinary Pathology 1990;27 96-102.

[7] Smith SH, Goldschmidt MH, McManus PM. A comparative review of melanocytic neoplasms. Veterinary Pathology 2002;39(6) 651-78.

[8] Spangler WL, Kass PH. The histologic and epidemiologic bases for prognostic considerations in canine melanocytic neoplasia. Veterinary Pathology 2006;43(2) 136-49.

[9] Trappler MC, Popovitch CA, Goldschmidt MH, Goldschmidt KH, Risbon RE. Scrotal tumors in dogs: A retrospective study of 676 cases (1986–2010). Canadian Veterinary Journal 2014;55.

[10] Ramos-Vara J, Beissenherz M, Miller M, Johnson G, Pace L, Fard A, Kottler S. Retrospective study of 338 canine oral melanomas with clinical, histologic, and immunohistochemical review of 129 cases. Veterinary Pathology 2000;37(6) 597-608.

[11] Kim D, Royal A, Villamil J. Disseminated melanoma in a dog with involvement of leptomeninges and bone marrow. Veterinary Pathology 2009;46(1) 80-3.

[12] Lacroux C, Raymon-Letron I, Bourges-Abella N, Lucas MN, Deviers A, Serra F, Degorce-Rubiales F, Delverdier M. Study of canine cutaneous melanocytic tumours: evaluation of histological and immunohistochemical prognostic criteria in 65 cases. Revue Médicine Véterinaire 2012;163(8-9) 393-401.

[13] Smedley RC, Spangler WL, Esplin DG, Kitchell BE, Bergman PJ, Ho HY, Bergin IL, Kiupel M. Prognostic markers for canine melanocytic neoplasms: a comparative review of the literature and goals for future investigation. Veterinary Pathology 2011;48(1) 54-72.

[14] Morrison WB. Tumors of the Skin and Subcutis. In: Morrison WB. (ed.) Cancer in Dogs and Cats: Medical and Surgical Management. University of Minnesota: Williams & Wilkins; 1998. p 499-500.

[15] Millanta F, Fratini F, Corazza M, Castagnaro M, Zappulli V, Poli A. Proliferation activity in oral and cutaneous canine melanocytic tumors: correlation with histological parameters, location, and clinical behaviour. Research in Veterinary Sciences 2002;73 45-51.

[16] Sulaimon SS, Kitchell BE, Ehrhart EJ. Immunohistochemical Detection of Melanoma-specific Antigens in Spontaneous Canine Melanoma. Journal of Comparative Pathology 2002;127(2–3) 162-8.

[17] Banks W, Morris E. Results of radiation treatment of naturally occurring animal tumors. Journal of the American Veterinary Medical Association 1975;166(11) 1063.

[18] Frimberger AE, Moore AS, Cincotta L, Cotter SM, Foley JW. Photodynamic therapy of naturally occurring tumors in animals using a novel benzophenothiazine photosensitizer. Clinical Cancer Research 1998;4(9) 2207-18.

[19] Gillette EL. Hyperthermia effects in animals with spontaneous tumors. National Cancer Institute monograph 1982;61 361-4.

[20] Marmor JB, Pounds D, Hahn N, Hahn GM. Treating spontaneous tumors in dogs and cats by ultrasound-induced hyperthermia. International Journal of Radiation Oncology Biology Physics 1978;4(11–12) 967-73.

[21] Westberg S, Sadeghi A, Svensson E, Segall T, Dimopoulou M, Korsgren O, Hemminki A, Loskog AS, Totterman TH, von Euler H. Treatment efficacy and immune stimu-

lation by AdCD40L gene therapy of spontaneous canine malignant melanoma. J Immunother 2013;36(6) 350-8.

[22] Dow SW, Elmslie RE, Willson AP, Roche L, Gorman C, Potter TA. In vivo tumor transfection with superantigen plus cytokine genes induces tumor regression and prolongs survival in dogs with malignant melanoma. Journal of Clinical Investigation 1998;101(11) 2406.

[23] MacEwen EG, Kurzman ID, Vail DM, Dubielzig RR, Everlith K, Madewell BR, Rodriguez CO, Phillips B, Zwahlen CH, Obradovich J. Adjuvant therapy for melanoma in dogs: results of randomized clinical trials using surgery, liposome-encapsulated muramyl tripeptide, and granulocyte macrophage colony-stimulating factor. Clinical Cancer Research 1999;5(12) 4249-58.

[24] Bergman PJ, McKnight J, Novosad A, Charney S, Farrelly J, Craft D, Wulderk M, Jeffers Y, Sadelain M, Hohenhaus AE, Segal N, Gregor P, Engelhorn M, Riviere I, Houghton AN, Wolchok JD. Long-Term Survival of Dogs with Advanced Malignant Melanoma after DNA Vaccination with Xenogeneic Human Tyrosinase: A Phase I Trial. Clinical Cancer Research 2003;9(4) 1284-90.

[25] Vail DM, Withrow SJ. Chapter 18 - Tumors of the Skin and Subcutaneous Tissues. In: Withrow SJ, Vail DM. editors. Withrow & MacEwen's Small Animal Clinical Oncology (Fourth Edition). Saint Louis: W.B. Saunders; 2007. p 375-401.

[26] Smedley R, Spangler W, Esplin D, Kitchell B, Bergman P, Ho H-Y, Bergin I, Kiupel M. Prognostic Markers for Canine Melanocytic Neoplasms A Comparative Review of the Literature and Goals for Future Investigation. Veterinary Pathology 2011;48(1) 54-72.

[27] Schultheiss PC. Histologic Features and Clinical Outcomes of Melanomas of Lip, Haired Skin, and Nail Bed Locations of Dogs. Journal of Veterinary Diagnostic Investigation 2006;18(4) 422-5.

[28] Orkin M, Schwartzman RM. A Comparative Study of Canine and Human Dermatology. The Journal of Investigative Dermatology 1959;32 451-66.

[29] de Camargo LP, Conceição LG, dos Santos Costa PR. Neoplasias melanocíticas cutâneas em cães: estudo retrospectivo de 68 casos (1996-2004). Brazilian Journal of Veterinary Research and Animal Science 2008;45(2) 138-52.

[30] Goldschmidt M, Hendrick M. Tumors of the skin and soft tissues. Tumors in Domestic Animals, Fourth Edition 2008 45-117.

[31] Spangler W, Kass P. The histologic and epidemiologic bases for prognostic considerations in canine melanocytic neoplasia. Veterinary Pathology 2006;43(2) 136-49.

[32] Junqueira L, Carneiro J. Pele e Anexos. Histologia Básica. Rio de Janeiro, RJ, Brazil 2004. p 359-70.

[33] Marks R. Epidemiology of melanoma. Clinical and Experimental Dermatology 2000;25(6) 459-63.

[34] Valentine B, McManus P, Knox A. Malignant transformation of a giant congenital pigmented nevus (hamartoma) in a dog. Veterinary Dermatology (United Kingdom) 1999.

[35] Conroy JD. Melanocytic Tumors of Domestic Animals: With Special Reference to Dogs. Archives of Dermatology 1967;96(4) 372-80.

[36] Mulligan R. Melanoblastic tumors in the dog. American Journal of Veterinary Research 1961;22 345-51.

[37] Koenig A, Bianco S, Fosmire S, Wojcieszyn J, Modiano J. Expression and significance of p53, rb, p21/waf-1, p16/ink-4a, and PTEN tumor suppressors in canine melanoma. Veterinary Pathology 2002;39(4) 458-72.

[38] Dobson JM. Breed-predispositions to cancer in pedigree dogs. International Scholarly Research Notices 2013;2013.

[39] Hsu M-Y, Meier FE, Nesbit M, Hsu J-Y, Van Belle P, Elder DE, Herlyn M. E-cadherin expression in melanoma cells restores keratinocyte-mediated growth control and down-regulates expression of invasion-related adhesion receptors. The American Journal of Pathology 2000;156(5) 1515-25.

[40] Meier F, Satyamoorthy K, Nesbit M, Hsu M-Y, Schittek B, Garbe C, Herlyn M. Molecular events in melanoma development and progression. Front Biosci 1998;3(D) 1005-10.

[41] Seiter S, Schadendorf D, Herrmann K, Schneider M, Rösel M, Arch R, Tilgen W, Zöller M. Expression of CD44 variant isoforms in malignant melanoma. Clinical Cancer Research 1996;2(3) 447-56.

[42] Goldschmidt MH, Hendrick MJ. Tumors of the Skin and Soft Tissues. In: M. DJ. (ed.) Tumors in Domestic Animals. Fourth Edition ed. Iowa State: Iowa State Press; 2002. p 78-83.

[43] Gross TL, Ihrke PJ, Walder EJ, Affolter VK. Melanocytic tumors. In: Gross TL, Ihrke PJ, Walder EJ, Affolter VK. editors. Skin Diseases of the Dog and Cat: Blackwell Science Ltd; 2005. p 813-36.

[44] Campagne C, Jule S, Alleaume C, Bernex F, Ezagal J, Chateau-Joubert S, Estrada M, Aubin-Houzelstein G, Panthier JJ, Egidy G. Canine melanoma diagnosis: RACK1 as a potential biological marker. Veterinary Pathology 2013;50(6) 1083-90.

[45] Ginn PE, Mensett JEKL, Rukich PM. The skin and appendages. In: Grant M. (ed.) Jubb, Kennedy & Palmer's Pathology of Domestic Animals. Ontario, Canada: Grant, M.; 2007. p 759-60.

[46] Friedrichs KR, Young KM. Diagnostic cytopathology in clinical oncology. Withrow and MacEwen's Small Animal Clinical Oncology 2013 111.

[47] Daskalopoulou D, Gourgiotou K, Thodou E, Vaida S, Markidou S. Rapid cytological diagnosis of primary skin tumours and tumour-like conditions. Acta Dermato-Venereologica 1997;77(4) 292-5.

[48] Dey P, Mallik M, Gupta S, Vasishta R. Role of fine needle aspiration cytology in the diagnosis of soft tissue tumours and tumour-like lesions. Cytopathology 2004;15(1) 32-7.

[49] Simeonov RS. The accuracy of fine-needle aspiration cytology in the diagnosis of canine skin and subcutaneous masses. Comparative Clinical Pathology 2012;21(2) 143-7.

[50] Ghisleni G, Roccabianca P, Ceruti R, Stefanello D, Bertazzolo W, Bonfanti U, Caniatti M. Correlation between fine-needle aspiration cytology and histopathology in the evaluation of cutaneous and subcutaneous masses from dogs and cats. Veterinary Clinical Pathology 2006;35(1) 24-30.

[51] Liu W, Bennet M, Helm T. Canine melanoma: a comparison with human pigmented epithelioid melanocytoma. International Journal of Dermatology 2011;50 1542-5.

[52] Cangul IT, van Garderen E, van der Linde-Sipman JS, van den Ingh TS, Schalken JA. Canine balloon and signet-ring cell melanomas: a histological and immunohistochemical characterization. Journal of Comparative Pathology 2001;125(2-3) 166-73.

[53] Goldschmidt MH, Dustan RW, Stannard AA, von Tscharner C, Walder EJ, Yager JA. Melanocytic tumors and tumor-like lesions. In: Goldschmidt MH, Dustan RW, Stannard AA, von Tscharner C, Walder EJ, Yager JA. editors. Washington DC: Armed Forces Institute of Pathology; 1998. p 38-48.

[54] Millanta F, Fratini F, Corazza M, Castagnaro M, Zappulli V, Poli A. Proliferation activity in oral and cutaneous canine melanocytic tumours: correlation with histological parameters, location, and clinical behaviour. Research in Veterinary Sciences 2002;73(1) 45-51.

[55] Laprie C, Abadie J, Amardeilh MF, Net JLLE, Lagadic M, Delverdier M. MIB-1 immunoreactivity correlates with biologic behaviour in canine cutaneous melanoma. Veterinary Dermatology 2001;12(3) 139-47.

[56] De los Monteros AE, de las Mulas JM, Fernández A, Orós J, Rodríguez F. Immunohistopathologic Characterization of a Dermal Melanocytoma-Acanthoma in a German Shepherd Dog. Veterinary Pathology 2000;37(3) 268-71.

[57] USDA licenses DNA vaccine for treatment of melanoma in dogs. Journal of American Veterinary Medical Association 2010;236(5) 495.

[58] Koenig A, Wojcieszyn J, Weeks BR, Modiano JF. Expression of S100a, vimentin, NSE, and melan A/MART-1 in seven canine melanoma cells lines and twenty-nine retrospective cases of canine melanoma. Veterinary Pathology 2001;38(4) 427-35.

[59] Sulaimon S, Kitchell B, Ehrhart E. Immunohistochemical detection of melanoma-specific antigens in spontaneous canine melanoma. Journal of Comparative Pathology 2002;127(2-3) 162-8.

[60] Ramos-Vara JA, Beissenherz ME, Miller MA, Johnson GC, Pace LW, Fard A, Kottler SJ. Retrospective study of 338 canine oral melanomas with clinical, histologic, and immunohistochemical review of 129 cases. Veterinary Pathology 2000;37(6) 597-608.

[61] Sandusky GE, Jr., Carlton WW, Wightman KA. Immunohistochemical staining for S100 protein in the diagnosis of canine amelanotic melanoma. Veterinary Pathology 1985;22(6) 577-81.

[62] Smedley RC, Lamoureux J, Sledge DG, Kiupel M. Immunohistochemical diagnosis of canine oral amelanotic melanocytic neoplasms. Veterinary Pathology 2011;48(1) 32-40.

[63] Rieger E, Hofmann-Wellenhof R, Soyer HP, Kofler R, Cerroni L, Smolle J, Kerl H. Comparison of proliferative activity as assessed by proliferating cell nuclear antigen (PCNA) and Ki-67 monoclonal antibodies in melanocytic skin lesions. A quantitative immunohistochemical study. Journal of Cutaneous Pathology 1993;20(3) 229-36.

[64] Millanta F, Fratini F, Corazza M, Castagnaro M, Zappulli V, Poli A. Proliferation activity in oral and cutaneous canine melanocytic tumours: correlation with histological parameters, location, and clinical behaviour. Research in Veterinary Sciences 2002;73(1) 45-51.

[65] Gerdes J, Schwab U, Lemke H, Stein H. Production of a mouse monoclonal antibody reactive with a human nuclear antigen associated with cell proliferation. International Journal of Cancer 1983;31(1) 13-20.

[66] Gerdes J, Li L, Schlueter C, Duchrow M, Wohlenberg C, Gerlach C, Stahmer I, Kloth S, Brandt E, Flad HD. Immunobiochemical and molecular biologic characterization of the cell proliferation-associated nuclear antigen that is defined by monoclonal antibody Ki-67. American Journal of Pathology 1991;138(4) 867-73.

[67] Laprie C, Abadie J, Amardeilh MF, Net JL, Lagadic M, Delverdier M. MIB-1 immunoreactivity correlates with biologic behaviour in canine cutaneous melanoma. Veterinary Dermatology 2001;12(3) 139-47.

[68] Roels S, Tilmant K, Ducatelle R. PCNA and Ki67 proliferation markers as criteria for prediction of clinical behaviour of melanocytic tumours in cats and dogs. Journal of Comparative Pathology 1999;121(1) 13-24.

[69] Grollino MG, Cavallo D, Di Silverio F, Rocchi M, De Vita R. Interphase cytogenetics and flow cytometry analyses of renal tumours. Anticancer Research 1993;13(6A) 2239-44.

[70] Yamal JM, Cox D, Hittelman WN, Boiko I, Malpica A, Guillaud M, MacAulay C, Follen M, Vlastos AT. Quantitative histopathology and chromosome 9 polysomy in a clinical trial of 4-HPR. Gynecology Oncology 2004;94(2) 296-306.

[71] Kronenwett U, Castro J, Roblick UJ, Fujioka K, Ostring C, Faridmoghaddam F, Laytragoon-Lewin N, Tribukait B, Auer G. Expression of cyclins A, E and topoisomerase II alpha correlates with centrosome amplification and genomic instability and influences the reliability of cytometric S-phase determination. BMC Cell Biology 2003;4 8.

[72] Sidoni A, Cavaliere A, D'Amico GA, Brachelente G, Bucciarelli E. Biopathological significance of single cell DNA aneuploidy measured by static cytometry in breast cancer. Breast 2001;10(4) 325-9.

[73] Li R, Sonik A, Stindl R, Rasnick D, Duesberg P. Aneuploidy vs. gene mutation hypothesis of cancer: recent study claims mutation but is found to support aneuploidy. Proceedings of the National Academy of Sciences USA 2000;97(7) 3236-41.

[74] Postier RG, Lerner MR, Lightfoot SA, Vannarath R, Lane MM, Hanas JS, Brackett DJ. DNA ploidy and markovian analysis of neoplastic progression in experimental pancreatic cancer. Journal of Histochemistry Cytochemistry 2003;51(3) 303-9.

[75] Elkowitz D, Daum F, Markowitz J, Proccaccino J, Boas E, Cuomo J, Kahn E. Risk factors for carcinoma of the pelvic ileal pouch/anal canal in ulcerative colitis. Annals of Clinical & Laboratory Science 2004;34(2) 143-9.

[76] Cohen C. Image cytometric analysis in pathology. Human Pathology 1996;27(5) 482-93.

[77] Nordemar S, Hogmo A, Lindholm J, Tani E, Sjostrom B, Auer G, Munck-Wikland E. The clinical value of image cytometry DNA analysis in distinguishing branchial cleft cysts from cystic metastases of head and neck cancer. Laryngoscope 2002;112(11) 1983-7.

[78] Harada K, Nishizaki T, Ozaki S, Kubota H, Okamura T, Ito H, Sasaki K. Cytogenetic alterations in pituitary adenomas detected by comparative genomic hybridization. Cancer Genetics and Cytogenetics 1999;112(1) 38-41.

[79] Frazier KS, Hines ME, 2nd, Hurvitz AI, Robinson PG, Herron AJ. Analysis of DNA aneuploidy and c-myc oncoprotein content of canine plasma cell tumors using flow cytometry. Veterinary Pathology 1993;30(6) 505-11.

[80] Lewis JE, Olsen KD, Sebo TJ. Carcinoma ex pleomorphic adenoma: pathologic analysis of 73 cases. Human Pathology 2001;32(6) 596-604.

[81] Johnson TS, Raju MR, Giltinan RK, Gillette EL. Ploidy and DNA distribution analysis of spontaneous dog tumors by flow cytometry. Cancer Research 1981;41(8) 3005-9.

[82] Bolon B, Calderwood Mays MB, Hall BJ. Characteristics of canine melanomas and comparison of histology and DNA ploidy to their biologic behavior. Veterinary Pathology 1990;27(2) 96-102.

[83] Roels SL, Van Daele AJ, Van Marck EA, Ducatelle RV. DNA ploidy and nuclear morphometric variables for the evaluation of melanocytic tumors in dogs and cats. American Journal of Veterinary Research 2000;61(9) 1074-9.

[84] Pilloni L, Bianco P, Difelice E, Cabras S, Castellanos ME, Atzori L, Ferreli C, Mulas P, Nemolato S, Faa G. The usefulness of c-Kit in the immunohistochemical assessment of melanocytic lesions. European Journal of Histochemistry 2011;55(2) e20.

[85] Yarden Y, Kuang WJ, Yang-Feng T, Coussens L, Munemitsu S, Dull TJ, Chen E, Schlessinger J, Francke U, Ullrich A. Human proto-oncogene c-kit: a new cell surface receptor tyrosine kinase for an unidentified ligand. EMBO Journal 1987;6(11) 3341-51.

[86] Gomes J, Queiroga FL, Prada J, Pires I. Study of c-kit immunoexpression in canine cutaneous melanocytic tumors. Melanoma Research 2012;22(3) 195-201.

[87] Foda HD, Zucker S. Matrix metalloproteinases in cancer invasion, metastasis and angiogenesis. Drug Discovery Today 2001;6(9) 478-82.

[88] Stamenkovic I. Extracellular matrix remodelling: the role of matrix metalloproteinases. Journal of Pathology 2003;200(4) 448-64.

[89] Szabo KA, Ablin RJ, Singh G. Matrix metalloproteinases and the immune response. Clinical and Applied Immunology Reviews 2004;4(5) 295-319.

[90] López-Otín C, Palavalli LH, Samuels Y. Protective roles of matrix metalloproteinases: From mouse models to human cancer. Cell Cycle 2009;8(22) 3657-62.

[91] Cauwe B, Van den Steen PE, Opdenakker G. The biochemical, biological, and pathological kaleidoscope of cell surface substrates processed by matrix metalloproteinases. Critical Reviews in Biochemistry and Molecular Biology 2007;42 113-85.

[92] Sternlicht MD, Werb Z. How matrix metalloproteinases regulate cell behavior. Cell and Developmental Biology 2001;17 463-516.

[93] Bergman RL. Matrix Metalloproteinases 2 and 9 in Normal Canine Cerebrospinal Fluid.Master thesis. Faculty of the Virginia Polytechnic Institute and State University 2001.

[94] Björklund M, Koivunen E. Gelatinase-mediated migration and invasion of cancer cells. Biochimica et Biophysica Acta (BBA) - Reviews on Cancer 2005;1755(1) 37-69.

[95] Visse R, Nagase H. Matrix Metalloproteinases and Tissue Inhibitors of Metalloproteinases. Circulation Research 2003;92(8) 827-39.

[96] Tonti Ga, Mannello F, Cacci E, Biagioni S. Neural stem cells at the crossroads: MMPs may tell the way. The International Journal of Developmental Biology 2009;53(1) 1-17.

[97] Handsley MM, Edwards DR. Metalloproteinases and their inhibitors in tumor angiogenesis. International Journal of Cancer 2005;115(6) 849-60.

[98] Galliera E, Tacchini L, Romanelli MM. Matrix metalloproteinases as biomarkers of disease: updates and new insights. Clin Chem Lab Med 2014.

[99] Chaudhary A, Singh M, Bharti A, Asotra K, Sundaram S, Mehrotra R. Genetic polymorphisms of matrix metalloproteinases and their inhibitors in potentially malignant and malignant lesions of the head and neck. Journal of Biomedical Science 2010;17(10).

[100] Joyce JA, Pollard JW. Microenvironmental regulation of metastasis. Nature Reviews Cancer 2009;9(4) 239-52.

[101] Mannello F, Medda V. Nuclear localization of Matrix metalloproteinases. Progress in Histochemistry and Cytochemistry 2012;47(1) 27-58.

[102] Kessenbrock K, Plaks V, Werb Z. Matrix Metalloproteinases: Regulators of the Tumor Microenvironment. Cell 2010;141(1) 52-67.

[103] Stamenkovic I. Matrix metalloproteinases in tumor invasion and metastasis. Seminars in Cancer Biology 2000;10(6) 415-33.

[104] Deryugina E, Quigley J. Matrix metalloproteinases and tumor metastasis. Cancer and Metastasis Reviews 2006;25(1) 9-34.

[105] Pires I, Gomes J, Prada J, Pereira D, Queiroga FL. MMP-2 and MMP-9 Expression in Canine Cutaneous Melanocytic Tumours: Evidence of a Relationship with Tumoural Malignancy2013. In: Lester D. (ed.) Recent Advances in the Biology, Therapy and Management of Melanoma. Rijeka: InTech; 2013.

[106] Docampo MJ, Cabrera J, Rabanal RM, Bassols A. Expression of matrix metalloproteinase-2 and -9 and membrane-type 1 matrix metalloproteinase in melanocytic tumors of dogs and canine melanoma cell lines. Am J Vet Res 2011;72(8) 1087-96.

[107] Le Bitoux MA, Stamenkovic I. Tumor-host interactions: the role of inflammation. Histochemical Cell Biology 2008;130(6) 1079-90.

[108] Guo C, Buranych A, Sarkar D, Fisher PB, Wang XY. The role of tumor-associated macrophages in tumor vascularization. Vascular Cell 2014;6(1) 2.

[109] Owen JL, Mohamadzadeh M. Macrophages and chemokines as mediators of angiogenesis. Frontiers Physiology 2013;4 159.

[110] Vinogradov S, Warren G, Wei X. Macrophages associated with tumors as potential targets and therapeutic intermediates. Nanomedicine (Lond) 2014;9(5) 695-707.

[111] Chanmee T, Ontong P, Konno K, Itano N. Tumor-associated macrophages as major players in the tumor microenvironment. Cancers (Basel) 2014;6(3) 1670-90.

[112] Brocker EB, Zwadlo G, Suter L, Brune M, Sorg C. Infiltration of primary and metastatic melanomas with macrophages of the 25F9-positive phenotype. Cancer Immunology & Immunotherapy 1987;25(2) 81-6.

[113] Bianchini F, Massi D, Marconi C, Franchi A, Baroni G, Santucci M, Mannini A, Mugnai G, Calorini L. Expression of cyclo-oxygenase-2 in macrophages associated with cutaneous melanoma at different stages of progression. Prostaglandins & Other Lipid Mediators 2007;83(4) 320-8.

[114] Pires I, Prada J, Coelho L, Garcia A, Queiroga FL. Tumour-Associated Macrophages (TAMs) and Cox-2 Expression in Canine Melanocytic Lesions. In: Murph M. (ed.) Melanoma in the Clinic - Diagnosis, Management and Complications of Malignancy. Rijeka: InTech; 2011.

[115] Carvalho MI, Pires I, Prada J, Queiroga FL. T-lymphocytic infiltrate in canine mammary tumours: clinic and prognostic implications. In Vivo 2011;25(6) 963-9.

[116] Kim JH, Yu CH, Yhee JY, Im KS, Sur JH. Lymphocyte infiltration, expression of interleukin (IL) -1, IL-6 and expression of mutated breast cancer susceptibility gene-1 correlate with malignancy of canine mammary tumours. J Comp Pathol 2010;142(2-3) 177-86.

[117] Monteiro P. Factores de prognóstico em melanomas em caninos. UTAD Vila Real; 2013.

[118] Makrilia N, Kollias A, Manolopoulos L, Syrigos K. Cell adhesion molecules: role and clinical significance in cancer. Cancer Investigation 2009;27(10) 1023-37.

[119] Patel SD, Chen CP, Bahna F, Honig B, Shapiro L. Cadherin-mediated cell-cell adhesion: sticking together as a family. Current Opinion Structural Biology 2003;13(6) 690-8.

[120] Santos M. Estudo da Immunoexpressão da caderina E em Tumores Melanocíticos do Cão. UTAD Vila Real; 2012.

[121] Han JI, Kim Y, Kim DY, Na KJ. Alteration in E-cadherin/beta-catenin expression in canine melanotic tumors. Veterinary Pathology 2013;50(2) 274-80.

[122] O'Banion MK, Winn VD, Young DA. cDNA cloning and functional activity of a glucocorticoid-regulated inflammatory cyclooxygenase. Proceedings of the National Academy of Sciences USA 1992;89(11) 4888-92.

[123] Williams CS, DuBois RN. Prostaglandin endoperoxide synthase: why two isoforms? Am J Physiol 1996;270(3 Pt 1) G393-400.

[124] Hla T, Bishop-Bailey D, Liu CH, Schaefers HJ, Trifan OC. Cyclooxygenase-1 and -2 isoenzymes. International Journal Biochemical Cell Biology 1999;31(5) 551-7.

[125] Dubois RN, Abramson SB, Crofford L, Gupta RA, Simon LS, Van De Putte LB, Lipsky PE. Cyclooxygenase in biology and disease. FASEB Journal 1998;12(12) 1063-73.

[126] Paglia D, Dubielzig RR, Kado-Fong HK, Maggs DJ. Expression of cyclooxygenase-2 in canine uveal melanocytic neoplasms. American Journal of Veterinary Research 2009;70(10) 1284-90.

[127] Pires I, Garcia A, Prada J, Queiroga FL. COX-1 and COX-2 expression in canine cutaneous, oral and ocular melanocytic tumours. Journal of Comparative Pathololology 2010;143(2-3) 142-9.

[128] Mohammed SI, Khan KN, Sellers RS, Hayek MG, DeNicola DB, Wu L, Bonney PL, Knapp DW. Expression of cyclooxygenase-1 and 2 in naturally-occurring canine cancer. Prostaglandins Leukocyt Essential Fatty Acids 2004;70(5) 479-83.

[129] Martinez CM, Penafiel-Verdu C, Vilafranca M, Ramirez G, Mendez-Gallego M, Buendia AJ, Sanchez J. Cyclooxygenase-2 expression is related with localization, proliferation, and overall survival in canine melanocytic neoplasms. Veterinary Pathology 2011;48(6) 1204-11.

[130] Thomas KA. Vascular endothelial growth factor, a potent and selective angiogenic agent. Journal Biology Chemestry 1996;271(2) 603-6.

[131] Robinson CJ, Stringer SE. The splice variants of vascular endothelial growth factor (VEGF) and their receptors. Journal Cell Science 2001;114(Pt 5) 853-65.

[132] Folkman J, D'Amore PA. Blood vessel formation: what is its molecular basis? Cell 1996;87(7) 1153-5.

[133] Risau W. Mechanisms of angiogenesis. Nature 1997;386(6626) 671-4.

[134] Ferrara N, Keyt B. Vascular endothelial growth factor: basic biology and clinical implications. EXS 1997;79 209-32.

[135] Ferrara N, Davis-Smyth T. The biology of vascular endothelial growth factor. Endocrine Reviews 1997;18(1) 4-25.

[136] Marneros AG. Tumor angiogenesis in melanoma. Hematology Oncology Clinics of North America 2009;23(3) 431-46.

[137] Einspahr JG, Thomas TL, Saboda K, Nickolof BJ, Warneke J, Curiel-Lewandrowski C, Ranger-Moore J, Duckett L, Bangert J, Fruehauf JP, Alberts DS. Expression of vascular endothelial growth factor in early cutaneous melanocytic lesion progression. Cancer 2007;110(11) 2519-27.

[138] Papetti M, Herman IM. Mechanisms of normal and tumor-derived angiogenesis. American Journa Physiology Cell Physiology 2002;282(5) C947-70.

[139] Mittal K, Ebos J, Rini B. Angiogenesis and the tumor microenvironment: vascular endothelial growth factor and beyond. Seminars Oncology 2014;41(2) 235-51.

[140] Benazzi C, Al-Dissi A, Chau CH, Figg WD, Sarli G, de Oliveira JT, Gartner F. Angiogenesis in spontaneous tumors and implications for comparative tumor biology. Scientific World Journal 2014;2014 919570.

[141] Ruhrberg C. Growing and shaping the vascular tree: multiple roles for VEGF. Bioessays 2003;25(11) 1052-60.

[142] Hoeben A, Landuyt B, Highley MS, Wildiers H, Van Oosterom AT, De Bruijn EA. Vascular endothelial growth factor and angiogenesis. Pharmacological Reviews 2004;56(4) 549-80.

[143] Goel HL, Mercurio AM. VEGF targets the tumour cell. Nature Reviews Cancer 2013;13(12) 871-82.

[144] Baldwin ME, Stacker SA, Achen MG. Molecular control of lymphangiogenesis. Bioessays 2002;24(11) 1030-40.

[145] Nagy JA, Vasile E, Feng D, Sundberg C, Brown LF, Detmar MJ, Lawitts JA, Benjamin L, Tan X, Manseau EJ, Dvorak AM, Dvorak HF. Vascular permeability factor/vascular endothelial growth factor induces lymphangiogenesis as well as angiogenesis. Journal Experimental Medicine 2002;196(11) 1497-506.

[146] Gabrilovich D, Ishida T, Oyama T, Ran S, Kravtsov V, Nadaf S, Carbone DP. Vascular endothelial growth factor inhibits the development of dendritic cells and dramatically affects the differentiation of multiple hematopoietic lineages in vivo. Blood 1998;92(11) 4150-66.

[147] Ohm JE, Gabrilovich DI, Sempowski GD, Kisseleva E, Parman KS, Nadaf S, Carbone DP. VEGF inhibits T-cell development and may contribute to tumor-induced immune suppression. Blood 2003;101(12) 4878-86.

[148] Ohm JE, Carbone DP. VEGF as a mediator of tumor-associated immunodeficiency. Immunology Research 2001;23(2-3) 263-72.

[149] Hattori K, Dias S, Heissig B, Hackett NR, Lyden D, Tateno M, Hicklin DJ, Zhu Z, Witte L, Crystal RG, Moore MA, Rafii S. Vascular endothelial growth factor and angiopoietin-1 stimulate postnatal hematopoiesis by recruitment of vasculogenic and hematopoietic stem cells. Journal Experimental Medice 2001;193(9) 1005-14.

[150] Xie K, Wei D, Shi Q, Huang S. Constitutive and inducible expression and regulation of vascular endothelial growth factor. Cytokine Growth Factor Rev 2004;15(5) 297-324.

[151] Taylor KH, Smith AN, Higginbotham M, Schwartz DD, Carpenter DM, Whitley EM. Expression of vascular endothelial growth factor in canine oral malignant melanoma. Veterinary Comparative Oncology 2007;5(4) 208-18.

[152] Simonetti O, Lucarini G, Brancorsini D, Nita P, Bernardini ML, Biagini G, Offidani A. Immunohistochemical expression of vascular endothelial growth factor, matrix met-

alloproteinase 2, and matrix metalloproteinase 9 in cutaneous melanocytic lesions. Cancer 2002;95(9) 1963-70.

[153] Bayer-Garner IB, Hough AJ, Jr., Smoller BR. Vascular endothelial growth factor expression in malignant melanoma: prognostic versus diagnostic usefulness. Modern Pathology 1999;12(8) 770-4.

[154] Brychtova S, Bezdekova M, Brychta T, Tichy M. The role of vascular endothelial growth factors and their receptors in malignant melanomas. Neoplasma 2008;55(4) 273-9.

[155] Vacca A, Ria R, Ribatti D, Bruno M, Dammacco F. Angiogenesis and tumor progression in melanoma. Recenti Prog Med 2000;91(11) 581-7.

[156] Wang Y, Yao X, Ge J, Hu F, Zhao Y. Can Vascular Endothelial Growth Factor and Microvessel Density Be Used as Prognostic Biomarkers for Colorectal Cancer? A Systematic Review and Meta-Analysis. ScientificWorldJournal 2014;2014 102736.

[157] Nico B, Benagiano V, Mangieri D, Maruotti N, Vacca A, Ribatti D. Evaluation of microvascular density in tumors: pro and contra. Histology Histopathology 2008;23(5) 601-7.

[158] Fanelli M, Locopo N, Gattuso D, Gasparini G. Assessment of tumor vascularization: immunohistochemical and non-invasive methods. International Journal Biological Markers 1999;14(4) 218-31.

[159] Cuitino MC, Massone AR, Idiart JR. Lack of prognostic significance of angiogenesis in canine melanocytic tumours. Journal of Comparative Pathology 2012;147(2-3) 147-52.

[160] Mukaratirwa S, Chikafa L, Dliwayo R, Moyo N. Mast cells and angiogenesis in canine melanomas: malignancy and clinicopathological factors. Veterinary Dermatology 2006;17(2) 141-6.

Section 3

Therapeutic Approaches Against Disease

Chapter 8

Emerging Drug Combination Approaches in Melanoma Therapy

Jin Wang, Duane D. Miller and Wei Li

Additional information is available at the end of the chapter

http://dx.doi.org/10.5772/59360

1. Introduction

The FDA approvals of ipilimumab targeting the cytotoxic T lymphocyte-associated antigen 4 (CTLA-4), pembrolizumab targeting the programmed cell death protein 1 (PD-1), BRAF inhibitors vemurafenib and dabrafenib, and MEK inhibitor trametinib represent significant milestones in more effective treatment of advanced melanoma. However, it is clear that the use of these single-agent therapies have limitation clinically. For example, ipilimumab only showed 4.5% objective response rate when used alone in a Phase II clinical trial [1]. The efficacy of vemurafenib lasts only 6.7 months before the disease relapses especially in patients with metastatic melanoma [2]. Therefore, rational combination approaches are strongly preferred in order to improve the overall patient progression-free survival (PFS), overcome or delay the development of multi-drug resistance and reduce the incidents of side effects [3-6].

In this chapter, we will summarize the emerging combination therapy approaches from both clinical trial and preclinical research in the past five years.

2. Combination of kinase inhibitors for melanoma treatment

2.1. Combined inhibitions targeting components within the Mitogen-Activated Protein Kinase (MAPK) signaling pathway

2.1.1. Targeting BRAF: Mechanism of action, toxicity and drug resistance

BRAF is a serine/threonine growth signal transduction protein kinase from RAF family which plays important roles in the RAS/RAF/MEK/ERK pathway and directs cell division, proliferation and secretion [7]. BRAF inhibitors (BRAFi) are ATP-competitive ligands which inactivate the function of BRAF protein by either stabilizing the inactive form of kinase domain (sorafenib) or preferentially inhibit the active form of the kinase (vemurafenib, dabrafenib) [8, 9]. Various mutations of *BRAF* gene have been identified in cancers including melanoma, colorectal and ovarian cancer. Around 60% of human melanoma adopted the T1799A transversion in exon 15, which lead to $BRAF^{V600E}$ mutation and the over-activated monomer phosphorylation for $BRAF^{V600E}$ [9, 10]. The two FDA approved BRAFi (Vemurafenib and dabrafenib) selectively and potently block the activation of $BRAF^{V600E}$ and thus inhibit the MAPK signaling pathway. These drugs show very high clinical efficacy in metastatic melanoma patients harboring the $BRAF^{V600E}$ mutation [11-13]. Interestingly, in a clinical study which treated 43 patients with any V600 BRAF mutation including the rare V600R variant, five out of the six melanoma patients having V600R mutation had clinical response to the therapy of vemurafenib or dabrafenib (response rate 86%) [14].

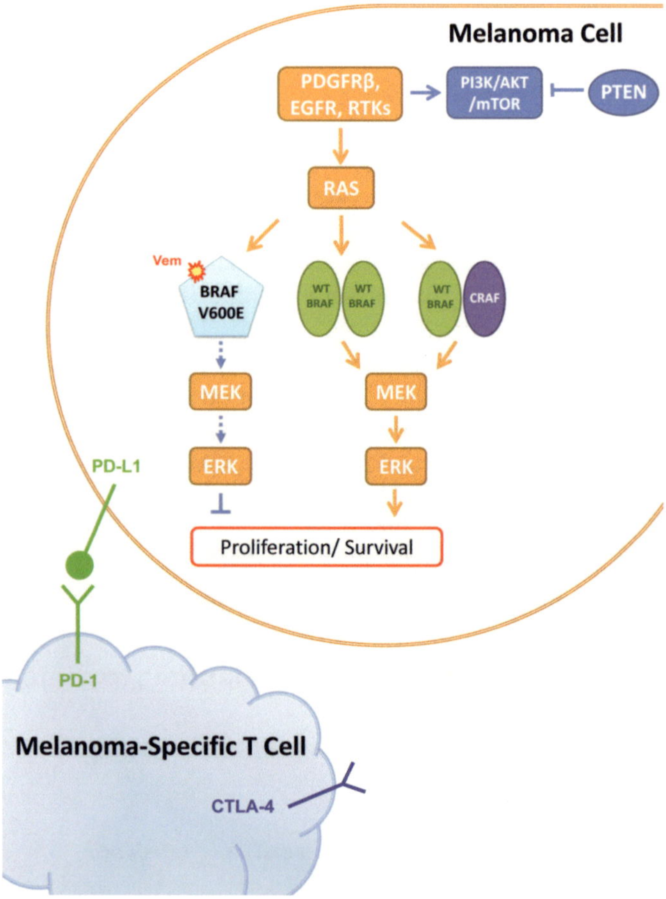

Figure 1. The mechanisms of BRAF inhibitor vemurafenib (Vem) action, toxicity and the interaction between melanoma cells with T lymphocytes.

However, wide type BRAF melanoma tumors do not respond to vemurafenib or dabrafenib inhibition, although they are sensitive to the MEK inhibitors [9]. Paradoxically, in cells with RAS mutation and wild-type BRAF, treatment with vemurafenib or dabrafenib will promote the formation of BRAF-CRAF heterodimer and lead to the activation of subsequent MEK/ERK signaling and cell proliferation as shown in Figure 1 [5]. This mechanism is used to explain the observation of typical clinical side effects associated with the use of vemurafenib: nearly 25% of patients developed skin lesions and even cutaneous squamous cell carcinoma (CSCC). In addition, *in vitro* study has revealed that vemurafenib inhibits multiple off-target kinases including c-Jun N-terminal kinase (JNK), suppresses JNK-dependent apoptosis, and generates CSCC toxicity [15].

2.1.2. Mechanisms of resistance to BRAF inhibition

In general, due to alternative pathway activations and inter-and intra-patients melanoma genetic heterogeneity, various mechanisms of resistance to BRAF inhibition have been identified [10, 16-19]. As we mentioned before, melanoma tumors bearing wide type BRAF are intrinsically resistant to vemurafenib and dabrafenib. Tumor micro-environment also contributes to the innate resistance to BRAF inhibition in melanoma. For example, stromal cells secrete hepatocyte growth factor (HGF), which activates the HGF-receptor MET, MAPK and PI3K-AKT pathways [20].

Eventually, nearly all BRAF mutated melanoma tumors develop acquired drug resistance upon treatment with BRAF inhibitors. The disease progression arises as early as two-month continuous treatment [18, 19]. The mechanisms of acquired resistance to BRAF inhibition can be generalized into two categories: $BRAF^{V600E}$-bypass mechanisms and MAPK-bypass mechanisms.

First, the $BRAF^{V600E}$-bypass mechanisms reactivate MAPK signaling and lead to ERK-dependent tumor cell survival and proliferation (Figure 2A). COT, which is coded by gene *MAP3K8*, is a MEK kinase. The overexpression of COT or amplification of *MAP3K8* directly activates MEK signaling without the participation of RAF protein [21]. The mutant of $MEK1^{C121S}$ increases catalytic capability and circumvents BRAF to activate basal level of ERK phosphorylation [22]. Before the treatment of vemurafenib or dabrafenib, melanoma cells with $BRAF^{V600E}$ mutation have over-activated monomer BRAF/MEK/ERK cascade which forms an ERK-dependent negative feedback loop. This negative feedback loop reduces the expression of the active RAS-GTP. In the presence of vemurafenib or dabrafenib, ERK phosphorylation level is rapidly reduced and the feed-back suppression on RAS activation is abolished (Figure 1). Therefore, eventually the ERK cascade level is restored through RAS over-activation. NRAS mutants including $NRAS^{Q61K}$ and $NRAS^{Q61R}$ can drive ERK activation through ARAF or CRAF homo-or hetero-dimers which are alternative MEK activators [23]. The combinations of BRAF inhibition plus MEK or ERK inhibition have showed efficacy of overcoming the resistance through these $BRAF^{V600E}$-bypass mechanisms [24-26], leading to the recent FDA approval of dabrafenib plus trametinib combination therapy for advanced melanoma.

Second, the MAPK-bypass mechanisms allow melanoma cells to escape from the cytotoxicity of BRAF or MEK inhibition through the activation of ERK-independent survival pathways

(Figure 2B). The PI3K-AKT signaling pathway can be activated through the overexpression of receptor tyrosine kinases (RTKs), for example, insulin-like growth factor 1 (IGF-1) receptor (IGF-1R) and platelet-derived growth factor receptor beta (PDGFRβ) [27]. The elevated levels of IGF-1R, PDGFRβ or HGF can also stimulate another receptor tyrosine kinase, MET, and increase the activity of PI3K. Phosphatase tensin (PTEN) is a negative regulator of PI3K. The PTEN loss-of-function mutation induces the resistance of BRAF inhibition and reduces the PFS of dabrafenib therapy in melanoma patients due to the PI3K activation [28]. Moreover, the upregulation of cyclin D1 can activate cyclin-dependent kinase 4 (CDK4) and 6 (CDK6) and make melanoma cells less dependent on MAPK signaling in cell cycle progressing [29].

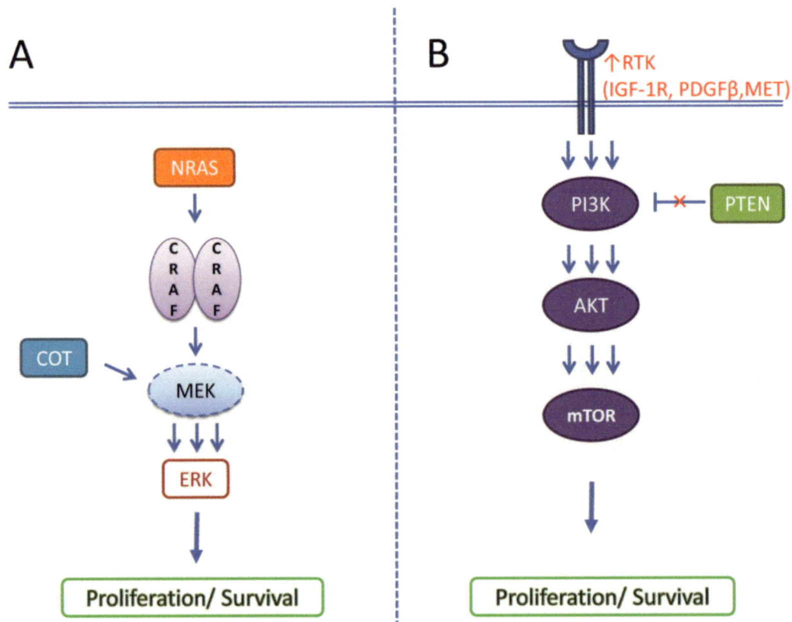

Figure 2. The mechanisms of acquired resistance to BRAF inhibition.

Additionally, Jaehyuk Choi *et al* has reported a $BRAF^{L505H}$ mutation which changes an amino acid residue in BRAF-vemurafenib interface and causes the resistance to vemurafenib treatment *in vitro* [30]. Since vemurafenib is a substrate of the ATP-binding cassette sub-family G member 2 (ABCG2), the overexpression of ABCG2 in $BRAF^{V600E}$ melanoma cell lines has caused the increasing of vemurafenib efflux *in vitro* [31]. The elucidation on the mechanism of acquired-resistance to BRAFi opens a door to rationally design and explore the proper combination strategies to overcome or delay the development of BRAFi resistance.

2.1.3. Targeting MEK: Mechanism of action, toxicity and resistance

Trametinib, which is approved by FDA in May 2013 as a monotherapy agent against advanced melanoma with $BRAF^{V600E}$ and $BRAF^{V600K}$ mutations, is a first-in-class, orally available, allosteric (non-ATP-competitive) MEK1/MEK2 inhibitor (MEKi) [32, 33]. It selectively inhibits

MEK, the down-stream kinase protein of RAF in the RAS-RAF-MEK-ERK pathway. As a result, melanoma cells with acquired resistance to BRAFi are commonly cross-resistant to MEKi such as trametinib or selumetinib, another selective allosteric MEKi [24, 34]. This mechanism explains the clinical trial results in which trametinib monotherapy fails to significantly benefit patients who have already developed acquired BRAFi resistance [35]. In contrast to the use of a BRAFi, no CSCC side effects are observed among the patients received trametinib treatment in clinical trials [13, 32]. However, similar to the use of vemurafenib, disease progression occurs within 6-7 months in patients receiving single-agent trametinib treatment [36]. Nevertheless, a retrospective analysis of 23 patients, who were first treated with MEKi and upon progression with a selective BRAFi, shows that the median time to progression (TTP) has been prolonged to 8.9 months from 4.8 months using a single-agent MEKi or 4.4 months for a single-agent BRAFi treatment, respectively [37]. However, a recent clinical trial indicated that if melanoma patients were treated with a BRAFi first then MEKi therapy, no confirmed response was observed [35]. This indicates that optimal treatment schedule and sequence is important for the melanoma therapy targeting the MAPK pathway.

2.1.4. Drug combination targeting MAPK pathway: From lab bench to clinical practice

Given that the mechanisms of tumor cells develop resistance to BRAFi partially by reactivating the ERK cascade and side effects such as CSCC are RAF-dependent, combining BRAFi with MEKi has attracted lots of research interest in order to further block the MAPK signaling pathway. *In vitro* and murine models first show the synergistic anti-proliferation and anti-tumor growth effects using the combined BRAFi and MEKi treatment [9, 27, 38, 39]. Further, this combination overcomes the acquired resistance to BRAFi [27, 38] in both cellular based assay and mouse xenograft models. In addition, the combined inhibition of BRAF-MEK suppresses the paradoxical BRAFi-induced MAPK signal elevation in melanoma cells and reduces the incidences of skin lesions in a rat model [9].

When it comes to the clinical trial data, the combined inhibition of BRAF-MEK has presented significant improvements of major patient benefits (PFS and overall survival). A phase I/II trial (ClinicalTrials.gov, NCT1072175) investigated the combination of oral dabrafenib (150 mg twice per day) plus oral trametinib (1 or 2 mg daily) (combination 150/1 and 150/2) versus monotherapy of dabrafenib (150 mg twice per day) over 108 metastatic melanoma patients bearing either V600E (92 patients) or V600K (16 patients) BRAF mutation [12, 36]. Median PFS in combination 150/2 group reached 9.4 months, compared to 5.8 months in the dabrafenib monotherapy group (hazard ratio 0.39, 95% confidence interval 0.25 to 0.62). The incidence of CSCC adverse events among combination 150/2 group is non-significantly lower than that among monotherapy group (7% versus 19%, P=0.09). But more frequent cases of pyrexia which is not common in trametinib single treatment have been reported in combination 150/2 group (71%, with recurrent rate 79%), as compared with dabrafenib monotherapy group (26%) [40]. These promising data lead to an accelerated FDA approval of the combination of dabrafenib (BRAFi) and trametinib (MEKi) for the treatment of unresectable or metastatic melanoma patients with BRAF V600E or V600K mutation, although further phase III studies with recruitment of more patients comparing the combination therapy with dabrafenib or vemurafenib single treatment (ClinicalTrials.gov, NCT01584648, NCT01597908) are still being assessed.

In addition, several ongoing phase I/II clinical trials now have shown that generally the combination of other BRAFi and MEKi is well tolerated in patients with or without receiving BRAFi treatment before (ClinicalTrials.gov, NCT01271803 vemurafenib (BRAFi)+cobimetinib (MEKi), NCT01543698 LGX818 (BRAFi)+MEK162 (MEKi)) [41-43] and overall response rate has increased comparing to the monotherapy groups, although the anti-tumor efficacy data haven't been released.

2.2. Combination targeted therapy using Phosphatidylinositol 3-Kinase (PI3K)/AKT/ mammalian Target of Rapamycin (mTOR) inhibitors

The activation of PI3K/AKT/mTOR pathway have been widely proved to be one of the major mechanisms of intrinsic or acquired resistance to both DNA-methylation agents (e.g. dacarbazine) and targeted BRAF inhibitor therapy (Figure 2). Some cell lines that are cross-resistant to both BRAFi and MEKi, are still sensitive to the inhibition of AKT/mTOR [34]. On the other hand, mechanistic study revealed evidences of a negative crosstalk between RAF/MEK/ERK and PI3K/AKT/mTOR pathways through RAS kinase. Therefore, when the downstream mTOR function is blocked, PI3K will be able to activate MAPK pathway via a switch of RAS [44, 45]. These investigations suggest a promising combination strategy of targeting MAPK pathway together with PI3K/AKT/mTOR cascade. Several preclinical studies widely proved that in MAPK inhibition sensitive melanoma cell lines, co-targeting PI3K/AKT/mTOR effectively induces cancer cell apoptosis with down-regulated anti-apoptotic BCL-2 family proteins [34, 46-48]. Such a co-targeting strategy can also postpone the emergence of acquired resistance to BRAFi dabrafenib mediated by PTEN mutation or disruption [49, 50]. Further, the dual inhibition of two pathways has successfully overcome NRAS mutation mediated resistance to MAPK blockade *in vitro* and induced xenograft tumor regression *in vivo* [34, 38, 51]. Finally, the combination of vemurafenib (BRAFi) or selumetinib (MEKi) with BEZ235 (dual PI3K and mTOR1/2 inhibitor) has been shown to overcome the PDGFRβ-driven resistance to MAPK pathway inhibition [52].

A series of Phase I studies have evaluated the clinical relevance of the combination therapy which co-targets PI3K/AKT/mTOR and RAF/MEK/ERK pathways in terms of the incidence on severe side effect and anti-tumor efficacy in 236 patients. These patients have advanced cancers including melanoma, colorectal, pancreatic and non-small cell lung cancers. Results from three combination groups (AKTi MK2206+MEKi selumetinib, NCT01021748; AKTi GSK2141795+MEKi trametinib, NCT01138085; mTOR inhibitor everolimus+MEKi trametinib, NCT 00955773) are compared to the single treatment groups [53]. Overall, the combination therapy did not provide significant increase of tumor control rate (64.6% for combination, 52.7% for monotherapy, P=0.16), although all five colorectal patients with co-activation of both pathways in combination group achieved tumor regression to varied extent between 2% and 64%. However, this combination strategy causes significant higher rates of drug-related grade III and above side effects (53.9% for combination, 18.1% for monotherapy, $P < 0.001$). Furthermore, two clinical trials which involve the combination therapy of BRAFi or MEKi with AKTi

DNE3 recently have been terminated due to the safety concerns of the toxic properties of DNE3 (ClinicalTrials.gov, NCT02087254 and NCT02095652). Nevertheless, in another ongoing phase I/II trial which measures the safety and efficacy of a well-tolerated pan-PI3K inhibitor BKM120 combined with vemurafenib therapy, preliminary data reveals that a vemurafenib-refractory melanoma patient with PTEN expression achieved a 35.9% reduction in target tumor (ClinicalTrials.gov, NCT01512251) [54]. In general, drug-related toxicity is one of the major issues for this cross-pathway targeted combination therapy and patients genetic profiling is very important to achieve the maximum objective response.

2.3. Combining targeted therapy with anti-angiogenic agents

Melanoma is a vascular tumor. The abnormal expression of the epidermal growth factor (EGF) family protein and the up-regulation of EGFR-mediated alternative survival pathway have critically shaped the response of melanoma to the current chemotherapy agents [55-58]. In a recent study by Sun *et al*, six out of sixteen melanoma cell lines display acquired EGFR expression after the development of resistance to BRAFi and MEKi [59]. Even before the FDA approval of BRAFi and MEKi, the combination of bevacizumab, a recombinant human monoclonal antibody VEGF inhibitor, with a specific chemotherapy agent (for example, fluorouracil [60] or fotemustine[61]), has become a first-line treatment for metastatic melanoma patients. Clinical trials that study the combination of anti-angiogenic agents with cytotoxic agents have achieved promising anti-tumor activity, although tolerability issues exist [62]. VEGF blockage has been shown to enhance the efficacy of a GM-CSF-secreting immunotherapy *in vitro* [63]. In addition, a VEGF receptor-2 inhibitor, semaxanib, prolonged both the complete and partial response time of an immunomodulatory drug, thalidomide, over 10 recurrent metastasis melanoma patients without showing significant drug-drug interaction toxicity in a phase II trial [64].

Along with the rapid development of targeted melanoma therapeutics, the combined inhibition of VEGFR plus PDGFR or mTOR has shown synergy anti-tumor effects on mouse models of B16 metastatic melanoma without increasing toxicity [65, 66]. A large-scale, unbiased drug screening study, which aims to discover effective genotype selective combinatorial therapeutics of vemurafenib-resistant BRAF and RAS mutant melanoma, identifies a triple BRAF+EGFR +AKT inhibition as highly effective approach [3]. In the year of 2010, combination of bevacizumab with an mTOR inhibitor, everolimus, was evaluated in a phase II trial for patients with metastatic melanoma [67]. The treatment was well tolerated in most patients. Seven out of fifty-seven patients (12%) receiving combination therapy have shown major responses, although the median PFS was only 4 months. This year (2014), in a phase II trial that combines bevacizumab and sorafenib, which is an inhibitor of both RAF kinase and VEGFR-2/PDGFRβ signaling, no objective tumor responses are seen in all the fourteen patients receiving treatment [68, 69]. Interestingly, the median TTP of patients with low VEGF (<300 pg/ml) was longer than that of patients with high VEGF (50 weeks versus 15 weeks, P=0.02). Therefore, the levels of VEGF in patients do influence the tumor progression profile (ClinicalTrials.gov, NCT00387751).

2.4. Combination therapy using targeted therapy with versatile chemotherapy agents

Since the abnormally activated (phosphorylation) of ERK and AKT constitutively exist in melanoma cells and promote the disease progression especially metastasis, blocking ERK or AKT pathway can sensitize the metastatic melanoma to the apoptosis induced by chemotherapeutic agents including cisplatin, temozolomide, DTIC and arsenite [70-72]. With the understanding of tumor biology about the programmed cell apoptosis and the rapid development of agents that can trigger the cell death process in melanoma, the combination of a MAPK inhibitor with a BCL-2 inhibitor (ABT-737 [73] or navitoclax [74]), or a MDM2 antagonist nutlin-3 [75], has synergistically induced apoptosis of melanoma *in vitro* and suppressed xenograft tumor growth *in vivo*. A comparative analysis on the samples collected from patients receiving vemurafenib or dabrafenib/trametinib combination treatment showed that BCL-2 expression level is closely related to the onset of MAPK inhibition resistance [74]. Clinical trials are being conducted to investigate the combination of BCL-2 inhibitor (BH3 mimetics) navitoclax and vemurafenib [74].

Due to the heterogenetic characteristics of melanoma disease, Vultur A *et al* [76] recently report that MEK or BRAF inhibition can potentially strengthen the invasion property of human melanoma cells by about 20%. As a result, co-inhibiting kinases that are actively involved in cell invasion process, such as RTK, STAT3 and Src, together with MEK inhibition has effectively abolished the invasive phenotype and further caused the tumor cell death in a 3D matrix model.

Metformin, a biguanide oral anti-diabetic drug, has been discovered with antitumor activity in various cancer types including melanoma. Although the exact mechanisms remain to be elucidated, accumulating data suggest that metformin can activate AMP-activated protein kinase (AMPK) and thus increase the activities of VEGF and ERK in $BRAF^{V600E}$ mutated melanoma cells [77]. AMPK negatively regulates malignant cell proliferation and viability [78]. The combination of vemurafenib and metformin has shown synergistic anti-proliferative effects on six out of eleven tested $BRAF^{V600E}$ melanoma cell lines [79]. Pilot clinical studies that evaluate the safety and efficacy of metformin combination therapies (plus dabrafenib or trametinib) are now recruiting patients (ClinicalTrials.gov, NCT0184000, NCT02143050).

Unlike the cutaneous melanoma, over-activation of MAPK pathway in uveal melanoma is associated GNAQ or GNA11 mutations instead of BRAF or RAS mutations [80]. Protein kinase C (PKC) inhibitors such as enzastaurin or AEB071 induce apoptosis in GNAQ-mutant but not in GNAQ wild type uveal melanoma cells [81]. The level of ERK phosphorylation also decreases in these cells when they are treated using PKC inhibitors [81]. Chen *et al.* has recently confirmed the synergy of the combination using a PKC inhibitor with a MEKi (PD0325901 or MEK162) in GNAQ/11 mutant uveal melanoma cells [82].

Understanding the mechanisms of resistance to MAPK inhibition in melanoma can lead to rational combination designs in order to overcome acquired drug resistance to BRAF inhibitors. For example, our lab recently identified a synergistic combination in which a novel tubulin inhibitor ABI-274 combined with vemurafenib could overcome the acquired vemurafenib-resistance [83]. This combination treatment effectively arrested the vemurafenib-resistant melanoma cells in both G_0/G_1 and G_2/M phases and induced strong apoptosis through the down-regulation of AKT phosphorylation. In addition, the combination of a MEKi (TAK-733) with an Hsp90 inhibitor (ganetespib) induces tumor regressions in vemurafenib-resistant xenograft models also through the depletion of AKT signaling [84]. With the finding that up-regulated cyclin D1 expression is critical for the survival of vemurafenib-resistant cells, a selective inhibitor of cyclin dependent kinase (CDK) 4/6, LY2835219, has been reported to overcome the reactivation of MAPK signaling in vemurafenib-resistant BRAF^{V600E} melanoma [85].

3. Combinations involving immunotherapy in melanoma treatment

3.1. Combined blockade of immuno-checkpoints

Given the unsatisfactory results of cytokine-based melanoma immunotherapy (recombinant interferon-α 2b and high dose interleukin-2) in the past decade, the development and approval of ipilimumab (anti-cytotoxic T lymphocyte-associated antigen 4 (CTLA-4) monoclonal antibody) in 2013 have marked a breakthrough of immune-checkpoints blockade therapy [86]. CTLA-4 (CD152) expresses on the surface of active T-lymphocytes and inhibits the initial T-cell proliferation and migration to the tumor tissue [87]. CTLA-4 antibodies preferentially target the suppressive regulatory T cells and prevent them from being hijacked by tumors [88]. In a double-blinded phase III study in 676 patients with pretreated and refractory metastatic melanoma, ipilimumab at the dose of 3 mg/kg achieved a median OS of 10 months [86]. In a meta-Kaplan-Meier-analysis of data collected from 1,861 melanoma patients in a clinical trial, a plateau of survival curve starts from around 3 years after ipilimumab treatment with follow-up extends as long as ten years, indicating a long-term survival benefits of ipilimumab therapy (ClinicalTrials.gov, NCT01844505). In addition, ipilimumab showed good tolerance and efficacy in several other clinical trials in which it was combined with a standard chemotherapy agent such as dacarbazine, fotemustine or temozolomide [89].

Another success of immune-check point blockade strategy is the development of anti-programmed death-1 (PD-1) antibodies, represented by pembrolizumab (MK-3475) and nivolumab [90, 91]. Pembrolizumab, as the first-in-class PD-1 inhibitor, has obtained FDA approval in September 2014 for patients with advanced or unresectable melanoma. The cDNA of PD-1 (CD279) is first cloned in programmed death T cells although PD-1 itself does not directly induce apoptosis. PD-1 is over-expressed on the surface of dysfunctional activated T-cells and contributes to the maintenance of T cell dysfunction (exhaust) phenotype and proliferation disability in the tumor site [92]. Two counter receptors of PD-1 have been identified: PD-L1 and PD-L2. PD-L1 is more frequently and exclusively expressed in various tumor cells; therefore, antibodies targeting PD-L1 (MPDL3280A and BMS-936559) also have anti-tumor activity in advanced cancer including melanoma [91, 93]. The PD-1-PD-L1 ligation retards the recognition and destroying of tumor cells by CD8+cytotoxic T-lymphocytes [87]. As a result, blocking PD-1 or PD-L1 will reverse the cancer cell immune escape. Because both CTLA-4 and PD-1 are key negative receptors that cooperatively modulate the adaptive immune response in tumor progression, their combination has been shown to be synergistic in B16 melanoma tumors without overt toxicity [94].

In a cohort phase I trial that studied the concurrent administration of ipilimumab and nivolumab to 53 patients with advanced, treatment-resistant melanoma, more than 80% tumor reduction was observed in 30% patients after 12 weeks treatment at the maximum tolerated dose. Twenty-one out of fifty-three patients had objective responses and over 80% of these patients had tumor regression. Grade 3/4 adverse events are diagnosed in 53% patients but the toxicities are manageable with immune-suppressants [95]. Consequential trials with more enrollment number of patients are necessary to further evaluate the safety and efficacy of this promising double immune-checkpoints blockage therapy comparing with each of its mono-therapy regiments.

Finally, combinatorial clinical trials using ipilimumab with other immunotherapy agents have shown some favorable therapeutic benefits. For example, combination of ipilimumab with peginterferon α-2b (pegylated interferon α-2b) in patients with unresectable melanoma both demonstrated significant increase of response rate and OS comparing with the monotherapy arm [96, 97] in recent phase I trials.

3.2. Combined therapy inhibiting both immuno-checkpoint and MAPK signaling pathway

Checkpoint blockade immunotherapy and MAPK targeted chemotherapy have distinct clinical profiles. For example, targeted therapy has relative higher initial response rate (~60% for BRAFi) with rapid onset of effect, but its efficacy restrictively rely on the continuous treatment and the therapeutic response is usually not durable due to the quick development of acquired drug resistance. In contrast, immunotherapy has much a lower response rate (4.5% for ipilimumab), delayed onset of effect and difficulty in predicting patient outcome, but it has shown potentially durable responses and long-term survival benefit even off treatment. In addition, since the MAPK pathway is not required in the process of anti-tumor immune response, blocking MAPK signaling should not interfere with the efficacy of checkpoint blockade immunotherapy. Therefore, it seems very rational that the combination of a MAPKi and an immunotherapy agent such as ipilimumab or pembrolizumab can maximize the therapeutic benefits in advance melanoma.

Interestingly, BRAF and MEK inhibition displayed an "endogenous vaccine-like" effects in melanoma cells [98]. Cytotoxic agents like BRAFi induce tumor cell death and promote the uptake and presentation of tumor antigens to the effector immune cells (T cells and B cells) through antigen-presenting cells [54]. MEK inhibition, $BRAF^{V600E}$ RNA silencing or BRAF inhibition by PLX4720 increases the CD4+ and CD8+ lymphocytes mediated T-cell infiltration and reduce the level of immune-suppressants including IL-6, IL-10 or VEGF [99-101] in mice. The expression of PD-L1 is found to be elevated in BRAFi-resistant melanoma cells and it is mediated through the off-target activity of BRAFi in JUN and STAT3 signaling [102]. However, Vella *et al* has published a paper in 2014 and stated that they have not found any impact of dabrafenib treatment on T lymphocytes. trametinib alone or in combination with dabrafenib has suppressed T lymphocyte proliferation, cytokine secretion and antigen-specific expansion

http://dx.doi.org/10.5772/59360

in their isolated T lymphocyte and monocyte-derived dendritic cells. These findings should be carefully tested *in vivo* to evaluate the clinical relevance [103].

As for the clinical practice, dose-limiting hepatotoxicity issues have led to the premature termination of the first phase I study on combination of ipilimumab with vemurafenib (ClinicalTrials.gov, NCT01400451). This signified the complexity of adverse effect in combined therapy of immune-regulating agents and kinase inhibitors. Another phase I study of ipilimumab plus dabrafenib, or ipilimumab plus the combination of dabrafenib with trametinib is still active and a phase II study is exploring the safety and efficacy of sequential administration of vemurafenib followed by ipilimumab (ClinicalTrials.gov, NCT01767454, NCT01673854). The data of these most recent trials will be released in the near future.

4. Conclusions

Extensive efforts and remarkable progresses have been made to discover and investigate rational approaches in combination melanoma therapy since the recent approval of MAPKi and immune checkpoints blockade antibodies. A number of new targeted or immune drugs for metastatic melanoma are currently under commercial development or late stage clinical trials, some of which will likely be approved in the next few years. Quality of life for many melanoma patients has been dramatically increased. However, significant challenges still remain. While some clinical evidence has really raised the expectation of survivals for patients with advanced melanoma, the benefits of combination therapy are usually accompanied by limitations. Comprehensive genetic profile and tailored patient matching is essential for targeted therapy, while biomarkers are critical to predict the patient immunotherapy response. Drug-related toxicity for combination treatment usually is not a simple one-plus-one situation, and potential drug-drug interactions, especially the combination of a targeted agent with an immunotherapeutic agent must be carefully evaluated in order to achieve both fast and durable responses. Adverse effects should be closely monitored and potential alternative dosing regiments is worth further exploration. Optimized dose schedule may help to delay the resistance development and reduce the frequency of adverse effect. For example, intermittent doses of BRAFi was able to enhance the tolerance in combination with immunotherapy, decrease the paradoxical MAPK activation, which might be the main cause of severe toxicity in clinical trial [104]. Solid evidence of synergistic combination in preclinical research must be established before clinical trial conduction. In fact, with the relatively large number of available targeted agents and immunotherapeutic agents for metastatic melanoma, the huge number of possible drug combinations coupled with dosing sequences or schedules already presents a significant challenge in designing proper clinical trials. To test all the possible drug combinations along with different dosing sequences clinically will not only have low benefits to patients, but is also a huge financial burden to the society. Carefully designed, predictive preclinical studies will be essential to provide critical supports for rational prioritization of clinical trials using drug combinations. Finally, clear understandings of various combination mechanisms and patient genetic profiles are critically important for the development of new combination approaches, prediction of expected therapy response and potential side effects.

With the rapid advances in this field, it is likely that optimal combination treatments will great improve the management of advanced melanoma in cancer patients.

Abbreviations

AMPK: 5' adenosine monophosphate-activated protein kinase

BRAF: B-Raf protein

BRAFi: BRAF inhibitor

CDK: Cyclin dependent kinase

CR: Complete response

CTLA-4: Cytotoxic T lymphocyte-associated antigen 4

ERK: Extracellular signal-regulated kinase

HR: Hazard ratio

JNK: c-Jun N-terminal kinase

MAPK: Mitogen-activated protein kinase

MEKi: MEK inhibitor

MHC: Membrane histocompatibility complex

mTOR: Mammalian target of rapamycin

ORR: Overall response rate

OS: Overall survival

PD-1: Programmed cell death 1

PD-L1: Programmed cell death 1 ligand 1

PDGFR: Platete-derived growth factor receptor

PFS: Progression-free survival

PI3K: Phosphoinositide 3-kinase

PKC: Protein kinase C

PR: Partial response

RTKs: Receptor tyrosine kinases

TCR: T cell receptor

VEGF: Vascular endothelial growth factor

http://dx.doi.org/10.5772/59360

VEGFR: Vascular endothelial growth factor receptor

Acknowledgements

This work was supported by NIH grants R01CA148706. The content is solely the responsibility of the authors and does not necessarily represent the official views of the National Institutes of Health. Jin Wang acknowledges the support of the Alma and Hal Reagan Fellowship.

Author details

Jin Wang, Duane D. Miller* and Wei Li

*Address all correspondence to: dmiller@uthsc.edu or wli@uthsc.edu

Department of Pharmaceutical Sciences, College of Pharmacy. The University of Tennessee Health Science Center, Memphis, TN, USA

References

[1] Hersh, E.M.; O'Day, S.J.; Powderly, J.; Khan, K.D.; Pavlick, A.C.; Cranmer, L.D.; Samlowski, W.E.; Nichol, G.M.; Yellin, M.J.; Weber, J.S., A phase II multicenter study of ipilimumab with or without dacarbazine in chemotherapy-naive patients with advanced melanoma. *Investigational new drugs,* 2011, *29,* (3), 489-498.

[2] Sosman, J.A.; Kim, K.B.; Schuchter, L.; Gonzalez, R.; Pavlick, A.C.; Weber, J.S.; McArthur, G.A.; Hutson, T.E.; Moschos, S.J.; Flaherty, K.T.; Hersey, P.; Kefford, R.; Lawrence, D.; Puzanov, I.; Lewis, K.D.; Amaravadi, R.K.; Chmielowski, B.; Lawrence, H.J.; Shyr, Y.; Ye, F.; Li, J.; Nolop, K.B.; Lee, R.J.; Joe, A.K.; Ribas, A., Survival in BRAF V600-mutant advanced melanoma treated with vemurafenib. *The New England journal of medicine,* 2012, *366,* (8), 707-714.

[3] Al-Lazikani, B.; Workman, P., Unpicking the combination lock for mutant BRAF and RAS melanomas. *Cancer discovery,* 2013, *3,* (1), 14-19.

[4] Hu-Lieskovan, S.; Robert, L.; Homet Moreno, B.; Ribas, A., Combining Targeted Therapy With Immunotherapy in BRAF-Mutant Melanoma: Promise and Challenges. *Journal of clinical oncology : official journal of the American Society of Clinical Oncology,* 2014, *32,* (21), 2248-2254.

[5] Nijenhuis, C.M.; Haanen, J.B.; Schellens, J.H.; Beijnen, J.H., Is combination therapy the next step to overcome resistance and reduce toxicities in melanoma? *Cancer treatment reviews,* 2013, *39,* (4), 305-312.

[6] Voskoboynik, M.; Arkenau, H.T., Combination therapies for the treatment of advanced melanoma: a review of current evidence. *Biochemistry research international,* 2014, *2014,* 307059.

[7] Wan, P.T.; Garnett, M.J.; Roe, S.M.; Lee, S.; Niculescu-Duvaz, D.; Good, V.M.; Jones, C.M.; Marshall, C.J.; Springer, C.J.; Barford, D.; Marais, R.; Cancer Genome, P., Mechanism of activation of the RAF-ERK signaling pathway by oncogenic mutations of B-RAF. *Cell,* 2004, *116,* (6), 855-867.

[8] Tsai, J.; Lee, J.T.; Wang, W.; Zhang, J.; Cho, H.; Mamo, S.; Bremer, R.; Gillette, S.; Kong, J.; Haass, N.K.; Sproesser, K.; Li, L.; Smalley, K.S.; Fong, D.; Zhu, Y.L.; Marimuthu, A.; Nguyen, H.; Lam, B.; Liu, J.; Cheung, I.; Rice, J.; Suzuki, Y.; Luu, C.; Settachatgul, C.; Shellooe, R.; Cantwell, J.; Kim, S.H.; Schlessinger, J.; Zhang, K.Y.; West, B.L.; Powell, B.; Habets, G.; Zhang, C.; Ibrahim, P.N.; Hirth, P.; Artis, D.R.; Herlyn, M.; Bollag, G., Discovery of a selective inhibitor of oncogenic B-Raf kinase with potent antimelanoma activity. *Proceedings of the National Academy of Sciences of the United States of America,* 2008, *105,* (8), 3041-3046.

[9] King, A.J.; Arnone, M.R.; Bleam, M.R.; Moss, K.G.; Yang, J.; Fedorowicz, K.E.; Smitheman, K.N.; Erhardt, J.A.; Hughes-Earle, A.; Kane-Carson, L.S.; Sinnamon, R.H.; Qi, H.; Rheault, T.R.; Uehling, D.E.; Laquerre, S.G., Dabrafenib; preclinical characterization, increased efficacy when combined with trametinib, while BRAF/MEK tool combination reduced skin lesions. *PloS one,* 2013, *8,* (7), e67583.

[10] Solit, D.B.; Rosen, N., Towards a unified model of RAF inhibitor resistance. *Cancer discovery,* 2014, *4,* (1), 27-30.

[11] Hooijkaas, A.; Gadiot, J.; Morrow, M.; Stewart, R.; Schumacher, T.; Blank, C.U., Selective BRAF inhibition decreases tumor-resident lymphocyte frequencies in a mouse model of human melanoma. *Oncoimmunology,* 2012, *1,* (5), 609-617.

[12] Menzies, A.M.; Long, G.V., Dabrafenib and trametinib, alone and in combination for BRAF-mutant metastatic melanoma. *Clinical cancer research : an official journal of the American Association for Cancer Research,* 2014, *20,* (8), 2035-2043.

[13] Carlino, M.S.; Gowrishankar, K.; Saunders, C.A.; Pupo, G.M.; Snoyman, S.; Zhang, X.D.; Saw, R.; Becker, T.M.; Kefford, R.F.; Long, G.V.; Rizos, H., Antiproliferative effects of continued mitogen-activated protein kinase pathway inhibition following acquired resistance to BRAF and/or MEK inhibition in melanoma. *Molecular cancer therapeutics,* 2013, *12,* (7), 1332-1342.

[14] Klein, O.; Clements, A.; Menzies, A.M.; O'Toole, S.; Kefford, R.F.; Long, G.V., BRAF inhibitor activity in V600R metastatic melanoma. *European journal of cancer,* 2013, *49,* (5), 1073-1079.

[15] Vin, H.; Ojeda, S.S.; Ching, G.; Leung, M.L.; Chitsazzadeh, V.; Dwyer, D.W.; Adelmann, C.H.; Restrepo, M.; Richards, K.N.; Stewart, L.R.; Du, L.; Ferguson, S.B.; Chakravarti, D.; Ehrenreiter, K.; Baccarini, M.; Ruggieri, R.; Curry, J.L.; Kim, K.B.; Ciurea, A.M.; Duvic, M.; Prieto, V.G.; Ullrich, S.E.; Dalby, K.N.; Flores, E.R.; Tsai, K.Y., BRAF inhibitors suppress apoptosis through off-target inhibition of JNK signaling. *eLife,* 2013, *2,* e00969.

[16] Roesch, A., Tumor heterogeneity and plasticity as elusive drivers for resistance to MAPK pathway inhibition in melanoma. *Oncogene,* 2014.

[17] Yancovitz, M.; Litterman, A.; Yoon, J.; Ng, E.; Shapiro, R.L.; Berman, R.S.; Pavlick, A.C.; Darvishian, F.; Christos, P.; Mazumdar, M.; Osman, I.; Polsky, D., Intra-and inter-tumor heterogeneity of BRAF(V600E))mutations in primary and metastatic melanoma. *PloS one,* 2012, *7,* (1), e29336.

[18] Little, A.S.; Smith, P.D.; Cook, S.J., Mechanisms of acquired resistance to ERK1/2 pathway inhibitors. *Oncogene,* 2013, *32,* (10), 1207-1215.

[19] Tentori, L.; Lacal, P.M.; Graziani, G., Challenging resistance mechanisms to therapies for metastatic melanoma. *Trends in pharmacological sciences,* 2013, *34,* (12), 656-666.

[20] Straussman, R.; Morikawa, T.; Shee, K.; Barzily-Rokni, M.; Qian, Z.R.; Du, J.; Davis, A.; Mongare, M.M.; Gould, J.; Frederick, D.T.; Cooper, Z.A.; Chapman, P.B.; Solit, D.B.; Ribas, A.; Lo, R.S.; Flaherty, K.T.; Ogino, S.; Wargo, J.A.; Golub, T.R., Tumour micro-environment elicits innate resistance to RAF inhibitors through HGF secretion. *Nature,* 2012, *487,* (7408), 500-504.

[21] Johannessen, C.M.; Boehm, J.S.; Kim, S.Y.; Thomas, S.R.; Wardwell, L.; Johnson, L.A.; Emery, C.M.; Stransky, N.; Cogdill, A.P.; Barretina, J.; Caponigro, G.; Hieronymus, H.; Murray, R.R.; Salehi-Ashtiani, K.; Hill, D.E.; Vidal, M.; Zhao, J.J.; Yang, X.; Alkan, O.; Kim, S.; Harris, J.L.; Wilson, C.J.; Myer, V.E.; Finan, P.M.; Root, D.E.; Roberts, T.M.; Golub, T.; Flaherty, K.T.; Dummer, R.; Weber, B.L.; Sellers, W.R.; Schlegel, R.; Wargo, J.A.; Hahn, W.C.; Garraway, L.A., COT drives resistance to RAF inhibition through MAP kinase pathway reactivation. *Nature,* 2010, *468,* (7326), 968-972.

[22] Wagle, N.; Emery, C.; Berger, M.F.; Davis, M.J.; Sawyer, A.; Pochanard, P.; Kehoe, S.M.; Johannessen, C.M.; Macconaill, L.E.; Hahn, W.C.; Meyerson, M.; Garraway, L.A., Dissecting therapeutic resistance to RAF inhibition in melanoma by tumor genomic profiling. *Journal of clinical oncology : official journal of the American Society of Clinical Oncology,* 2011, *29,* (22), 3085-3096.

[23] Poulikakos, P.I.; Zhang, C.; Bollag, G.; Shokat, K.M.; Rosen, N., RAF inhibitors transactivate RAF dimers and ERK signalling in cells with wild-type BRAF. *Nature,* 2010, *464,* (7287), 427-430.

[24] Gowrishankar, K.; Snoyman, S.; Pupo, G.M.; Becker, T.M.; Kefford, R.F.; Rizos, H., Acquired resistance to BRAF inhibition can confer cross-resistance to combined

BRAF/MEK inhibition. *The Journal of investigative dermatology,* 2012, *132,* (7), 1850-1859.

[25] Carlino, M.S.; Todd, J.R.; Gowrishankar, K.; Mijatov, B.; Pupo, G.M.; Fung, C.; Snoyman, S.; Hersey, P.; Long, G.V.; Kefford, R.F.; Rizos, H., Differential activity of MEK and ERK inhibitors in BRAF inhibitor resistant melanoma. *Molecular oncology,* 2014, *8,* (3), 544-554.

[26] Sanchez-Laorden, B.; Viros, A.; Girotti, M.R.; Pedersen, M.; Saturno, G.; Zambon, A.; Niculescu-Duvaz, D.; Turajlic, S.; Hayes, A.; Gore, M.; Larkin, J.; Lorigan, P.; Cook, M.; Springer, C.; Marais, R., BRAF inhibitors induce metastasis in RAS mutant or inhibitor-resistant melanoma cells by reactivating MEK and ERK signaling. *Science signaling,* 2014, *7,* (318), ra30.

[27] Su, F.; Bradley, W.D.; Wang, Q.; Yang, H.; Xu, L.; Higgins, B.; Kolinsky, K.; Packman, K.; Kim, M.J.; Trunzer, K.; Lee, R.J.; Schostack, K.; Carter, J.; Albert, T.; Germer, S.; Rosinski, J.; Martin, M.; Simcox, M.E.; Lestini, B.; Heimbrook, D.; Bollag, G., Resistance to selective BRAF inhibition can be mediated by modest upstream pathway activation. *Cancer research,* 2012, *72,* (4), 969-978.

[28] Nathanson, K.L.; Martin, A.M.; Wubbenhorst, B.; Greshock, J.; Letrero, R.; D'Andrea, K.; O'Day, S.; Infante, J.R.; Falchook, G.S.; Arkenau, H.T.; Millward, M.; Brown, M.P.; Pavlick, A.; Davies, M.A.; Ma, B.; Gagnon, R.; Curtis, M.; Lebowitz, P.F.; Kefford, R.; Long, G.V., Tumor genetic analyses of patients with metastatic melanoma treated with the BRAF inhibitor dabrafenib (GSK2118436). *Clinical cancer research : an official journal of the American Association for Cancer Research,* 2013, *19,* (17), 4868-4878.

[29] Smalley, K.S.; Lioni, M.; Dalla Palma, M.; Xiao, M.; Desai, B.; Egyhazi, S.; Hansson, J.; Wu, H.; King, A.J.; Van Belle, P.; Elder, D.E.; Flaherty, K.T.; Herlyn, M.; Nathanson, K.L., Increased cyclin D1 expression can mediate BRAF inhibitor resistance in BRAF V600E-mutated melanomas. *Molecular cancer therapeutics,* 2008, *7,* (9), 2876-2883.

[30] Choi, J.; Landrette, S.F.; Wang, T.; Evans, P.; Bacchiocchi, A.; Bjornson, R.; Cheng, E.; Stiegler, A.L.; Gathiaka, S.; Acevedo, O.; Boggon, T.J.; Krauthammer, M.; Halaban, R.; Xu, T., Identification of PLX4032-resistance mechanisms and implications for novel RAF inhibitors. *Pigment cell & melanoma research,* 2014, *27,* (2), 253-262.

[31] Wu, C.P.; Sim, H.M.; Huang, Y.H.; Liu, Y.C.; Hsiao, S.H.; Cheng, H.W.; Li, Y.Q.; Ambudkar, S.V.; Hsu, S.C., Overexpression of ATP-binding cassette transporter ABCG2 as a potential mechanism of acquired resistance to vemurafenib in BRAF(V600E) mutant cancer cells. *Biochemical pharmacology,* 2013, *85,* (3), 325-334.

[32] Flaherty, K.T.; Robert, C.; Hersey, P.; Nathan, P.; Garbe, C.; Milhem, M.; Demidov, L.V.; Hassel, J.C.; Rutkowski, P.; Mohr, P.; Dummer, R.; Trefzer, U.; Larkin, J.M.; Utikal, J.; Dreno, B.; Nyakas, M.; Middleton, M.R.; Becker, J.C.; Casey, M.; Sherman, L.J.; Wu, F.S.; Ouellet, D.; Martin, A.M.; Patel, K.; Schadendorf, D.; Group, M.S., Im-

proved survival with MEK inhibition in BRAF-mutated melanoma. *The New England journal of medicine,* 2012, *367,* (2), 107-114.

[33] Wright, C.J.; McCormack, P.L., Trametinib: first global approval. *Drugs,* 2013, *73,* (11), 1245-1254.

[34] Atefi, M.; von Euw, E.; Attar, N.; Ng, C.; Chu, C.; Guo, D.; Nazarian, R.; Chmielowski, B.; Glaspy, J.A.; Comin-Anduix, B.; Mischel, P.S.; Lo, R.S.; Ribas, A., Reversing melanoma cross-resistance to BRAF and MEK inhibitors by co-targeting the AKT/mTOR pathway. *PloS one,* 2011, *6,* (12), e28973.

[35] Kim, K.B.; Kefford, R.; Pavlick, A.C.; Infante, J.R.; Ribas, A.; Sosman, J.A.; Fecher, L.A.; Millward, M.; McArthur, G.A.; Hwu, P.; Gonzalez, R.; Ott, P.A.; Long, G.V.; Gardner, O.S.; Ouellet, D.; Xu, Y.; DeMarini, D.J.; Le, N.T.; Patel, K.; Lewis, K.D., Phase II study of the MEK1/MEK2 inhibitor Trametinib in patients with metastatic BRAF-mutant cutaneous melanoma previously treated with or without a BRAF inhibitor. *Journal of clinical oncology : official journal of the American Society of Clinical Oncology,* 2013, *31,* (4), 482-489.

[36] Flaherty, K.T.; Infante, J.R.; Daud, A.; Gonzalez, R.; Kefford, R.F.; Sosman, J.; Hamid, O.; Schuchter, L.; Cebon, J.; Ibrahim, N.; Kudchadkar, R.; Burris, H.A., 3rd; Falchook, G.; Algazi, A.; Lewis, K.; Long, G.V.; Puzanov, I.; Lebowitz, P.; Singh, A.; Little, S.; Sun, P.; Allred, A.; Ouellet, D.; Kim, K.B.; Patel, K.; Weber, J., Combined BRAF and MEK inhibition in melanoma with BRAF V600 mutations. *The New England journal of medicine,* 2012, *367,* (18), 1694-1703.

[37] Goldinger, S.M.; Zimmer, L.; Schulz, C.; Ugurel, S.; Hoeller, C.; Kaehler, K.C.; Schadendorf, D.; Hassel, J.C.; Becker, J.; Hauschild, A.; Dummer, R.; Dermatology Cooperative Oncology, G., Upstream mitogen-activated protein kinase (MAPK) pathway inhibition: MEK inhibitor followed by a BRAF inhibitor in advanced melanoma patients. *European journal of cancer,* 2014, *50,* (2), 406-410.

[38] Greger, J.G.; Eastman, S.D.; Zhang, V.; Bleam, M.R.; Hughes, A.M.; Smitheman, K.N.; Dickerson, S.H.; Laquerre, S.G.; Liu, L.; Gilmer, T.M., Combinations of BRAF, MEK, and PI3K/mTOR inhibitors overcome acquired resistance to the BRAF inhibitor GSK2118436 dabrafenib, mediated by NRAS or MEK mutations. *Molecular cancer therapeutics,* 2012, *11,* (4), 909-920.

[39] Nakamura, A.; Arita, T.; Tsuchiya, S.; Donelan, J.; Chouitar, J.; Carideo, E.; Galvin, K.; Okaniwa, M.; Ishikawa, T.; Yoshida, S., Antitumor activity of the selective pan-RAF inhibitor TAK-632 in BRAF inhibitor-resistant melanoma. *Cancer research,* 2013, *73,* (23), 7043-7055.

[40] Lee, C.I.; Menzies, A.M.; Haydu, L.E.; Azer, M.; Clements, A.; Kefford, R.F.; Long, G.V., Features and management of pyrexia with combined dabrafenib and trametinib in metastatic melanoma. *Melanoma research,* 2014.

[41] Ribas, A.; Gonzalez, R.; Pavlick, A.; Hamid, O.; Gajewski, T.F.; Daud, A.; Flaherty, L.; Logan, T.; Chmielowski, B.; Lewis, K.; Kee, D.; Boasberg, P.; Yin, M.; Chan, I.; Musib,

L.; Choong, N.; Puzanov, I.; McArthur, G.A., Combination of vemurafenib and cobimetinib in patients with advanced BRAF(V600)-mutated melanoma: a phase 1b study. *The lancet oncology,* 2014, *15,* (9), 954-965.

[42] Kefford, R.; Miller, W.H.; Tan, D.S.W.; Sullivan, R.J.; Long, G.; Dienstmann, R.; Tai, W.M.D.; Flaherty, K.; Stutvoet, S.; Schumacher, K.M.; Wandel, S.; De Parseval, L.A.; Tabernero, J., Preliminary results from a phase Ib/II, open-label, dose-escalation study of the oral BRAF inhibitor LGX818 in combination with the oral MEK1/2 inhibitor MEK162 in BRAF V600-dependent advanced solid tumors. *Journal of Clinical Oncology,* 2013, 31, (15_supplement), abstract 9029.

[43] Dummer, R.; Robert, C.; Nyakas, M.; McArthur, G.A.; Kudchadkar, R.R.; Gomez-Roca, C.; Sullivan, R.J.; Flaherty, K.; Murer, C.; Michel, D.; Tang, Z.W.; De Parseval, L.A.; Delord, J.P., Initial results from a phase I, open-label, dose escalation study of the oral BRAF inhibitor LGX818 in patients with BRAF V600 mutant advanced or metastatic melanoma. *Journal of Clinical Oncology,* 2013, *31,* (15).

[44] Carracedo, A.; Pandolfi, P.P., The PTEN-PI3K pathway: of feedbacks and cross-talks. *Oncogene,* 2008, *27,* (41), 5527-5541.

[45] Villanueva, J.; Vultur, A.; Lee, J.T.; Somasundaram, R.; Fukunaga-Kalabis, M.; Cipolla, A.K.; Wubbenhorst, B.; Xu, X.; Gimotty, P.A.; Kee, D.; Santiago-Walker, A.E.; Letrero, R.; D'Andrea, K.; Pushparajan, A.; Hayden, J.E.; Brown, K.D.; Laquerre, S.; McArthur, G.A.; Sosman, J.A.; Nathanson, K.L.; Herlyn, M., Acquired resistance to BRAF inhibitors mediated by a RAF kinase switch in melanoma can be overcome by cotargeting MEK and IGF-1R/PI3K. *Cancer cell,* 2010, *18,* (6), 683-695.

[46] Lasithiotakis, K.G.; Sinnberg, T.W.; Schittek, B.; Flaherty, K.T.; Kulms, D.; Maczey, E.; Garbe, C.; Meier, F.E., Combined inhibition of MAPK and mTOR signaling inhibits growth, induces cell death, and abrogates invasive growth of melanoma cells. *The Journal of investigative dermatology,* 2008, *128,* (8), 2013-2023.

[47] Niessner, H.; Beck, D.; Sinnberg, T.; Lasithiotakis, K.; Maczey, E.; Gogel, J.; Venturelli, S.; Berger, A.; Mauthe, M.; Toulany, M.; Flaherty, K.; Schaller, M.; Schadendorf, D.; Proikas-Cezanne, T.; Schittek, B.; Garbe, C.; Kulms, D.; Meier, F., The farnesyl transferase inhibitor lonafarnib inhibits mTOR signaling and enforces sorafenib-induced apoptosis in melanoma cells. *The Journal of investigative dermatology,* 2011, *131,* (2), 468-479.

[48] Khalili, J.S.; Yu, X.; Wang, J.; Hayes, B.C.; Davies, M.A.; Lizee, G.; Esmaeli, B.; Woodman, S.E., Combination small molecule MEK and PI3K inhibition enhances uveal melanoma cell death in a mutant GNAQ-and GNA11-dependent manner. *Clinical cancer research : an official journal of the American Association for Cancer Research,* 2012, *18,* (16), 4345-4355.

[49] Lassen, A.; Atefi, M.; Robert, L.; Wong, D.J.; Cerniglia, M.; Comin-Anduix, B.; Ribas, A., Effects of AKT inhibitor therapy in response and resistance to BRAF inhibition in melanoma. *Molecular cancer,* 2014, *13,* 83.

[50] Byron, S.A.; Loch, D.C.; Wellens, C.L.; Wortmann, A.; Wu, J.; Wang, J.; Nomoto, K.; Pollock, P.M., Sensitivity to the MEK inhibitor E6201 in melanoma cells is associated with mutant BRAF and wildtype PTEN status. *Molecular cancer,* 2012, *11,* 75.

[51] Posch, C.; Moslehi, H.; Feeney, L.; Green, G.A.; Ebaee, A.; Feichtenschlager, V.; Chong, K.; Peng, L.; Dimon, M.T.; Phillips, T.; Daud, A.I.; McCalmont, T.H.; LeBoit, P.E.; Ortiz-Urda, S., Combined targeting of MEK and PI3K/mTOR effector pathways is necessary to effectively inhibit NRAS mutant melanoma in vitro and in vivo. *Proceedings of the National Academy of Sciences of the United States of America,* 2013, *110,* (10), 4015-4020.

[52] Shi, H.; Kong, X.; Ribas, A.; Lo, R.S., Combinatorial treatments that overcome PDGFRbeta-driven resistance of melanoma cells to V600EB-RAF inhibition. *Cancer research,* 2011, *71,* (15), 5067-5074.

[53] Shimizu, T.; Tolcher, A.W.; Papadopoulos, K.P.; Beeram, M.; Rasco, D.W.; Smith, L.S.; Gunn, S.; Smetzer, L.; Mays, T.A.; Kaiser, B.; Wick, M.J.; Alvarez, C.; Cavazos, A.; Mangold, G.L.; Patnaik, A., The clinical effect of the dual-targeting strategy involving PI3K/AKT/mTOR and RAS/MEK/ERK pathways in patients with advanced cancer. *Clinical cancer research : an official journal of the American Association for Cancer Research,* 2012, *18,* (8), 2316-2325.

[54] Frederick, D.T.; Piris, A.; Cogdill, A.P.; Cooper, Z.A.; Lezcano, C.; Ferrone, C.R.; Mitra, D.; Boni, A.; Newton, L.P.; Liu, C.W.; Peng, W.Y.; Sullivan, R.J.; Lawrence, D.P.; Hodi, F.S.; Overwijk, W.W.; Lizee, G.; Murphy, G.F.; Hwu, P.; Flaherty, K.T.; Fisher, D.E.; Wargo, J.A., BRAF Inhibition Is Associated with Enhanced Melanoma Antigen Expression and a More Favorable Tumor Microenvironment in Patients with Metastatic Melanoma. *Clinical Cancer Research,* 2013, *19,* (5), 1225-1231.

[55] Lev, D.C.; Ruiz, M.; Mills, L.; McGary, E.C.; Price, J.E.; Bar-Eli, M., Dacarbazine causes transcriptional up-regulation of interleukin 8 and vascular endothelial growth factor in melanoma cells: a possible escape mechanism from chemotherapy. *Molecular cancer therapeutics,* 2003, *2,* (8), 753-763.

[56] Ghosh, S.; Maity, P., Augmented antitumor effects of combination therapy with VEGF antibody and cisplatin on murine B16F10 melanoma cells. *International immunopharmacology,* 2007, *7,* (13), 1598-1608.

[57] Sini, P.; Samarzija, I.; Baffert, F.; Littlewood-Evans, A.; Schnell, C.; Theuer, A.; Christian, S.; Boos, A.; Hess-Stumpp, H.; Foekens, J.A.; Setyono-Han, B.; Wood, J.; Hynes, N.E., Inhibition of multiple vascular endothelial growth factor receptors (VEGFR) blocks lymph node metastases but inhibition of VEGFR-2 is sufficient to sensitize tu-

mor cells to platinum-based chemotherapeutics. *Cancer research,* 2008, *68,* (5), 1581-1592.

[58] Terheyden, P.; Hofmann, M.A.; Weininger, M.; Brocker, E.B.; Becker, J.C., Anti-vascular endothelial growth factor antibody bevacizumab in conjunction with chemotherapy in metastasising melanoma. *Journal of cancer research and clinical oncology,* 2007, *133,* (11), 897-901.

[59] Sun, C.; Wang, L.; Huang, S.; Heynen, G.J.; Prahallad, A.; Robert, C.; Haanen, J.; Blank, C.; Wesseling, J.; Willems, S.M.; Zecchin, D.; Hobor, S.; Bajpe, P.K.; Lieftink, C.; Mateus, C.; Vagner, S.; Grernrum, W.; Hofland, I.; Schlicker, A.; Wessels, L.F.; Beijersbergen, R.L.; Bardelli, A.; Di Nicolantonio, F.; Eggermont, A.M.; Bernards, R., Reversible and adaptive resistance to BRAF(V600E) inhibition in melanoma. *Nature,* 2014, *508,* (7494), 118-122.

[60] Motl, S., Bevacizumab in combination chemotherapy for colorectal and other cancers. *American journal of health-system pharmacy : AJHP : official journal of the American Society of Health-System Pharmacists,* 2005, *62,* (10), 1021-1032.

[61] Del Vecchio, M.; Mortarini, R.; Canova, S.; Di Guardo, L.; Pimpinelli, N.; Sertoli, M.R.; Bedognetti, D.; Queirolo, P.; Morosini, P.; Perrone, T.; Bajetta, E.; Anichini, A., Bevacizumab plus fotemustine as first-line treatment in metastatic melanoma patients: clinical activity and modulation of angiogenesis and lymphangiogenesis factors. *Clinical cancer research : an official journal of the American Association for Cancer Research,* 2010, *16,* (23), 5862-5872.

[62] Kottschade, L.A.; Suman, V.J.; Perez, D.G.; McWilliams, R.R.; Kaur, J.S.; Amatruda, T.T., 3rd; Geoffroy, F.J.; Gross, H.M.; Cohen, P.A.; Jaslowski, A.J.; Kosel, M.L.; Markovic, S.N., A randomized phase 2 study of temozolomide and bevacizumab or nab-paclitaxel, carboplatin, and bevacizumab in patients with unresectable stage IV melanoma : a North Central Cancer Treatment Group study, N0775. *Cancer,* 2013, *119,* (3), 586-592.

[63] Li, B.; Lalani, A.S.; Harding, T.C.; Luan, B.; Koprivnikar, K.; Huan Tu, G.; Prell, R.; VanRoey, M.J.; Simmons, A.D.; Jooss, K., Vascular endothelial growth factor blockade reduces intratumoral regulatory T cells and enhances the efficacy of a GM-CSF-secreting cancer immunotherapy. *Clinical cancer research : an official journal of the American Association for Cancer Research,* 2006, *12,* (22), 6808-6816.

[64] Mita, M.M.; Rowinsky, E.K.; Forero, L.; Eckhart, S.G.; Izbicka, E.; Weiss, G.R.; Beeram, M.; Mita, A.C.; de Bono, J.S.; Tolcher, A.W.; Hammond, L.A.; Simmons, P.; Berg, K.; Takimoto, C.; Patnaik, A., A phase II, pharmacokinetic, and biologic study of semaxanib and thalidomide in patients with metastatic melanoma. *Cancer chemotherapy and pharmacology,* 2007, *59,* (2), 165-174.

[65] Hasumi, Y.; Klosowska-Wardega, A.; Furuhashi, M.; Ostman, A.; Heldin, C.H.; Hellberg, C., Identification of a subset of pericytes that respond to combination therapy

targeting PDGF and VEGF signaling. *International journal of cancer. Journal international du cancer,* 2007, *121,* (12), 2606-2614.

[66] O'Reilly, T.; Lane, H.A.; Wood, J.M.; Schnell, C.; Littlewood-Evans, A.; Brueggen, J.; McSheehy, P.M., Everolimus and PTK/ZK show synergistic growth inhibition in the orthotopic BL16/BL6 murine melanoma model. *Cancer chemotherapy and pharmacology,* 2011, *67,* (1), 193-200.

[67] Hainsworth, J.D.; Infante, J.R.; Spigel, D.R.; Peyton, J.D.; Thompson, D.S.; Lane, C.M.; Clark, B.L.; Rubin, M.S.; Trent, D.F.; Burris, H.A., 3rd, Bevacizumab and everolimus in the treatment of patients with metastatic melanoma: a phase 2 trial of the Sarah Cannon Oncology Research Consortium. *Cancer,* 2010, *116,* (17), 4122-4129.

[68] Mahalingam, D.; Malik, L.; Beeram, M.; Rodon, J.; Sankhala, K.; Mita, A.; Benjamin, D.; Ketchum, N.; Michalek, J.; Tolcher, A.; Wright, J.; Sarantopoulos, J., Phase II study evaluating the efficacy, safety, and pharmacodynamic correlative study of dual anti-angiogenic inhibition using bevacizumab in combination with sorafenib in patients with advanced malignant melanoma. *Cancer chemotherapy and pharmacology,* 2014, *74,* (1), 77-84.

[69] Mittal, K.; Koon, H.; Elson, P.; Triozzi, P.; Dowlati, A.; Chen, H.; Borden, E.C.; Rini, B.I., Dual VEGF/VEGFR inhibition in advanced solid malignancies: Clinical effects and pharmacodynamic biomarkers. *Cancer biology & therapy,* 2014, *15,* (8), 975-981.

[70] Mirmohammadsadegh, A.; Mota, R.; Gustrau, A.; Hassan, M.; Nambiar, S.; Marini, A.; Bojar, H.; Tannapfel, A.; Hengge, U.R., ERK1/2 is highly phosphorylated in melanoma metastases and protects melanoma cells from cisplatin-mediated apoptosis. *The Journal of investigative dermatology,* 2007, *127,* (9), 2207-2215.

[71] Ivanov, V.N.; Hei, T.K., Combined treatment with EGFR inhibitors and arsenite upregulated apoptosis in human EGFR-positive melanomas: a role of suppression of the PI3K-AKT pathway. *Oncogene,* 2005, *24,* (4), 616-626.

[72] Sinnberg, T.; Lasithiotakis, K.; Niessner, H.; Schittek, B.; Flaherty, K.T.; Kulms, D.; Maczey, E.; Campos, M.; Gogel, J.; Garbe, C.; Meier, F., Inhibition of PI3K-AKT-mTOR signaling sensitizes melanoma cells to cisplatin and temozolomide. *The Journal of investigative dermatology,* 2009, *129,* (6), 1500-1515.

[73] Keuling, A.M.; Andrew, S.E.; Tron, V.A., Inhibition of p38 MAPK enhances ABT-737-induced cell death in melanoma cell lines: novel regulation of PUMA. *Pigment cell & melanoma research,* 2010, *23,* (3), 430-440.

[74] Frederick, D.T.; Salas Fragomeni, R.A.; Schalck, A.; Ferreiro-Neira, I.; Hoff, T.; Cooper, Z.A.; Haq, R.; Panka, D.J.; Kwong, L.N.; Davies, M.A.; Cusack, J.C.; Flaherty, K.T.; Fisher, D.E.; Mier, J.W.; Wargo, J.A.; Sullivan, R.J., Clinical profiling of BCL-2 family members in the setting of BRAF inhibition offers a rationale for targeting de novo resistance using BH3 mimetics. *PloS one,* 2014, *9,* (7), e101286.

[75] Ji, Z.; Kumar, R.; Taylor, M.; Rajadurai, A.; Marzuka-Alcala, A.; Chen, Y.E.; Njauw, C.N.; Flaherty, K.; Jonsson, G.; Tsao, H., Vemurafenib synergizes with nutlin-3 to deplete survivin and suppresses melanoma viability and tumor growth. *Clinical cancer research : an official journal of the American Association for Cancer Research,* 2013, *19,* (16), 4383-4391.

[76] Vultur, A.; Villanueva, J.; Krepler, C.; Rajan, G.; Chen, Q.; Xiao, M.; Li, L.; Gimotty, P.A.; Wilson, M.; Hayden, J.; Keeney, F.; Nathanson, K.L.; Herlyn, M., MEK inhibition affects STAT3 signaling and invasion in human melanoma cell lines. *Oncogene,* 2014, *33,* (14), 1850-1861.

[77] Martin, M.J.; Hayward, R.; Viros, A.; Marais, R., Metformin accelerates the growth of BRAF V600E-driven melanoma by upregulating VEGF-A. *Cancer discovery,* 2012, *2,* (4), 344-355.

[78] Woodard, J.; Platanias, L.C., AMP-activated kinase (AMPK)-generated signals in malignant melanoma cell growth and survival. *Biochemical and biophysical research communications,* 2010, *398,* (1), 135-139.

[79] Niehr, F.; von Euw, E.; Attar, N.; Guo, D.; Matsunaga, D.; Sazegar, H.; Ng, C.; Glaspy, J.A.; Recio, J.A.; Lo, R.S.; Mischel, P.S.; Comin-Anduix, B.; Ribas, A., Combination therapy with vemurafenib (PLX4032/RG7204) and metformin in melanoma cell lines with distinct driver mutations. *Journal of translational medicine,* 2011, *9,* 76.

[80] Sagoo, M.S.; Harbour, J.W.; Stebbing, J.; Bowcock, A.M., Combined PKC and MEK inhibition for treating metastatic uveal melanoma. *Oncogene,* 2014.

[81] Wu, X.; Zhu, M.; Fletcher, J.A.; Giobbie-Hurder, A.; Hodi, F.S., The protein kinase C inhibitor enzastaurin exhibits antitumor activity against uveal melanoma. *PloS one,* 2012, *7,* (1), e29622.

[82] Chen, X.; Wu, Q.; Tan, L.; Porter, D.; Jager, M.J.; Emery, C.; Bastian, B.C., Combined PKC and MEK inhibition in uveal melanoma with GNAQ and GNA11 mutations. *Oncogene,* 2013.

[83] Wang, J.; Chen, J.; Miller, D.D.; Li, W., Synergistic combination of novel tubulin inhibitor ABI-274 and vemurafenib overcome vemurafenib acquired resistance in BRAFV600E melanoma. *Molecular cancer therapeutics,* 2014, *13,* (1), 16-26.

[84] Acquaviva, J.; Smith, D.L.; Jimenez, J.P.; Zhang, C.; Sequeira, M.; He, S.; Sang, J.; Bates, R.C.; Proia, D.A., Overcoming acquired BRAF inhibitor resistance in melanoma via targeted inhibition of Hsp90 with ganetespib. *Molecular cancer therapeutics,* 2014, *13,* (2), 353-363.

[85] Yadav, V.; Burke, T.F.; Huber, L.; Van Horn, R.D.; Zhang, Y.; Buchanan, S.G.; Chan, E.M.; Starling, J.J.; Beckmann, R.P.; Peng, S.B., The CDK4/6 Inhibitor LY2835219 Overcomes Vemurafenib Resistance Resulting from MAPK Reactivation and Cyclin D1 Upregulation. *Molecular cancer therapeutics,* 2014.

[86] Hodi, F.S.; O'Day, S.J.; McDermott, D.F.; Weber, R.W.; Sosman, J.A.; Haanen, J.B.; Gonzalez, R.; Robert, C.; Schadendorf, D.; Hassel, J.C.; Akerley, W.; van den Eertwegh, A.J.; Lutzky, J.; Lorigan, P.; Vaubel, J.M.; Linette, G.P.; Hogg, D.; Ottensmeier, C.H.; Lebbe, C.; Peschel, C.; Quirt, I.; Clark, J.I.; Wolchok, J.D.; Weber, J.S.; Tian, J.; Yellin, M.J.; Nichol, G.M.; Hoos, A.; Urba, W.J., Improved survival with ipilimumab in patients with metastatic melanoma. *The New England journal of medicine,* 2010, *363,* (8), 711-723.

[87] Srivastava, N.; McDermott, D., Update on benefit of immunotherapy and targeted therapy in melanoma: the changing landscape. *Cancer management and research,* 2014, *6,* 279-289.

[88] Riley, J.L., Combination checkpoint blockade--taking melanoma immunotherapy to the next level. *The New England journal of medicine,* 2013, *369,* (2), 187-189.

[89] Maio, M.; Di Giacomo, A.M.; Robert, C.; Eggermont, A.M., Update on the role of ipilimumab in melanoma and first data on new combination therapies. *Current opinion in oncology,* 2013, *25,* (2), 166-172.

[90] Topalian, S.L.; Hodi, F.S.; Brahmer, J.R.; Gettinger, S.N.; Smith, D.C.; McDermott, D.F.; Powderly, J.D.; Carvajal, R.D.; Sosman, J.A.; Atkins, M.B.; Leming, P.D.; Spigel, D.R.; Antonia, S.J.; Horn, L.; Drake, C.G.; Pardoll, D.M.; Chen, L.; Sharfman, W.H.; Anders, R.A.; Taube, J.M.; McMiller, T.L.; Xu, H.; Korman, A.J.; Jure-Kunkel, M.; Agrawal, S.; McDonald, D.; Kollia, G.D.; Gupta, A.; Wigginton, J.M.; Sznol, M., Safety, activity, and immune correlates of anti-PD-1 antibody in cancer. *The New England journal of medicine,* 2012, *366,* (26), 2443-2454.

[91] Shah, D.J.; Dronca, R.S., Latest advances in chemotherapeutic, targeted, and immune approaches in the treatment of metastatic melanoma. *Mayo Clinic proceedings,* 2014, *89,* (4), 504-519.

[92] Perez-Gracia, J.L.; Labiano, S.; Rodriguez-Ruiz, M.E.; Sanmamed, M.F.; Melero, I., Orchestrating immune check-point blockade for cancer immunotherapy in combinations. *Current opinion in immunology,* 2014, *27,* 89-97.

[93] Brahmer, J.R.; Tykodi, S.S.; Chow, L.Q.; Hwu, W.J.; Topalian, S.L.; Hwu, P.; Drake, C.G.; Camacho, L.H.; Kauh, J.; Odunsi, K.; Pitot, H.C.; Hamid, O.; Bhatia, S.; Martins, R.; Eaton, K.; Chen, S.; Salay, T.M.; Alaparthy, S.; Grosso, J.F.; Korman, A.J.; Parker, S.M.; Agrawal, S.; Goldberg, S.M.; Pardoll, D.M.; Gupta, A.; Wigginton, J.M., Safety and activity of anti-PD-L1 antibody in patients with advanced cancer. *The New England journal of medicine,* 2012, *366,* (26), 2455-2465.

[94] Curran, M.A.; Montalvo, W.; Yagita, H.; Allison, J.P., PD-1 and CTLA-4 combination blockade expands infiltrating T cells and reduces regulatory T and myeloid cells within B16 melanoma tumors. *Proceedings of the National Academy of Sciences of the United States of America,* 2010, *107,* (9), 4275-4280.

[95] Wolchok, J.D.; Kluger, H.; Callahan, M.K.; Postow, M.A.; Rizvi, N.A.; Lesokhin, A.M.; Segal, N.H.; Ariyan, C.E.; Gordon, R.A.; Reed, K.; Burke, M.M.; Caldwell, A.;

Kronenberg, S.A.; Agunwamba, B.U.; Zhang, X.; Lowy, I.; Inzunza, H.D.; Feely, W.; Horak, C.E.; Hong, Q.; Korman, A.J.; Wigginton, J.M.; Gupta, A.; Sznol, M., Nivolumab plus ipilimumab in advanced melanoma. *The New England journal of medicine,* 2013, *369,* (2), 122-133.

[96] Kudchadkar, R.R.; Gibney, G.T.; Weber, J.; Chen, A.; Smith, K.; Merek, S., A phase IB study of ipilimumab with peginterferon alfa-2b in patients with unresectable melanoma. *Journal of Clinical Oncology,* 2013, *31,* (15).

[97] Hodi, F.S.; Lee, S.J.; McDermott, D.F.; Rao, U.N.M.; Butterfield, L.H.; Tarhini, A.A.; Leming, P.D.; Puzanov, I.; Kirkwood, J.M.; Grp, E.C.O., Multicenter, randomized phase II trial of GM-CSF (GM) plus ipilimumab (Ipi) versus ipi alone in metastatic melanoma: E1608. *Journal of Clinical Oncology,* 2013, *31,* (15).

[98] Kwong, M.L.; Neyns, B.; Yang, J.C., Adoptive T-cell transfer therapy and oncogene-targeted therapy for melanoma: the search for synergy. *Clinical cancer research : an official journal of the American Association for Cancer Research,* 2013, *19,* (19), 5292-5299.

[99] Wilmott, J.S.; Long, G.V.; Howle, J.R.; Haydu, L.E.; Sharma, R.N.; Thompson, J.F.; Kefford, R.F.; Hersey, P.; Scolyer, R.A., Selective BRAF Inhibitors Induce Marked T-cell Infiltration into Human Metastatic Melanoma. *Clinical Cancer Research,* 2012, *18,* (5), 1386-1394.

[100] Donia, M.; Fagone, P.; Nicoletti, F.; Andersen, R.S.; Hogdall, E.; Straten, P.T.; Andersen, M.H.; Svane, I.M., BRAF inhibition improves tumor recognition by the immune system: Potential implications for combinatorial therapies against melanoma involving adoptive T-cell transfer. *Oncoimmunology,* 2012, *1,* (9), 1476-1483.

[101] Liu, C.; Peng, W.; Xu, C.; Lou, Y.; Zhang, M.; Wargo, J.A.; Chen, J.Q.; Li, H.S.; Watowich, S.S.; Yang, Y.; Tompers Frederick, D.; Cooper, Z.A.; Mbofung, R.M.; Whittington, M.; Flaherty, K.T.; Woodman, S.E.; Davies, M.A.; Radvanyi, L.G.; Overwijk, W.W.; Lizee, G.; Hwu, P., BRAF inhibition increases tumor infiltration by T cells and enhances the antitumor activity of adoptive immunotherapy in mice. *Clinical cancer research : an official journal of the American Association for Cancer Research,* 2013, *19,* (2), 393-403.

[102] Jiang, X.; Zhou, J.; Giobbie-Hurder, A.; Wargo, J.; Hodi, F.S., The activation of MAPK in melanoma cells resistant to BRAF inhibition promotes PD-L1 expression that is reversible by MEK and PI3K inhibition. *Clinical cancer research : an official journal of the American Association for Cancer Research,* 2013, *19,* (3), 598-609.

[103] Vella, L.J.; Pasam, A.; Dimopoulos, N.; Andrews, M.; Knights, A.; Puaux, A.L.; Louahed, J.; Chen, W.; Woods, K.; Cebon, J.S., MEK inhibition, alone or in combination with BRAF inhibition, affects multiple functions of isolated normal human lymphocytes and dendritic cells. Cancer immunology research, 2014, 2, (4), 351-360.

[104] Ribas, A.; Hodi, F.S.; Callahan, M.; Konto, C.; Wolchok, J., Hepatotoxicity with combination of vemurafenib and ipilimumab. The New England journal of medicine, 2013, 368, (14), 1365-1366.

Chapter 9

New Insights in Cutaneous Melanoma Immune-Therapy — Tackling Immune-Suppression and Specific Anti-Tumoral Response

Monica Neagu and Carolina Constantin

Additional information is available at the end of the chapter

http://dx.doi.org/10.5772/59494

1. Introduction

In this chapter the maturity of immune-therapy in cancer, with emphasis on melanoma will be discussed.

The heterogeneity of melanoma tumour regarding primary and metastatic variants will be argued. Therefore the mutational heterogeneity of this type of tumor triggers complex immune-therapy approach. Notions such as *Immune-therapy* will be tackled, meaning targeting immune elements like immune suppression and using immune drugs like monoclonal antibodies against targets that can or not be immune elements. The chapter will end with the importance of designing complex immune-therapies like abolishing the immune-suppression and enhancing the specific anti-tumoral effect.

Physiologically, the immune system can recognize cells that display an aberrant proliferation like neoplasia. The immune system is equipped with cells that can destroy cancer cells them during their early development. Years ago, when the theory of immunoediting was initiated [1], immunosurveillance was defined as a complex pathway that supervises and controls the elimination of transformed self cells/tissue. When the immune system cannot properly control these aberrantly proliferating cells, and the equilibrium is deregulated, tumour cells escape and form a clinically significant tumoral tissue [2].

In cancer immune-therapy, several approaches that aim to start and sustain the immune response and eventually elicit an immunological memory were lately tackled. The therapy armentarium that started the "bumpy road" from bench to bedside comprises cancer vaccines, adoptive T cell therapy, anti-tumor antibodies, immune checkpoint blockade and/or various immune combinations. Some of the conclusions of the last Congress of SITC (*Society for*

Immunotherapy of Cancer) is that combining these above mentioned immune approaches with other immunomodulators (e.g. cytokines, cyclic dinucleotides) and/or indoleamine 2,3-dioxygenase (IDO) inhibitors can increase the efficacy of immunotherapy [3] and hopefully replace in the future routine approaches such as chemotherapy/radiotherapy.

Early diagnosed stages of melanoma are resolved mainly by surgery and large margin excision, but for advanced stages, systemic therapies, whether chemotherapy, immune-therapy or combined ones have had very low efficacy. Advanced melanoma remains a continuous clinical provocation for the physicians who use therapeutical approaches with low response rates, unmanageable toxicities, and reduced efficacy.

One of the main *molecular hurdles* in cutaneous melanoma is the heterogeneity of tumors. A tumoral tissue has cells with different characteristics in terms of proliferation, invasiveness and pheno/genotype. In melanoma, aggressiveness has a distinct cellular genotype and in the tumor dynamic development, cells go through several phenotype switching [4]. Specific genetic expression studies have identified more than 100 genes over-expressed in cells with a higher proliferative capacity or in cells that were committed to invade tissues [5].

Recently, a study was published on single melanoma cells and the report shows that there are 114 genes expression that could distinguish the proliferative and invasive phenotype of cells. Among these genes, regulatory networks were found along with genes that encode for pluripotency factor (e.g. POUF51); all these genes were found associated with cell's tumorigenic potential. Authors report that among the regulatory network genes, MITF (microphthalmia-associated transcription factor) is one of the key players in the heterogeneous character of tumour cells populations. Moreover, the heterogeneity of cells depends on the 2D or 3D status of the cell cultures, thus TPBG (trophoblast glycoprotein) is expressed in a melanoma cell line, 501Mel, only in 3D cultures [4]. In the same way, in 1205Lu melanospheres, PI3K/AKT (phosphatidylinositol 3' –kinase/protein kinase B) signaling pathway is enhanced [4], while DAPK1 (death-associated protein kinase 1) expression is decreased in 501Mel experimental tumors, finding that is in line with the hypermethylated gene promoter associated to melanoma [6]. This study emphasizes that when transformed melanocytes start to organize in growing tumors, the heterogeneity of the cellular populations' increases, the tumoral tissue having MITF-low/negative cells [4, 7]. In experimental tumour spheres, cells that grow on the exterior layers have an active proliferation, while in the interior of the tumour, due to hypoxic conditions, cells are arrested in the G1 phase [8]. The overall mechanism is that 3D growth enhances tumour-initiating properties [9].

Cell's heterogeneity is important from the immunological point of view. Tumour heterogeneous tissues have different expression of tumor antigens, thus any type of therapy that addresses only one tumour epitope is proned to have low efficacy. This is the rationale to investigate tumor antigens and evaluate the patient's immune responses prior to any immune-therapy [10].

Extensive studies performed by large groups of researchers and extended networks like *Melanoma Research Networks* established in Europe, Canada, and New Zeeland have provided seminal scientific information regarding melanoma's immune biology. All these insights have led to an actual scientific leap by the development of the first immune-therapies that proved efficacy in advanced melanoma treatment. Therefore drugs that aim intracellular pathways such as mitogen-activated protein kinase (MAPK) pathway, or antibodies that aim CTLA4 (cytotoxic T lymphocyte-associated protein 4), or PD1/PD1-L (programmed cell death 1/ programmed cell death 1 ligand) have recently followed the bench to bedside path [11]. Building upon the early success of these therapies, trials involving new classes of drugs and combinations of these drugs are underway [12].

Starting from 2011, metastatic melanoma beneficiated from four new approved drugs, all these drugs proving in clinical trials the improvement of patient's survival. From this four drugs, one is a B-Raf enzyme inhibitor (vemurafenib), one is an inhibitor of the associated enzyme B-Raf (dabrafenib), and one is a MEK inhibitor (trametinib); the only one that is an actual immune-therapy, is an anti-CTLA-4 (ipilimumab) antibody [13]. Therefore searching new efficacious immune-therapies in this disease is still an open subject of intense research.

This chapter summarizes the main achievements gathered in the last 3 years regarding immune-therapy as the ultimate approach for melanoma treatment.

2. Reducing specific immune-suppression

Until recently, the approved therapy armentarium in advanced melanoma was comprising only dacarbazine (DTIC), hydroxyurea, while the only approved immune agent was high-dose interleukin-2 (IL-2) [14]. These drugs cannot provide satisfactory overall survival (OS) rates in advanced stages. After searching various combination of immune-therapies, from vaccination [15] to drugs that inhibit immune-signaling pathways [16], in 2011 FDA approved, ipilimumab and vemurafenib, agents that significantly increased OS and long-term improvement in advanced melanoma [17].

In this case, monoclonal antibodies (mAbs) as immune-therapy agents have the intrinsic role to establish an antineoplastic action through stimulation of a specific immune response. This action can be performed by inducing *de novo* primary response and/or by eliciting an already existing antitumor action, but repressed in these patients.

The most advanced, in terms of positive research results, were the immune-related drugs that abrogated the immune –suppression such as CTLA4 or PD-1. Other mAbs were designed to aim toward stimulation of co-stimulatory receptors, molecules that are expressed by antigen presenting cells (APC); the aimed molecules were CD40 or OX40 (member 4 tumor necrosis factor receptor superfamily) or GITR (TNFRSF18), expressed on activated T lymphocytes.

Tremelimumab, also an anti CTLA4 mAb, is being evaluated in solid tumors. Nivolumab, an anti PD-1 mAb is also in the evaluation phase. This year (2014) clinical trials assessing OX40- and GITR-activating mAbs were initiated as well [18].

2.1. Anti-CTLA-4 antibodies

Activated T lymphocytes express transiently CTLA-4 transmembrane protein, while on T regulatory lymphocytes (Tregs) this protein is expressed constitutively. Two possible mechanisms are known accounting for CTLA-4 immune-suppressive effect. One of the mechanisms is the competitive binding to B7-1 and B7-2 in the detriment of the normal binding to CD28, delivering thus an immune-suppressive signal [19]. Actually CTLA-4 competes with the binding of CD28 to B7, thus hindering a normal activation. The other possible mechanism is that cells expressing CTLA-4, endocytose the appropriate ligands of other cells, as such, CD28 cannot trigger activation [20].

Overall in cancer research, drugs that aim B7 family can enhance the therapeutic panel and thorough studies are further needed for elucidating these regulatory pathways [21].

The particular action of monoclonal anti-CTLA-4 antibody is to link to CTLA-4, blocking the inhibitory immune-suppressive signal, T cell can perform thus its activation pathways, proliferate while infiltrating the tumors, and in the end, set off tumour apoptosis. Designed to bind to CTLA-4, ipilimumab was approved by FDA in 2011 for advanced melanoma [22] and in the same year the European Commission issued a marketing authorization for ipilimumab [23].This type of immune-drug aims to downregulate the inhibitory activity of T-lymphocytes leading to the normal activation of T cells by allowing the binding of CD28 to B7, this costimulatory process participates to the main coupling of MHC (major histocompatibility complex) that presents the tumour antigen to TCR (T cell receptor). Re-establishing these physiological molecular interactions, T-cells can mount an efficient antitumor immune response (Figure 1) [24]. CTLA-4 expressed on T cells is omnipresent and is not dependent upon the tumour's particularities, thus the drug's action should not be dependent on tumor's characteristics.

EMA recommendation after analyzing the post-phase III results extended clinical trials [25,17] is a dose of intravenously 3 mg/kg ipilimumab over a 90 min period, this procedure needs to be repeated every 3 weeks; overall four doses should be administered [23]. If the patients are treated in combination with DTIC it is recommended that a dose of 10 mg/kg should be used [25,17].

The actual clinical results of using this immune-therapy showed that patients with advanced melanoma increased their median OS to 10 months when compared to the 6 months OS in gp100 melanoma vaccine. When comparing OS in patients treated with ipilimumab in combination with DTIC, OS was 11 months, while DTIC monotherapy just 9 months.

As stated above ipilimumab's action is not dependent on specific and individual tumor cell mutations, hence it can be efficient in different patients and stages [26, 27]. The beneficial clinical results regarding OS were registered as independent of various parameters such as age, gender, stage and/or previous therapy regimens.

Investigating the patients survival curves it has been shown that there are groups surviving more than 4 years [28], and that their clinical response was durable during the follow-up [29]. Durability is an important differentiating criterion when recommending first-line therapy with immunomodulators in comparison to the duration obtained in kinase inhibitors treatment.

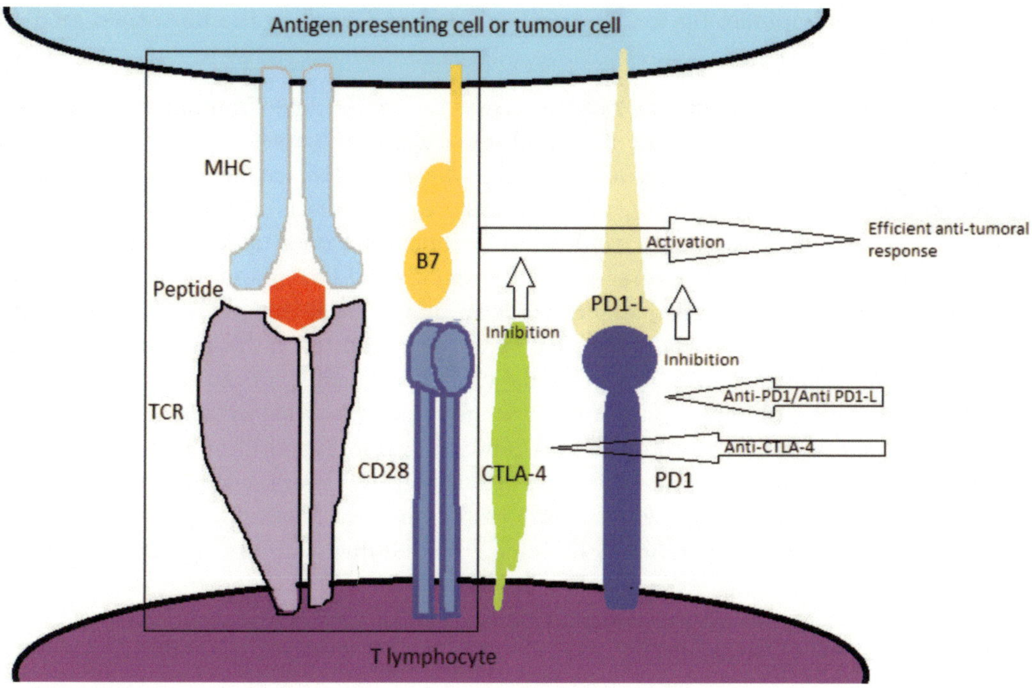

Figure 1. Main immune-suppression molecular mechanisms that can be overridden by therapeutical monoclonal antibodies targeting CTLA-4 and PD1.

As we are focusing on an immune therapy and as *immune memory* is a characteristic of this process, it was a logic approach to see what the effects are when ipilimumab gets another round of therapy. The National Comprehensive Cancer Network (NCCN) recommendation show that ipilimumab re-treatment can be done when the first round induced intolerable toxicity and/or for patients relapsing after the first therapy or proving at least 3 months stable disease [30]. Adverse reaction during re-treatment are similar to those for the first approach (see below) and no actual predisposition was noted regarding first encountered toxicity with the re-treatment one. Authors report that retreatment with ipilimumab is a feasible therapy and, currently a phase II trial (http://trialsunited.com/studies/NCT01709162) focuses on the immune response parameters in ipilimumab re-treatment [31].

Non-cutaneous melanomas were also therapeutic targets for ipilimumab therapy. Thus, in an Australian study published in 2014 over 100 patients were followed after ipilimumab therapy. Median OS for mucosal and uveal melanoma patients was half of that registered in cutaneous melanoma patients. This report underlines the severities of adverse effects, even death-related to therapy cases, thus administration and follow-up by an experienced clinical team is extremely necessary in this type of clinical trials [32].

Stage IV patients presenting brain metastasis were another therapy target group as blood-brain barrier is permeable to activated T lymphocytes, cells capable of inducing a local immune response [33]. In a large study comprising over 800 patients with brain metastasis treated with ipilimumab, up to 25% survived at least 1 year, as the un-treated median OS is only 5 months [34].

Adverse reactions in ipilimumab therapy are associated with hyper-immune reactions, but these can be solved by the physician using additional classic therapies. Over 10% of patients experienced gastrointestinal deregulations (e.g. diarrhea, nausea, vomiting, decreased appetite and abdominal pain), rash, pruritus, fatigue. Side-effects are manageable by the physician and, seldom, the severity can lead to treatment discontinuation (www.ema.europa.eu). These immune-related adverse effects (irAEs) are mild to moderate toxicity and are experienced by around 60% of the patients, while around 15% developed grade 3 or 4 toxicity [25]. Endocrine system – related adverse effects were also reported in this therapy; in patients group receiving ipilimumab, 8% have experienced hypophysitis and 6% hypothyroidism/thyroiditis. Combined therapy, ipilimumab and nivolumab, induce in 22% of the patients thyroiditis or hypothyroidism and in 9% hypophysitis. Authors report hormone replacement as adjuvant therapy and immediate initiation of this therapy reverses symptoms [35]. If the ipilimumab therapy is combined with vemurafenib, important hepatotoxicity was reported, thus caution should be taken when combining immune-therapy with this B-Raf enzyme inhibitor [36].

2.2. Anti-PD-1 or PD-1L antibodies

2.2.1. *Nivolumab*

In July 2014, the first human monoclonal antibody against programmed death receptor-1 was announced as approved in Japan-*Nivolumab* [37]. As shown above in Figure 1, it targets a negative regulatory molecule that sustains immunosuppression. After accomplishing phase I and II clinical trials, around 25% of stage III and IV patients had a good clinical response when 2 mg/kg intravenous nivolumab was administered every 3 weeks. The clinical outcome was very optimistic in this study, patients did not progress in their disease for a median of 172 days, and at the time of publication (July 2014) median OS was still not achieved.

Nivolumab displayed a good tolerability profile; grade 3 or 4 adverse effects were reported in les than 18 % of patients, mainly an increased γ-glutamyl transferase [38].

Another group studying T lymphocyte interaction with tumour cell, interaction mediated by PD-1 receptor linking to PD-L 1, has shown that in phase I/II studies this antibody can lead to tumor regression and can enhance OS in various cancers including skin melanoma. Studying antibodies that target PD-1 or PD-1L (e.g. nivolumab, MK-3475, pidilizumab, MPDL3280A, BMS-936559, MEDI4736, MSB0010718C) the authors show that the positive clinical response goes to a maximum of 50% response rate when antibodies against PD-1 combined with anti-CTLA-4 were used. The clinical responses start early upon treatment and continue after the treatment is finished [39].

Another study published in 2014 searched to evaluate the survival of patients upon discontinuation of the therapy. After enrolling over 100 patients with advanced melanoma, the authors concluded that the median OS was 16.8 months [40].

Melanoma patients along with other cancer diagnosed patients were treated with anti-PD-1 (nivolumab). This early-phase clinical trial published in 2014 aimed to elucidate the link between PD-1, PD-L1, and PD-L2 expression, immune cell infiltration and the clinical efficacy of this therapy. The degree of PD-L1 expression depicted on tumor cells was associated with its receptor PD-1 expressed by lymphocytes. The other ligand of PD-1, PD-L2 corroborated with PD-L1 expression. The expression of PD-L1 on the tumors was correlated with the clinical efficacy of the anti-PD-1 therapy, and the found best correlation when compared to other studied factors, such as PD-1 expression and/or TIL (tumor infiltrating lymphocytes). The study concludes that, when achieving maximum efficacy with novilumab, tumor PD-L1 expression is the base of anti-PD-1 therapeutical blockade [41].

In 2013, results from phase I clinical trials, of nivolumab and MK-3475 (anti-PD-1 and anti-PD-L1 antibodies) were released. For MK-3475 an objective response of 38 % with only 13 % of the patients reporting grade 3/4 toxicities was shown [42]. These results were probably the ground for further approval (see below).

Phase III clinical trails are on-going and, it seems that PD-1-PD-L1 triggers a sequence of intracellular signaling that brings important clinical benefits [43].

Adverse effects in this type of therapy are of low grade, the physician can impose a good patient management [39] and long-term safety is acceptable [40].

2.2.2. *Pembrolizumab*

In September 2014, FDA granted accelerated approval to pembrolizumab (formerly known as MK-3475), an antibody targeting PD-1, to be used following ipilimumab therapy. A recently published report showed the efficacy and safety results of this antibody at two doses (2 mg/kg and 10 mg/kg) given every 21 days. The enrolled patients that received the therapy were refractory to ipilimumab therapy. Similar safety profiles were reported whether patients were treated with 2 mg/kg or 10 mg/kg and authors show that no drug-related deaths were registered [44]. Another published study had similar results with the difference that the response rate between patients with or without prior ipilimumab treatment were not statistically different. Positive clinical outcome was registered with the overall median progression-free survival exceeding 7 months. Patients with advanced melanoma, prior refractory to ipilimumab, proved in this study a high rate of tumor regression [45].

Drug-related adverse effects were fatigue in one third of the patients and around 20% of them experienced pruritus and rash. Grade 3 fatigue was the single drug-related grade 3 to 4 adverse effect in 3% of the patients [44].

The positive results in a difficult to manage patients, like the ones refractory to ipilimumab, probably accelerated this drug authorization with two months ahead of its planned approval and the clinical study is still on going [46].

After ipilimumab approval, finding another antibody that could be used as immune-therapy for blocking an immune checkpoint like PD-1 and PD-1L gained an intense research frenzy in the last years.Therapeutical approaches that use immunomodulatory drugs have completely different mode of action in comparison to the well-known chemotherapeutical procedures. From this point of view investigating the intimate mechanisms that underlie their effect is of outmost importance because it can reveal new signaling molecules, future to be drug targets. Moreover biomarkers that can clinically predict the patient response could optimize the approach and personalize the immune-therapy [47].

2.3. Biomarkers for clinical benefit prediction

In the last couple of years there is a less abundant literature focusing on predictive and/or prognostic biomarkers in the immune-therapy of cutaneous melanoma. Biomarkers that were published lately range from classic serum LDH, to membrane molecules and circulating cells without any *clear-cut biomarker* that could predict the immune-therapy efficacy.

In the last year researchers were focusing on biomarkers that can predict immune-therapy with ipilimumab outcome. Thus some studies show that ipilimumab therapy was correlated with an increase in peripheral blood absolute lymphocyte count when patients had a good clinical outcome in terms of OS. More specifically OS was 11.9 months for patients that had more than 1,000 lymphocyte count / μL peripheral blood in comparison to OS of 1.4 months in patients with lower counts [48, 49]. These results were confirmed this year when increased absolute lymphocyte count was associated with increased progression free survival (PFS) but not with OS. Any other parameters including classic serum LDH did not relate to OS or PFS [32].

Another cell biomarker, forkhead box P3 (FoxP3) expressed by T-regs, was correlated with positive clinical outcome in advanced melanoma patients [50].

Correlations were investigated regarding circulatory myeloid-derived suppressor cells (MDSC) in treated patients. Authors report that circulatory MDSC with Lin(-) CD14(+) HLA-DR(-) phenotype are increased in patients compared to normal. After surgically removing the tumour and subjecting patients' to ipilimumab treatment, this immune parameter did not change. Then again, an interesting finding was that patients could be stratified in the ipilimumab-responders and non-responders based on the lower and respectively higher concentration of circulatory MDSC, thus pinpointing these cells as possible predictive markers of response to ipilimumab. This candidate immune-marker did not correlate with baseline serum LDH, but showed higher values in severe metastasis compared to localized metastasis to skin and/or to lymph nodes [51].

As to the possible efficacy biomarkers for nivolumab therapy, in a phase I clinical trial, stage III or IV patients were followed after this therapy by several biomarkers evaluation. This recent study reports that high circulatory T lymphocytes with NY-ESO-1 and MART-1-specific CD8(+) phenotype are associated with disease progression. After therapy, increased circulatory Tregs and decreased antigen-specific T cells are the two immune biomarkers that were found associated with disease progression. The expression of PD-L1 on the tumor did not correlate with the clinical response [52].

2.4. Animal models studying immune-therapy mechanisms

There are few studies focusing on animal models that bring new data regarding the intimate cellular mechanisms in immune-therapy. Having in mind the fact that these recent immune-therapies are limited to certain groups of patients, the published animal models searched for the resistance mechanisms that could hinder this therapy.

In 2013, the role of IDO upon an experimental anti CTLA-4 blockade was shown. Authors used IDO knockout mice and showed that, upon treatment with anti-CTLA-4 antibody, B16 melanoma was growing more slowly and that, the animals' overall survival increased compared to normal mice expressing IDO. The mechanisms were similar when the animal model was treated with anti PD-1/ anti-PD-L1 and GITR. The authors show in this animal model that CTLA-4 and IDO inhibitors converge and that the inhibitory role of IDO can be the background mechanisms accounting for the resistance to anti-CTLA-4 therapy. Moreover, the process is T lymphocyte dependent and, if this resistance is overridden, effector T cells are found increased in tumour infiltration, the effector-to-regulatory T cell ratio increases as well [53]. The molecular mechanisms of IDO expression are intimately related to the immune response. Several years ago it was reported that IDO expression is controlled by T activated lymphocytes through their secreted cytokines. IL-13 can repress the induction of IDO mediated by IFN-gamma [54]. Regarding possible emerging therapies, authors report that fludarabine that hinders the up-regulation of IDO in a T lymphocytes dependent manner, can be tested as a pre-treatment drug for melanoma patients. These patients can receive afterwards immuno-therapies that would have been less efficient when IDO was over-expressed [55].

Using animal models, new emerging therapies can be discovered, overriding the resistance to immune-therapies in certain patients groups.

3. Dendritic cells pulsed with specific antigens as inductors of specific immune-response

Treatment paradigms aim to include naturally occurring dendritic cells subsets in a single vaccine. The studies that are in the pre-clinical phases show synergistic effects between various antigen-presenting cells. We will present different types of methodologies to pulse dendritic cells, starting with mere cultivation of dendritic cells in total tumour lysates and ending with newer technologies such as electroporation mRNA-pulsed dendritic cells. Recently, the first clinical trials released their results and showed increased survival rates and broader anti-cancer immune responses. These new clinical findings will be presented.

In just a short period of time, the cancer immunotherapy field has gained new combatants through sipuleucel-T FDA approval, first DC immunovaccine for metastatic prostate cancer patients, followed closely by ipilimumab, an antibody specific to CTLA-4 as major target in metastatic melanoma [56]. Due to its clear tumor immunogenicity, melanoma treatment could be handled from an immunotherapeutic viewpoint. However, an important issue in melanoma immunovaccine success is the highly heterogeneous composition of antigens expressed within tumor site along with different genetic patterns of melanoma patients [57]. Deciphering this complex (intra)tumor heterogeneity of melanoma is directly linked to the possibility for clearly identifying, targeting and manageing drug-resistant cell subpopulations from the tumour site [58]. The genetic profile of melanoma patient is one of the foremost rationales for an autologous whole cell vaccine acting more efficiently in treating the micrometastasis than would an allogeneic designed one.

Revisiting the melanoma vaccines, it was pointed out that a preponderant cytokine-driven therapy activates a robust antitumoral T-cell mediated response representing a class of individualized auto-vaccination formula, surmounting thus the melanoma intratumoral heterogeneity [57]. Assembling a cancer vaccine aims to activate a specific anti-tumor immune response and/or to better access the tumor-associated antigens. In cutaneous melanoma, the pattern of tumor specific and tumor associated antigens is both large and heterogeneous, making melanoma immunogenicity exploitable in therapeutic approaches. Therefore, the plenty of discovered or yet hidden melanoma tumor antigens could open the way for vaccination of patients groups with the same vaccine type [59]. Being explored with synthetic peptides, whole tumor cells, cellular lysates or autologous immunovaccine, dendritic cells (DCs) take advantages in treatment or even in prevention approaches of cancer [60].

Dendritic cell in melanoma immunotherapy undergo a sequential number of actions. Thus, loading DCs with a tumor antigen and a specific adjuvant will induce the maturation state which involves antigens processing by proteasomal degradation and presenting the resulted peptides to T cells *via* MHC complex to stimulate further CD4+ cells, CD8+ cells as well as phagocytes and NK cells or, in certain activation conditions, induce Tregs that hamper antitumor responses [61].

3.1. Dendritic cells subsets

In malignant skin, the principal subsets of DC responsible for Ag-specific T cell immune response comprise *epidermal* (Langerhans cells) and *dermal* cell populations. The primary tumor site and the sentinel lymph nodes endure the immune-suppression generated by melanoma, this immune site being the field where T cells should start the fight against melanoma while being armed by activated DC to engender anti-melanoma immunity [62]. As in case of tumor associated macrophages, under the influence of tumor milieu DC are versatile players which could become *tumor-associated DC* enhancing Immune-suppression by sustaining T cell regulatory activity [63] (Table 1). Upon electrochemotherapy of tumor cells, for example, a relatively new approach to deliver better an antitumor drug, melanoma inflammatory infiltrate contains beside dermal DC, *plasmacytoid* DC cells for capturing tumor antigens to further elicit, along with dermal and Langerhans cells, a T cell antitumor response [64].

DCs subsets	Uptake receptors evaluated for immunotherapy of DC		
	Antigen uptake receptors	**Unique receptors**	**TLR receptors**
LC/dermal DC	FcR; DEC205; CD40; DCIR	Langerin	TLR-3
pDC	FcR; DEC205; CD40; DCIR	CD303; CD123; BDCA-2	TLR-7; TLR-9 specific to pDC
MoDC	FcR; DEC205; CD11c; CD40; DCIRDC-SIGN; MR		TLR-4; 8; 3; 7.

Table 1. DCs subsets and receptors for immunovaccine (LC – Langerhans cell; pDC - plasmacytoid-derived DC; MoDC – monocyte-derived DC; DEC205 – C-type lectin receptor on DC; BDCA-2 – blood dendritic cell antigen, specific to pDC subset; DCIR - dendritic cell immunoreceptor; DC-SIGN - dendritic cell specific ICAM-3 grabbing non-integrin; MR – mannose receptor; TLR – toll-like receptor)

http://dx.doi.org/10.5772/59494

3.2. Exploring dendritic cells in melanoma immunovaccine

As skin is an abundant cellular immune network and hence an accessible portal for therapeutical approaches, DC cells remain an attractive target in melanoma therapy both as *ex-vivo*-generated or *in-vivo*-DC-targeting immunovaccine blueprint [65]. Peripheral blood and Langerhans cells are the main sources for DCs immunotherapy. Langerhans cells and monocyte-derived DCs elicit immune responses in comparable levels although the cytokine stimulation conditions are different. The initial therapeutical attempts with DCs vaccination was based on *ex-vivo* generated monocyte-derived DC pulsed with tumor lysates, peptide or tumor antigens which led to a tumor regression rate of 3-7%, having also a lower toxicity compared with standard therapeutical procedures [66]. In melanoma, DC derived from CD34+ progenitors prove better results compared with monocyte-DC vaccine in spite of the known heterogeneity of tumor antigens [10].

3.2.1. Loading DC with tumor associated-antigens

Loading effector immune cells with antigenic peptides or a whole tumor-associated antigen (TAA) was initially designed as an immune vaccination system with T lymphocytes *via* MHC molecules recognition. Due to possible issues related to molecule stability and/or delivery route, resulting in an ineffective antigen presentation, these approaches could fail in clinic due to a low response rate in patients. Using DC as tool for intracellular delivery of such tumor antigenic peptides, the process of antigen presentation to T cells could be improved [67]. Moreover, the Th1/Th2 balance could be regulated by such modified DC. Therefore, DCs loaded with MART-126-35 melanoma peptide were used in combination with anti-CTLA4 monoclonal antibody (tremelimumab) in advanced melanoma patients. Upon therapy, high levels of pro-inflammatory Th1 invariant natural killer T cells (iNKT) CD8(+) was associated with positive clinical responses, indicating that antitumor T cell activity could be immunomodulated *via* iNKT cells by peptide-pulsed DCs [68]. In another recent study, high-risk stage III melanoma patients with lymph node resection were vaccinated with DC loaded with MHC I melanoma peptides respective to the patient's haplotype. The peptide pulsed DCs were well tolerated and elicited immune specific responses to melanoma antigens or/and IFN-γ-producing CD8+ cell response to melanoma peptides in 15 of 22 patients. The three-year overall survival rate was 68.2% vs. 25.7% in the control patients group [69].

Monocyte-derived DCs could be loaded in different conditions with a mixture of peptides, tumor lysates or even with a single tumor peptide such as from Mage-3A1. For 8 of 11 patients enrolled in the study it was registered an increase of Mage-3A1-specific (CD8+) T cells, with regression of a few metastases for 6 advanced melanoma patients; a lack of Mage 3A1 expression was observed in some non-regressed areas of melanoma [70]. Even immature DCs could be exploited in vaccination, thus DCs generated from CD34+ progenitor cells were cytokines-stimulated and pulsed *in vitro* with a pool of melanoma derived peptides [71].

Engineered DCs loaded with peptides or antigens could be delivered by lymphatic nodes or intradermally; the last type being the optimum method for generating T cell antitumor immunity [72].

3.2.2. DC electroporation with mRNA

Cellular electroporation is a transfection method to efficiently introduce mRNA encoding for a certain biomolecule in order to express at high level that specific antigen. A main advantage of mRNA transfection is the prolongation of the exposure and an accurate antigens processing. This approach was translated for DCs as a promising opportunity to facilitate access to tumor antigens and thus priming the T cell specific antitumor melanoma response, being applicable even in advanced stages of melanoma [73].

In the last few years, mRNA was proposed as an innovative vehicle for antigen delivery appropriate for cancer vaccination purposes. DCs were evaluated as the most suitable immune cells for mRNA transfection due to their professional quality in processing and presenting antigens for inducing specific immune responses by T cells. mRNA as an antigen delivery tool could generate a whole antigenic protein with all epitopes ready to be viewed by MHC molecules; last but not least, the interest mRNA molecule could be produced in large quantities with high purity.

The successful use of *ex vivo* mRNA-modified DCs for melanoma immunotherapy rely on DCs cellular subtype involved, the proper cellular activation and path of delivery [74]. The DCs *subtype* electroporated with mRNA in cancer vaccination purposes accounts for vaccination efficiency. pDCs cells loaded with melanoma antigenic peptides and further activated at CD40L elicit T cytotoxic anti-melanoma responses [75]. The cellular *activation* method of DC counts for CTL full activity and subsequently inhibition of Tregs. Engagement of TLR in DC activation proves to be a good approach in immunovaccine. Moreover, transfection with mRNA and activation of DC cells is the fundament of the TriMix mRNA set encoding for CD40L, CD70 and active form of TLR4. Thus in one clinical study with TriMix-DCs intradermally administrated, the efficacy of procedure was registered by means of the skin infiltrating CD8+ lymphocytes monitored by IL-12p70 as a marker of successful inoculation of the DC product [76]. The *delivery way* of modified DCs was compared in several clinical studies. The best way to target the lymph nodes in melanoma site by modified mRNA DCs is intradermic inoculation associated with an increased number of T cells although intranodally delivery reveal a higher number of DC. One recent study refers to DC electroporated with mRNA for gp100/tyrosinase antigens and injected in regional lymph nodes of melanoma patients prior to local surgery. The mRNA for electroporated melanoma antigen was immunohistochemically detected in T cells populations from both the primary and the adjacent lymph node concomitantly with a CD8+ T lymphocyte responses registered in 7 of 11 patients subjected to immunovaccination [77]. Some promising results in terms of safety, feasibility and immunogenic properties were obtained in patients with advanced cutaneous melanoma in a pilot study were DC were co-electroporated with mRNA encoding for CD40L, TLR4 and CD70 as a autologous TriMix-DC formula combined with IFN-α-2b sequential administration [76].

The foremost parameter to be monitored for immunovaccine efficacy is the induction or the enhancement of melanoma anti-tumor immune response. Several technologies like ELISPOT technique allows quantifying the precise number of active immune cells by counting antigen-specific cells that secrete a particular anti-tumor cytokine e.g. IFN-γ [59]. Since 2006, clinical studies with tumor mRNA transfected DCs administrated usually intradermic in patients with metastatic melanoma, detect an immunological T cell response with promising results at least for disease stabilization. In addition, advanced melanoma patients were treated intradermic with DCs simultaneously co-electroporated for 4 tumor antigens – Mage A3, Mage C2, Tyrosinase and gp100/DC-LAMP followed by TriMix mRNA single or in combination with additional therapy like IFNa-2b. In both clinical set-ups, the CD4/CD8 T cell responses were enhanced [74].

Recently, a small study on seven melanoma patients involved DCs from peripheral blood mononuclear cells pulsed with gp100 peptides and maturated further *in vitro* with a cocktail of CD40L and INF-γ. It was noted a direct correlation between the clinical responses and levels of IL-12 produced by modified DCs. The highest levels of IL-12 were registered in one patient with complete remission. DCs from non-responding patients were unable to produce IL-12 without additional stimulation with TLR agonist, observation that induced a modification of the *in vitro* maturation protocol and thus contributed to the improvement of the clinical outcome [78].

4. Translating up-dated knowledge to clinics — Therapeutical future scenery

There is a recent trend that advises as first therapy a BRAF inhibitor in *advanced* stages, because, time-wise, these patients cannot build an effective immune response while in patients with less advanced stages, immune-therapy will lead to a better outcome whether the patient presents or not a BRAF mutation [79].

In the clinical management of melanoma it is certain that immune-therapy is one of the pillars. Among this new therapeutical approaches, MEK inhibitors can overcome the resistance induced by BRAF inhibitors [79, 80]. has shown in phase 3 clinical studies, an improved [81].

Combination of these antibodies with the new anti-CTLA4 drug induces an astonishing 80% or more tumor regression in patients (http://www.clinicaltrials.gov/show/NCT01783938; http://trialsunited.com/studies/NCT01024231/) [82]. Newer therapeutical combination of ipilimumab with oncolytic immunotherapy with GM-CSF-expressing engineered herpes simplex virus, have shown in phase 3 clinical studies an improved OS in advanced melanoma [83].

On-going studies seek to establish the clinical boundaries of NK adoptive transfer in melanoma. Last year a study was published searching to rationalize the clinical trial framework [84] as the prior published results of a pilot trial showed no tumor regression in spite of the increased concentration of circulating autologous NK cells persistence [85].

Immunotherapy is the only therapeutical "light" that can increase OS in advanced melanomas. Eliciting an efficient immune response takes a certain amount of time in order to have an efficient anti-tumoral response, but as *immunological memory* is installed, the effect of immune-therapy persists in the absence of further immune-treatment.

We strongly believe, taking into account our experience in melanoma patients follow-up [86, 87] that immune-therapy is a major therapy weapon, increasing survival in advanced melanomas. The only draw-back is that, in order to develop its full efficacy, immune-therapy takes time, and this time interval can be up to 2–4 months. Thus, an early diagnostic in the metastatic stage would make a huge difference for a positive clinical outcome [88].

Besides imaging-based follow-up, immune parameters should complete the panel of investigation. New data regarding circulatory MDSC can enhance this panel and prospective clinical trials should soon validate them. Resistance to immune-therapy, like IDO expression opens new therapeutical avenues aiming at immune checkpoints and combining specific antibodies with IDO inhibitors.

5. Conclusion

The immune system is still not fully explored in this type of skin cancer [89, 90], thus new insights in tumour microenvironment and the involvement of innate immunity cells could enhance the panel of new therapeutical targets.

Balancing antitumor efficacy and reconstitution of a proper functioning immune system are processes aimed by immune-therapy in cutaneous melanoma. Owing to cutaneous melanoma immunogenic outline, this disease treatment could be addressed from an immunotherapeutic viewpoint. As we are facing the great success of having the first immune-therapy approved drug in melanoma, there is an open research combat of targeting personalized/individual antigens or undifferentiating antigens-stem-like to tackle the aggressive character of this disease.

Acknowledgements

The study was financed by the following Research Projects: PN-II-PT-PCCA-2013-4-1407, PN-II-ID-PCE-2011-3-0918 and PN.09.33-01.01/2009.

Author details

Monica Neagu* and Carolina Constantin

*Address all correspondence to: neagu.monica@gmail.com

Immunobiology Laboratory, Victor Babes National Institute of Pathology, Bucharest, Romania

References

[1] Dunn GP, Bruce AT, Ikeda H, et al. Cancer Immunoediting: From Immunosurveillance To Tumor Escape. Nature Immunology 2002; 3 991–998

[2] Dunn GP, Old LJ, Schreiber RD. The Immunobiology Of Cancer Immunosurveillance And Immunoediting. Immunity 2004; 21 137–148

[3] Raval RR, Sharabi AB, Walker AJ, Drake CG, Padmanee Sharma P. Tumor Immunology And Cancer Immunotherapy: Summary Of The 2013 SITC Primer. Journal for Immunotherapy of Cancer 2014; 2 14

[4] Ennen M, Keime C, Kobi D, Mengus G, Lipsker D, Thibault-Carpentier C, Davidson I. Single-Cell Gene Expression Signatures Reveal Melanoma Cell Heterogeneity. Oncogene 2014; doi: 10.1038/onc.2014.262. [Epub ahead of print]

[5] Widmer DS, Cheng PF, Eichhoff OM, Belloni BC, Zipser MC, Schlegel NC et al. Systematic Classification Of Melanoma Cells By Phenotype-Specific Gene Expression Mapping. Pigment Cell Melanoma Research 2012; 25 343–353

[6] Liu S, Ren S, Howell P, Fodstad O, Riker AI. Identification Of Novel Epigenetically Modified Genes In Human Melanoma Via Promoter Methylation Gene Profiling. Pigment Cell Melanoma Research 2008; 21 545–558

[7] Thurber AE, Douglas G, Sturm EC, Zabierowski SE, Smit DJ, Ramakrishnan SN et al. Inverse Expression States Of The BRN2 And MITF Transcription Factors In Melanoma Spheres And Tumour Xenografts Regulate The NOTCH Pathway. Oncogene 2011; 30 3036–3048

[8] Haass NK, Beaumont KA, Hill DS, Anfosso A, Mrass P, Munoz MA, Kinjyo I, Weninger W. Real-Time Cell Cycle Imaging During Melanoma Growth, Invasion, And Drug Response. Pigment Cell Melanoma Research 2014; 27(5) 764-776

[9] Perego M, Tortoreto M, Tragni G, Mariani L, Deho P, Carbone A et al. Heterogeneous Phenotype of Human Melanoma Cells with In Vitro and In Vivo Features of Tumor-Initiating Cells. The Journal of Investigative Dermatology 2010; 130 1877–1886

[10] Md. Selim Ahmed, Yong-Soo Bae. Dendritic Cell-Based Therapeutic Cancer Vaccines: Past, Present And Future. Clinical and Experimental Vaccine Research 2014;3 113-116

[11] Khattak M, Fisher R, Turajlic S, Larkin J. Targeted Therapy And Immunotherapy In Advanced Melanoma: An Evolving Paradigm. Therapeutic Advances in Medical Oncology 2013; 5 105–118

[12] Menzies AM, Long GV. New Combinations And Immunotherapies For Melanoma: Latest Evidence And Clinical Utility. Therapeutic Advances in Medical Oncology 2013; 5(5) 278–285

[13] Saraceni MM, Khushalani NI, Jarkowski A 3rd. Immunotherapy in Melanoma: Recent Advances and Promising New Therapies. Journal of Pharmacy Practice. 2014 Mar 27. Epub ahead of print]

[14] Garbe C, Eigentler TK, Keilholz U, Hauschild A, Kirkwood JM. Systematic Review Of Medical Treatment In Melanoma: Current Status And Future Prospects. Oncologist 2011;16(1) 5-24

[15] Slingluff CL JrPetroni GR, Olson W, Czarkowski A, Grosh WW, et al. Helper T-Cell Responses and Clinical Activity of a Melanoma Vaccine with Multiple Peptides from MAGE and Melanocytic Differentiation Antigens. Journal of Clinical Oncology 2008; 26, 4973-4980

[16] Bernardo-Faura M, Massen S, Falk CS, Brady NR, Eils R. Data-Derived Modeling Characterizes Plasticity of MAPK Signaling in Melanoma. PLOS Computational Biology 2014; 10(9) e1003795. doi:10.1371/journal.pcbi.1003795

[17] Robert C, Thomas L, Bondarenko I, et al. Ipilimumab Plus Dacarbazine for Previously Untreated Metastatic Melanoma. The New England Journal of Medicine 2011;364(26) 2517-2526

[18] Aranda F, Vacchelli E, Eggermont A, Galon J, Fridman WH, Zitvogel L, Kroemer G, Galluzzi L. Trial Watch: Immunostimulatory Monoclonal Antibodies in Cancer Therapy. Oncoimmunology 2014; 3(1) e27297

[19] Salama AK, Hodi FS. Cytotoxic T-Lymphocyte-Associated Antigen-4. Clinical Cancer Research 2011; 17 4622–4628

[20] Qureshi OS et al. Trans-Endocytosis Of CD80 And CD86: A Molecular Basis for the Cell-Extrinsic Function of CTLA-4. Science 2011; 332 600–603

[21] Ceeraz S, EC, Noelle RJ. B7 family checkpoint regulators in immune regulation and disease. Trends in Immunology 2013; 34 (11) 556-563

[22] Yervoy (ipilimumab) prescribing Information. Bristol-Myers Squibb Co. Revised December 2013. Available at: http://packageinserts.bms.com/pi/pi_yervoy.pdf. (accessed August 2014).

[23] Hanaizi Z, van Zwieten-Boot B, Calvo G, Sancho Lopez A, van Dartel M, Camarero J, Abadie E, Pignatti F. The European Medicines Agency Review of Ipilimumab (Yervoy) for the Treatment of Advanced (Unresectable Or Metastatic) Melanoma In Adults who Have Received Prior Therapy: Summary of the scientific assessment of the Committee for Medicinal Products for Human Use, European Journal of Cancer 2012; 48(2) 237–242

[24] Tarhini A, Lo E, Minor DR. Releasing the brake on the immune system: ipilimumab in melanoma and other tumors. Cancer Biotherapy and Radiopharmaceuticals 2010; 25(6) 601-613

[25] Hodi FS, O'Day SJ, McDermott DF, et al. Improved survival with ipilimumab in patients with metastatic melanoma. The New England Journal of Medicine 2010; 363(8) 711-723

[26] Wolchok JD, Weber JS, Maio M, et al. Four-Year Survival Rates for Patients with Metastatic Melanoma who Received Ipilimumab in Phase II Clinical Trials. Annals of Oncology 2013; 24(8) 2174-2180

[27] Eggermont AM. Can Immuno-Oncology Offer a Truly Pan-Tumour Approach to Therapy? Annals of Oncology 2012; 23(Suppl 8) viii53-57

[28] Olszanski AJ. Current and Future Roles of Targeted Therapy and Immunotherapy in Advanced Melanoma. Journal of Managed Care Pharmacy JMCP 2014; 20(4) 346-356

[29] Prieto PA, Yang JC, Sherry RM, et al. CTLA-4 Blockade with Ipilimumab: Long-Term Follow-Up of 177 Patients with Metastatic Melanoma. Clinical Cancer Research 2012;18(7) 2039-2047

[30] National Comprehensive Cancer Network website. NCCN Clinical Practice Guidelines in Oncology. Melanoma v2.2014. (Available at: http://www.nccn.org/professionals/physician_gls/pdf/melanoma.pdf)

[31] Robert C, Schadendorf D, Messina M, Hodi FS, O'Day S, for the MDX010-20 investigators. Efficacy and Safety of Retreatment with Ipilimumab in Patients with Pretreated Advanced Melanoma who Progressed After Initially Achieving Disease Control. Clinical Cancer Research 2013;19(8) 2232-2239

[32] Alexander M, Mellor JD, McArthur G, Kee D. Ipilimumab in Pretreated Patients with Unresectable Or Metastatic Cutaneous, Uveal And Mucosal Melanoma. Medical Journal of Australia 2014; 201(1) 49-53

[33] [Becher B, Bechmann I, Greter M. Antigen Presentation In Autoimmunity And CNS Inflammation: How T Lymphocytes Recognize The Brain. Journal of molecular medicine (Berlin, Germany) 2006; 84(7) 532-543

[34] Eigentler TK, Figl A, Krex D, et al. on behalf of the Dermatologic Cooperative Oncology Group and the National Interdisciplinary Working Group on Melanoma. Number Of Metastases, Serum Lactate Dehydrogenase Level, And Type Of Treatment Are Prognostic Factors In Patients With Brain Metastases Of Malignant Melanoma. Cancer 2011;117(8) 1697-1703

[35] Ryder M, Callahan M, Postow MA, Wolchok J, Fagin JA. Endocrine-Related Adverse Events Following Ipilimumab In Patients With Advanced Melanoma: A Comprehensive Retrospective Review From A Single Institution. Endocrine-related cancer 2014; 21(2) 371-381

[36] Ribas A, Hodi FS, Callahan M, Konto C, Wolchok J. Hepatotoxicity With Combination Of Vemurafenib And Ipilimumab. The New England Journal of Medicine 2013; 368(14) 1365-1366

[37] Nivolumab Receives Manufacturing and Marketing Approval in Japan for the Treatment of Unresectable Melanoma http://www.esmo.org/Oncology-News/Nivolumab-Receives-Manufacturing-and-Marketing-Approval-in-Japan-for-the-Treatment-of-Unresectable-Melanoma

[38] Deeks ED. Nivolumab: A Review Of Its Use In Patients With Malignant Melanoma. Drugs 2014;74(11) 1233-1239

[39] Lu J, Lee-Gabel L, Nadeau MC, Ferencz TM, Soefje SA. Clinical Evaluation Of Compounds Targeting PD-1/PD-L1 Pathway For Cancer Immunotherapy. Journal of oncology pharmacy practice: official publication of the International Society of Oncology Pharmacy Practitioners 2014; pii: 1078155214538087 [Epub ahead of print]

[40] Topalian SL, Sznol M, McDermott DF, et al. Survival, Durable Tumor Remission, and Long-Term Safety In Patients With Advanced Melanoma Receiving Nivolumab. Journal of Clinical Oncology 2014; 32(10) 1020-1030. doi: 10.1200/JCO.2013.53.0105.

[41] Taube JM, Klein A, Brahmer JR, Xu H, Pan X, Kim JH, Chen L, Pardoll DM, Topalian SL, Anders RA. Association of PD-1, PD-1 Ligands, and Other Features of the Tumor Immune Microenvironment with Response to Anti-PD-1 Therapy. Clinical Cancer Research 2014 Apr 8. [Epub ahead of print]

[42] Hamid O, Sosman JA, Lawrence DP, Sullivan RJ, Ibrahim N, Kluger HM, et al. Clinical activity, safety, and biomarkers of MPDL3280A, an engineered PD-L1 antibody in patients with locally advanced or metastatic melanoma (mM). 2013 ASCO Annual Meeting (May 31-June 4, 2013, Chicago, IL. 31(15suppl) 9010

[43] Mamalis A, Garcha M, Jagdeo J. Targeting the PD-1 pathway: a promising future for the treatment of melanoma. Archives of dermatological research 2014; 306(6) 511-519

[44] Robert C, Ribas A, Wolchok JD, Hodi FS, Hamid O, Kefford R, et al. Anti-programmed-death-receptor-1 treatment with pembrolizumab in ipilimumab-refractory advanced melanoma: a randomised dose-comparison cohort of a phase 1 trial. Lancet. 2014; 384(9948):1109-17

[45] Hamid O, Robert C, Daud A, Hodi FS, Hwu WJ, Kefford R, et al.Safety and tumor responses with lambrolizumab (anti-PD-1) in melanoma. N Engl J Med. 2013;369(2): 134-44.

[46] ClinicalTrials.gov identifier: NCT01295827

[47] Naidoo J, Page DB, Wolchok JD. Immune checkpoint blockade. Hematology/Oncology Clinics of North America 2014; 28(3) 585-600

[48] Ku GY, Yuan J, Page DB, et al. Single-Institution Experience With Ipilimumab In Advanced Melanoma Patients In The Compassionate Use Setting: Lymphocyte Count After 2 Doses Correlates With Survival. Cancer 2010;116(7) 1767–1775

[49] Berman DM, Wolchok J, Weber J, et al. Association Of Peripheral Blood Absolute Lymphocyte Count (ALC) And Clinical Activity In Patients (Pts) With Advanced

Melanoma Treated With Ipilimumab. Journal of Clinical Oncology 2009; 27(Suppl 15) Abstr 3020

[50] Hamid O, Chasalow SD, Tsuchihashi Z, et al. Association Of Baseline And On-Study Tumor Biopsy Markers With Clinical Activity In Patients (Pts) With Advanced Melanoma Treated With Ipilimumab. Journal of Clinical Oncology 2009; 27(Suppl 15) Abstr 9008

[51] Meyer C, Cagnon L, Costa-Nunes CM, Baumgaertner P, Montandon N, Leyvraz L, Michielin O, Romano E, Speiser DE. Frequencies Of Circulating MDSC Correlate With Clinical Outcome Of Melanoma Patients Treated With Ipilimumab. Cancer Immunology, Immunotherapy 2014; 63(3) 247-257

[52] Weber JS, Kudchadkar RR, Yu B, Gallenstein D, Horak CE, Inzunza HD, et al. Safety, efficacy, and biomarkers of nivolumab with vaccine in ipilimumab-refractory or -naive melanoma. Journal of Clinical Oncology 2013; 31(34) 4311-438

[53] Holmgaard RB, Zamarin D, Munn DH, Wolchok JD, Allison JP. Indoleamine 2,3-Dioxygenase Is A Critical Resistance Mechanism In Antitumor T Cell Immunotherapy Targeting CTLA-4. The Journal of Experimental Medicine 2013; 210(7) 1389-1402

[54] Godin-Ethier J, Pelletier S, Hanafi LA, Gannon PO, Forget MA, et al. Human activated T lymphocytes modulate IDO expression in tumors through Th1/Th2 balance. The Journal of Immunology 2009; 183 7752–7760

[55] Hanafi L-A, Gauchat D, Godin-Ethier J, et al. Fludarabine Downregulates Indoleamine 2,3-Dioxygenase in Tumors via a Proteasome-Mediated Degradation Mechanism, PLOS ONE 2014; 9(6) e99211

[56] Iversen TZ, Andersen MH, Svane IM. The Targeting of IDO-Mediated Immune Escape in Cancer. Basic & Clinical Pharmacology & Toxicology 2014; doi: 10.1111/bcpt. 12320.

[57] Elias EG, Sharma BK. Melanoma Vaccines, Revisited a Review, Update. G Ital Dermatol Venereol. 2014 Jul 31. [Epub ahead of print]

[58] Seftor EA, Seftor RE, Weldon DS, Kirsammer GT, Margaryan NV, Gilgur A, Hendrix MJ. Melanoma Tumor Cell Heterogeneity: A Molecular Approach to Study Subpopulations Expressing the Embryonic Morphogen Nodal. Semininars in Oncology 2014;41(2) 259-266. doi: 10.1053/j.seminoncol.2014.02.001.

[59] Butterfield LH, Buffo MJ. Immunologic Monitoring of Cancer Vaccine Trials Using the ELISPOT assay. Methods in Molecular Biology 2014;1102 71-82. doi: 10.1007/978-1-62703-727-3_5

[60] Ahmed MS, Bae YS. Dendritic cell-based therapeutic cancer vaccines: past, present and future. Clin Exp Vaccine Res. 2014 Jul;3(2):113-6. doi: 10.7774/cevr.2014.3.2.113.

[61] Shtivelman E, Davies MQ, Hwu P, Yang J, Lotem M, Oren M, Flaherty KT, Fisher DE. Pathways And Therapeutic Targets In Melanoma. Oncotarget 2014; 5(7) 1701-1752

[62] Oosterhoff D, Sluijter BJ, Hangalapura BN, de Gruijl TD. The Dermis as A Portal For Dendritic Cell-Targeted Immunotherapy Of Cutaneous Melanoma. Current Topics in Microbiology and Immunology 2012; 351 181-220.

[63] Benencia F, Muccioli M, Alnaeeli M. Perspectives On Reprograming Cancer-Associated Dendritic Cells For Anti-Tumor Therapies. Frontiers in Oncology 2014; 4 72. doi: 10.3389/fonc.2014.00072. eCollection 2014.

[64] Gerlini G, Di Gennaro P, Borgognoni L. Enhancing Anti-Melanoma Immunity By Electrochemotherapy and In Vivo Dendritic-Cell Activation. Oncoimmunology 2012;1(9) 1655-1657

[65] Palucka K, Banchereau J. Cancer Immunotherapy via Dendritic Cells. Nature Reviews Cancer 2012;12 265-277

[66] Butterfield LH. Dendritic Cells In Cancer Immunotherapy Clinical Trials: Are We Making Progress? Frontiers in Immunology 2013;4 454.

[67] Li H, Ma W. Intracellular Delivery Of Tumor Antigenic Peptides In Biodegradable-Polymer Adjuvant For Enhancing Cancer Immunotherapy. Current Medicinal Chemistry. 2014; 21(21) 2357-2366

[68] Ibarrondo FJ, Yang OO, Chodon T, Avramis E, Lee Y, Sazegar H, et al. Natural Killer T Cells In Advanced Melanoma Patients Treated With Tremelimumab. PLoS One 2013; 8(10) e76829. doi: 10.1371/journal.pone.0076829. eCollection 2013

[69] Markowicz S, Nowecki ZI, Rutkowski P, Lipkowski AW, Biernacka M, Jakubowska-Mucka A, et al. Adjuvant vaccination with melanoma antigen-pulsed dendritic cells in stage III melanoma patients. Medical Oncology 2012; 29(4) 2966-2977

[70] Thurner B, Haendle I, Roder C, Dieckmann D, Keikavoussi P, Jonuleit H, et al. Vaccination With Mage-3A1 Peptide-Pulsed Mature, Monocyte-Derived Dendritic Cells Expands Specific Cytotoxic T Cells And Induces Regression Of Some Metastases In Advanced Stage IV Melanoma. The Journal of experimental medicine. 1999; 190(11) 1669-1678

[71] Mackensen A, Herbst B, Chen JL, Kohler G, Noppen C, Herr W, et al. Phase I Study In Melanoma Patients Of A Vaccine With Peptide-Pulsed Dendritic Cells Generated In Vitro From CD34(+) Hematopoietic Progenitor Cells. International journal of cancer Journal international du cancer 2000; 86(3) 385-392

[72] Lesterhuis WJ, de Vries IJ, Schreibelt G, Lambeck AJ, Aarntzen EH, Jacobs JF, Scharenborg NM, van de Rakt MW, de Boer AJ, Croockewit S, van Rossum MM, Mus R, Oyen WJ, Boerman OC, Lucas S, Adema GJ, et al. Route Of Administration Modulates The Induction Of Dendritic Cell Vaccine-Induced Antigen-Specific T Cells In

Advanced Melanoma Patients. Clinical cancer research: an official journal of the American Association for Cancer Research 2011; 17(17) 5725-5735

[73] Aarntzen EH, Schreibelt G, Bol K, Lesterhuis WJ, Croockewit AJ, de Wilt JH, van Rossum MM, Blokx WA, Jacobs JF, Duiveman-de Boer T, Schuurhuis DH, Mus R, Thielemans K, de Vries IJ, Figdor CG, Punt CJ, et al. Vaccination With Mrna-Electroporated Dendritic Cells Induces Robust Tumor Antigen-Specific CD4+ And CD8+ T Cells Responses In Stage III And IV Melanoma Patients. Clinical cancer research: an official journal of the American Association for Cancer Research 2012; 18(19) 5460-5470

[74] Van Lint S, Heirman C, Thielemans K, Breckpot K. mRNA: From A Chemical Blueprint for Protein Production to an Off-The-Shelf Therapeutic. Human vaccines & immunotherapeutics 2013; 9(2) 265-274

[75] Salio M, Cella M, Vermi W, Facchetti F, Palmowski MJ, Smith CL, et al. Plasmacytoid Dendritic Cells Prime IFN-Gamma-Secreting Melanoma-Specific CD8 Lymphocytes And Are Found In Primary Melanoma Lesions. European Journal of Immunology 2003; 33 1052–1062

[76] Wilgenhof S, Van Nuffel AM, Corthals J, Heirman C, Tuyaerts S, Benteyn D, et al. Therapeutic vaccination with an autologous mRNA electroporated dendritic cell vaccine in patients with advanced melanoma. Journal of Immunotherapy 2011; 34 448-456

[77] Schuurhuis DH, Verdijk P, Schreibelt G, Aarntzen EH, Scharenborg N, de Boer A, van de Rakt MW, Kerkhoff M, Gerritsen MJ, Eijckeler F, Bonenkamp JJ, Blokx W, van Krieken JH, Boerman OC, Oyen WJ, Punt CJ, Figdor CG, Adema GJ, de Vries IJ. In Situ Expression of Tumor Antigens by Messenger RNA-Electroporated Dendritic Cells in Lymph Nodes of Melanoma Patients. Cancer Research 2009; 69(7) 2927-2934

[78] Carreno BM, Becker-Hapak M, Huang A, Chan M, Alyasiry A, Lie WR, Aft RL, Cornelius LA, Trinkaus KM and Linette GP. IL-12p70-Producing Patient DC Vaccine Elicits Tc1-Polarized Immunity. The Journal of Clinical Investigation 2013; 123(8)3383-3394

[79] Flaherty KT, Robert C, Hersey P, et al., for the METRIC Study Group. Improved Survival With MEK Inhibition In BRAF-Mutated Melanoma. The New England Journal of Medicine 2012; 367(2) 107-114

[80] Falchook GS, Lewis KD, Infante JR, et al. Activity of the Oral MEK Inhibitor Trametinib in Patients with Advanced Melanoma: A Phase 1 Dose Escalation Trial. The Lancet Oncology 2012; 13(8) 782-789

[81] Brahmer JR, Tykodi SS, Chow LQ, et al. Safety And Activity Of Anti-PD-L1 Antibody In Patients With Advanced Cancer. The New England Journal of Medicine 2012; 366(26) 2455-2465

[82] Wolchok JD, Kluger H, Callahan MK, et al. Nivolumab Plus Ipilimumab In Advanced Melanoma. The New England Journal of Medicine 2013; 369(2) 122-133

[83] Kaufman HL, Ruby CE, Hughes T, Slingluff CL Jr. Current Status of Granulocyte-Macrophage Colony-Stimulating Factor in the Immunotherapy of Melanoma. Journal for ImmunoTherapy of Cancer 2014; 13(2) 11

[84] Besser MJ1, Shoham T, Harari-Steinberg O, Zabari N, Ortenberg R, Yakirevitch A, Nagler A, Loewenthal R, Schachter J, Markel G. Development of allogeneic NK cell adoptive transfer therapy in metastatic melanoma patients: in vitro preclinical optimization studies. PLoS One 2013; 8(3) e57922

[85] Parkhurst MR, Riley JP, Dudley ME, Rosenberg SA. Adoptive Transfer Of Autologous Natural Killer Cells Leads To High Levels Of Circulating Natural Killer Cells But Does Not Mediate Tumor Regression. Clinical Cancer Research 2011; 17(9) 6287–6297

[86] Neagu M, Constantin C, Manda G et al. Biomarkers Of Metastatic Melanoma. Biomarkers In Medicine 2009; 3(1) 71-89

[87] Neagu M, Constantin C, Zurac S. Immune Parameters In Prognosis And Therapy Monitoring Of Cutaneous Melanoma Patients - Experience, Role And Limitations. BioMed Research International, special issue Molecular Biomarkers: Tools of Medicine (MBTM) 2013; 2013 Article ID 107940

[88] Gore M. Introduction Optimal approach for melanoma. European Journal of Cancer Supplements 2013; 11(2), 80

[89] Neagu M. The Immune System-A Hidden Treasure for Biomarker Discovery in Cutaneous Melanoma In: Makowski G.S. (ed.) Advances In Clinical Chemistry. Book Series: Advances in Clinical Chemistry; 2012. p89-140

[90] Neagu M, Constantin C, Tanase C. Immune-Related Biomarkers For Diagnosis/Prognosis And Therapy Monitoring Of Cutaneous Melanoma. Expert Review Of Molecular Diagnostics 2011; 10(7) 897-919

Chapter 10

Can Redirected T Cells Outsmart Aggressive Melanoma? The Promise and Challenge of Adoptive Cell Therapy

Jennifer Makalowski and Hinrich Abken

Additional information is available at the end of the chapter

http://dx.doi.org/10.5772/59255

1. Introduction

1.1. The challenge to induce lasting remission in late stage melanoma

In early stages of the disease surgical resection of melanoma lesions is a curative option; a 10-year-survival rate of 75-85% can be achieved in stage I or II of the disease. However, stage III or IV melanoma is associated with low survival rates of less than 1 year upon diagnosis [1]. The poor prognosis in advanced stages of the disease is thought to be particularly due to the properties of melanoma cells to systemically spread into various organs, to form micro-metastases beyond the detection limit of current imaging procedures [2, 3] and to give rise to relapse of the disease. This is even the case after initially complete response to therapy and after more than a decade from initial treatment. Durable remission is so far only achieved in pre-defined patient subsets despite the development of novel drugs and major improvements in therapeutic regimens [4-6]. This unsatisfactory situation is thought to be due to the extra-ordinary property of melanoma cells to persist in "dormancy" for long periods of time which is associated with their resistance to chemo-and radiotherapy [7-10]. Taken together, durable cure from melanoma requires eliminating single melanoma cells in a highly specific and efficient fashion even in dormant micro-metastatic lesions.

In this situation recruiting the cellular immune defense machinery to detect and destroy individual melanoma cells is a powerful alternative to conventional therapeutic regimens. The hope is sustained by the supportive effect of high dose interleukin-2 (IL-2) [11] and anti-cytotoxic T-lymphocyte-associated antigen-4 (CTLA-4) antibody [12] as well as interferon (IFN) α-2b to prolong the disease-free survival even in late stages of the disease. However, the response rate is quite low and frequently not curative over time [13, 14].

A number of strategies for sharpening the immune cell response against melanoma are currently explored, some of these with remarkable success. In particular, the adoptive transfer of tumor infiltrating lymphocytes (TILs), isolated from melanoma biopsies and amplified to therapeutic relevant numbers ex vivo, produced encouraging phase II results [15, 16]. In a further development, patients' blood T cells are genetically engineered with pre-defined specificity for melanoma-associated antigens making adoptive cell therapy with melanoma specific T cells possible. In this contribution we will discuss the rationale for adoptive cell therapy of melanoma, evidence for efficacy and current challenges to achieve long-term remission. Upcoming strategies in melanoma stem cell targeting are also discussed.

2. Adoptive therapy with ex vivo amplified TILs can induce regression of melanoma

An effective immune response can control melanoma. This notion is supported by the observation that spontaneous and complete melanoma regressions can occur and that immune compromised patients suffer from a higher frequency of melanoma [17, 18]. The conclusion is moreover sustained by the clinical observation that treatment with high dose IL-2 produces an objective response even in late stage melanoma, some patients with long-term complete response for years [11, 19]. Although about 16%, the response rate is remarkable compared to the low and short-lived response rates of classical therapeutic regimens.

First described in 1969 [20], melanoma is infiltrated by T cells of both effector and helper cell origin which can be expanded to high numbers ex vivo in the presence of IL-2. Pioneered by the NCI-Surgery Branch, such tumor infiltrating T cells (TILs) were selected for melanoma reactivity by incubation on feeder cells expressing melanoma-associated antigens [21] and re-administered in substantial numbers together with high dose IL-2 to the patient (Figure 1). Initial trials produced an objective response rate of 11/20 patients [22] which is remarkable since TILs are obviously capable to fight melanoma even in late stage patients who experienced multiple lines of therapy. Responses, however, were of short duration and TILs did not persist for longer period in the peripheral blood after administration. Subsequent trials identified that the key to successful TIL therapy was the number of TILs administered to the patient, the activity of those cells against melanoma and the rapidity of T cell amplification ex vivo [23, 24]. During the subsequent years the initial protocols were optimized with respect to these and other issues and adopted according to GMP standards [25]; a number of trials are currently open in various centers (Table 1).

Persistence of administered TILs in circulation was substantially improved by depletion of the lymphoid compartment of the patient prior to adoptive cell therapy [26-28]. Such pre-conditioning by non-myeloablative chemotherapy had the effect that cytokines sustaining lymphocyte amplification including IL-7 and IL-15 were present in augmented levels ("cytokine sink"). Moreover, space for transferred lymphocytes was created and suppressor cells including regulatory T cells were depleted which additionally helped to improve engraftment of adoptively transferred T cells.

http://dx.doi.org/10.5772/59255

Target antigen	Adoptively transferred T cells and additional treatment	NCT ID	Center
	TILs, IL-2 in variable doses	NCT00001832	NIH
	TILs vs. lymphokine-activated killer (LAK) cells	NCT00002535	StLMC
	TILs, high dose IL-2	NCT00096382	NIH
	TILs, low dose IL-2 s.c.	NCT00200577	NUH
	TILs with vs. without IL-2	NCT00314106	NIH
	TILs, high dose IL-2 with or without dendritic cell immunization	NCT00338377	MDACC
	TILs, high dose IL-2	NCT00604136	HMC
	TILs, high dose IL-2	NCT00863330	AHC
	TILs, high dose IL-2	NCT00937625	HUH
	TILs, high dose IL-2	NCT01005745	MOFFITT
	TILs, low dose IL-2 and intra-tumoral injection of IFN-γ producing adenovirus	NCT01082887	NUH
	TILs, high dose IL-2	NCT01659151	MOFFITT
	TILs, high dose IL-2	NCT01701674	MOFFITT
	TILs, high dose IL-2	NCT01807182	FHCRC
	"re-stimulated"(autologous DCs &anti-CD3 antibody) TILs, low dose IL-2	NCT01883297	UHN
	TILs, low dose IL-2	NCT01883323	UHN
	TILs, dendritic cell vaccination with NY-ESO-1	NCT01946373	KUH
	TILs, high vs. low dose IL-2	NCT01995344	CHNHSFT
	4-1BB selected TILs	NCT02111863	NIH
	"young" TILs, high dose IL-2	NCT00287131	SMC
	"young" TILs with or without CD4+ T cell depletion, high dose IL-2	NCT00513604	NIH
	"young" CD8+ TILs, high dose IL-2	NCT01118091	NIH
	"young" TILs, high dose IL-2	NCT01319565	NIH
	"young" TILs, high dose IL-2	NCT01369875	NIH
	"young" TILs, IL-15	NCT01369888	NIH
	"young" TILs	NCT01468818	NIH
	"young" TILs, high dose IL-2, BRAF kinase inhibitor	NCT01585415	NIH
	"young" TILs, with or without high dose IL-2	NCT01814046	NIH
	"young" TILs, anti-CTLA-4 antibody	NCT01988077	SMC
	"young" TILs, high dose IL-2 with standard vs. low dose chemotherapy	NCT01993719	NIH

Aurora Health Care; **CHNHSFT**, Christie Hospital NHS Foundation Trust; **FHCRC**, Fred Hutchinson Cancer Research Center; **HMC**, Hadassah Medical Center; **HUH**, Herlev University Hospital (Copenhagen); **KUH,** Karolinska University Hospital; **MDACC**, M.D. Anderson Cancer Center; **MOFFITT**, H. Lee Moffitt Cancer Center and Research Institute; **MUH**, Mie University Hospital; **NIH**, National Institutes of Health; **NUH**, Nantes University Hospital; **SMC**, Sheba Medical Center; **StLMC**, St. Luke's Medical Center; **UC**, University of California; **UHN,** University Health Network (Toronto)

Table 1. Adoptive cell therapy with tumor infiltrating lymphocytes (TILs) in patients with melanoma

There are still some issues to be addressed, for instance whether clinically most potent TILs can be defined by phenotype and whether these cells can be selectively expanded. There is a common sense that for therapeutic efficacy in the long-term the functional activity of T cells needs to be preserved without signs of exhaustion which is particularly crucial when T cells experienced extensive amplification ex vivo. In the further development of the procedure, TILs were only selected with respect to their proliferative capacities which is independent of their antigen specificity and represents a furthermore simplification of the standard protocol (Figure 1) [29-31]. Those so-called "young TILs" after short-term ex vivo expansions passed through fewer cell division cycles prior to infusion and are thereby in a maturation stage less prone to terminal differentiation and senescence [32]. Those protocols do not further select TILs for their melanoma reactivity based on the observation that infusion of ex vivo activated, IFN-γ^+TILs produced no superior therapeutic efficacy compared to non-responding TILs [16]. These modifications in the protocol resulted in improved persistence of young TILs [33] and about 50% response rates [27, 29, 34], so far in non-randomized trials (Table 1). A series of recent clinical trials with TILs following different lympho-conditioning regimes resulted in objective responses in 56% and complete responses in 22% of patients at the Surgery Branch [35]. Current TIL trials at various centers reproduced objective response rates of 40-50% in melanoma patients, a significant portion of patients free of disease 3-5 years after treatment [36, 37]. Of note, TILs can have anti-tumor activity also towards brain metastases as shown in a NCI trial with 7/17 complete and 6/17 partial remissions [38] sustaining the hope that adoptive cell therapy may be effective towards metastases which are otherwise not accessible.

While most trials apply non-separated TILs, administration of isolated CD8$^+$T cell clones with specificity for Melan-A and gp100 mediated only moderate benefit, required IL-2 and did not persist for longer times [39]. Those CD8$^+$T cells which persisted long-term acquired a phenotype of central memory-type T cells in vivo [40]. It is therefore assumed that CD8$^+$TILs require help of CD4$^+$cells for prolonged persistence making application of non-separated T cell populations more suitable.

Not only the stage of maturation but also the recruitment of T cells through chemokine gradients is crucial for therapeutic success. A recent prospective-retrospective hypothesis-driven analysis revealed that coordinate over-expression of CXCL9, CXCL10, CXCL11, CCL5 in melanoma is associated with responsiveness to treatment after TIL therapy [41].

Melanoma-reactive T cells need to persist in circulation to ensure therapeutic success of TIL therapy [42, 43]. This is reflected by the median survival of patients treated with Melan-A specific TILs of 53.5 months compared to 3.5 months for patients who received TILs of unknown specificity [44]. Some trials are initiated using melanoma specific patient's T cells from the peripheral blood for adoptive cell therapy of melanoma (Table 2). MART-1 or gp100 specific T cell clones isolated and amplified ex vivo produced a 50% response rate [45], however, technical difficulties limit a broad application of such specific T cells since melanoma reactive T cells in the peripheral blood of melanoma patients are extremely rare.

http://dx.doi.org/10.5772/59255

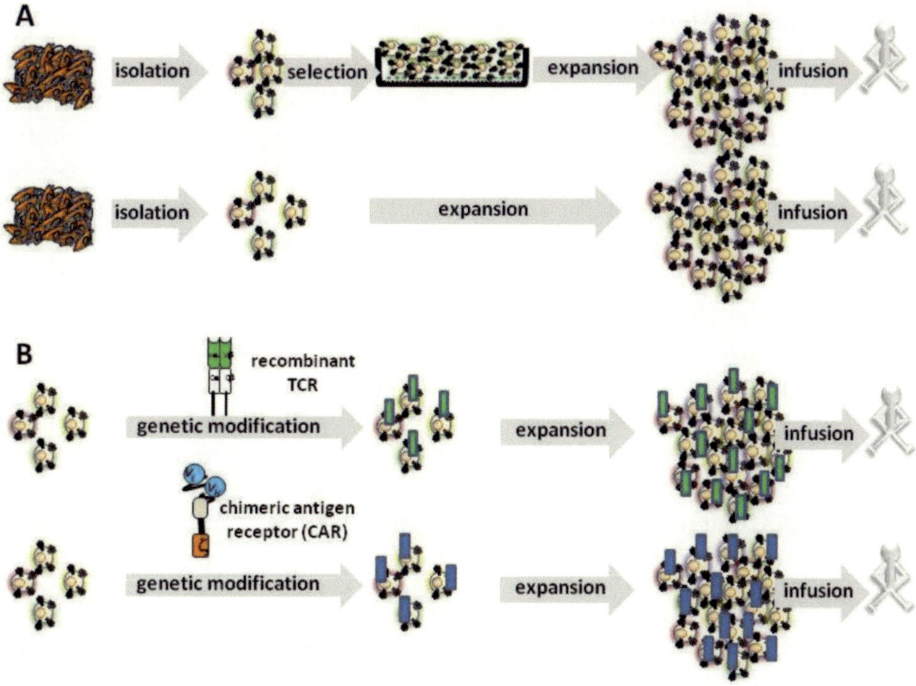

Figure 1. T cells used in adoptive cell therapy of melanoma. (A) Tumor infiltrating T cells (TILs) are isolated from melanoma biopsies, selected for reactivity towards melanoma cells, amplified in the presence of IL-2 to clinically relevant numbers and infused to the patient. Alternatively, TILs are expanded without prior selection for melanoma reactivity using a short-term amplification protocol ("young TILs"). (B) T cells from the peripheral blood of melanoma patients are genetically modified by retro- or lentivirus transduction to express a recombinant T cell receptor (TCR) or a chimeric antigen receptor (CAR), specific for a melanoma associated antigen, amplified and administered to the patient.

Target antigen	Adoptively transferred T cells	NCT ID	Center
MAGE-1 or MAGE-3	melanoma specific CD8+ T cells	NCT00045149	FHCRC
Tyrosinase	tyrosinase specific CD8+ T cells	NCT00002786	FHCRC
MART-1	MART-1 specific CD8+ T cells with or without high dose IL-2	NCT01495572	NIH
MART-1	MART-1 specific CD8+ T cells	NCT00512889	DFCI
MART-1	MART-1 specific T cells	NCT00720031	NUH
MART-1	MART-1 specific CD8+ T cells	NCT00324623	CHUV
MART-1	MART-1 specific TILs, high dose IL-2	NCT00924001	NIH
MART-1	MART-1 specific CD8+ T cells, low dose IL-2	NCT01106235	FHCRC
NY-ESO-1	NY-ESO-1 specific CD8+ T cells, low dose IL-2, anti-CTLA-4 antibody	NCT00871481	FHCRC

CHUV, Centre Hospitalier Universitaire Vaudois; **DFCI**, Dana-Farber Cancer Institute; **FHCRC**, Fred Hutchinson Cancer Research Center; **NIH**, National Institutes of Health; **NUH**, Nantes University Hospital

Table 2. Adoptive cell therapy with autologous, antigen specific T cells in patients with melanoma

3. T cells with engineered anti-melanoma specificity

The success of melanoma antigen specific T cells from peripheral blood strengthened efforts to obtain melanoma-specific T cell clones by genetic engineering of patient's T cells from the peripheral blood. In particular, the molecular cloning of the TCR from melanoma-reactive T cells enabled the engraftment of melanoma specificity to any T cell (Figure 1) [46-49]. A TCR with specificity for gp100 was cloned from melanoma reactive TILs and transferred by retrovirus-mediated gene transfer into blood T cells which thus obtained redirected specificity for gp100$^+$cells in addition to their parental specificity. TCR engineered T cells recognized gp100$^+$melanoma cells, secreted pro-inflammatory cytokines including IFN-γ and lysed gp100$^+$melanoma cells [50, 51]. By the same strategy, blood T cells were modified with the TCR specific for other melanoma associated antigens (Table 3). Using T cells modified with a gp100 specific TCR objective response was induced in 19% of patients, most responses were persistent [49]. Melanoma regression was also obtained in 5/11 melanoma patients after transfer of T cells modified with a TCR that recognizes NY-ESO-1, a protein encoded by a member of the cancer/ germline family of genes [52, 53].

Melanoma regression was obtained in about 30% of patients after cell therapy with MART-1 specific T cells [49, 52, 54-56]. As a side effect, patients suffered from vitiligo and destruction of melanocytes in the eye and ear indicating that T cells with engineered specificity can target rare and healthy cells even with the cognate antigen at low levels. In a recent trial, patients were treated with T cells engineered with an anti-MAGE-A3 TCR [57]. While 5/9 patients experienced melanoma regression, three of them had mental status changes and two lapsed into coma and died. Histology revealed necrotizing leukoencephalopathy which is likely due to the recognition of previously unknown epitopes of MAGE-A9/A12, the latter expressed in the brain.

Prolonged clinical remission was observed when engineered T cells persisted in the circulation for longer times; TCR modified T cells were recorded in the blood for more than a year after initiation of treatment [56, 58]. Moreover, TCR engineered T cells were capable to penetrate the blood-brain barrier and to induce regression of brain metastases [57] giving hope that patients with metastases at otherwise incurable sites may benefit from adoptive cell therapy. However, tumor cells may become invisible to TCR modified T cells due to repression of the MHC complex [60], β2 microglobulin mutation [61], and deficiencies in the antigen processing machinery [60, 62], all of them resulting in diminished antigen presentation and less TCR-mediated T cell activation.

Engineering T cells with a recombinant TCR may produce a safety hazard when the transgenic αβ TCR forms hetero-dimers with the respective α and β TCR chains of the endogenous TCR. Such mis-pairing of TCR chains can induce severe auto-reactivity as a result in gain of an unpredictable specificity [63, 64]. The situation was technically solved by different means including replacing the human by the homologous murine constant moieties of the TCR [65] and by inserting additional cysteine bridges [66] to facilitate preferential pairing of the recombinant TCR αβ chains in the presence of the physiologic αβ TCR. These and other

http://dx.doi.org/10.5772/59255

technical difficulties of the TCR strategy promoted the development of an artificial "all-in-one" receptor molecule to redirect T cells in an antigen-restricted fashion as summarized below.

Target antigen	Adoptively transferred T cells	NCT ID	Center
	IL-12 engineered TILs	NCT01236573	NIH
	IL-2 engineered TILs	NCT00062036	NIH
	CXCR2 and NGFR transduced TILs, high dose IL-2	NCT01740557	MDACC
	TGF-Beta resistant (DNRII) and NGFR transduced TILs, high dose IL-2	NCT01955460	MDACC
gp-100	anti-gp-100 TCR engineered CD8+ cells, anti-gp-100 TCR engineered TILs, high dose IL-2	NCT00085462	NIH
gp-100	anti-gp-100 TCR engineered T cells, high dose IL-2 plus gp-100 vaccination	NCT00610311	NIH
gp-100 & MART-1	anti-gp-100 TCR & anti-MART-1 TCR engineered T cells high dose IL-2 Peptide Immunization	NCT00923195	NIH
MAGE-A3	anti-MAGE-A3/12 TCR engineered T cells, high dose IL-2	NCT01273181	NIH
MAGE-A3	anti-MAGE-A3 TCR engineered T cells, high dose IL-2	NCT02153905	NIH
MAGE-A3	anti-MAGE-A3-DP4 TCR engineered CD4+ cells, high dose IL-2	NCT02111850	NIH
MAGE-A4	anti-MAGE-A4 TCR engineered T cells	NCT02096614	MUH
MAGE-A4	anti-MAGE-A4 TCR engineered T cells	NCT01694472	TMUCIH
MART-1	anti-MART-1 TCR engineered T cells, IL-2, peptide immunization	NCT00091104	NIH
MART-1	anti-MART-1 TCR engineered T cells, IL-2, MART-1 peptide pulsed dendritic cells	NCT00910650	UC
MART-1	anti-MART-1 TCR engineered T cells, high dose IL-2, peptide immunization	NCT00612222	NIH
MART-1	anti-MART-1 TCR T cells vs. anti-MART-1 TCR TILs, high dose IL-2	NCT00509288	NIH
MART-1	anti-MART-1 TCR engineered T cells, low dose IL-2, peptide immunization	NCT00706992	NIH
NY-ESO-1	anti-NY-ESO-1 TCR engineered T cells, high dose IL-2	NCT00670748	NIH
NY-ESO-1	anti-NY ESO-1 mTCR engineered T cells, high dose IL-2	NCT01967823	NIH
NY-ESO-1	anti-NY ESO-1 TCR CD62L+ T cells, high dose IL-2	NCT02062359	NIH
NY-ESO-1	anti-NY-ESO-1 TCR engineered T cells	NCT01350401	Adaptimmune
NY-ESO-1	anti-NY-ESO-1 TCR engineered T cells, cotransduced with IL-12 cDNA	NCT01457131	NIH
p53	anti-p53 TCR engineered T cells, high dose IL-2, p53 peptide pulsed dendritic cells	NCT00704938	NIH
p53	anti-p53 TCR engineered T cells, high dose IL-2	NCT00393029	NIH
tyrosinase	anti-tyrosinase(368-376) TCR engineered T cells	NCT01586403	LU
GD2	3rd generation anti-GD2 CAR engineered T cells	NCT02107963	NIH
VEGFR2	anti-VEGFR2 CAR engineered CD8+ T cells, low dose IL-2	NCT01218867	NIH

LU, Loyola University (Chicago); MDACC, M.D. Anderson Cancer Center; MUH, Mie University Hospital; NIH, National Institutes of Health; TMUCIH, Tianjin Medical University Cancer Institute and Hospital; UC, University of California;

Table 3. Adoptive cell therapy with engineered antigen specific T cells in patients with melanoma

4. CAR T cells with engineered specificity for melanoma

In order to link antigen recognition with the downstream signaling machinery of the TCR, Zelig Eshhar (Weizmann Institute of Science) reported a chimeric antigen receptor (CAR) molecule, also named immunoreceptor, which is composed in the extracellular moiety of a single chain fragment of variable region (scFv) antibody for binding and in the intracellular moiety of the CD3ζ endodomain to initiate T cell activation [67]. The coding sequence of such recombinant receptor molecule is transferred by retro- or lentiviral transduction into T cells in vitro (Figure 1) [68]. CAR engineered T cells, also nick-named "T-bodies", recognize their new target by CAR binding and become activated to secrete pro-inflammatory cytokines, to amplify and to lyse the cognate target cells. Since the binding domain is derived from an antibody the CAR recognizes the target in a MHC-independent fashion which makes major differences to TCR mediated T cell recognition. For instance, the CAR recognizes its target independently of the individual HLA subtype and CAR T cells are not affected by MHC repression and loss of HLA molecules on target cells which frequently occurs during tumor progression. However, recognition by CARs is restricted to target antigens on the cell surface; intracellular antigens like transcription factors are not visible to CAR T cells. Despite that limitation, a nearly infinite variety of targets can be recognized including those which are not classical T cell targets like carbohydrates and gangliosides [69].

Full and lasting T cell activation requires two complementary signals, one provided by the TCR/CD3 and the other by co-receptors the prototype of which is CD28. Prolonged T cell activation, however, requires costimulation and autocrine factors, in particular IL-2 which is only secreted upon TCR and simultaneous CD28 signaling. The lack of appropriate costimulation in the tumor lesion provides the rationale for combining the intracellular CD3ζ with the CD28 signaling domain in one polypeptide chain of a "second generation" CAR (Figure 2). A CAR with combined CD28-CD3ζ signaling domain provides both the primary CD3ζ and the required costimlatory signal when engaging the cognate target. CARs with a costimulatory domain clearly provide clinical benefit and improved T cell persistence compared to CARs with the CD3ζ domain only [70-72]. Other costimulatory moieties, such as 4-1BB (CD137) and OX40 (CD134), also provide full T cell activation when linked to CD3ζ in a CAR; the individual costimulory domains have different impact on T cell effector functions [73]. These and other costimulatory domains were furthermore combined in so-called "3rd generation" CARs which provide advantage for matured effector T cells in terminal differentiation but less in younger stages of T cell development [74]. A number of additional modifications of the CAR design were explored in order to improve T cell persistence and activation and finally the anti-tumor response [75, 76].

While the antibody domain defines the target specificity of the CAR, a plethora of antigens can potentially be used as target for the adoptive cell therapy of melanoma. T cells engineered for targeting melanoma-associated antigens include CARs with specificity for HMW-MAA, also known as MCSP [77, 78], melanotransferrin [79], and the gangliosides GD2 [80] and GD3 [81]. Trials are currently recruiting; to our best knowledge no published data are so far available.

During the last years spectacular efficacy was achieved with CAR T cells in phase I trials for the treatment of lymphoma/leukemia [82, 83]. Clinical response and prolonged T cell activation was accompanied by a "cytokine storm", which occurred even weeks after initial T cell administration; the side effect can clinically be managed by treatment with a neutralizing anti-IL-6 antibody without affecting the anti-tumor efficacy.

The enthusiasm in CAR T cell therapy, however, was dampened by reports on serious adverse events and fatalities after CAR T cell administration [84, 85]. Targeting ErbB2 produced respiratory failure which is thought to be due to low levels of antigen on a number of healthy cells which are sufficient to trigger "on-target-off-organ" T cell activation [86]. This and other serious adverse events emphasize a careful evaluation of potential targets and the necessity for T cell dose escalation studies to balance anti-tumor efficacy and auto-immunity [75, 87, 88].

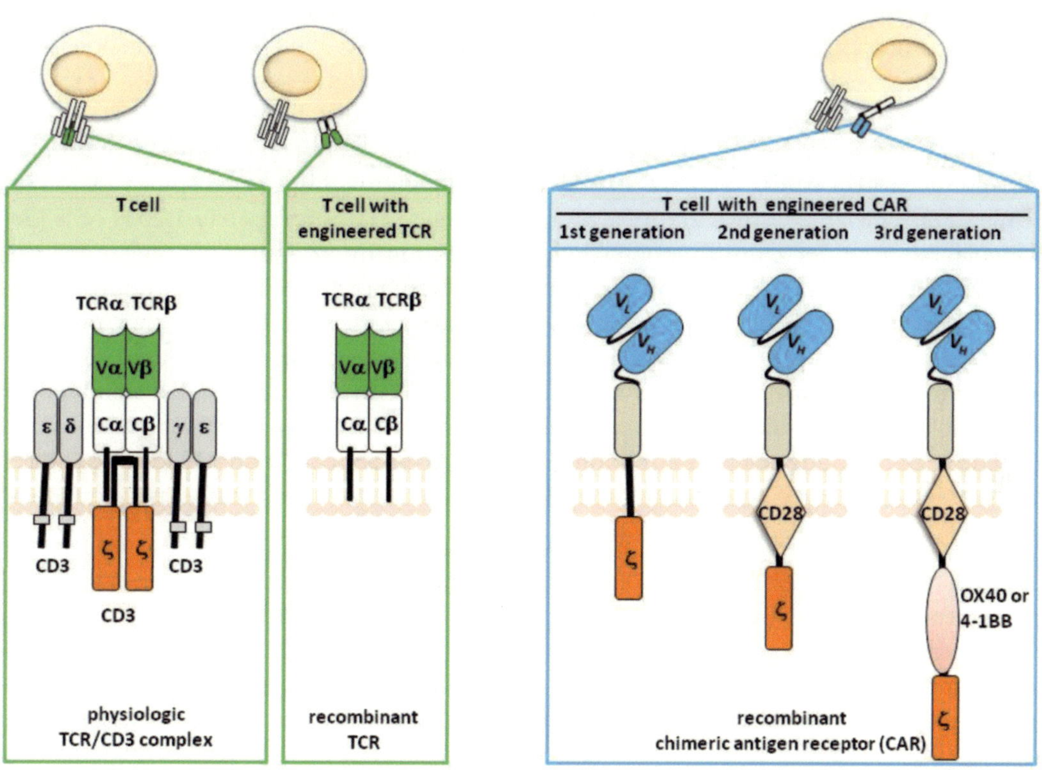

Figure 2. T cells with engineered specificity. T cells physiologically recognize their target by the T cell receptor (TCR) complex which is composed of the TCR α and β chain for recognition and the CD3 chains for signaling. The variable regions of each TCR chain ($V\alpha$ and $V\beta$) together bind to the MHC presented antigen, $C\alpha$ and $C\beta$ represent the constant domains. T cells can be genetically engineered with defined specificity by expression of recombinant TCR $\alpha\beta$ chains of known specificity. In contrast to the TCR, the chimeric antigen receptor (CAR) is one polypeptide chain composed of a single chain fragment of variable region (scFv) antibody for antigen recognition, the extracellular spacer domain, a trans-membrane domain and the intracellular CD3ζ ("first generation" CAR), the CD28-CD3ζ ("second generation" CAR), or the CD28-OX40-CD3ζ ("third generation" CAR) signaling chain.

5. "Melanoma stem cells": Target cells to achieve long-term remission?

Despite the tremendous cellular and phenotypic heterogeneity in tumor lesions, cancer is thought to be initiated and maintained by so-called cancer stem cells (CSCs). Such pluripotent stem cells are of low abundance, induce tumors upon transplantation under limiting dilution conditions, resist radiation and chemotherapy, and drive self-renewal and a-symmetric differentiation into a variety of cell types. Residual CSCs are thought to initiate cancer relapse even after years of "dormancy", which can be more than a decade after surgical treatment of the primary lesion [89]. While the concept of the hierarchical organization in driving tumor progression was initially drawn upon deciphering hematological malignancies, basically the same organization was subsequently reported for other solid cancers including mammary, prostate, pancreatic, colon carcinoma and glioma [90-94].

Transplantation of melanoma cell subsets into recipient mice under limiting dilution conditions also revealed that a defined subset of cancer cells, and not every cell from the same biopsy, can induce tumors of same histology as the parental tumor [90, 95-97]. One conclusion is that melanoma is organized in a hierarchical manner originating from a particular initiator cell, the cancer stem cell, which gives rise to the described diversity of cells in an established lesion. Melanoma initiating cells were described by various, but not common markers, including the transporter protein ABCB5 [95], CD20 [97], or the nerve growth factor receptor CD271 [98]. While CD271$^+$melanoma cells are present in a frequency of approximately 1/2000 cells [98], transplantation under more rigorous conditions, i.e., ideally of one single melanoma cell, revealed that nearly every fourth randomly taken melanoma cell (1/2-1/15) can induce tumors in the host animal. This observation, however, questioned the validity of the stem cell paradigm for melanoma [99, 100]. Subsequent studies made clear that the potential to induce melanoma is not closely associated with a particular phenotype and that the number of potential CSCs in melanoma may not necessarily be low. If nearly every melanoma cell is capable to re-program to a tumor initiating cell under certain conditions, blocking stem cell properties in melanoma will reduce tumor initiation and growth in a transplantation model finally resulting in melanoma ablation [101].

Once the tumor lesion is established, a minor subset of cancer cells seems to take over to control malignant progression. Evidence for this hypothesis was provided from a pre-clinical model [79] which asked whether all or a defined subset of melanoma cells in an established xeno-transplanted lesion need to be eliminated to cause tumor regression. Such melanoma sustaining cell may be, but not must be identical to melanoma stem cells identified by transplantation assays.

Evidence for a particular targetable melanoma cell subset which sustains tumor progression was provided by the observation that elimination of CD20$^+$melanoma cells by adoptive transfer of CAR T cells completely eradicated xeno-transplanted melanoma. Those human melanoma biopsies contained a subset of CD20$^+$melanoma cells which constituted about 1-2% of melanoma cells and which are present in different histological melanoma types and tumor stages. A caveat is that in approximately 20% of melanoma samples analyzed so far, no CD20$^+$melanoma cells were detected by histological screening; CD20-specific CAR T cells did not induce regression of those transplanted tumor lesions. Interestingly, CD20 re-expression in a random subpopulation of those tumor cells by genetic modification did not render the tumor lesion sensitive for eradication indicating that CD20 expression per se is not sufficient but requires additional capabilities to sustain melanoma progression [79].

There are additionally clinical observations that sustain the notion of $CD20^+$cells in promoting melanoma progression. Firstly, a patient with stage III/IV metastatic, refractory melanoma and 2% $CD20^+$melanoma cells who received intra-lesional injections of the anti-CD20 therapeutic antibody rituximab experienced lasting remission accompanied by a decline of the melanoma serum marker S-100 to physiological levels and a switch of a T helper-2 to a more pro-inflammatory T helper-1 response [102]. Although anecdotic, data provide the first clinical evidence that targeted elimination of $CD20^+$melanoma cells can produce regression of chemotherapy-refractory melanoma. Secondly, in a small pilot trial, stage IV melanoma patients without evidence of disease by way of surgery, chemo-and/or radiation therapy received the anti-CD20 antibody systemically for a 2 year period [103]. Data suggest a benefit of anti-CD20 therapy in overall and recurrence-free survival; a caveat being that the number of patients is still small for definitive conclusions.

Currently, the hierarchical stem cell model in the maintenance of an established melanoma is supported by some experimental evidence [79], whereas a body of information on melanoma initiation by transplantation of single melanoma cells sustains the stochastic model [99, 100], although not confirmed by others [98]. The most determining proof of the stem cell hypothesis, however, will be the successful melanoma elimination by targeting stem cells or stem cell properties. For the development of such therapeutic strategies several aspects need to be taken into account.

First, standard therapy will rapidly de-bulk the tumor lesion and the remaining melanoma stem cells, which are more chemo-and radiation resistant, will drive relapse of the disease. Since those melanoma initiating cells are merely in a "dormant" state and replicate less frequently than the majority of melanoma cells in the same lesion, anti-proliferative strategies by classical chemotherapeutic drugs are unlikely efficient. Transporter systems including ABCB5, which is highly expressed by melanoma stem cells [95], additionally contribute to chemotherapy resistance; the chemotherapy and/or radiation itself may promote expression of those transporter systems and survival of those resistant cells which finally contributes to relapse of the disease.

Second, if clinical progression correlates with the prevalence of $CD20^+$melanoma cells, targeted elimination of those melanoma cells requires to meet the fact that those target cells are a small minority. Targeted elimination, e.g., by CD20 redirected cytotoxic T cells or by CD20-specific therapeutic antibodies like Rituxan™ (rituximab) or Arzerra™ (ofatumumab), will be required to obtain substantial efficacy.

Third, the extraordinary functional and phenotypic plasticity of melanoma cells may make it necessary to have the therapeutic agent in place for a longer time. In their pre-clinical model, Schmidt and colleagues [79] used CAR T cells which persist for long-term acting as an antigen-specific guardian as long as target cells are present. Since repetitive re-stimulation sustains the persistence and amplification of CAR T cells, cellular therapy has a major advantage compared to pharmaceutical drugs with a comparable short half-life. CAR T cells can moreover provide antigen-specific memory with defined specificity [104], potentially contributing to control melanoma in the long-term.

6. Production of engineered T cells for clinical application

Application of adoptive cell therapy to clinical use requires efficient production of cells according to good manufacturing practice (GMP). This particularly applies to patient's T cells which are ex vivo genetically modified. The vector used for T cell modification is of major relevance with respect to the efficiency and stability in modification. Crucial steps in this process are the stable integration of the genetic vector, the site of integration to avoid insertion mutagenesis, and the resistance of the vector to genetic repression. To date, most clinical trials were performed employing retroviral or lentiviral vectors which fulfill some but not all of these requirements. Recently, other vector systems including RNA modification are alternatively utilized and it is expected that these systems will be explored in parallel in the near future.

The way of stimulating the T cells ex vivo for genetic modification and subsequent amplification is crucial for both the success in transduction and the functional capacities of modified cells. T cells are commonly activated by TCR/CD3 stimulation in addition to IL-2 [105]; most protocols use anti-CD3 and anti-CD28 magnetic beads [83, 106] which can be easily eliminated during the production process. IL-2 is replaced by other cytokines such as IL-7 and IL-15 to obtain a T cell population with a more naive and central memory phenotype [107]. Alternatively, cell lines were engineered, so-called "artificial APCs", which are modified with the various co-stimulating molecules to mimic the physiological stimulation and to provide the required signals [108]. However, difficulties in adopting those cells to GMP standard prevent their broad application in large scale production processes.

For the production itself, static culture systems in flasks or gas permeable bags are traditionally used. Due to their amplification at low cell densities (0.25-1x10^6 cells per ml), high culture volumes are required to obtain clinically relevant T cell numbers which is more easily achieved by non-static systems including the WAVE-Bioreactor or the G-Rex100 device [83, 106, 109]. In order to produce engineered T cells for a large number of patients it will be required to manufacture cells in a closed system and to produce multiple batches in parallel in the same clean room facility without the risk of batch contamination.

7. Challenges and promise in the adoptive cell therapy of melanoma

To date, approximately half of the melanoma patients benefit from adoptive cell therapy with TILs. Specifically targeted T cells may further improve the therapeutic response. Despite substantial success, the strategy still has major challenges which need to be addressed in the near future.

Significant numbers of effector T cells have to accumulate in the targeted tumor lesion which is mediated by a network of chemokines. Adoptively transferred T cells use these networks to accumulate at the tumor site; melanoma cells secrete a number of chemokines including CXCL1 to attract lymphocytes. However, early imaging studies revealed that melanoma-specific T cells massively infiltrate the lungs, spleen and liver with only some accumulation at the tumor site before the cells decline to undetectable levels in circulation [110-112]. To improve tumor targeting TILs were engineered with CXCR2, the receptor for melanoma secreted CXCL1, which resulted in improved anti-tumor activity in a mouse model [113]. The strategy is currently being explored in an early phase I trial (Table 3) [113].

Since tumor eradication requires a beneficial T cell-to-target cell ratio, higher numbers of tumor-specific T cells applied per dose likely increase the clinical efficacy. The optimal dose of T cells, however, is still a matter of discussion and requires empiric evaluation. A number of trials, in particular applying TILs, administered up to 10^{10} cells per dose [27]. Such high doses in turn require extended expansions of T cells ex vivo with the risk of loss of the "young" phenotype and gain of more matured T cells. Highly expanded T cells become hypo-responsive to CD28 costimulation and rapidly enter activation induced cell death, in particular upon IL-2 driven expansion [114]. With respect to more potent effector functions short-term amplification protocols are envisioned for both TILs and engineered T cells. This may be achieved by T cell amplification in the presence of IL-15 and IL-21 and/or by 4-1BB co-stimulation [115].

On the other hand, administration of about 10^5 engineered T cells induced remarkable therapeutic efficacy in recent trials targeting $CD19^+$ leukemia [83]. Since the T cells substantially amplify in vivo upon antigen encounter, the capacity of cells to amplify under appropriate conditions is more relevant than the applied cell number.

Once targeted in sufficient numbers to the tumor tissue, a major challenge is the tumor selectivity of redirected T cells. While the TCR and the CAR is specific for a particular target, in most cases the targeted antigen is not exclusively expressed by cancer but also by healthy cells, although sometimes at lower levels [116, 117]. MART-1, frequently expressed by the majority of melanoma cells, is also expressed by melanocytes. Targeting such type of antigen frequently produces vitiligo, sometimes also inner ear toxicity with a certain degree of deafness [49]. Since nearly all "tumor-associated antigens" which are frequently used as targets for adoptive cell therapy are self-antigens, strategies are needed to minimize such off-target toxicities. Among these, low-avidity TCRs or CARs or combinatorial antigen recognition by two CARs are currently explored.

Melanoma cells may become invisible to TILs or TCR modified T cells due to down-regulation of their MHC components or due to deficiencies in antigen processing. However, melanoma cells may still be visible to CAR T cells which recognized their target by their antibody-derived binding domain in a MHC independent fashion. On the other hand, TCR T cells are capable to recognize cross-presented antigen, for instance tumor antigen presented by stroma cells, which is invisible to CAR T cells but helps to destroy the tumor lesion in the long-term [118, 119].

Consequently, a TCR-like CAR aims at combining the benefits of TCR and CAR redirected T cells. This is performed by using a single chain antibody with TCR-like specificity for recognizing MHC presented antigen. T cells with such a TCR-like CAR were successfully redirected in a MHC restricted fashion towards NY-ESO-1 and MAGE-A1, respectively [120, 121].

The redirected T cell activation depends on the amount of target antigen and binding affinity. Compared to TILs and TCR modified T cells, CAR T cells bind with extraordinary high affinity by their antibody-derived CAR binding domain. A furthermore increase in affinity by affinity maturation does not necessarily improve CAR redirected T cell activation [120, 122]; CD28 costimulation does not add to the affinity dependent activation threshold, however, prolongs T cell persistence and resistance to apoptosis [123]. Targeting cancer cells also depends on the amount of target antigen in addition to the binding affinity. Low affinity CARs require abundant antigen levels for efficient activation of engineered T cells while high affinity CARs are likewise effective against low antigen levels on target cells. In this context, the selectivity in targeting melanoma cells versus healthy cells needs to be discussed not only with respect to the targeted antigen itself but also to antigen amount and binding affinity.

Amplification and persistence of adoptively transferred cells correlates with clinical outcome in some trials [124]. T cells will persist in detectable numbers as long as targeted antigen is present, however, will contract to undetectable levels and disappear from circulation when no target is furthermore present. To enable survival of CAR T cells in the long-term, Epstein-Barr virus (EBV)-specific T cells were used as effector cells and modified with a tumor-specific CAR. The rationale is that EBV specific T cells are maintained in a sizable population in circulation by recognizing EBV antigens by their physiological TCR. The strategy is sustained by the first clinical observation that EBV-specific T cells engineered with an anti-GD2 CAR showed benefit over non-virus-specific, CAR engineered T cells in the treatment of neuroblastoma (NCT00085930) [124]. Other trials use EBV or CMV specific, autologous T cells engineered with a first or second generation CAR, for instance directed against HER2/neu (ErbB2) (NCT01109095), CD30 (NCT01192464), or CD19 (NCT00709033; NCT01475058; NCT01430390; NCT00840853; NCT01195480).

The T cell subset matters, adoptively transferred $CD8^+$T cell clones poorly persist [125] and need help of $CD4^+$cells. Prolonged T cell anti-tumor response also requires resistance to repression in the tumor tissue. A number of efforts are currently undertaken to counteract tumor associated T cell repression, in particular mediated by Treg cells and checkpoint mediators. In animal models, CD28 costimulation without induction of IL-2 secretion protects a CAR redirected T cell response from Treg cell repression [126]. On the other hand, repetitive T cell stimulation upregulates CTLA-4 which acts as negative regulator to return the T cell to a resting stage. Administration of a CTLA-4 blocker, e.g., ipilimumab antibody, may prolong the anti-tumor activation of transferred T cells, although it is not locally restricted and will likewise affect all T cells [127, 128]. Expression profiling of TCR-engineered T cells demonstrates overexpression of multiple inhibitory receptors in persisting lymphocytes, including PD-1 and CD160, the latter associated with decreased reactivity of TCR T cells in a ligand independent manner [129]. Essentially the same was observed for CAR T cells [130]. These analyses point to a multi-factorial T cell repression in the tumor tissue; there is more than one uni-directional strategy needed to sustain the T cell anti-tumor response in the long-term.

A major hurdle of specific immunotherapy in general is the tremendous heterogeneity of cancer cells within the same lesion. Low or loss of target antigen expression negatively affects the long-term therapeutic efficacy of an antigen-redirected approach. This is supported by several reports which document a relapse of antigen-loss tumor metastases after adoptive therapy with melanoma-reactive T cell clones [39,131, 132]. A solution may be the use of polyclonal T cells with specificities for various melanoma antigens or T cells modified with different CARs recognizing different antigens; however, target-negative tumor cells will not be recognized. On the other hand, pro-inflammatory cytokines secreted by redirected T cells upon activation can attract a second wave of innate immune cells which in turn may eradiate the antigen-negative tumor cells. At least in an animal model, antigen-negative melanoma cells are indeed eliminated when co-inoculated with antibody-targeted cytokines [133]. T cells engineered with induced expression of transgenic IL-12 can attract innate immune cells including macrophages into the tumor tissue which eliminate antigen-negative tumor cells in the same lesion, at least in an immune competent animal model [134]. Such "TRUCK" cells ("T cells redirected for unrestricted cytokine killing") may pave a novel way to deliver transgenic cell products to pre-defined, target lesions.

Combination of adoptive cell therapy with pathway inhibitors may improve the efficacy in melanoma cell elimination, in particular in disseminated stages of the disease. Metastatic melanoma patients with the B-raf activating mutation V600E benefit from a small molecule drug, PLX4032 or vemurafenib, which inhibits the mitogen-activated protein kinase (MAPK) pathway. Treatment with vemurafenib is accompanied by increased T cell infiltrations in the melanoma lesions [135, 136] which may contribute to the therapeutic effect and may be improved by co-administration of melanoma-specific T cells.

While adoptive cell therapy is mostly performed with modified or non-modified T cells, other cells like monocytes, macrophages as well as NK cells can also be redirected by CARs in an antigen-specific fashion [137-141, 144]. In contrast to T cells, NK cells can be rapidly activated and exhibit high cytotoxic potential and continuously growing NK cell lines such as NK-92 can be used for adoptive cancer immunotherapy [142]. CD3ζ chain CARs trigger cytolytic activities of NK cells which has been shown for CARs with various specificities [138, 141, 143-147]. Similar to T cells, the anti-tumor activity was improved by adding 4-1BB or 2B4 (CD244) costimulatory domains [148, 149]. Since NK cells cannot provide IL-2 or IL-15 required for amplification, CAR modified NK cells were additionally engineered to release IL-15 which sustains NK cell expansion and CAR-mediated cytotoxicity in the absence of IL-2 [150]. Despite these and other advances during the last years, experience with CAR engineered primary NK cells in clinical trials is still limited; whether redirected cells of the innate immune system are more advantageous in melanoma elimination than modified T cells has moreover to be explored in clinical trials.

Acknowledgements

Work in the author's laboratory was supported by the Deutsche Forschungsgemeinschaft, Bonn, Deutsche Krebshilfe, Bonn, Else Kröner-Fresenius-Stiftung, Bad Homburg v.d.H., Wilhelm Sander-Stiftung, München, the European Union (European Regional Development Fund-Investing in your future), the German federal state North Rhine-Westphalia (NRW), and the Fortune program of the Medical Faculty of the University of Cologne.

Author details

Jennifer Makalowski[1,2] and Hinrich Abken[1,2*]

*Address all correspondence to: hinrich.abken@uk-koeln.de

1 Center for Molecular Medicine Cologne (CMMC), University of Cologne, Germany

2 Dept. I Internal Medicine, University Hospital Cologne, Cologne, Germany

References

[1] Garbe C, Peris K, Hauschild A, Saiag P, Middleton M, Spatz A, Grob J-J, Malvehy J, Newton-Bishop J, Stratigos A, Pehamberger H, Eggermont A. Diagnosis and treatment of melanoma: European consensus-based interdisciplinary guideline. European Journal of Cancer 2010;46(2) 270-283.

[2] Denninghoff VC, Kahn AG, Falco J, Curutchet HP, Elsner B. Sentinel lymph node: detection of micrometastases of melanoma in a molecular study. Molecular Diagnosis 2004;8(4) 253-258.

[3] Bedikian AY, Wei C, Detry M, Kim KB, Papadopoulos NE, Hwu WJ, Homsi J, Davies M, McIntyre S, Hwu P. Predictive Factors for the Development of Brain Metastasis in Advanced Unresectable Metastatic Melanoma. American Journal of Clinical Oncology 2010;34(6) 603-610.

[4] Chapman PB, Hauschild A, Robert C, Haanen JB, Ascierto P, Larkin J, Dummer R, Garbe C, Testori A, Maio M, Hogg D, Lorigan P, Lebbe C, Jouary T, Schadendorf D, Ribas A, O'Day SJ, Sosman JA, Kirkwood JM, Eggermont AM, Dreno B, Nolop K, Li J, Nelson B, Hou J, Lee RJ, Flaherty KT. Improved survival with vemurafenib in melanoma with BRAF V600E mutation. The New England Journal of Medicine 2011;364 (26) 2507-2516.

[5] Carter RD, Krementz ET, Hill GJ 2nd, Metter GE, Fletcher WS, Golomb FM, Grage TB, Minton JP, Sparks FC. DTIC (nsc-45388) and combination therapy for melanoma.

I. Studies with DTIC, BCNU (NSC-409962), CCNU (NSC-79037), vincristine (NSC-67574), and hydroxyurea (NSC-32065). Cancer Treat Rep. 1976;60(5) 601-609.

[6] Flaherty KT, Puzanov I, Kim KB, Ribas A, McArthur GA, Sosman JA, O'Dwyer PJ, Lee RJ, Grippo JF, Nolop K, Chapman PB. Inhibition of mutated, activated BRAF in metastatic melanoma. The New England Journal of Medicine 2010;363(9) 809-819.

[7] Leiter U, Eigentler TK, Forschner A, Pflugfelder A, Weide B, Held L, Meier F, Garbe C. Excision guidelines and follow-up strategies in cutaneous melanoma: Facts and controversies. Clinics in Dermatology 2010;28(3) 311-315.

[8] Bradbury PA, Middleton MR. DNA repair pathways in drug resistance in melanoma. Anti-cancer Drugs 2004;15(5) 421-426.

[9] Pak BJ, Chu W, Lu SJ, Kerbel RS, Ben-David Y. Lineage-specific mechanism of drug and radiation resistance in melanoma mediated by tyrosinase-related protein 2. Cancer Metastasis Reviews 2001;20(1-2) 27-32.

[10] Pak BJ, Lee J, Thai BL, Fuchs SY, Shaked Y, Ronai Z, Kerbel RS, Ben-David Y. Radiation resistance of human melanoma analysed by retroviral insertional mutagenesis reveals a possible role for dopachrome tautomerase. Oncogene 2004;23(1) 30-38.

[11] Atkins MB, Lotze MT, Dutcher JP, Fisher RI, Weiss G, Margolin K, Abrams J, Sznol M, Parkinson D, Hawkins M, Paradise C, Kunkel L, Rosenberg SA. High-dose recombinant interleukin 2 therapy for patients with metastatic melanoma: analysis of 270 patients treated between 1985 and 1993. Journal of Clinical Oncology 1999;17(7) 2105-2116.

[12] Hodi FS, O'Day SJ, McDermott DF, Weber RW, Sosman JA, Haanen JB, Gonzalez R, Robert C, Schadendorf D, Hassel JC, Akerley W, van den Eertwegh AJ, Lutzky J, Lorigan P, Vaubel JM, Linette GP, Hogg D, Ottensmeier CH, Lebbé C, Peschel C, Quirt I, Clark JI, Wolchok JD, Weber JS, Tian J, Yellin MJ, Nichol GM, Hoos A, Urba WJ. Improved survival with ipilimumab in patients with metastatic melanoma. The New England Journal of Medicine 2010;363(8) 711-723.

[13] Kirkwood JM, Ibrahim JG, Sondak VK, Richards J, Flaherty LE, Ernstoff MS, Smith TJ, Rao U, Steele M, Blum RH. High-and low-dose interferon alfa-2b in high-risk melanoma: first analysis of intergroup trial E1690/S9111/C9190. Journal of Clinical Oncology 2000;18(12) 2444-2458.

[14] Kirkwood JM, Strawderman MH, Ernstoff MS, Smith TJ, Borden EC, Blum RH. Interferon alfa-2b adjuvant therapy of high-risk resected cutaneous melanoma: the Eastern Cooperative Oncology Group Trial EST 1684. Journal of Clinical Oncology 1996;14(1) 7-17.

[15] Galluzzi L, Vacchelli E, Eggermont A, Fridman WH, Galon J, Sautès-Fridman C, Tartour E, Zitvogel L, Kroemer G. Trial Watch: Adoptive cell transfer immunotherapy. Oncoimmunology 2012;1(3) 306-315.

[16] Bernatchez C, Radvanyi LG, Hwu P. Advances in the treatment of metastatic melanoma: adoptive T-cell therapy. Seminars in Oncology 2012;39(2) 215-226.

[17] Grulich AE, van Leeuwen MT, Falster MO, Vajdic CM. Incidence of cancers in people with HIV/AIDS compared with immunosuppressed transplant recipients: a meta-analysis. Lancet 2007;370(9581) 59-67.

[18] Nathanson. Spontaneous regression of malignant melanoma: a review of the literature on incidence, clinical features, and possible mechanisms. National Cancer Institute Monograph 1976;44 67-76.

[19] Rosenberg SA, Yang JC, Topalian SL, Schwartzentruber DJ, Weber JS, Parkinson DR, Seipp CA, Einhorn JH, White DE. Treatment of 283 consecutive patients with metastatic melanoma or renal cell cancer using high-dose bolus interleukin 2. The journal of the American Medical Association 1994;271(12) 907-913.

[20] Clark WH Jr, From L, Bernardino EA, Mihm MC. The histogenesis and biologic behavior of primary human malignant melanomas of the skin. Cancer Research 1969;29(3) 705-727.

[21] Vignard V, Lemercier B, Lim A, Pandolfino MC, Guilloux Y, Khammari A, Rabu C, Echasserieau K, Lang F, Gougeon ML, Dreno B, Jotereau F, Labarriere N. Adoptive transfer of tumor-reactive Melan-A-specific CTL clones in melanoma patients is followed by increased frequencies of additional Melan-A-specific T cells. Journal of Immunology 2005;175(7) 4797-4805.

[22] Rosenberg SA, Packard BS, Aebersold PM, Solomon D, Topalian SL, Toy ST, Simon P, Lotze MT, Yang JC, Seipp CA, et al. Use of tumor-infiltrating lymphocytes and interleukin-2 in the immunotherapy of patients with metastatic melanoma. N. Engl. J. Med. 1988;319(25), 1676–1680.

[23] Clemente CG, Mihm MC Jr, Bufalino R, Zurrida S, Collini P, Cascinelli N. Prognostic value of tumor infiltrating lymphocytes in the vertical growth phase of primary cutaneous melanoma. Cancer 1996;77(7) 1303-1310.

[24] Burton AL, Roach BA, Mays MP, Chen AF, Ginter BA, Vierling AM, Scoggins CR, Martin RC, Stromberg AJ, Hagendoorn L, McMasters KM. Prognostic significance of tumor infiltrating lymphocytes in melanoma. The American Surgeon 2011;77(2) 188-192.

[25] Hinrichs CS, Rosenberg SA. Exploiting the curative potential of adoptive T-cell therapy for cancer. Immunological Reviews Adoptive Immunotherapy for Cancer 2014; 257(1) 56–71.

[26] Dudley ME, Wunderlich JR, Robbins PF, Yang JC, Hwu P, Schwartzentruber DJ, Topalian SL, Sherry R, Restifo NP, Hubicki AM, Robinson MR, Raffeld M, Duray P, Seipp CA, Rogers-Freezer L, Morton KE, Mavroukakis SA, White DE, Rosenberg SA.

Cancer regression and autoimmunity in patients after clonal repopulation with antitumor lymphocytes. *Science* 2002;298(5594) 850–854.

[27] Dudley ME, Wunderlich JR, Yang JC, Sherry RM, Topalian SL, Restifo NP, Royal RE, Kammula U, White DE, Mavroukakis SA, Rogers LJ, Gracia GJ, Jones SA, Mangiameli DP, Pelletier MM, Gea-Banacloche J, Robinson MR, Berman DM, Filie AC, Abati A, Rosenberg SA. Adoptive cell transfer therapy following non-myeloablative but lymphodepleting chemotherapy for the treatment of patients with refractory metastatic melanoma. Journal of Clinical Oncology 2005;23(10) 2346-2357.

[28] Dudley ME, Yang JC, Sherry R, Hughes MS, Royal R, Kammula U, Robbins PF, Huang J, Citrin DE, Leitman SF, Wunderlich J, Restifo NP, Thomasian A, Downey SG, Smith FO, Klapper J, Morton K, Laurencot C, White DE, Rosenberg SA. Adoptive cell therapy for patients with metastatic melanoma: evaluation of intensive myeloablative chemoradiation preparative regimens. Journal of Clinical Oncology 2008;26(32) 5233-5239.

[29] Besser MJ, Shapira-Frommer R, Treves AJ, Zippel D, Itzhaki O, Hershkovitz L, Levy D, Kubi A, Hovav E, Chermoshniuk N, Shalmon B, Hardan I, Catane R, Markel G, Apter S, Ben-Nun A, Kuchuk I, Shimoni A, Nagler A, Schachter J. Clinical responses in a phase II study using adoptive transfer of short-term cultured tumor infiltration lymphocytes in metastatic melanoma patients. Clinical Cancer Research 2010;16(9) 2646-2655.

[30] Tran KQ, Zhou J, Durflinger KH, Langhan MM, Shelton TE, Wunderlich JR, Robbins PF, Rosenberg SA, Dudley ME. Minimally cultured tumor-infiltrating lymphocytes display optimal characteristics for adoptive cell therapy. J. Immunother 2008;31(8) 742–751.

[31] Dudley ME, Gross CA, Langhan MM, Garcia MR, Sherry RM, Yang JC, Phan GQ, Kammula US, Hughes MS, Citrin DE, Restifo NP, Wunderlich JR, Prieto PA, Hong JJ, Langan RC, Zlott DA, Morton KE, White DE, Laurencot CM, Rosenberg SA. CD8+enriched "young" tumor infiltrating lymphocytes can mediate regression of metastatic melanoma. Clinical Cancer Research 2010;16(24) 6122-6131.

[32] Itzhaki O, Hovav E, Ziporen Y, Levy D, Kubi A, Zikich D, Hershkovitz L, Treves AJ, Shalmon B, Zippel D, Markel G, Shapira-Frommer R, Schachter J, Besser MJ. Establishment and large-scale expansion of minimally cultured "young" tumor infiltrating lymphocytes for adoptive transfer therapy. Journal of Immunology 2011;34(2) 212-220.

[33] Shen X, Zhou J, Hathcock KS, Robbins P, Powell DJ Jr, Rosenberg SA, Hodes RJ. Persistence of tumor infiltrating lymphocytes in adoptive immunotherapy correlates with telomere length. Journal of Immunology 2007;30(1) 123-129.

[34] Besser MJ, Shapira-Frommer R, Treves AJ, Zippel D, Itzhaki O, Schallmach E, Kubi A, Shalmon B, Hardan I, Catane R, Segal E, Markel G, Apter S, Nun AB, Kuchuk I, Shimoni A, Nagler A, Schachter J. Minimally cultured or selected autologous tumor-

infiltrating lymphocytes after a lympho-depleting chemotherapy regimen in metastatic melanoma patients. Journal of Immunotherapy 2009;32(4) 415-423.

[35] Rosenberg SA, Yang JC, Sherry RM, Kammula US, Hughes MS, Phan GQ, Citrin DE, Restifo NP, Robbins PF, Wunderlich JR, Morton KE, Laurencot CM, Steinberg SM, White DE, Dudley ME. Durable complete responses in heavily pretreated patients with metastatic melanoma using T-cell transfer immunotherapy. Clin Cancer Res 2011;17(13) 4550–4557.

[36] Radvanyi LG, Bernatchez C, Zhang M, Fox PS, Miller P, Chacon J, Wu R, Lizee G, Mahoney S, Alvarado G, Glass M, Johnson VE, McMannis JD, Shpall E, Prieto V, Papadopoulos N, Kim K, Homsi J, Bedikian A, Hwu WJ, Patel S, Ross MI, Lee JE, Gershenwald JE, Lucci A, Royal R, Cormier JN, Davies MA, Mansaray R, Fulbright OJ, Toth C, Ramachandran R, Wardell S, Gonzalez A, Hwu P. Specific lymphocyte subsets predict response to adoptive cell therapy using expanded autologous tumor-infiltrating lymphocytes in metastatic melanoma patients. Clin Cancer Res 2012;18 (24) 6758–6770.

[37] Itzhaki O, Hovav E, Ziporen Y, Levy D, Kubi A, Zikich D, Hershkovitz L, Treves AJ, Shalmon B, Zippel D, Markel G, Shapira-Frommer R, Schachter J, Besser MJ. Establishment and large-scale expansion of minimally cultured "young" tumor infiltrating lymphocytes for adoptive transfer therapy. J Immunother 2011;34(2) 212–220.

[38] Hong JJ, Rosenberg SA, Dudley ME, Yang JC, White DE, Butman JA, Sherry RM. Successful treatment of melanoma brain metastases with adoptive cell therapy. Clin Cancer Res 2006;16(19), 4892–4898.

[39] Yee C, Thompson JA, Byrd D, Riddell SR, Roche P, Celis E, Greenberg PD. Adoptive T cell therapy using antigen-specific CD8+T cell clones for the treatment of patients with metastatic melanoma: in vivo persistence, migration, and antitumor effect of transferred T cells. Proc Natl Acad Sci USA (2002);99(25) 16168–16173.

[40] Inozume T, Hanada K, Wang QJ, Ahmadzadeh M, Wunderlich JR, Rosenberg SA, Yang JC. (2010) Selection of CD8+PD-1+lymphocytes in fresh human melanomas enriches for tumor-reactive T cells. J Immunother(2010); 33(9) 956–964.

[41] Bedognetti D, Spivey TL, Zhao Y, Uccellini L, Tomei S, Dudley ME, Ascierto ML, De Giorgi V, Liu Q, Delogu LG, Sommariva M, Sertoli MR, Simon R, Wang E, Rosenberg SA, Marincola FM. CXCR3/CCR5 pathways in metastatic melanoma patients treated with adoptive therapy and interleukin-2. British Journal of Cancer 2013;109(9) 2412–2423.

[42] Vignard V, Lemercier B, Lim A, Pandolfino MC, Guilloux Y, Khammari A, Rabu C, Echasserieau K, Lang F, Gougeon ML, Dreno B, Jotereau F, Labarriere N. Adoptive transfer of tumor-reactive Melan-A-specific CTL clones in melanoma patients is followed by increased frequencies of additional Melan-A-specific T cells. Journal of Immunology 2005;175(7) 4797-4805.

[43] Kawakami Y, Eliyahu S, Jennings C, Sakaguchi K, Kang X, Southwood S, Robbins PF, Sette A, Appella E, Rosenberg SA. Recognition of multiple epitopes in the human melanoma antigen gp100 by tumor-infiltrating T lymphocytes associated with in vivo tumor regression. Journal of Immunology 1995;154(8) 3961-39618.

[44] Benlalam H, Vignard V, Khammari A, Bonnin A, Godet Y, Pandolfino MC, Jotereau F, Dreno B, Labarrière N. Infusion of Melan-A/Mart-1 specific tumor-infiltrating lymphocytes enhanced relapse-free survival of melanoma patients. Cancer Immunology Immunotherapy 2007;56(4) 515-526.

[45] Khammari A, Labarrière N, Vignard V, Nguyen JM, Pandolfino MC, Knol AC, Quéreux G, Saiagh S, Brocard A, Jotereau F, Dreno B. Treatment of metastatic melanoma with autologous Melan-A/MART-1-specific cytotoxic T lymphocyte clones. The Journal of Investigative Dermatology 2009;129(12) 2835-2842.

[46] Johnson LA, Heemskerk B, Powell DJ Jr, Cohen CJ, Morgan RA, Dudley ME, Robbins PF, Rosenberg SA. Gene transfer of tumor-reactive TCR confers both high avidity and tumor reactivity to nonreactive peripheral blood mononuclear cells and tumor-infiltrating lymphocytes. Journal of Immunology 2006;177(9) 6548-6559.

[47] Zhao Y, Zheng Z, Khong HT, Rosenberg SA, Morgan RA. Transduction of an HLA-DP4-restricted NY-ESO-1-specific TCR into primary human CD4+lymphocytes. Journal of Immunology 2006;29(4) 398-406.

[48] Frankel TL, Burns WR, Peng PD, Yu Z, Chinnasamy D, Wargo JA, Zheng Z, Restifo NP, Rosenberg SA, Morgan RA. Both CD4 and CD8 T cells mediate equally effective in vivo tumor treatment when engineered with a highly avid TCR targeting tyrosinase. Journal of Immunology 2010;184(11) 5988-5998.

[49] Johnson LA, Morgan RA, Dudley ME, Cassard L, Yang JC, Hughes MS, Kammula US, Royal RE, Sherry RM, Wunderlich JR, Lee CC, Restifo NP, Schwarz SL, Cogdill AP, Bishop RJ, Kim H, Brewer CC, Rudy SF, VanWaes C, Davis JL, Mathur A, Ripley RT, Nathan DA, Laurencot CM, Rosenberg SA. Gene therapy with human and mouse T-cell receptors mediates cancer regression and targets normal tissues expressing cognate antigen. Blood 2009;114(3) 535-546.

[50] Schaft N, Willemsen RA, de Vries J, Lankiewicz B, Essers BW, Gratama JW, Figdor CG, Bolhuis RL, Debets R, Adema GJ. Peptide fine specificity of anti-glycoprotein 100 CTL is preserved following transfer of engineered TCR alpha beta genes into primary human T lymphocytes. Journal of Immunology 2003;170(4) 2186-2194.

[51] Morgan RA, Dudley ME, Yu YY, Zheng Z, Robbins PF, Theoret MR, Wunderlich JR, Hughes MS, Restifo NP, Rosenberg SA. High efficiency TCR gene transfer into primary human lymphocytes affords avid recognition of melanoma tumor antigen glycoprotein 100 and does not alter the recognition of autologous melanoma antigens. Journal of Immunology 2003;171(6) 3287-3295.

[52] Robbins PF, Morgan RA, Feldman SA, Yang JC, Sherry RM, Dudley ME, Wunderlich JR, Nahvi AV, Helman LJ, Mackall CL, Kammula US, Hughes MS, Restifo NP, Raf-

feld M, Lee CC, Levy CL, Li YF, El-Gamil M, Schwarz SL, Laurencot C, Rosenberg SA. Tumor regression in patients with metastatic synovial cell sarcoma and melanoma using genetically engineered lymphocytes reactive with NY-ESO-1. Journal of Clinical Oncology 2011;29(7) 917-924.

[53] Zhang G, Wang L, Cui H, Wang X, Zhang G, Ma J, Han H, He W, Wang W, Zhao Y, Liu C, Sun M, Gao B. Anti-melanoma activity of T cells redirected with a TCR-like chimeric antigen receptor. Sci Rep. 2014;4 3571.

[54] Hughes MS, Yu YY, Dudley ME, Zheng Z, Robbins PF, Li Y, Wunderlich J, Hawley RG, Moayeri M, Rosenberg SA, Morgan RA. Transfer of a TCR gene derived from a patient with a marked antitumor response conveys highly active T-cell effector functions. Human Gene Therapy 2005;16(4) 457-472.

[55] Willemsen R, Ronteltap C, Heuveling M, Debets R, Bolhuis R. Redirecting human CD4+T lymphocytes to the MHC class I-restricted melanoma antigen MAGE-A1 by TCR alphabeta gene transfer requires CD8alpha. Gene Therapy 2005; 12(2) 140-146.

[56] Morgan RA, Dudley ME, Wunderlich JR, Hughes MS, Yang JC, Sherry RM, Royal RE, Topalian SL, Kammula US, Restifo NP, Zheng Z, Nahvi A, de Vries CR, Rogers-Freezer LJ, Mavroukakis SA, Rosenberg SA. Cancer Regression in Patients After Transfer of Genetically Engineered Lymphocytes. Science. 2006;314(5796) 126-129.

[57] Morgan RA, Chinnasamy N, Abate-Daga D, Gros A, Robbins PF, Zheng Z, Dudley ME, Feldman SA, Yang JC, Sherry RM, Phan GQ, Hughes MS, Kammula US, Miller AD, Hessman CJ, Stewart AA, Restifo NP, Quezado MM, Alimchandani M, Rosenberg AZ, Nath A, Wang T, Bielekova B, Wuest SC, Akula N, McMahon FJ, Wilde S, Mosetter B, Schendel DJ, Laurencot CM, Rosenberg SA. Cancer regression and neurological toxicity following anti-MAGE-A3 TCR gene therapy. J Immunother 2013;36(2) 133-151.

[58] Coccoris M, Swart E, de Witte MA, van Heijst JW, Haanen JB, Schepers K, Schumacher TN. Long-term functionality of TCR-transduced T cells in vivo. Journal of Immunology 2008; 180(10) 6536-6543.

[59] Rosenberg SA, Yannelli JR, Yang JC, Topalian SL, Schwartzentruber DJ, Weber JS, Parkinson DR, Seipp CA, Einhorn JH, White DE. Treatment of patients with metastatic melanoma with autologous tumor-infiltrating lymphocytes and interleukin 2. Journal of the National Cancer Institute 1994;86(15) 1159–1166.

[60] Seliger B. Molecular mechanisms of MHC class I abnormalities and APM components in human tumors. Cancer Immunology Immunotherapy 2008;57(11) 1719-1726.

[61] Sigalotti L, Fratta E, Coral S, Tanzarella S, Danielli R, Colizzi F, Fonsatti E, Traversari C, Altomonte M, Maio M. Intratumor heterogeneity of cancer/testis antigens expression in human cutaneous melanoma is methylation-regulated and functionally reverted by 5-aza-2'-deoxycytidine. Cancer Research 2004;64(24) 9167-9171.

[62] Vitale M, Pelusi G, Taroni B, Gobbi G, Micheloni C, Rezzani R, Donato F, Wang X, Ferrone S. HLA class I antigen down-regulation in primary ovary carcinoma lesions: association with disease stage. Clinical Cancer Research 2005;11(1) 67-72.

[63] Coccoris M, Straetemans T, Govers C, Lamers C, Sleijfer S, Debets R. T cell receptor (TCR) gene therapy to treat melanoma: lessons from clinical and preclinical studies. Expert Opinion on Biological Therapy 2010;10(4) 547-562.

[64] Bendle GM, Linnemann C, Hooijkaas AI, Bies L, de Witte MA, Jorritsma A, Kaiser AD, Pouw N, Debets R, Kieback E, Uckert W, Song JY, Haanen JB, Schumacher TN. Lethal graft-versus-host disease in mouse models of T cell receptor gene therapy. Nature Medicine 2010; 16(5) 565-570.

[65] Cohen CJ, Zhao Y, Zheng Z, Rosenberg SA, Morgan RA. Enhanced antitumor activity of murine-human hybrid T-cell receptor (TCR) in human lymphocytes is associated with improved pairing and TCR/CD3 stability. Cancer Research 2006;66(17) 8878-8886.

[66] Kuball J, Dossett ML, Wolfl M, Ho WY, Voss RH, Fowler C, Greenberg PD. Facilitating matched pairing and expression of TCR chains introduced into human T cells. Blood 2007;109(6) 2331-2338.

[67] Eshhar Z, Waks T, Gross G, Schindler DG. Specific activation and targeting of cytotoxic lymphocytes through chimeric single chains consisting of antibody-binding domains and the gamma or zeta subunits of the immunoglobulin and T-cell receptors. Proceedings of the National Academy of Sciences of the United States of America 1993;90(2) 720-724.

[68] Cheadle EJ, Sheard V, Hombach, AA, Chmielewski M, Riet T, Berrevoets C, Schooten E, Lamers C, Abken H, Debets R, Gilham DE. Chimeric antigen receptors for T-cell based therapy. Methods Mol Biol 2012;907 645-666.

[69] Hombach A, Heuser C, Sircar R, Tillmann T, Diehl V, Kruis W, Pohl C, Abken H. T cell targeting of TAG72+tumor cells by a chimeric receptor with antibody-like specificity for a carbohydrate epitope. Gastroenterol 1997;113(4), 1163 – 1170.

[70] Hombach A, Abken H. Costimulation tunes tumor-specific activation of redirected T cells in adoptive immunotherapy," Cancer Immunology Immunotherapy 2007;56(5)731-737.

[71] ClinicalTrials.gov A service of the U.S. National Institutes of Health. Trial ID: NCT00586391 http://clinicaltrials.gov/ct2/results?term=NCT+00586391

[72] ClinicalTrials.gov A service of the U.S. National Institutes of Health. Trial ID: NCT00709033 http://clinicaltrials.gov/ct2/results?term=NCT+00709033

[73] Hombach AA, Abken H. Costimulation by chimeric antigen receptors revisited the T cell antitumor response benefits from combined CD28-OX40 signalling. International Journal of Cancer 2011;129(12) 2935-2944.

[74] Hombach AA, Chmielewski M, Rappl G, Abken H. Adoptive immunotherapy with redirected T cells produces CCR7-cells that are trapped in the periphery and benefit from combined CD28-OX40 costimulation. Hum Gene Ther 2013;24(3) 259-269.

[75] Bridgeman JS, Hawkins RE, Hombach AA, Abken H, Gilham DE.Building better chimeric antigen receptors for adoptive T cell therapy. Current Gene Therapy 2010; 10(2) 77-90.

[76] Gilham DE, Debets R, Pule M, Hawkins RE, Abken H. CAR-T cells and solid tumors: tuning T cells to challenge an inveterate foe. Trends in Molecular Medicine 2012;18(7) 377-384.

[77] Reinhold U, Liu L, Lüdtke-Handjery HC, Heuser C, Hombach A, Wang X, Tilgen W, Ferrone S, Abken H. Specific lysis of melanoma cells by receptor grafted T cells is enhanced by anti-idiotypic monoclonal antibodies directed to the scFv domain of the receptor. The Journal of Investigative Dermatology 1999;112(5) 744-750.

[78] Burns WR, Zhao Y, Frankel TL, Hinrichs CS, Zheng Z, Xu H, Feldman SA, Ferrone S, Rosenberg SA, Morgan RA. A high molecular weight melanoma-associated antigen-specific chimeric antigen receptor redirects lymphocytes to target human melanomas. Cancer Research 2010;70(8) 3027-3033.

[79] Schmidt P, Kopecky C, Hombach A, Zigrino P, Mauch C, Abken H. Eradication of melanomas by targeted elimination of a minor subset of tumor cells. Proceedings of the National Academy of Sciences of the United States of America 2011;108(6) 2474-2479.

[80] Yvon E, Del Vecchio M, Savoldo B, Hoyos V, Dutour A, Anichini A, Dotti G, Brenner MK. Immunotherapy of metastatic melanoma using genetically engineered GD2-specific T cells. Clinical Cancer Research 2009;15(18) 5852-5860.

[81] Lo AS, Ma Q, Liu DL, Junghans RP. Anti-GD3 chimeric sFv-CD28/T-cell receptor zeta designer T cells for treatment of metastatic melanoma and other neuroectodermal tumors. Clinical Cancer Research 2010;16(10) 2769-2780.

[82] Kalos M, Levine BL, Porter DL, Katz S, Grupp SA, Bagg A, June CH. T cells with chimeric antigen receptors have potent antitumor effects and can establish memory in patients with advanced leukemia. Science Translational Medicine 2011;3(95) 95ra73.

[83] Porter DL, Levine BL, Kalos M, Bagg A, June CH. Chimeric antigen receptor-modified T cells in chronic lymphoid leukemia. The New England Journal of Medicine 2011;365(8) 725-733.

[84] Lamers CH, Sleijfer S, Vulto AG, Kruit WH, Kliffen M, Debets R, Gratama JW, Stoter G, Oosterwijk E. Treatment of metastatic renal cell carcinoma with autologous T-lymphocytes genetically retargeted against carbonic anhydrase IX: first clinical experience. Journal of Clinical Oncology 2006; 24(3) 20-22.

[85] Brentjens R, Yeh R, Bernal Y, Riviere I, Sadelain M. Treatment of chronic lymphocytic leukemia with genetically targeted autologous T cells: case report of an unforeseen adverse event in a phase I clinical trial. Molecular Therapy 2010;18(4) 666-668.

[86] Morgan RA, Yang JC, Kitano M, Dudley ME, Laurencot CM, Rosenberg SA. Case report of a serious adverse event following the administration of T cells transduced with a chimeric antigen receptor recognizing ERBB2. Molecular Therapy 2010;8(4) 843-851.

[87] Hawkins RE, Gilham DE, Debets R, Eshhar Z, Taylor N, Abken H, Schumacher TN, ATTACK Consortium. Development of adoptive cell therapy for cancer: a clinical perspective. Human Gene Therapy 2010;21(6) 665-672.

[88] Büning H, Uckert W, Cichutek K, Hawkins RE, Abken H. Do CARs need a driver's license? Adoptive cell therapy with chimeric antigen receptor-redirected T cells has caused serious adverse events. Human Gene Therapy 2010;21(9) 1039-1042.

[89] Zhou BB, Zhang H, Damelin M, Geles KG, Grindley JC, Dirks PB. Tumour-initiating cells: challenges and opportunities for anticancer drug discovery. Nature Reviews Drug Discovery 2009;8(10) 806-823.

[90] Al-Hajj M, Wicha MS, Benito-Hernandez A, Morrison SJ, Clarke MF. Prospective identification of tumorigenic breast cancer cells. Proceedings of the National Academy of Sciences of the United States of America 2003;100(7) 3983-3988.

[91] Dalerba P, Dylla SJ, Park IK, Liu R, Wang X, Cho RW, Hoey T, Gurney A, Huang EH, Simeone DM, Shelton AA, Parmiani G, Castelli C, Clarke MF. Phenotypic characterization of human colorectal cancer stem cells. Proceedings of the National Academy of Sciences of the United States of America 2007;104(24) 10158-10163.

[92] Singh SK, Clarke ID, Terasaki M, Bonn VE, Hawkins C, Squire J, Dirks PB. Identification of a cancer stem cell in human brain tumors. Cancer Research 2003;63(18) 5821-5828.

[93] Ricci-Vitiani L, Lombardi DG, Pilozzi E, Biffoni M, Todaro M, Peschle C, De Maria R. Identification and expansion of human colon-cancer-initiating cells. Nature 2007;445(7123) 111-115.

[94] Li C, Heidt DG, Dalerba P, Burant CF, Zhang L, Adsay V, Wicha M, Clarke MF, Simeone DM. Identification of pancreatic cancer stem cells. Cancer Research 2007;67(3) 1030-1037.

[95] Schatton T, Murphy GF, Frank NY, Yamaura K, Waaga-Gasser AM, Gasser M, Zhan Q, Jordan S, Duncan LM, Weishaupt C, Fuhlbrigge RC, Kupper TS, Sayegh MH, Frank MH. Identification of cells initiating human melanomas. Nature. 2008;451(7176) 345-349.

[96] Zabierowski SE, Herlyn M. Melanoma stem cells: the dark seed of melanoma. Journal of Clinical Oncology 2008;26(17) 2890-2894.

[97] Fang D, Nguyen TK, Leishear K, Finko R, Kulp AN, Hotz S, Van Belle PA, Xu X, Elder DE, Herlyn M. A tumorigenic subpopulation with stem cell properties in melanomas. Cancer Research 2005;65(20) 9328-9337.

[98] Boiko AD, Razorenova OV, van de Rijn M, Swetter SM, Johnson DL, Ly DP, Butler PD, Yang GP, Joshua B, Kaplan MJ, Longaker MT, Weissman IL. Human melanoma-initiating cells express neural crest nerve growth factor receptor CD271. Nature 2010;466(7302) 133-137.

[99] Quintana E, Shackleton M, Sabel MS, Fullen DR, Johnson TM, Morrison SJ. Efficient tumour formation by single human melanoma cells. Nature 2008;456(7222) 593-598.

[100] Quintana E, Shackleton M, Foster HR, Fullen DR, Sabel MS, Johnson TM, Morrison SJ. Phenotypic Heterogeneity among Tumorigenic Melanoma Cells from Patients that Is Reversible and Not Hierarchically Organized. Cancer Cell 2010;18(5) 510-523.

[101] Shakhova O, Zingg D, Schaefer SM, Hari L, Civenni G, Blunschi J, Claudinot S, Okoniewski M, Beermann F, Mihic-Probst D, Moch H, Wegner M, Dummer R, Barrandon Y, Cinelli P, Sommer L. Sox10 promotes the formation and maintenance of giant congenital naevi and melanoma. Nat Cell Biol 2012;14(8) 882-890.

[102] Schlaak M, Schmidt P, Bangard C, Kurschat P, Mauch C, Abken H. Regression of metastatic melanoma in a patient by antibody targeting of cancer stem cells. Oncotarget 2012;3(1) 22-30.

[103] Pinc A, Somasundaram R, Wagner C, Hörmann M, Karanikas G, Jalili A, Bauer W, Brunner P, Grabmeier-Pfistershammer K, Gschaider M, Lai CY, Hsu MY, Herlyn M, Stingl G, Wagner SN. Targeting CD20 in melanoma patients at high risk of disease recurrence. Mol Ther 2012;20(5) 1056-1062.

[104] Chmielewski M, Rappl G, Hombach AA, Abken H. T cells redirected by a CD3ζ chimeric antigen receptor can establish self-antigen-specific tumour protection in the long term. Gene Ther. 2013;20(2) 177-186.

[105] Kershaw MH, Westwood JA, Parker LL, Wang G, Eshhar Z, Mavroukakis SA, White DE, Wunderlich JR, Canevari S, Rogers-Freezer L, Chen CC, Yang JC, Rosenberg SA, Hwu P.A phase I study on adoptive immunotherapy using gene-modified T cells for ovarian cancer. Clin Cancer Res 2006;12(20.1) 6106-6115.

[106] Brentjens RJ, Davila ML, Riviere I, Park J, Wang X, Cowell LG, Bartido S, Stefanski J, Taylor C, Olszewska M, Borquez-Ojeda O, Qu J, Wasielewska T, He Q, Bernal Y, Rijo IV, Hedvat C, Kobos R, Curran K, Steinherz P, Jurcic J, Rosenblat T, Maslak P, Frattini M, Sadelain M. CD19-targeted T cells rapidly induce molecular remissions in adults with chemotherapy-refractory acute lymphoblastic leukemia. Sci Transl Med. 2013;5(177) 177ra38.

[107] Kaneko S, Mastaglio S, Bondanza A, Ponzoni M, Sanvito F, Aldrighetti L, Radrizzani M, La Seta-Catamancio S, Provasi E, Mondino A, Nagasawa T, Fleischhauer K, Russo V, Traversari C, Ciceri F, Bordignon C, Bonini C. IL-7 and IL-15 allow the generation

of suicide gene-modified alloreactive self-renewing central memory human T lymphocytes. Blood 2009; 113(5) 1006-1015.

[108] Suhoski MM, Golovina TN, Aqui NA, Tai VC, Varela-Rohena A, Milone MC, Carroll RG, Riley JL, June CH. Engineering artificial antigen-presenting cells to express a diverse array of co-stimulatory molecules. Mol Ther 2007;15(5) 981-988.

[109] Vera JF, Brenner LJ, Gerdemann U, Ngo MC, Sili U, Liu H, Wilson J, Dotti G, Heslop HE, Leen AM, Rooney CM. Accelerated production of antigen-specific T cells for preclinical and clinical applications using gas-permeable rapid expansion cultureware (G-Rex). J Immunother 2010;33(3) 305-315.

[110] Meidenbauer N, Marienhagen J, Laumer M, Vogl S, Heymann J, Andreesen R, Mackensen A. Survival and tumor localization of adoptively transferred Melan-A-specific T cells in melanoma patients. Journal of Immunology 2003;170(4) 2161-2169.

[111] Griffith KD, Read EJ, Carrasquillo JA, Carter CS, Yang JC, Fisher B, Aebersold P, Packard BS, Yu MY, Rosenberg SA. In vivo distribution of adoptively transferred indium-111-labeled tumor infiltrating lymphocytes and peripheral blood lymphocytes in patients with metastatic melanoma. Journal of the National Cancer Institute 1989;81(22) 1709-1717.

[112] Fisher B, Packard BS, Read EJ, Carrasquillo JA, Carter CS, Topalian SL, Yang JC, Yolles P, Larson SM, Rosenberg SA. Tumor localization of adoptively transferred indium-111 labeled tumor infiltrating lymphocytes in patients with metastatic melanoma. Journal of Clinical Oncology 1989;7(2) 250-261.

[113] Peng W, Ye Y, Rabinovich BA, Liu C, Lou Y, Zhang M, Whittington M, Yang Y, Overwijk WW, Lizée G, Hwu P. Transduction of tumor-specific T cells with CXCR2 chemokine receptor improves migration to tumor and antitumor immune responses. Clinical Cancer Research 2010;16(22) 5458-5468.

[114] Li Y, Liu S, Hernandez J, Vence L, Hwu P, Radvanyi L.MART-1-specific melanoma tumor-infiltrating lymphocytes maintaining CD28 expression have improved survival and expansion capability following antigenic restimulation in vitro. Journal of Immunology 2010;184(1) 452-465.

[115] Hernandez-Chacon JA, Li Y, Wu RC, Bernatchez C, Wang Y, Weber JS, Hwu P, Radvanyi LG. Costimulation through the CD137/4-1BB pathway protects human melanoma tumor-infiltrating lymphocytes from activation-induced cell death and enhances antitumor effector function. Journal of Immunology 2011;34(3) 236-250.

[116] Offringa R. Antigen choice in adoptive T-cell therapy of cancer. Current Opinion in Immunology 2009;21(2) 190-199.

[117] Overwijk WW, Theoret MR, Finkelstein SE, Surman DR, de Jong LA, Vyth-Dreese FA, Dellemijn TA, Antony PA, Spiess PJ, Palmer DC, Heimann DM, Klebanoff CA, Yu Z, Hwang LN, Feigenbaum L, Kruisbeek AM, Rosenberg SA, Restifo NP. Tumor

regression and autoimmunity after reversal of a functionally tolerant state of self-reactive CD8+T cells. The Journal of Experimental Medicine 2003;198(4) 569-580.

[118] Spiotto MT, Rowley DA, and Schreiber H. "Bystander" elimination of antigen loss variants in established tumors. Nature Medicine 2004; 10(3) 294-298.

[119] Schüler T, Blankenstein T. Cutting edge: CD8+effector T cells reject tumors by direct antigen recognition but indirect action on host cells. Journal of Immunology 2003;170(9) 4427-4431.

[120] Stewart-Jones G, Wadle A, Hombach A, Shenderov E, Held G, Fischer E, Kleber S, Nuber N, Stenner-Liewen F, Bauer S, McMichael A, Knuth A, Abken H, Hombach AA, Cerundolo V, Jones EY, Renner C. Rational development of high-affinity T-cell receptor-like antibodies. Proceedings of the National Academy of Sciences of the United States of America 2009;106(14) 5784-5788.

[121] Willemsen RA, Debets R, Hart E, Hoogenboom HR, Bolhuis RL, Chames P. A phage display selected fab fragment with MHC class I-restricted specificity for MAGE-A1 allows for retargeting of primary human T lymphocytes. Gene Therapy 2001;8(21) 1601-1608.

[122] Chmielewski M, Hombach A, Heuser C, Adams GP, Abken H.T cell activation by antibody-like immunoreceptors: increase in affinity of the single-chain fragment domain above threshold does not increase T cell activation against antigen-positive target cells but decreases selectivity. Journal of Immunology 2004; 173(12) 7647-7653.

[123] Chmielewski M, Hombach AA, Abken H. CD28 cosignalling does not affect the activation threshold in a chimeric antigen receptor-redirected T-cell attack. Gene Therapy 2011;18(1) 62-72.

[124] Pule MA, Savoldo B, Myers GD, Rossig C, Russell HV, Dotti G, Huls MH, Liu E, Gee AP, Mei Z, Yvon E, Weiss HL, Liu H, Rooney CM, Heslop HE, Brenner MK. Virus-specific T cells engineered to coexpress tumor-specific receptors: persistence and antitumor activity in individuals with neuroblastoma Nature Medicine 2008;14(11) 1264-1270.

[125] Antony PA, Piccirillo CA, Akpinarli A, Finkelstein SE, Speiss PJ, Surman DR, Palmer DC, Chan CC, Klebanoff CA, Overwijk WW, Rosenberg SA, Restifo NP. CD8+T cell immunity against a tumor/self-antigen is augmented by CD4+T helper cells and hindered by naturally occurring T regulatory cells. Journal of Immunology 2005;174(5) 2591-2601.

[126] Kofler DM, Chmielewski M, Rappl G, Hombach A, Riet T, Schmidt A, Hombach AA, Wendtner CM, Abken H. CD28 costimulation Impairs the efficacy of a redirected t-cell antitumor attack in the presence of regulatory t cells which can be overcome by preventing Lck activation. Mol Ther 2011;19(4) 760-767.

[127] [127]Leach DR, Krummel MF, Allison JP. Enhancement of antitumor immunity by CTLA-4 blockade. Science 1996;271(5256) 1734-1736.

[128] [128]Pedicord VA, Montalvo W, Leiner IM, Allison JP. Single dose of anti-CTLA-4 enhances CD8+T-cell memory formation, function, and maintenance. Proc Natl Acad Sci USA 2011;108(1) 266-271.

[129] Abate-Daga D, Hanada K, Davis JL, Yang JC, Rosenberg SA, Morgan RA. Expression profiling of TCR-engineered T cells demonstrates overexpression of multiple inhibitory receptors in persisting lymphocytes. Blood 2013;122(8) 1399-1410.

[130] Moon EK, Wang LC, Dolfi DV, Wilson CB, Ranganathan R, Sun J, Kapoor V, Scholler J, Puré E, Milone MC, June CH, Riley JL, Wherry EJ, Albelda SM. Multifactorial T-cell Hypofunction That Is Reversible Can Limit the Efficacy of Chimeric Antigen Receptor-Transduced Human T cells in Solid Tumors. Clin Cancer Res 2014;20(16) 4262-4273.

[131] Mackensen A, Meidenbauer N, Vogl S, Laumer M, Berger J, Andreesen R. Phase I study of adoptive T-cell therapy using antigen-specific CD8+T cells for the treatment of patients with metastatic melanoma. Journal of Clinical Oncology 2006;24(31) 5060-5069.

[132] Lozupone F, Rivoltini L, Luciani F, Venditti M, Lugini L, Cova A, Squarcina P, Parmiani G, Belardelli F, Fais S. Adoptive transfer of an anti-MART-1(27-35)-specific CD8+T cell clone leads to immunoselection of human melanoma antigen-loss variants in SCID mice. European Journal of Immunology 2003;33(2) 556-566.

[133] Becker JC, Varki N, Gillies SD, Furukawa K, Reisfeld RA. An antibody-interleukin 2 fusion protein overcomes tumor heterogeneity by induction of a cellular immune response," Proceedings of the National Academy of Sciences of the United States of America 1996;93(15) 7826-7831.

[134] Chmielewski M, Kopecky C, Hombach AA, Abken H. IL-12 release by engineered T cells expressing chimeric antigen receptors can effectively Muster an antigen-independent macrophage response on tumor cells that have shut down tumor antigen expression. Cancer Research 2011;71(17) 5697-5706.

[135] Boni A, Cogdill AP, Dang P, Udayakumar D, Njauw CN, Sloss CM, Ferrone CR, Flaherty KT, Lawrence DP, Fisher DE, Tsao H, Wargo JA. Selective BRAFV600E inhibition enhances T-cell recognition of melanoma without affecting lymphocyte function. Cancer Research 2010;70(13) 5213-5219.

[136] Wilmott JS, Long GV, Howle JR, Haydu LE, Sharma RN, Thompson JF, Kefford RF, Hersey P, Scolyer RA. Selective BRAF inhibitors induce marked T-cell infiltration into human metastatic melanoma. Clinical Cancer Research 2012;18(5) 1386-1394.

[137] Pegram HJ, Jackson JT, Smyth MJ, Kershaw MH, Darcy PK. Adoptive transfer of gene-modified primary NK cells can specifically inhibit tumor progression in vivo. Journal of Immunology 2008;181(5) 3449-3455.

[138] Kruschinski A, Moosmann A, Poschke I, Norell H, Chmielewski M, Seliger B, Kiessling R, Blankenstein T, Abken H, Charo J. Engineering antigen-specific primary human NK cells against HER-2 positive carcinomas," Proceedings of the National Academy of Sciences of the United States of America 2008;105(45) 17481-17486.

[139] Boissel L, Betancur-Boissel M, Lu W, Krause DS, Van Etten RA, Wels WS, Klingemann H. Retargeting NK-92 cells by means of CD19-and CD20-specific chimeric antigen receptors compares favorably with antibody-dependent cellular cytotoxicity. Oncoimmunology 2013;2(10) e26527.

[140] Jiang H, Zhang W, Shang P, Zhang H, Fu W, Ye F, Zeng T, Huang H, Zhang X, Sun W, Man-Yuen Sze D, Yi Q, Hou J. Transfection of chimeric anti-CD138 gene enhances natural killer cell activation and killing of multiple myeloma cells. Mol Oncol 2014;8(2) 297-310.

[141] Boissel L, Betancur M, Wels WS, Tuncer H, Klingemann H. Transfection with mRNA for CD19 specific chimeric antigen receptor restores NK cell mediated killing of CLL cells. Leuk Res 2009; 33(9), 1255-1259.

[142] Klingemann HG. Cellular therapy of cancer with natural killer cells-where do we stand? Cytotherapy 2013;15(10) 1185-1194.

[143] Müller T, Uherek C, Maki G, Chow KU, Schimpf A, Klingemann HG, Tonn T, Wels WS. Expression of a CD20-specific chimeric antigen receptor enhances cytotoxic activity of NK cells and overcomes NK-resistance of lymphoma and leukemia cells. Cancer Immunol Immunother 2008;57(3) 411-423.

[144] Chu J, Deng Y, Benson DM, He S, Hughes T, Zhang J, Peng Y, Mao H, Yi L, Ghoshal K, He X, Devine SM, Zhang X, Caligiuri MA, Hofmeister CC, Yu J. CS1-specific chimeric antigen receptor (CAR)-engineered natural killer cells enhance In Vitro and In Vivo anti-tumor activity against human multiple myeloma. Leukemia 2014;28(4) 917-927.

[145] Uherek C, Tonn T, Uherek B, Becker S, Schnierle B, Klingemann HG, Wels W. Retargeting of natural killer-cell cytolytic activity to ErbB2-expressing cancer cells results in efficient and selective tumor cell destruction. Blood 2002;100(4) 1265-1273.

[146] Tavri S, Jha P, Meier R, Henning TD, Müller T, Hostetter D, Knopp C, Johansson M, Reinhart V, Boddington S, Sista A, Wels WS, Daldrup-Link HE. Optical imaging of cellular immunotherapy against prostate cancer. Mol Imaging2009;8(1) 15-26.

[147] Esser R, Müller T, Stefes D, Kloess S, Seidel D, Gillies SD, Aperlo-Iffland C, Huston JS, Uherek C, Schönfeld K, Tonn T, Huebener N, Lode HN, Koehl U, Wels WS. NK cells engineered to express a GD2-specific antigen receptor display built-in ADCC-

like activity against tumour cells of neuroectodermal origin. J Cell Mol Med 2012;16(3) 569-581.

[148] Imai C, Iwamoto S, Campana D. Genetic modification of primary natural killer cells overcomes inhibitory signals and induces specific killing of leukemic cells. Blood 2005;106(1) 376-383.

[149] Altvater B, Landmeier S, Pscherer S, Temme J, Schweer K, Kailayangiri S, Campana D, Juergens H, Pule M, Rossig C. 2B4 (CD244) signaling by recombinant antigen-specific chimeric receptors costimulates natural killer cell activation to leukemia and neuroblastoma cells. Clin Cancer Res2009;15(15) 4857-4866.

[150] Sahm C, Schönfeld K, Wels WS. Expression of IL-15 in NK cells results in rapid enrichment and selective cytotoxicity of gene-modified effectors that carry a tumor-specific antigen receptor. Cancer Immunol Immunother 2012;61(9) 1451-1461.

Chapter 11

Toxicities of New Drugs for Melanoma Treatment and their Management

Paola Savoia and Paolo Fava

Additional information is available at the end of the chapter

http://dx.doi.org/10.5772/59860

1. Introduction

Advanced melanoma is a highly aggressive tumor with a low response rate to the majority of pharmacological agents.

Among conventional cytotoxic chemotherapies, dacarbazine (DTIC) is the only FDA-approved alkylating agent, at present; its clinical efficacy is pretty low with 5–10% responsiveness, which is generally short-lived. Carmustine, temozolomide and other chemotherapic agents (taxanes and platinum-analogs) showed similar efficacy in metastatic settings [1, 2].

Adjuvant immunotherapy for stage III melanoma is mainly based on interferon-α2b (IFN-α2b) even if its efficacy is quite limited. In fact, only about the 20% of patients showed an improvement in relapse-free survival as demonstrated in randomized observation-controlled trials without a clear effect on overall survival [3]. FDA approved high-dose interleukin-2 (IL-2) for the treatment of advanced stage melanoma, on the basis of its ability to elicit durable responses in a small percentage of patients [4, 5]. However, the durable response rate is only 10-20% and toxicities associated with IL-2 are quite severe.

Recently, molecular targeted therapies have radically changed the management of metastatic melanoma. Anti-CTLA-4 monoclonal antibodies (Ipilimumab) and B-Raf inhibitors are the first examples of this new kind of drugs, the firsts approved with both overall survival and progression-free survival benefits in respect of the standard chemotherapic agent dacarbazine [6-10].

Ipilimumab targets the anti-cytotoxic T-lymphocyte antigen-4, a key immune-checkpoint molecule that down-regulates some pathways of T-cell activation. Ipilimumab inactivating the CTLA-4 inhibitory signal, enhance the immune system response against melanoma cells. Several randomized phases II and III trials demonstrated a statistically significant improvement in overall survival in patients with metastatic melanoma treated with Ipilimumab alone or in combination with dacarbazine. The efficacy of Ipilimumab was confirmed both in treated and untreated metastatic melanoma patients [6, 9, 11]. Furthermore, re-treatment with Ipilimumab can re-establish disease control in a percentage of patients who progress after achieving an objective response or stable disease after the first treatment course [6, 9, 11-13].

As a consequence of this peculiar mechanism of action, Ipilimumab may determine the development of autoimmune conditions and exacerbate a series of immune-related adverse events, which will be described in the next section of this review.

Vemurafenib is a low molecular weight molecule (489.9 Da), orally available, which belongs to the new generation inhibitors of B-Raf as well as of other members of the RAF kinase family (including the products of ARAF, BRAF and CRAF genes). The BRAF protein is a part of the RAS/RAF/MEK/ERK signaling pathway, which is a key regulator of melanoma cell growth. In cells expressing the pro-oncogenic BRAF-V600E, BRAF-V600D and BRAF-V600R genes, Vemurafenib inhibits both phosphorylated ERK (pERK) and pMEK in a dose-dependent manner, resulting in a reduction of tumour growth and even in tumour regression in in vitro studies and xenograft transplant models. Several clinical trials have confirmed and extended these preclinical observations and, to date, RAF inhibitors represent the emerging standard of care for metastatic melanoma harboring the BRAF-V600E mutation, with clinical responsiveness in more than 90% of these patients [1, 14]. In particular, results from a phase III clinical trial of patiente expressing the BRAF-V600E mutated isoform affected by unresectable or metastatic melanoma showed a median overall survival significantly higher for Vemurafenib-treated patients,in comparison to those treated with dacarbazine (13.2 vs 9.9 months, respectively).

Even if the toxicity of this treatment is normally considered to be acceptable, Vemurafenib triggers the onset of a wide spectrum of systemic and cutaneous toxicities which can impact patient's quality of life in a significant way [15-17]. The adverse effects, which will be detailed later, are dose-dependent and related to the alteration of the cell-signaling pathway in response to B-Raf inhibition in cells expressing the wild-type BRAF gene [18].

2. Ipilimumab toxicities

The onset of immune-related adverse events (irAEs) during the treatment with Ipilimumab is consequent to action on the immune system. Actually, CTLA-4 blockage removes CTLA4-mediated downregulation of the immune response, leading thus to a large spectrum of autoimmune–inflammatory side effects with a dose-dependent mechanism [19]. These irAEs are described both at the currently approved 3mg/kg dose and at the investigational 10mg/kg dose and may affect a number of organs and systems, including the eye, the skin, the gut and the endocrine system.

In a retrospective analysis of phase I–III Ipilimumab trials on patients with advanced melanomas, the occurrence of irAEs of any grade was a quite common phenomenon, regarding about 60% of the patients [20]. Nevertheless, Ipilimumab can be considered a safe drug: irAEs-related deaths occurred only in about 1% of treated patients [20]. In these trials, the most common immune side effects were represented by enterocolitis, dermatitis, hepatitis, hypo-

http://dx.doi.org/10.5772/59860

physitis, and uveitis, usually with an early onset. More recent data obtained on an Italian multicentric expanded-access cohort reported an occurrence of irAEs of any grade in 33% of treated patients, with a median time of onset of 5 weeks. Most irAEs were low grade, whereas grade 3/4 irAEs were described in 6% of the cases and were most commonly represented by diarrhea, liver toxicity and fatigue/asthenia [21].

IrAE	Grade 1	Grade 2	Grade 3	Grade 4
Skin Toxicity	Mild to moderate localized rash or pruritus; papules/pustules covering <10%–30% of the body surface	Non localized rash (diffuse, ≥50% of skin surface)	Intense and widespread (>30% of body surface) skin rash; skin sloughing of <10%–30% of the body surface; epidermal or mucus membrane detachment	Stevens–Johnson syndrome, toxic epidermal necrolysis, or rash complicated by full-thickness dermal ulceration, or necrotic, bullous, or hemorrhagic manifestations
Diarrhea	Increase of <4 stools per day over baseline; mild increase in ostomy output compared with baseline	Increase of 4–6 stools per day over baseline; Intra venous fluids indicated <24 hours; moderate increase in ostomy output compared to baseline; not interfering with activities of daily living	Increase of ≥7 stools per day over baseline; incontinence; Intra venous fluids >24hours; hospitalization; severe increase in ostomy output compared with baseline; interfering with activities of daily living	Life-threatening diarrhea, causing severe hemodynamic alterations and even collapse
Liver toxicity	Asymptomatic or mild symptoms; clinical or diagnostic observations only; intervention not indicated	AST or ALT >2.5 to ≤5.0 × ULN and/or total bilirubin >1.5 to ≤3.0× ULN	AST or ALT >5× ULN and/or total bilirubin >3.0× ULN	Moderate to severe encephalopathy with abnormal plasma levels of ammonia, bilirubin, lactic dehydrogenase, and alkaline phosphatase
Endocrine toxicity	Asymptomatic; clinical or diagnostic observations only; intervention not indicated	Moderate symptoms; medical intervention indicated	Severe symptoms; hospitalization indicated	Adrenal crisis: severe dehydration, hypotension, or shock. Life-threatening consequences

Modified from Weber J, et al. J Clin Oncol 30 (21), 2012: 2691-2697[23].

Table 1. Most common Immunorelated Edverse events and their grade:

IrAE	Grade 1	Grade 2	Grade 3	Grade 4
Skin Toxicity	Antihistamines and topical corticosteroids; if no response, consider oral corticosteroids	Antihistamines and topical corticosteroids if no response, consider oral corticosteroids	High-dose systemic corticosteroid therapy	High-dose systemic corticosteroid therapy; antibiotics if indicated and definitive discontinuation of Ipilimumab
Diarrhea	Anti-diarrhea drugs, loperamide and diphenoxylate Patient hydration	Anti-diarrhea drugs Loperamide and diphenoxylate. Patient hydration	Hospitalization, patients hydration and systemic corticosteroids	Hospitalization, patient hydration, and systemic corticosteroids. Definitive discontinuation of Ipilimumab
Liver toxicity	Monitoring of LFTs	Withhold Ipilimumab dose and check LFTs every day for 3 consecutive days; if LFT improvement to grade 1, resume routine monitoring of LFTs and continue Ipilimumab If no improvement in the LFTs, administer corticosteroid treatment and skip the next Ipilimumab dose until event resolves	Withhold Ipilimumab dose and check LFTs every day for 3 consecutive days; if LFT improvement to grade 1, resume routine monitoring of LFTs and continue Ipilimumab If no improvement in LFTs, administer corticosteroid treatment and skip the next Ipilimumab dose until event resolves	High dose of intravenous corticosteroids Definitive discontinuation of Ipilimumab
Endocrine toxicity	Abnormal endocrine workup, grade 1 or 2 endocrine toxicity without adrenal crisis May resolve spontaneously If no spontaneous resolution, consider low–moderate dose Of systemic corticosteroids Consider temporary Ipilimumab suspension	Symptoms suggestive of hypophysitis require prompt corticosteroid therapy. Temporary Ipilimumab suspension	Intravenous corticosteroids Hormone replacement Hydration Electrolyte replacement Temporary Ipilimumab suspension	Intravenous corticosteroids Hormone replacement Hydration Electrolyte replacement Definitive discontinuation of Ipilimumab

Modified from Weber J, et al. J Clin Oncol 30 (21), 2012: 2691-2697 [23].

Table 2. Most common immunorelated adverse events and their management:

http://dx.doi.org/10.5772/59860

In phase I-III studies, irAE resolution time varied from 4.3 to 7.7 weeks, whereas in patients included in the expanded-access projects ranged from 0.1 to 11.1 weeks (median 1.7 weeks). When grade 3/4 irAE were separately analyzed the median resolution time was 1.1 weeks (range, 0.1–3.4 weeks) [20, 21]. Despite some early findings, no relationship seems to exist between clinical benefit and irAEs onset in treated patients.

Grade 1/2 events take advantage from symptomatic treatments and the use of topical steroids, whereas early administration of high-dose systemic corticosteroids is mandatory for the right management of grade 3/4 irAEs. Specific guidelines to manage irAEs are available [19, 22]. In literature are available guidelines to manage Ipilimumab side effects (see Table 1 and 2) [23].

3. Cutaneous side effects from Ipilimumab

Systemic side effects from Ipilimumab are usually dose-related. However, the incidence and severity of pruritus or skin reactions appear independent of Ipilimumab dosage, as demonstrated by a meta-analysis of the studies in which Ipilimumab was administered as monotherapy at different doses (3 mg/kg vs 10 mg/kg),

Commonly used targeted anticancer agents (e.g. erlotinib, cetuximab, panitumumab, vandetanib, pertuzumab) usually induce a characteristic papulopustular (acneiform) rash in 68% to 75% of treated patients. Conversely, Ipilimumab-induced maculo-papular rash are more similar to those commonly seen with traditional drugs (ie, antibiotics, non steroidal anti-inflammatory drugs) or shows clinical characteristics mimicking atopic dermatitis [22].

From a recent meta-analysis performed on 19 studies from 1998-2011, which included several trials testing Ipilimumab (as monotherapy or in combination at various doses in randomized multi-arm and single-arm studies) [24], emerged that the overall incidence of all-grade rash was 24.3%. The overall incidence of high-grade rash was 2.4%, with a relative risk ranging from 0.7% to 11.8%. Interestingly, among 320 patients receiving 3 mg/kg and 440 receiving 10 mg/kg, there was no significant difference in terms of incidence of all-grade or high-grade rash between doses [24]. Skin irAEs have a shorter time of onset than those affecting other sites and usually develop 3-4 weeks after Ipilimumab initiation.

In our series of 57 patients treated with Ipilimumab, the incidence of cutaneous side effects was 10% (any grade). Ipilimumab-related skin lesion were erythematous, edematous or maculo-papular, often located on the trunk and extremities (Figure 1); vasculitic and purpuric lesions were also observed. Pruritus was present in almost half of the patients who showed skin reactions [unpublished data]. Some literature reports suggest that rash can coincide with the regression of subcutaneous disease and may be especially pronounced around nevi, suggesting the presence of an underlying inflammatory response against melanocytes [25-27]. The onset of vitiligo-like lesions during Ipilimumab treatment is also a finding related to an immune activation status of the host, and was a relatively common event in our experience [personal unpublished data], as well as in other case reports [28].

From a histological point of view, skin biopsies of Ipilimumab-related skin lesions showed a perivascular inflammatory infiltrate in the superficial dermis that extend to the epidermis with CD4+ and CD8+ T cells that are CD3+. Eosinophils may also be present [24-27].

4. Vemurafenib toxicities

Even if Vemurafenib is generally a safe and well-tolerated drug, a wide spectrum of toxic effects has been described [14-18, 29, 30]. The most common one is represented by arthralgia, which occurs in about 60% of patients. Most cases are mild to moderate, but about 5% of patients treated with Vemurafenib experienced a grade 3 arthralgia [14, 29]. These latter cases can be managed conservatively with non-steroidal anti-inflammatory drugs and acetaminophen; however, severe cases may require a short course of steroid treatment [31]

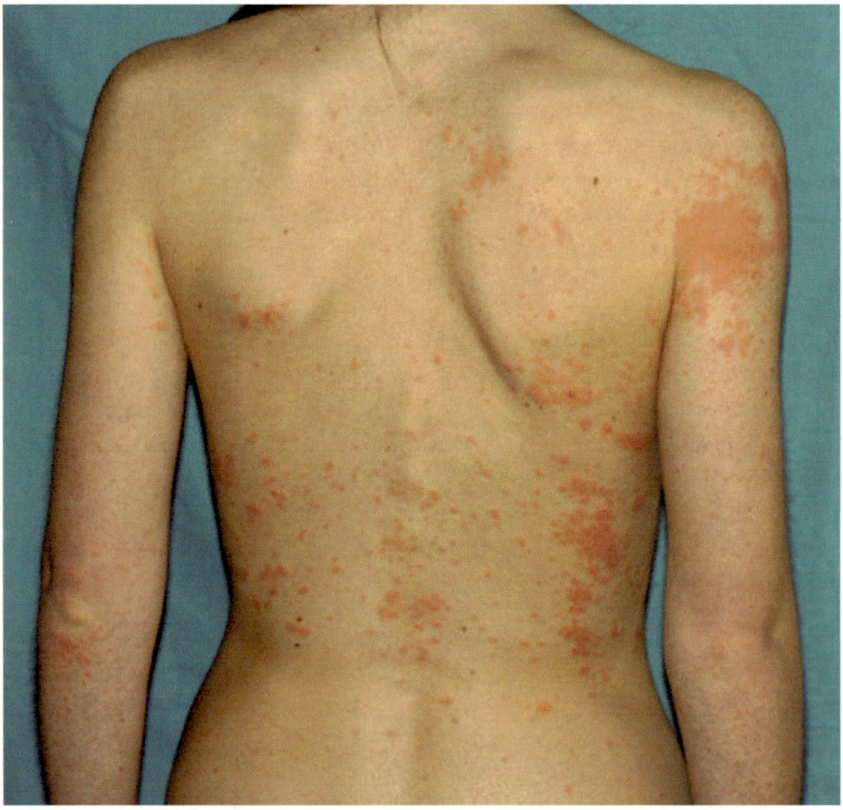

Figure 1. Erythemato-edematous rash in a patient treated with Ipilimumab

Liver enzymes should be monitored, since elevated liver enzymes have been documented in about 20% of treated patients;, usually resolving with a treatment suspension [14, 29, 31].

http://dx.doi.org/10.5772/59860

Only a relatively small percentage of patients (approximately 20%) experience nausea, which is normally responsive to oral antiemetics [31].

Quite unusual but potentially life-threatening side effects are related to alterations of the cardiac rhythm, including the prolongation of cardiac repolarization and arrhythmia, which occurs in about 8% of patients. Hence, the monitoring of cardiac activity is mandatory in all Vemurafenib-treated patients; however, the occurrence of absolute QTc values >500 ms [29, 31, 32] that require prompt clinical management is quite rare.

5. Cutaneous side effects from Vemurafenib

Cutaneous reactions are the most common side effects described during Vemurafenib treatment and impact significantly on patient's quality of life [15-17, 29]. As expected from the experience collected with other molecular targeted therapies, skin toxicity is related to the alteration of the wild-type BRAF signaling [18].

The cutaneous adverse reactions affect a percentage of treated patients from 75 to 90%, without difference of age and sex and can be classified according to the reaction pattern and time of appearance as follows:

5.1. Rash

Literature data report the onset of a maculo-papular eruption in about 50% of treated patients [14, 16, 18, 29]. Also in our experience, rash was the earliest and most frequent cutaneous side effect during Vemurafenib treatment (48% of treated patients of our series). From a clinical point of view, this rash could be similar to other drug-related exanthemas and it is characterized by the onset of maculae and follicular papules mainly distributed on the trunk and limbs (Figure 2); the head region is generally spared. Rush appears after a median time of 11 days (range 7-55 days), it is generally self-limiting and spontaneously resolve after a median of 18 days from the onset (range 2-95). In the majority of cases, it is asymptomatic, even if some patients reported pruritus [personal unpublished data].

Cases that underwent skin biopsy show an inflammatory lympho-histiocytic lichenoid infiltrate, even if keratinocytes activation should be observed [18]. The origin of this maculo-papular eruption is still unclear; however these features can explain the usefulness of topical steroids, as well as the anecdotic finding that rush did not occurred in patients receiving concomitant steroids for medical treatments related to other diseases.

Because of the self-limiting nature of this side effect, we recommend the routinely use of topical emollients; steroids should be limited to symptomatic cases. Patients also have to be informed about the frequency and benignity of this rash; however, persistent or clinically atypical exanthemas should be referred to an experienced dermatologist to avoid the risk of Steven-Johnson Syndrome /Toxic Epidermal Necrolysis (SJS/TEN) [33, 34].

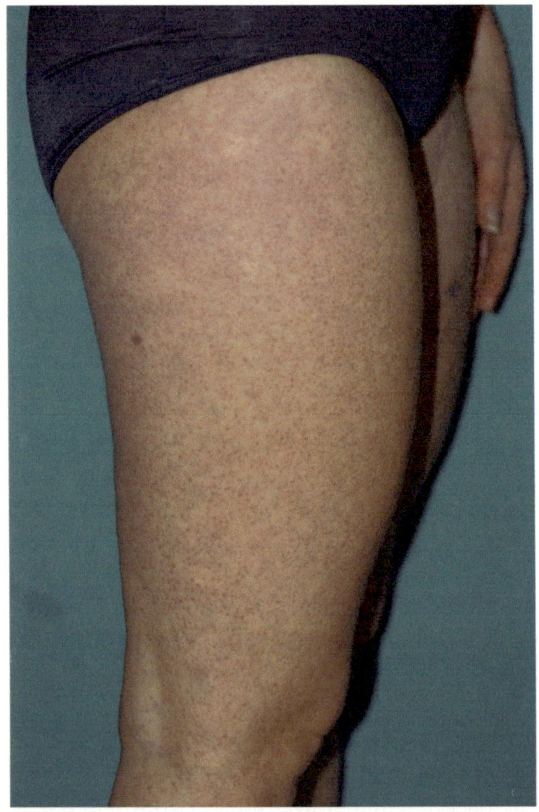

Figure 2. Maculae and follicular papules distributed on limbs in a patients treated with Vemurafenib

5.2. Warts

Viral warts represent the second most frequent cutaneous side effect of Vemurafenib [15-17] which affects about 41% of patients in our experience; median time of onset is 50 days from the initiation of treatment. Warts affect mainly the regions of the head and neck, less frequently the trunk and limbs (Figure 3). In our casistics, viral warts were the first cutaneous side effect in 13.7% of patients [unpublished data].

Histologically, Vemurafenib-dependent warts were indistinguishable from common viral warts [15, 19]; standard wart treatments (e.g. cryosurgery, keratolytic solutions, and diathermic coagulation) usually are very effective.

5.3. Hyperkeratosis

In a percentage of Vemurafenib-treated patients, the induction of a keratinocytic hyperproliferation without signs of apoptosis results in an increased epidermal thickness [28]. Plantar hyperkeratosis occurs mainly in areas under physical pressure, whereas diffuse hyperkeratotic follicular papules are observed mainly in the lower limbs and forearms (Figure 4). In our

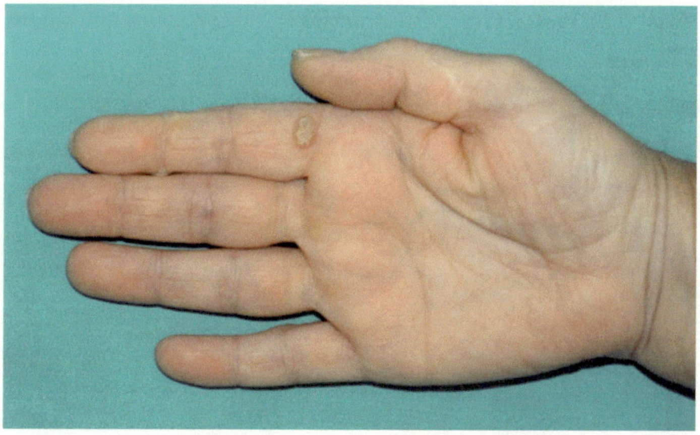

Figure 3. Disseminated viral warts in a patient treated with Vemurafenib

experience, the median onset time of localized and diffuse hyperkeratosis is 44 and 31 days, respectively.

Topical keratolytic and emollient treatment can reduce hyperkeratosis, even if a complete resolution of this side effect was observed only after Vemurafenib discontinuation.

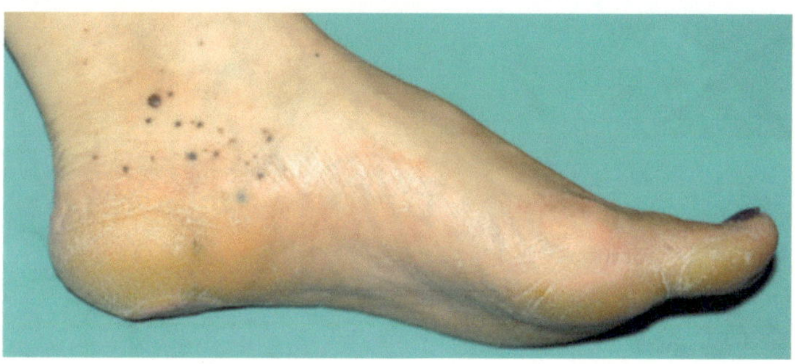

Figure 4. Plantar hyperkeratosis occurred in areas under physical pressure during Vemurafenib treatment

5.4. Photosensitivity

Photosensitivity is another common phenomenon in Vemurafenib-treated patients. Even if this side effect does not represent a life-threatening condition, it can impact on patients' quality of life and could be difficult to manage [14, 17, 29, 30]. Painful sunburns are an early phenomenon and may occur after few minutes of sun exposure; UVA seems to play a more prominent role than UVB. In our experience, sunburns were observed in 14% of patients, also after a few days of treatment (Figure 5). Patient phototype and intensity of sun exposure can concur in the onset of this phenomenon. In our series, all patients who developed sunburns during Vemurafenib treatment showed a photo type II [personal unpublished data].

Sun protection is mandatory in Vemurafenib-treated patients, and should be started together with BRAF inhibitor.

Actinic conjunctivitis is also described as an early as well as a very late side effect.

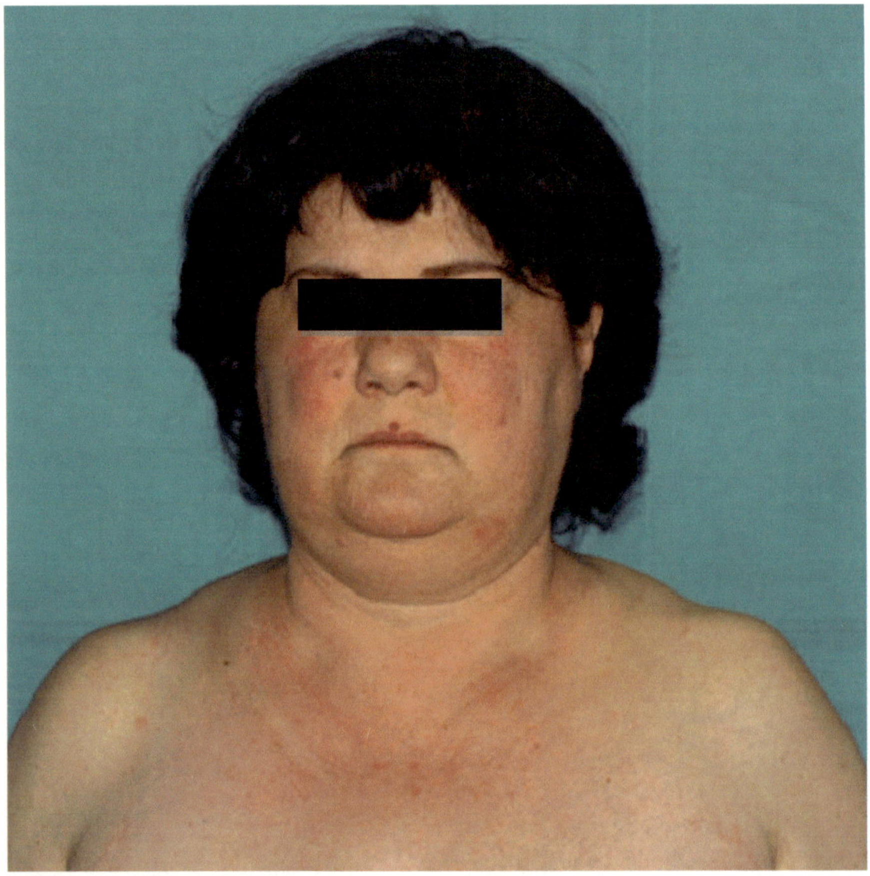

Figure 5. Painful sunburns developed after a few days of Vemurafenib treatment

5.5. Effluvium and hair changes

In our experience, effluvium occur in 17% of patient, after a median time of 88 days, usually without complete hair loss. Moreover, some patients experience a curling and ticking of the hair. Hair changes belong to the late onset side effects. All these phenomena could be explained by a paradoxical up-regulation of MAPK signaling [35-37].

5.6. Hands oedema and urticaria

A less frequent skin toxicity is represented by localized hand oedema, that developed in a few patients as an early side effect, usually within a month from the beginning of the treatment, in

http://dx.doi.org/10.5772/59860

the absence of other signs of localized or diffuse oedema. In these patients, laboratory tests did not show renal toxicity or hypoalbuminemia. Morevover, cases of urticarial episodes during the Vemurafenib treatment are described, particularly in patients with a personal history of atopia; normally, these episodes spontaneously resolve without drug suspension, and, hence, the relationship between Vemurafenib and urticaria remains to be ascertained [15-17, 29].

5.7. Skin cancer

The first reports of skin toxicity obtained from phase I-III clinical trials and expanded access studies showed the onset of squamous cell carcinomas (SCCs) in up to 31% of Vemurafenib-treated patients [30]. However, a pathology review of all lesions excised in phase II study revealed that 90% of reported SCCs were keratoacanthomas and the remaining 10%, well-differentiated squamous cell carcinomas. More recent reports stated that incidence of SCCs and keratoacanthomas is about 14-18%, respectively [18].

Literature data hypothesize that keratoacanthomas and SCCs develop as a consequence of pre-existing precancerous RAS mutations in keratinocytes of sun-exposed areas that are then activated by Vemurafenib through a paradoxical up-regulation of MAPK signaling [30, 35]. This mechanism could explain the keratinocytes proliferation that leads to keratosis pilaris-like lesions, palmo-plantar hyperkeratosis and hair changes in Vemurafenib-treated patients; notably, the same side effects are also observed during treatment with sorafenib and MEK inhibitors. Along this line, chemoprevention of cutaneous SCCs by the subministration of systemic retinoids has been reported to be successful in Vemurafenib-treated [28]. In our experience, also topical retinoid can significantly reduce the hyperkeratosis, with lower side effects (unpublished data).

6. Toxicity profiles of emerging BRAF inhibitors

The second-generation BRAFV600 inhibitor Dabrafenib has an acceptable safety profile. The percentage of patients that experience treatment-related side toxicities is lower respect to Vemurafenib and drug-related adverse events of grade ≥2 occur in about 5% of patients.

Clinical trials with Dabrafenib and Vemurafenib show several differences in type, grade and frequencies of toxicities [15-18, 38, 39]. Cutaneous toxicities such as rash, hyperkeratosis and the development of non-melanoma skin cancers are less frequent in Dabrafenib-treated patients than inr those treated with Vemurafenib. In particular, skin carcinomas occur in 19% of patients treated with Vemurafenib as opposed to 5% during treatment with dabrafenib. Patients included in the phase I and II trials with Dabrafenib do not experienced photosensitivity, which could therefore be considered a Vemurafenib-specific toxicity.

Non-cutaneous toxicities such as arthralgia and fatigue also occur at an increased rate and grade for patients treated with Vemurafenib, whereas pyrexia is a specific toxicity seen with dabrafenib. The mechanisms underlying Dabrafenib-associated pyrexia are poorly understood and require further investigation. However, this condition can be successfully treated with steroids. No patient included in clinical trials with Dabrafenib experience liver toxicity [38, 39].

The increased incidence of high class toxicities scored with Vemurafenib than with Dabrafenib is likely to be explained by a number of factors, including differences in drug dosage (the administered dose for Dabrafenib is lower than for Vemurafenib), RAF inhibitor potency, histopathologic assessment of cutaneous lesions, classification and reporting of toxicity. Moreover, the differences in phototype and exposure to exogenous risk factors for skin carcinomas of the different geographic populations enrolled in these studies could also play an important role.

7. Conclusions

The efficacy of new drugs for the treatment of metastatic melanoma is accompanied by a new spectrum of toxicities, very different from those caused by conventional chemotherapy, but not less important. Therefore, it is crucial that clinicians develop the necessary skills for the early detection and management of these toxicities, in order to limit the need of interruption or suspension of these treatment and to offer the best chance of disease control.

Author details

Paola Savoia* and Paolo Fava

*Address all correspondence to: paola.savoia@unito.it

Department of Medical Science, University of Turin, Italy

References

[1] Chapman, P.B., Einhorn, L.H., Meyers, M.L., Saxman, S., Destro, A.N., Panageas, K.S., Begg, C.B., Agarwala, S.S., Schuchter, L.M., Ernstoff, M.S., Houghton, A.N., Kirkwood, J.M. Phase III multicenter randomized trial of the Dartmouth regimen versus dacarbazine in patients with metastatic melanoma. J. Clin. Oncol. 1999; 17, 2745–51.

[2] Tarhini, A.A., Agarwala, S.S. Cutaneous melanoma: available therapy for metastatic disease. Dermatol. Ther. 2006; 19: 19–25

[3] Kirkwood JM, Manola J, Ibrahim J. Eastern cooperative oncology group. A pooled analysis of eastern cooperative oncology group and intergroup trials of adjuvant high-dose interferon for melanoma. Clin. Cancer Res. 1999; 10, 1670–7.

[4] Atkins, M.B., Lotze, M.T., Dutcher, et al. High-dose recombinant interleukin 2 therapy for patients with metastatic melanoma: analysis of 270 patients treated between 1985 and 1993. J Clin. Oncol 1999; 17: 2105-16.

[5] Atkins, M.B., Kunkel, L., Sznol, M., Rosenberg, S.A. High-dose recombinant interleukin-2 therapy in patients with metastatic melanoma: long-term survival update. Cancer J Sci.Am 2000; 6 (Suppl. 1), S11-4.

[6] Hodi FS, O'Day SJ, McDermott DF et al. Improved survival with Ipilimumab in patients with metastatic melanoma. N Engl J Med 2010; 363:711–23.

[7] Liu W, Kelly JW, Trivett M, et al. Distinct clinical and pathological features are associated with the BRAF(T1799A(V600E)) mutation in primary melanoma. J Invest Dermatol 2007; 127: 900–5.

[8] Long GV, Menzies AM, Nagrial AM, et al. Prognostic and clinicopathologic associations of oncogenic BRAF in metastatic melanoma. J Clin Oncol 2011; 29: 1239–46.

[9] Robert C, Thomas L, Bondarenko I et al. Ipilimumab plus dacarbazine for previously untreated metastatic melanoma. N Engl J Med 2011; 364:2517–26.

[10] Viros A, Fridlyand J, Bauer J, et al. Improving melanoma classification by integrating genetic and morphologic features. PLoS Med 2008; 5: e120.

[11] Hoos A, Ibrahim R, Korman A et al. Development of Ipilimumab: contribution to a new paradigm for cancer immunotherapy. Semin Oncol 2010;37: 533-46.

[12] Weber J, Thompson JA, Hamid O et al. A randomized, double-blind, placebo-controlled, phase II study comparing the tolerability and efficacy of Ipilimumab administered with or without prophylactic budesonide in patients with unresectable stage III or IV melanoma. Clin Cancer Res 2009;15:5591-8.

[13] Wolchok JD, Weber JS, Maio M et al. Four-year survival rates for patients with metastatic melanoma who received Ipilimumab in phase 2 trials [abstract P-20]. Presented at: Perspectives in Melanoma XV; September 16-17, 2011; New York, NY.

[14] Sosman JA, Kim KB, Schuchter L, et al. Survival in BRAF V600-mutant advanced melanoma treated with Vemurafenib. N Engl J Med 2012; 366: 707–14.

[15] Boyd KP, Vincent B, Andea A, et al. Nonmalignant cutaneous findings associated with Vemurafenib use in patients with metastatic melanoma. J Am Acad Dermatol 2012; 6:1375-79.

[16] Boussemart L, Routier E, Mateus C, et al. Prospective study of cutaneous side-effects associated with the BRAF inhibitor Vemurafenib: a study of 42 patients. Ann Oncol. 2013; 24:1691-97.

[17] Sinha R, Edmonds K, Newton-Bishop JA, et al. Cutaneous adverse events associated with Vemurafenib in patients with metastatic melanoma: practical advice on diagno-

sis, prevention and management of the main treatment-related skin toxicities. Br J Dermatol 2012; 167:987-94.

[18] Rinderknecht JD, Goldinger SM, Rozati S, et al. RASopathic skin eruptions during Vemurafenib therapy. PLoS One. 2013; 8:e58721

[19] Della Vittoria Scarpati G, Fusciello C, Perri F et al. 2014 Ipilimumab in the treatment of metastatic melanoma: management of adverse events. Onco Targets Ther. 2014 19;7:203-9

[20] Ibrahim R, Berman D, De Pril V, et al. Ipilimumab safety profile: summary of findings from completed trials in advanced melanoma. J Clin Oncol. 2011;29(Suppl):Abstract 8583.

[21] Ascierto P, Simeone E, Chiarion Sileni V et al. Clinical experience with Ipilimumab 3 mg/kg: real-world efficacy and safety data from an expanded access programme cohort. Journal of Translational Medicine 2014; 12:116.

[22] Lacouture, M, Wolchok J, Yosipovitch G, et al. Ipilimumab in patients with cancer and thecmanagement of dermatologic adverse events. J Am Acad Dermatol 2014; dx.doi.org/10.1016/j.jaad.2014.02.035.

[23] Weber J, et al. Management of immune-related adverse events and kinetics of response with Ipilimumab. J Clin Oncol 30 (21), 2012: 2691-2697.

[24] Attia P, Phan GQ,Maker AJ, et al. Autoimmunity correlates with tumor regression in patients with metastatic melanoma treated with antiecytotoxic T-lymphocyte antigen-4. J Clin Oncol 2005; 25:6043-53.

[25] Minkis K, Garden BC, Wu S, Pulitzer MP, Lacouture ME. The risk of skin rash associated with Ipilimumab in patients with cancer: a systematic review of literature and meta-analysis. J Am Acad Dermatol 2013;69:e121-8

[26] Klein O, Ebert LM, Nicholaou T, et al. Melan-A-specific cytotoxic T cells are associated with tumor regression and autoimmunity following treatment with anti-CTLA-4. Clin Cancer Res 2009;15:2507-13.

[27] Phan GQ, Yang JC, Sherry RM, et al. Cancer regression and autoimmunity induced by cytotoxic T lymphocyte-associated antigen 4 blockade in patients with metastatic melanoma. Proc Natl Acad Sci U S A 2003;100:8372-7.

[28] Choi JN. Dermatologic adverse events to chemotherapeutic agents, Part 2: BRAF inhibitors, MEK inhibitors, and Ipilimumab. Semin Cutan Med Surg. 2014; 33:40-8.

[29] Chapman PB, Hauschild A, Robert C et al. Improved survival with Vemurafenib in melanoma with BRAF V600E mutation. N Engl J Med 2011; 364:2507–16.

[30] Anforth R, Fernandez-Peñas P, Long GV. Cutaneous toxicities of RAF inhibitors. Lancet Oncol. 2013;14 :e11-8.

[31] Lemech C, Arkenau HT. Novel treatments for metastatic cutaneous melanoma and the management of emergent toxicities. Clin Med Insights Oncol. 2012;6:53-66

[32] Tsai KY, Nowroozi S, Kim KB. Drug safety evaluation of Vemurafenib in the treatment of melanoma. Expert Opin Drug Saf. 2013;12:767-75.

[33] Wantz M, Spanoudi-Kitrimi I, Lasek A, Lebas D, Quinchon JF, Modiano P Vemurafenib-induced toxic epidermal necrolysis].Ann Dermatol Venereol. 2014;141:215-8

[34] Minor DR, Rodvien R, Kashani-Sabet M. Successful desensitization in a case of Stevens-Johnson syndrome due to Vemurafenib. Melanoma Res. 2012;22:410-1.

[35] Hatzivassiliou G, Song K, Yen I, et al. RAF inhibitors prime wildtype RAF to activate the MAPK pathway and enhance growth. Nature 2010; 464:431–35.

[36] Poulikakos PI, Zhang C, Bollag G, et al. RAF inhibitors transactivate RAF dimers and ERK signalling in cells with wild-type BRAF. Nature 2010; 464:427–30

[37] Su F, Viros A, Milagre C, et al. RAS mutations in cutaneous squamous- cell carcinomas in patients treated with BRAF. N Engl J Med 2012; 366:207–15

[38] Long GV, Trefzer U, Davies MA, et al. Dabrafenib in patients with Val600Glu or Val600Lys BRAF-mutant melanoma metastatic to the brain (BREAK-MB): a multicentre, open-label, phase 2 trial. Lancet Oncol. 2012; 13:1087-95.

[39] Ascierto PA, Minor D, Ribas A, et al. Phase II trial (BREAK-2) of the BRAF inhibitor dabrafenib (GSK2118436) in patients with metastatic melanoma. J Clin Oncol. 2013; 31: 3205-11.

Section 4

Emerging Research on Melanoma

Chapter 12

Autotaxin – An Enzymatic Augmenter of Malignant Progression Linked to Inflammation

David N. Brindley, Matthew G.K. Benesch and
Mandi M. Murph

Additional information is available at the end of the chapter

http://dx.doi.org/10.5772/59013

1. Introduction

Malignant melanoma cells are incredibly hardy, stemming from their intrinsic defensive nature. These cells inherit unique characteristics, which allowed their non-malignant predecessors, melanocytes, to survive solar ultraviolet radiation and simultaneously provide protection to neighboring cells. Most other cell types would die after such harsh exposure. Unsurprisingly, melanoma cells, which survive ultraviolet radiation, are intrinsically resistant to most chemotherapy.

Although there are numerous molecular reasons for this reality, herein we focus on the causal role of autotaxin (ATX) in melanoma. ATX is a 125 kDa glycoprotein enzyme that was initially discovered in the serum-free medium of A2058 human melanoma cells by Stracke et al. in 1992 [1] (Figure 1). Today, we know much more about this glycoprotein enzyme and how it affects melanoma. Indeed, ATX is highly overexpressed among primary melanomas and metastatic melanomas, in comparison to melanoma *in situ* and in normal skin [2].

In fact, "autotaxin" derived its name based on its initial property as an "autocrine motility factor". The rationale is that A2058 melanoma cells secrete ATX into culture medium and then respond to it with self-stimulated random and directed motility. Even though the amount of ATX in conditioned medium is less than 0.005% of total protein, only miniscule amounts, detected in picomolar and nanomolar concentrations, are needed to promote motility. [1] This suggests a large role for a low-abundant secreted enzyme.

There are five alternatively-spliced isoforms of ATX that are catalytically active [3,4]. The original ATX protein described in 1992 is termed ATXα, whereas the most abundant isoform is ATXβ and is the same isoform responsible for plasma lysoPLD activity [5]. Full length ATX is synthesized as a pre-proenzyme and is secreted by the classical secretory pathway [6,7]. Secreted ATX binds to cell surface integrin or heparan sulfates through its somatomedin-B-like (SMB) domain. This surface binding is believed to localize LPA production adjacent to LPA receptors [8-12].

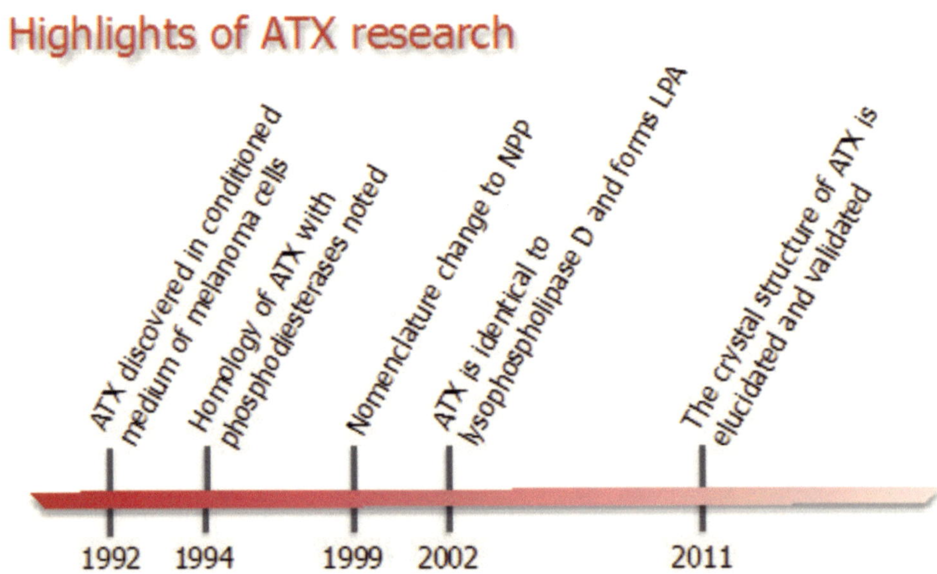

Figure 1. Major milestones in autotaxin (ATX) research. After the discovery of ATX in the conditioned medium of melanoma cells, it was not until a decade later that the enzyme was connected to lysophosphatidate. The elucidation of the crystal structure by two different groups caused a surge of novel inhibitors.

2. Multiple functions of ATX

In addition to the ability of ATX to stimulate motility, ATX also has ATPase, phosphodiesterase and ATP pyrophosphatase activities [13]. In other words, ATX releases nucleoside-5'-monophosphates from phosphodiester and pyrophosphate bonds [14], which is why it belongs to the family of ENPP (ectonucleotide pyrophosphatase/ phosphodiesterase) enzymes with ENPP1/PC-1, ENPP3/B10 [15], ENPP4 [14,16], ENPP6 [17], ENPP7 [18], and is also named ENPP2 (Table 1). Interestingly, all of the phosphodiesterase catalytic activity of ATX resides in one amino acid, threonine 210. Losing this phosphorylatable residue in the catalytic site results in a loss of phosphodiesterase activity and motility, but not ATP binding [19]. Theoretically, GTP, NAD, FAD, AMP and PPi are all susceptible to hydrolysis by ATX. However, the preferred substrate for ATX is lysophosphatidylcholine (LPC), which it converts to lysophosphatidate (LPA) (Figure 2). Since LPC concentrations in human plasma are greater than 200 μM, this should outcompete the hydrolysis of nucleotide phosphates and pyrophosphate, which are present in much lower concentrations.

http://dx.doi.org/10.5772/59013

Enzyme	Major Functions	Disease Association
ENPP1 / PC-1	Insulin signaling, glucose import, bone mineralization, immune response	Diabetes, obesity, stroke
ENPP2 / ATX	Vasculature formation, neural development, catalyzes lysophosphatidate production	Cancer, obesity, pulmonary fibrosis, arthritis, asthma, neuropathic pain, liver and colonic disorders
ENPP3 / B10	Basophil activation biomarker	Asthma, allergic reactions
ENPP4	Blood coagulant	Stroke
ENPP5	Putative neural glycoprotein	
ENPP6	Choline-specific hydrolysis of LPC, GPC and SPC	
ENPP7	Alkaline sphingomyelinase	

Table 1. Comparison between enzymes among the Ectonucleotide Pyrophosphatase/ Phosphodiesterase (ENPP) family

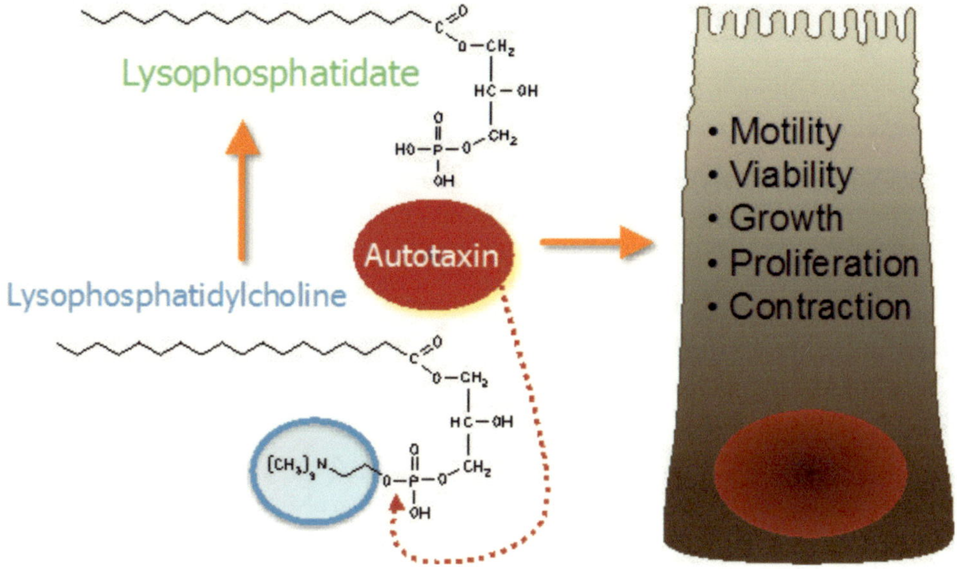

Figure 2. Autotaxin (ATX) catalyzes the biosynthesis of lysophosphatidiate (LPA). Since the lysophosphatidylcholine (LPC) concentrations in human circulation are >200 μM, ATX has abundantly available lipids to produce LPA. ATX hydrolyzes the choline head group from LPC to yield LPA. As a consequence of LPA signaling on cells, a multitude of various responses result, including motility, viability, growth, proliferation and contraction.

The ability of ATX to stimulate motility in melanoma cells can be modulated by chemical methods and genetic engineering. For example, ATX-meditated motility is inhibited by the PI3K inhibitors, wortmannin and LY294002, along with the catalytically inactive mutant of PI3K, PI3KK832R [20]. In addition, *ras*-transformed NIH3T3 cells become more motile and invasive in the presence of ATX. These cells also show enhanced colony formation in soft agar *in vitro* and produce significantly larger and metastatic tumors *in vivo* [21]. This suggests that while ATX alone may be insufficient to transform cells to a malignant phenotype, the presence of ATX significantly enhances malignant transformation among 'primed' cells.

3. Role as the main enzyme for the generation of extracellular LPA

The majority of LPA in the circulation is generated by ATX from the abundant LPC (>200 μM in human plasma) in the circulation. In fact, LPC is the major plasma phospholipid and it is bound to albumin [22]. Extracellular LPC is derived from two major routes of metabolism. The first is through the action of lecithin:cholesterol acyltransferase, which is present in plasma high-density lipoproteins. Lecithin:cholesterol acyltransferase, preferentially transfers unsaturated fatty acids from postion-2 of phosphatidylcholine to cholesterol, producing cholesterol ester and a mainly saturated LPC. However, a large proportion of circulating LPC is polyunsaturated [22] and this indicates another route for the production of extracellular LPC. Part of the polyunsaturated LPC is derived from secretion by hepatocytes, but it is possible that other cell types could produce polyunsaturated LPC. Since hepatocytes secrete a large quantity of arachidonoyl-LPC [22-26], it was originally postulated that this might represent a novel transport system for delivering choline and polyunsaturated fatty acids to the brain [22]. Although, this could still be true, we now know that LPC is an important substrate for ATX and that this is the major route for the production of extracellular LPA [27].

This predominant role of ATX in generating LPA is confirmed by circulating LPA concentrations that are 50% of normal levels among ATX heterozygous mice for a null-mutation for ATX [28,29]. Also, ATX inhibition produces a rapid decrease in plasma LPA of >95% [30-32]. The effects of ATX inhibition are more dramatic for the unsaturated species [33]. This is compatible with the substrate preference of ATX for unsaturated and polyunsaturated LPCs [34]. The crystal structures of ATX:LPA complexes show a hydrophobic pocket in the catalytic domain that is slightly U-shaped. This accommodates the kinked acyl chains of unsaturated fatty acids better than the linear conformations of saturated fatty acids [34].

Even though ATX is the major enzyme that generates LPA, other enzymes have a minor role in its biosynthesis. For example, saturated LPA species can also be derived through secretory phospholipase A_2, which hydrolyzes phosphatidate in microvesicles that are shed from cells during inflammation [35] and platelet aggregation [36]. In addition, LPA production by the Group VIA phospholipase A_2 (Ca^{2+}-independent) appears to be involved in the development of prostate cancers [37].

4. Crystal structure of ATX

The elucidation of the crystal structure of mouse and rat ATX revealed that the enzyme is composed of four domains [9,34]. The most important among these domains is the slightly U-shaped catalytic domain, which contains the enzyme's active site, a hydrophobic pocket and

http://dx.doi.org/10.5772/59013

hydrophobic channel. Although ATX can hydrolyze both nucleotides and lysophospholipid substrates, when the unique hydrophobic pocket engages lysophospholipids, nucleotides are unable to bind to the active site. In addition, lipid acyl chains form further interactions with this pocket that nucleotides do not, which is also why ATX has a higher affinity for lysophospholipids [38]. The unique shape of the catalytic domain also accommodates the kinked acyl chains of unsaturated fatty acids better than the linear conformations of saturated fatty acids [34], which further explains substrate specificity for ATX.

ATX is the only member of the ENPP enzyme family that contains a hydrophobic pocket for lysophospholipids, thus giving it a unique capability over other ENPPs. Interestingly, one amino acid, asparagine 230, is required for ATX to recognize phosphate moieties and produce lysophosphatidate. Mutating asparagine to alanine inhibited all production. [34] Other single-point mutations deep within the hydrophobic pocket are capable of altering binding selectivity and reducing some of ATX's activity [9].

Perhaps the most exciting biological implication arising from the structural resolution of ATX is its proposed role as a directed transporter of LPA. In other words, ATX does not appear to arbitrarily release lysophospholipids from its hydrophobic pocket and channel them into solution. Rather, ATX is hypothesized to directly transfer LPA to its receptors along the plasma membrane. The flat surface of ATX on the side of the channel entrance facing the cell presumably facilitates this purpose [34]. This insinuates a role for ATX as an indirect initiator of cell signaling through its guided transport of an agonist to its receptor. It also further explains early observations of ATX as a motility-stimulating factor, even though it was actually due to LPA.

5. ATX Inhibitors

ATX, as an extracellular enzyme, is a very attractive drug candidate for reducing the abundance of extracellular LPA and subsequent signaling. Indeed, even a transient knockdown of ATX using siRNA is sufficient to significantly reduce melanoma cell viability [2]. Furthermore, the advantage of inhibiting ATX is the attenuation of signaling by all LPA receptors. This is considerably advantageous over the use of individual receptor antagonists because there are at least six and possibly eight confirmed LPA receptors with extensive redundancy. The design of ATX inhibitors has been reviewed previously [39-41] and so we will focus only those inhibitors that show utility *in vivo*.

Among the first ATX inhibitors was L-histidine, which was reported to have an ATX binding affinity (K_i) of about 1 mM *in vitro*, with 10 mM concentrations required to block ATX-stimulated migration in melanoma cells by 90% [42]. L-histidine inhibits ATX non-competitively by chelating cations such as Zn^{2+}, which are required for optimum catalytic rates [42]. Later work showed L-histidine administered intraperitoneally to rats limits thioacetamide-induced liver fibrosis [43]. Although L-histidine is required mM concentrations for activity *in vitro*, the authors cited its importance because it was the first "proof-of-principle" that inhibiting ATX was achievable.

Few studies have focused on inhibiting ATX transcription. However, one study showed that cholera toxin inhibits the proliferation of human hepatocellular carcinoma cells *in vitro* by suppressing the production of ATX through a TNF-α-dependent mechanism [44]. Cholera toxin increases the expression of anti-inflammatory cytokines (IL-4 and IL-10), which suppress ATX mRNA levels [45]. Knockdown of ATX expression with siRNA decreased the effects of cholera-toxin in suppressing the growth of Hep3B and Huh7 HCC cells [44]. Also, oral administration of the anti-inflammatory steroid, prednisolone, decreased serum ATX levels in a dose-dependent manner in patients treated for autoimmune skin diseases [46]. It is uncertain if suppressing ATX activity contributed to symptom relief since tapering the prednisolone dosage caused a rebound in serum ATX levels independently of disease severity. Significantly, the authors proposed that serum ATX levels could be used as a marker of compliance and/or efficacy of steroid therapy [46]. In addition, rifampicin, which is an inhibitor of DNA-dependent RNA polymerase, can be used to lower ATX mRNA transcription in the treatment of cholestatic pruritus. Cessation of rifampicin treatment led to both reoccurrence of pruritus and a rebound of ATX levels to pretreatment levels [47]. All of the treatment options for decreasing ATX expression appear to be effective in only specific diseases. By contrast, ATX inhibitors are designed to block LPA production and therefore this approach should have greater utility in multiple pathologies.

Major criteria for the efficacy of any therapeutic agent is a favorable therapeutic index and good bioavailability and potency. Reports on competitive ATX inhibitors began around 2006. These consisted of carba analogs of cyclic phosphatidate (cPA) with a K_i of approximately 100 nM (Table 2). These compounds inhibited metastasis of melanoma cells, which were injected in the tail vein in mouse models [48] and they inhibited chronic inflammation-induced C-fiber stimulation in rat neuropathic pain models [49]. However, cyclic phosphatidate analogs are also weak agonists of LPA receptors, which limits their utility [39].

Compound	Class	*In vivo therapeutic effects*
cPA	Lipid	• inhibits B16F10 melanoma metastasis in mouse tail vein model [48] • inhibits C-fiber stimulation by chronic inflammation in rat neuropathic pain models [49]
BrP-LPA	Lipid	• reduces MDA-MB-231 orthotopic breast tumor growth in mice [50] • inhibits A549 lung metastasis in engineered 3D mouse xenografts [51] • radiosensitizes GL-261 mouse glioma models [52] reduces collagen-induced arthritis in mice [53]
GWJ-A-23	Lipid	• reduces allergen-induced asthmatic phenotype in ATX-transgenic mice [54] • reduces fibrosis in bleomycin-treated mice [55]
PF-8380	Non-Lipid	• inhibits inflammatory hyperalgesia in rat air-pouch models [30] • radiosensitizes glioblastoma multiforme heteotropic mouse models [56]
ONO-8430506	Non-Lipid	• reduces tumor growth and metastasis in 4T1/Balb/c syngeneic and orthotopic mouse model and is synergistic with doxorubicin [33,57] • reduces urethral tension in rat benign prostatic hyperplasia models [58]

Table 2. ATX inhibitors used to effect a therapeutic response *in vivo*

http://dx.doi.org/10.5772/59013

A series of lipid-mimetic ATX inhibitors were developed in 2009 based on α-bromophosphonates (BrP-LPA). The *anti*-BrP-LPA isomer had IC_{50} of 22 nM in plasma, which was more potent than for *syn*-BrP-LPA [50] (Table 2). BrP-LPA is also a pan-antagonist of $LPA_{1\text{-}3,}$ which is effective in decreasing to tumor growth in orthotopic xenograft models of breast cancer using MDA-MB-231 cells [50] and in metastasis of A549 lung cancer cells in nude mice [51]. We have also previously demonstrated that BrP-LPA is more effective than dacarbazine in reducing the viability of melanoma cells [59].

In addition to its efficacy against cancer cells, BrP-LPA had a radio-sensitizing effect on the tumor vasculature and delayed tumor growth by 7 days compared to radiation alone in a heterotopic murine glioma model using GL-261 cells [52]. This study was one of the first to demonstrate that ATX inhibitors can potential be used as an adjuvant therapy for cancer. A later report showed that BrP-LPA attenuated disease symptoms by diminishing synovial LPA signaling in a collagen-induced arthritis mouse model. Histological analysis of the joints showed a marked decrease in inflammation and synovial hyperplasia [53].

Several lipid-analogs of LPC, which have been used as ATX inhibitors, have relatively poor bioavailability, mainly because of the hydrophobic acyl tail [41]. This is illustrated by S32826, which is a benzyl phosphonic acid derivative (Figure 3). Despite having a very low nM IC_{50} *in vitro*, the long chain contributes to a very high lipophilicity and it cannot suppress circulating ATX activity for more than a few minutes [32]. Analogs of S32826, such as GWJ-A-23, were developed by shortening the hydrophobic chain and adding α-halo-or α-hydroxy-substituents to increase solubility. However, most of these compounds are less potent inhibitors of ATX compared to S32826 [60], but have been used in pulmonary studies of ATX [54,55]. Hence, much of the recent effort in discovering ATX inhibitors for use *in vivo* has concentrated on compounds that are more soluble and not based on lipid analogs.

There are numerous, small, non-lipid inhibitors of ATX that have been modified to increase potency [40,41]. These inhibitors tend to have better bioavailability because of decreased hydrophobicity and they are unlikely to be rapidly degraded by endogenous hydrolytic pathways [61]. One of these is PF-8380, which is a piperazinylbenzoxazolone derivative that was developed by Pfizer from compound library screening and optimization (Table 2). PF-8380 has an IC_{50} of 2.8 nM against recombinant human ATX and 101 nM for ATX in human whole blood. It was the first ATX inhibitor that was reported to decrease plasma LPA levels *in vivo* for an extended period [30]. In rat air-pouch models, 30 mg/kg PF-8380 inhibited inflammatory hyperalgesia with the same efficacy as 30 mg/kg naproxen, a routinely used nonsteroidal anti-inflammatory drug [30]. This dosage of PF-8380 produced a maximum decrease in LPA concentrations in plasma and also at the site of inflammation. Like BrP-LPA, PF-8380 had radio-sensitizing effects in a heterotopic mouse model of glioblastoma multiforme, delaying tumor growth by at least 20 days [52, 56]. In this study, inhibition of ATX by PF-8380 abrogated radiation-induced activation of Akt and subsequently decreased tumor vascularity and tumor growth [56]. Although we have *repeatedly* tested 30 mg/kg PF-8380 in animal models of melanoma, we have not observed a reduction of tumor growth (results not shown).

We have worked recently with another potent ATX inhibitor, which is a tetrahydrocarboline derivative (ONO-8430506) developed by Ono Pharmaceuticals Ltd. (Patent WO20120052227).

Oral dosing with 10 mg/kg ONO-8430506 suppressed plasma ATX activity as measured by choline release assay in the presence of 3 mM LPC by at least 90% at 6 h after administration in mice [33]. Plasma LPA levels were suppressed, especially the unsaturated species. C16:1-LPA and C20:5-LPA remained non-detectable at 6 and 24 h after ONO-8430506 administration. ONO-8430506 decreased the initial rate of tumor growth and subsequent lung metastasis by up to 60% in a syngeneic orthotopic model of breast cancer in BALB/c mice. This was accompanied by decreased concentrations of unsaturated LPA species in the breast tumors. These findings again confirm that ATX produces most of the extracellular LPA and that decreases in LPA concentrations in tissues mirror the decreases in plasma LPA levels following ATX inhibition [30, 33].

In other work, ONO-8430506 (30 mg/kg/day) decreased intra-urethral pressure and this was ascribed to urethral relaxation [58]. This work demonstrates the potential of ATX inhibition to decrease smooth muscle contraction by LPA. It also shows that ATX inhibition ameliorates urethral obstructive disease, such as benign prostatic hyperplasia.

6. Strategies to identify novel ATX inhibitors

So far, the most common technique for ATX inhibitor discovery and design is to screen libraries of compounds by using assays with ATX substrates such as Fluorescent Substrate-3 (FS-3). Inhibitors are then modified to increase potency. FS-3 is a fluorogenic substrate that is a doubly-labeled analogue of LPC. The fluorophore is quenched through intra-molecular energy transfer. Hydrolysis of FS-3 by ATX increases the fluorescent signal by removing the quencher [62]. The initial studies with this technique identified several inhibitors with an IC_{50} in the μM range [63, 64]. Later work with compounds designed from these studies developed nine pharmacophores for ATX inhibition and the results of these analyses were used to screen the National Cancer Institute's open chemical repository database to prioritize screening efforts [61]. This lead to the identification of several novel compounds with an IC_{50} in the high to low μM range [61, 65].

The identification of the crystal structure of ATX is also enabling structure-activity relationships to be established and more rational-design approaches towards optimizing inhibitor structures are now possible. The first study to report this approach was by Kawaguchi *et al.* who identified a thiazolone derivative from a 81,600-compound library, which inhibited ATX activity with an IC_{50} of 180 nM [66]. The authors proposed a series of side-chain modifications from the crystal structure of ATX complexed with this inhibitor. This led to the synthesis of a derivative compound, 3BoA, which has an IC_{50} of 13 nM [66]. More recent studies by Fells *et al.* combined large library screening results using the crystal structure of ATX with virtual screening tools to discover additional novel ATX inhibitors [67, 68]. This technique identified a common aromatic sulfonamide structural motif among potent inhibitors that targets the hydrophobic pocket of ATX. This accommodates the hydrocarbon tail of LPC/LPA [67, 68]. Similar techniques are expected to lead to the rapid development of ATX inhibitors for subsequent testing and development *in vivo*.

7. Physiological functions of ATX and LPA signaling

7.1. Vasculature system

Although studies *in vitro* detected no difference in the growth rate of *ras*-transformed NIH3T3 cells with or without ATX in culture, the growth rates in animals were significantly different, which suggested a role for ATX in blood vessel formation [21]. Indeed, Matrigel plugs of cells with ATX displayed extensive micro-aneurysms filled with red blood cells and more tumor cells, further corroborating this role. Furthermore, the ability of ATX to stimulate blood vessel formation in Matrigel plugs after 6 days was equivalent to VEGF, thus solidifying ATX as an angiogenesis-stimulating factor in the circulation [69].

Developmentally, the expression of ATX is indispensible. Beginning at 8.5 days, ATX expression is detectable in the early mouse embryo, within the floor plate of the neural tube [70]. Knocking out of ATX in mice causes embryonic lethality around 9.5 – 10.5 days with embryos exhibiting open, kinky neural tubes [28,71]. Although heartbeats are detected until 10.5 days *in utero*, contractions are weak, irregular and clearly abnormal. In addition, even the yolk sacs of ATX knockout embryos are irregular with a complete absence of blood vessels. [72] The role of ATX in vascular and neural development is also observed in zebrafish [72, 73]. ATX regulates the differentiation of oligodendrocytes in the hindbrain [74] and the correct left-right asymmetry for normal organ morphogenesis through Wnt-dependent pathways [75]. Taken together, these results definitively prove that the absence of ATX results in severe defects of the vasculature system and embryonic lethality. Organisms cannot develop without functional ATX expression.

Other groups have explored the parallel correlation by investigating the vasculature system when ATX is overexpressed in transgenic mice. Interestingly, ATX transgenic mice have an unusual susceptibility to bleeding and impaired platelet-dependent thrombus formation after injury [10]. Further studies have confirmed an important role for ATX in platelet activation through the production of LPA [76]. In addition, ATX binds to platelet β1-and β3-integrins, which localizes ATX to the cell surface of the appropriate microenvironment [11].

8. Adipose tissue regulation

An alternative, yet highly interesting function of ATX *in vivo* occurs in adipogenesis, obesity and the regulation of glucose homeostasis [77]. Foremost, ATX is expressed and secreted by adipose tissue. Its expression is also significantly upregulated during pre-adipocyte differentiation into adipocytes (adipogenesis) as well as in the adipose tissue of genetically obese diabetic mice [78]. In support of this finding, transgenic ATX mice accumulate more fat than littermates when they are fed a high-fat diet and thus, are more susceptible to diet-induced obesity [79]. Other work showed that ATX mRNA is upregulated in differentiating adipocytes but downregulated in hypertrophied adipocytes from obese mice [80]. Further, in humans, serum ATX levels and ATX mRNA expression in subcutaneous fat were negatively correlated with body mass index [80]. However this does not appear to be true if the subject is diabetic. Instead, these patients tend to have higher serum ATX levels [80]. In regards to the regulation of glucose metabolism, LPA produced by ATX is able to dose-dependently inhibit glucose-induced insulin secretion [77, 81]. Furthermore, knocking out the expression of ATX in adipose tissue results in a mouse with improved glucose tolerance [82].

9. Wound healing, tissue remodeling and inflammation

ATX and LPA facilitate critical processes necessary for skin re-epithelialization and wound healing. For example, among blister fluids, both ATX and LPA are produced and detected, originating *de novo* in the blister fluid and not from plasma. LPA is a potent activator of platelet aggregation and promotes keratinocyte migration, proliferation and differentiation. Thus, ATX and LPA facilitate critical processes necessary for skin re-epithelialization and wound healing [83]. ATX expression and LPA production are increased in rabbit aqueous humor following wounding by corneal freezing [84].

The range of physiological functions requiring ATX is quite diverse. For example, ATX and LPA signaling are involved in luteal tissue remodeling of regressing corpora lutea in rat ovaries. This occurs by recruiting phagocytes and proliferating fibroblasts, which are ultimately the factors involved in remodeling [85]. Other roles for ATX include hair follicle morphogenesis [86], bone mineralization [87] and myeloid differentiation in human bone marrow [88].

Another unique role of ATX occurs in response to oxidative stress in microglia, whereby ATX expression is increased. This protects microglia cells from damage by H_2O_2 and this effect is partially reversed by the mixed $LPA_{1/3}$ antagonist, Ki16425 [89]. Microglia cells overexpressing ATX show suppressed production of the pro-inflammatory cytokines, TNF-α and IL-6, and increases in the anti-inflammatory cytokine IL-10 upon treatment with lipopolysaccharide [90]. ATX is expressed in high endothelial venules in lymph nodes and other secondary lymphoid tissues [91]. This mediates lymphocyte extravasation, a process required for maintaining immune homeostasis [92, 93]. However, in chronically inflamed tissues, ATX mediates lymphocyte trafficking and increases cytokine production in response to repeated micro-injuries and incomplete tissue repair [94-96].

Interestingly, the catalytic activity of ATX has a dualistic role in wound healing. In this way, an ATX-like enzyme, SMaseD, is responsible for the pathology associated with venomous poisons through its dermonecrotic and hemolytic activities [97, 98]. In other words, the aberrant over-production of LPA by ATX cultivates an inappropriate immune response, similar to a wound that never heals, whereby overabundant inflammatory cytokines and chemokines are released. The damage is manifested in several ways, including the presence of severe dermonecrosis with blackened or missing skin appearing at the wounded site. The dermonecrosis can occur after envenomation by either *Loxosceles reclusa,* the brown recluse spider [97], or *Hemiscorpius lepturus,* a venomous scorpion [98]. Intriguingly, susceptibility to SMaseD is conferred by the LPA_1 receptor [99], suggesting a possible role for LPA receptor antagonists in this pathology.

http://dx.doi.org/10.5772/59013

As mentioned above, one of the main functions of ATX in adults is to repair damaged tissue. ATX is secreted in this situation partly in response to inflammation and the release of inflammatory cytokines. In normal wound healing, the production of LPA by ATX causes cells to migrate into the area of damage to effect wound repair and the formation of new blood vessels. In cases where the inflammation is not resolved, the process can result in tissue damage and fibrosis as in rheumatoid arthritis, atherosclerosis, organ fibrosis, diabetes and even obesity [100]. Cancer can be added to this list since it has been likened to "a wound that does not heal" [101]. The role of inflammatory cytokines in tumor progression [102-106] explains why inflammatory bowel disease and viral hepatitis can progress to cancer [107].

10. ATX in malignancy: Metastasis and angiogenesis

ATX is among the top 40 upregulated genes in metastatic cancer [108] and this is explained by the effects of LPA, which signals through at least six and putatively eight G-protein-coupled receptors. Through these receptors, LPA stimulates cell motility, cell survival/viability, cell proliferation, morphological changes, contraction, wound healing and invasion [109-118]. LPA achieves these effects by signaling through the relative activations of phosphatidylinositol 3-kinase (PI3K), $ERK_{1/2}$, mTOR, Ca^{2+}-transients, Rac, Rho and Ras [119].

The involvement of ATX and LPA in tumor progression affects multiple malignant processes and stages of tumor progression. For example, LPA increases the production of vascular endothelial growth factor, which stimulates angiogenesis [51, 120], a process required for tumor growth beyond 1 mm. However, in order for tumors to arise at all, tumor suppressors must be made ineffective. LPA levels can rise to 10 μM in the ascites fluid from advanced ovarian cancer patients [121]. Interestingly, LPA also decreases the abundance of the tumor suppressor, p53 [122], thus increasing cancer cell survival and proliferation, even in the presence of actinomycin D.

Pre-clinical models of disease and clinical pathology provide insight into the role of ATX and LPA receptors in cancer. For example, transgenic multiparous mice designed to overexpress ATX, LPA_1, LPA_2 or LPA_3 in mammary epithelium develop spontaneous metastatic mammary tumors as they age [123]. Women who express high levels of LPA_3 receptors in epithelial cells, or ATX in stromal cells, have larger breast tumors, nodal involvement, and higher stages of disease [124]. Since many early stage breast cancer patients are able to be cured using current treatment modalities, this suggests that the presence of ATX and/or LPA receptors has the ability to alter outcomes of malignancy.

The involvement of ATX and LPA in tumor progression can be understood in terms of a dysfunctional wound healing response. As mentioned above, one of the main functions of ATX in adults is to repair damaged tissue. ATX is secreted in this situation partly in response to inflammation and the release of inflammatory cytokines. In normal wound healing, the production of LPA by ATX causes cells to migrate into the area of damage to effect wound repair and the formation of new blood vessels. Cancer can be considered to be a case of unresolved inflammation and it has been likened to "a wound that does not heal" [101]. In fact, inflammation is now considered to be one of the "Hallmarks of Cancer" [125]. The secretion of ATX and increased LPA signaling should now be included as one of the inflammatory factors that drives tumor progression.

The role of ATX and LPA in this process is well illustrated in the case of work with mouse models of breast cancer. Most breast cancer cells do not themselves express ATX, but rather this is produced by fibroblasts within the breast tissue or by the surrounding adipose tissue [33] (Figure 3). The development of the breast tumor causes the release of inflammatory cytokines, which stimulate fibroblasts and adipose tissue to secrete ATX in a syngeneic orthotopic mouse model of breast cancer [33, 107]. This is part of a vicious cycle since LPA in turn stimulates the production of inflammatory cytokines [126-128]. This inflammatory cycle can be effectively blocked in a mouse by inhibiting ATX activity with ONO-8430506, which results in about a 60% decrease in tumor growth and lung metastasis.

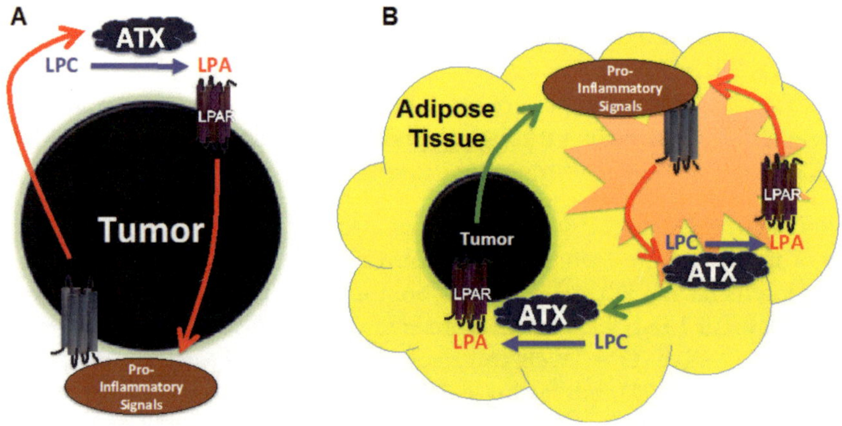

Figure 3. Proposed inflammatory-mediated models of ATX secretion. A) In cancer cells that overexpress ATX such as thyroid cancers, neuroblastomas and melanomas, autocrine-secreted ATX produces LPA, which signals through LPA receptors (LPARs) on the cancer cell surface. This signaling further increases the production of pro-inflammatory signals including growth factors, cytokines and chemokines. These molecules in turn can signal through specific receptors to increase ATX production. B) In breast cancer, a paracrine model of ATX secretion is possible since breast adipose tissue secretes high levels of ATX, whereas breast cancer cells normally produce negligible ATX. As the tumor grows, pro-inflammatory signals secreted by the tumor create an inflammatory environment within the surrounding adipose tissue (green arrows). This signaling increases ATX secretion and LPA production, which in turn can establish an autocrine feedback loop of increased pro-inflammatory signaling and ATX production (red arrows) within the adipose tissue. Increased ATX and LPA production can in turn contribute to tumor progression (green arrows). A combination of both autocrine and paracrine production of ATX is also possible when cancer cells produce significant quantities of ATX.

Although breast cancer cells do not do not express significant levels of ATX activity, this is not typical of other tumors where ATX activity is expressed in the cancer cells themselves. These cancers include thyroid [129], neuroblastomas [71, 130, 131] and melanomas [132-134]. However, in the case of melanomas, their normal predecessor cells, melanocytes, do not express ATX. Thus, the data suggests that ATX expression is acquired during the transition to malignancy in melanoma [2]. The secretion of inflammatory cytokines by cells in the tumor also produces a vicious cycle of ATX secretion and LPA production, which is a driving force

http://dx.doi.org/10.5772/59013

in tumor progression [107]. In the case of breast tumors, we propose that the ATX come from surrounding adipose tissue, whereas in thyroid tumors, neuroblastomas and melanomas, ATX is secreted by the cancer cells (Figure 3).

11. ATX in chemo-resistance

Another important role of ATX expression and LPA signaling in malignancy occurs during the acquisition and manifestation of chemo-resistance. LPA facilitates chemo-resistance to the cytotoxic effects mediated by Taxol [119, 135, 136], doxorubicin [57], actinomycin D [122] and carboplatin [137]. These effects are mediated by LPA partly through activation of survival and viability pathways, such as ERK and PI3K. In addition, we previously demonstrated that LPA signaling does not encompass the entire molecular mechanism and there are other proteins, like the Regulators of G-protein Signaling proteins, which play a more dominant role [138]. Indeed, in the absence of appropriate Regulators of G-protein Signaling proteins, cells exposed to LPA have increased capacity to acquire chemo-resistance.

As chemo-resistance is a complex process, there are other molecular mechanisms involved. For example, among chemo-resistant cells, increased expression of multidrug resistance transporters enables toxins, like chemotherapeutic drugs, to be exported out of cancer cells. This is particularly problematic in the case of renal cell carcinomas, for which cytotoxic chemotherapy is largely ineffective, but also occurs widely in malignancy.

Recent work shows that the activation of PI3K by through LPA_1 receptors increases the stability of the transcription factor Nrf2, which increases the expression of antioxidant genes and multidrug resistant transporters [57]. The expression of antioxidant genes protects cancer cells against the oxidative damage caused by chemotherapeutic agents. Also, the expression of multidrug resistant transporters enables toxic oxidative products and chemotherapeutic drugs to be exported out of cancer cells. These effects explain why inhibiting ATX activity and blocking LPA signaling improves the efficacy of doxorubicin as a chemotherapeutic agent [57]. Thus blocking ATX activity can provide a novel adjuvant therapy for improving the efficacy of existing chemotherapeutic agents.

ATX inhibition could also have a beneficial effect as an adjuvant for improving the effects of radiotherapy as discussed above. This is possible since LPA, through activation of LPA_2 receptors, also protects against radiation-induced cell death. This action depends on the depletion Siva-1, which is a pro-apoptotic signaling protein [139].

The function of ATX in aggravating resistance to chemotherapy and radiotherapy can be understood in terms of the vicious cycle of inflammation caused by repeated bouts of therapy as described above [140] (Figure 3). Cancer therapy itself causes damage to the tumor and surrounding tissue, which responds by producing inflammatory cytokines resulting in increased ATX production [107]. This explains why blocking this cycle by inhibiting LPA formation can improve the sensitivity to chemotherapy by attenuating the effects of increased Nrf2 expression.

12. ATX in melanoma

Although accumulating studies suggest that inhibiting ATX activity could provide a novel adjuvant therapy for improving the efficacy of existing chemotherapeutic agents, we have previously demonstrated a role for ATX inhibitors as monotherapy against advanced cutaneous melanoma [2,48,59]. After injecting B16F10 metastatic melanoma cells into the tail veins of C57/Bl6 mice, we observed a significant reduction in the number of lung nodules, which represent metastatic melanoma tumors, after treatment with a phosphonothionate analogue of carba cyclic phosphatidic acid, thio-ccPA 18:1 [2]. This compound was synthesized for improved metabolic stability and activity, based on our previous results [48]. In addition to being an inhibitor of ATX, thio-ccPA 18:1 is a direct antagonist of LPA_1 and LPA_3 receptors [141].

As mentioned previously, melanomas are notoriously resistant to chemotherapy. In light of the role of ATX/LPA signaling in melanoma, perhaps it should not be surprising that melanoma cells, which produce high quantities of ATX, are resistant to chemotherapy, since excessive LPA signaling contributes to this phenotype. Only a few chemotherapy agents are approved options against melanoma, these include dacarbazine and temozolomide. Thus, we compared these single agents against both the anti-BrP-LPA and the mixed diastereomers BrP-LPA on the viability of MeWo melanoma cells. Indeed, both BrP-LPA compounds were more effective single-agents at 10 μM and 100 μM than either dacarbazine or temozolomide, at concentration ranging from 10-1000 μM [59]. This suggests that targeted approaches against ATX in melanoma have potential and further results will be reported in due time.

Besides cutaneous melanoma, in a study on uveal melanoma, ATX was the only gene among 32 candidate genes whose expression was sufficient to distinguish classes representing metastasis and prognosis. Paradoxically, "underexpression" of ATX correlated with poor prognosis and metastatic death among 27 samples [132]. Based on the discussion provided above it is tempting to propose that melanocytes evolved to survive solar ultraviolet radiation and simultaneously provide protection to neighboring cells by producing ATX and thus providing LPA. However, with repeated DNA damage and incomplete repair from excessive UV radiation, melanocytes are malignantly transformed into melanoma cells. At this point, the increased production of ATX and signaling by inflammatory cytokines, which are meant to facilitate repair, could be subverted into promoting cancer progression.

13. Summary and conclusions

Advanced metastatic melanoma is an incurable disease in dire need of additional therapeutic options. Although many newly targeted inhibitors have extended the life of patients with *BRAF* mutations, they do not achieve cure due to chemo-resistance, and they are not applicable to patients with Wild-type B-Raf. Thus, additional therapeutics are desperately needed to treat this growing population. Herein we have summarized the current state of ATX inhibitors and what we currently know about the role of ATX in melanoma and malignancy.

The original ATX inhibitors had little utility *in vivo* because of the very low bioavailability. However, as described above, potent ATX inhibitors are now being developed, which are

http://dx.doi.org/10.5772/59013

effective *in vivo* for longer than 24 h. These inhibitors appear to be well tolerated by animals and the next stage is to take such inhibitors through Phase 1 clinical trials. These ATX inhibitors should be effective in improving the outcomes for which the ATX/LPA axis is involved. These include various forms of cancer whereby an ATX inhibitor could be used as a monotherapy or as an adjuvant to improve existing chemotherapies or radiation treatment. The ATX inhibitors should also be effective in improving the treatment of a variety of inflammatory conditions. These compounds deserve further examination.

Acknowledgements

This work was supported by research grants from the National Institutes of Health (1R15CA151006-01 American Recovery and Reinvestment Act and 1R15CA176653-01A1), a Research Scholar Grant 120634-RSG-11-269-01-CDD from the American Cancer Society and a Distinguished Scientist award from the Georgia Research Alliance to MMM. MGKB received a Vanier Canada Graduate Scholarship from the Government of Canada, a Killam Trust Award and an MD/PhD scholarship from Alberta Innovates-Health Solutions. DNB was supported by grants from the Canadian Breast Cancer Foundation, Women and Children's Health Research Institute of the University of Alberta and CIHR with the Alberta Cancer Foundation. DNB declares a conflict of interest in having received a consulting fee from Ono Pharmaceuticals.

Author details

David N. Brindley[1], Matthew G.K. Benesch[1] and Mandi M. Murph[2*]

*Address all correspondence to: mmurph@uga.edu

1 Signal Transduction Research Group, Department of Biochemistry, University of Alberta, Heritage Medical Research Center, Edmonton, Alberta, Canada

2 Department of Pharmaceutical and Biomedical Sciences, The University of Georgia, College of Pharmacy, Athens, Georgia, USA

References

[1] Stracke ML, Krutzsch HC, Unsworth EJ, Arestad A, Cioce V, Schiffmann E, Liotta LA (1992) Identification, purification, and partial sequence analysis of autotaxin, a novel motility-stimulating protein. J Biol Chem 267: 2524-2529.

[2] Altman MK, Gopal V, Jia W, Yu S, Hall H, Mills GB, McGinnis AC, Bartlett MG, Jiang G, Madan D, Prestwich GD, Xu Y, Davies MA, Murph MM (2010) Targeting melanoma growth and viability reveals dualistic functionality of the phosphonothionate analogue of carba cyclic phosphatidic acid. Mol Cancer 9: 140.

[3] Hashimoto T, Okudaira S, Igarashi K, Hama K, Yatomi Y, Aoki J (2012) Identification and biochemical characterization of a novel autotaxin isoform, ATXdelta, with a four-amino acid deletion. J Biochem 151: 89-97.

[4] Boutin JA, Ferry G (2009) Autotaxin. Cell Mol Life Sci 66: 3009-3021.

[5] Hausmann J, Perrakis A, Moolenaar WH (2013) Structure-function relationships of autotaxin, a secreted lysophospholipase D. Adv Biol Regul 53: 112-117.

[6] Jansen S, Stefan C, Creemers JW, Waelkens E, Van Eynde A, Stalmans W, Bollen M (2005) Proteolytic maturation and activation of autotaxin (NPP2), a secreted metastasis-enhancing lysophospholipase D. J Cell Sci 118: 3081-3089.

[7] Koike S, Keino-Masu K, Ohto T, Masu M (2006) The N-terminal hydrophobic sequence of autotaxin (ENPP2) functions as a signal peptide. Genes Cells 11: 133-142.

[8] Houben AJ, van Wijk XM, van Meeteren LA, van Zeijl L, van de Westerlo EM, Hausmann J, Fish A, Perrakis A, van Kuppevelt TH, Moolenaar WH (2013) The polybasic insertion in autotaxin alpha confers specific binding to heparin and cell surface heparan sulfate proteoglycans. J Biol Chem 288: 510-519.

[9] Hausmann J, Kamtekar S, Christodoulou E, Day JE, Wu T, Fulkerson Z, Albers HM, van Meeteren LA, Houben AJ, van Zeijl L, Jansen S, Andries M, Hall T, Pegg LE, Benson TE, Kasiem M, Harlos K, Kooi CW, Smyth SS, Ovaa H, Bollen M, Morris AJ, Moolenaar WH, Perrakis A (2011) Structural basis of substrate discrimination and integrin binding by autotaxin. Nat Struct Mol Biol 18: 198-204.

[10] Pamuklar Z, Federico L, Liu S, Umezu-Goto M, Dong A, Panchatcharam M, Fulkerson Z, Berdyshev E, Natarajan V, Fang X, van Meeteren LA, Moolenaar WH, Mills GB, Morris AJ, Smyth SS (2009) Autotaxin/lysopholipase D and lysophosphatidic acid regulate murine hemostasis and thrombosis. J Biol Chem 284: 7385-7394.

[11] Fulkerson Z, Wu T, Sunkara M, Kooi CV, Morris AJ, Smyth SS (2011) Binding of autotaxin to integrins localizes lysophosphatidic acid production to platelets and mammalian cells. J Biol Chem 286: 34654-34663.

[12] Wu T, Vander Kooi C, Shah P, Charnigo R, Huang C, Smyth SS, Morris AJ (2013) Integrin-mediated cell surface recruitment of autotaxin promotes persistent directional cell migration. FASEB J: 10.1096/fj.1013-229211.

[13] Clair T, Lee HY, Liotta LA, Stracke ML (1997) Autotaxin is an exoenzyme possessing 5'-nucleotide phosphodiesterase/ATP pyrophosphatase and ATPase activities. J Biol Chem 272: 996-1001.

[14] Albright RA, Chang WC, Robert D, Ornstein DL, Cao W, Liu L, Redick ME, Young JI, De La Cruz EM, Braddock DT (2012) NPP4 is a procoagulant enzyme on the surface of vascular endothelium. Blood 120: 4432-4440.

[15] Stefan C, Gijsbers R, Stalmans W, Bollen M (1999) Differential regulation of the expression of nucleotide pyrophosphatases/phosphodiesterases in rat liver. Biochim Biophys Acta 1450: 45-52.

[16] Albright RA, Ornstein DL, Cao W, Chang WC, Robert D, Tehan M, Hoyer D, Liu L, Stabach P, Yang G, De La Cruz EM, Braddock DT (2014) Molecular basis of purinergic signal metabolism by ectonucleotide pyrophosphatase/phosphodiesterases 4 and 1 and implications in stroke. J Biol Chem 289: 3294-3306.

[17] Sakagami H, Aoki J, Natori Y, Nishikawa K, Kakehi Y, Natori Y, Arai H (2005) Biochemical and molecular characterization of a novel choline-specific glycerophosphodiester phosphodiesterase belonging to the nucleotide pyrophosphatase/ phosphodiesterase family. J Biol Chem 280: 23084-23093.

[18] Duan RD, Bergman T, Xu N, Wu J, Cheng Y, Duan J, Nelander S, Palmberg C, Nilsson A (2003) Identification of human intestinal alkaline sphingomyelinase as a novel ecto-enzyme related to the nucleotide phosphodiesterase family. J Biol Chem 278: 38528-38536.

[19] Lee HY, Clair T, Mulvaney PT, Woodhouse EC, Aznavoorian S, Liotta LA, Stracke ML (1996) Stimulation of tumor cell motility linked to phosphodiesterase catalytic site of autotaxin. J Biol Chem 271: 24408-24412.

[20] Lee HY, Bae GU, Jung ID, Lee JS, Kim YK, Noh SH, Stracke ML, Park CG, Lee HW, Han JW (2002) Autotaxin promotes motility via G protein-coupled phosphoinositide 3-kinase gamma in human melanoma cells. FEBS Lett 515: 137-140.

[21] Nam SW, Clair T, Campo CK, Lee HY, Liotta LA, Stracke ML (2000) Autotaxin (ATX), a potent tumor motogen, augments invasive and metastatic potential of ras-transformed cells. Oncogene 19: 241-247.

[22] Brindley DN (1993) Hepatic secretion of lysphosphatidylcholine: a novel transport system for polyunsaturated fatty acids and choline. J Nutr Biochem 4: 442-449.

[23] Mangiapane EH, Brindley DN (1986) Effects of dexamethasone and insulin on the synthesis of triacylglycerols and phosphatidylcholine and the secretion of very-low-density lipoproteins and lysophosphatidylcholine by monolayer cultures of rat hepatocytes. Biochem J 233: 151-160.

[24] Graham A, Bennett AJ, McLean AA, Zammit VA, Brindley DN (1988) Factors regulating the secretion of lysophosphatidylcholine by rat hepatocytes compared with the synthesis and secretion of phosphatidylcholine and triacylglycerol. Effects of albumin, cycloheximide, verapamil, EGTA and chlorpromazine. Biochem J 253: 687-692.

[25] Graham A, Zammit VA, Brindley DN (1988) Fatty acid specificity for the synthesis of triacylglycerol and phosphatidylcholine and for the secretion of very-low-density lip-

oproteins and lysophosphatidylcholine by cultures of rat hepatocytes. Biochem J 249: 727-733.

[26] Graham A, Zammit VA, Christie WW, Brindley DN (1991) Sexual dimorphism in the preferential secretion of unsaturated lysophosphatidylcholine by rat hepatocytes but no secretion by sheep hepatocytes. Biochim Biophys Acta 1081: 151-158.

[27] Saulnier-Blache JS (2004) [Lysophosphatidic acid: a "bioactive" phospholipid]. Med Sci (Paris) 20: 799-803.

[28] van Meeteren LA, Ruurs P, Stortelers C, Bouwman P, van Rooijen MA, Pradere JP, Pettit TR, Wakelam MJ, Saulnier-Blache JS, Mummery CL, Moolenaar WH, Jonkers J (2006) Autotaxin, a secreted lysophospholipase D, is essential for blood vessel formation during development. Mol Cell Biol 26: 5015-5022.

[29] Tanaka M, Okudaira S, Kishi Y, Ohkawa R, Iseki S, Ota M, Noji S, Yatomi Y, Aoki J, Arai H (2006) Autotaxin stabilizes blood vessels and is required for embryonic vasculature by producing lysophosphatidic acid. J Biol Chem 281: 25822-25830.

[30] Gierse J, Thorarensen A, Beltey K, Bradshaw-Pierce E, Cortes-Burgos L, Hall T, Johnston A, Murphy M, Nemirovskiy O, Ogawa S, Pegg L, Pelc M, Prinsen M, Schnute M, Wendling J, Wene S, Weinberg R, Wittwer A, Zweifel B, Masferrer J (2010) A novel autotaxin inhibitor reduces lysophosphatidic acid levels in plasma and the site of inflammation. J Pharmacol Exp Ther 334: 310-317.

[31] Albers HM, Dong A, van Meeteren LA, Egan DA, Sunkara M, van Tilburg EW, Schuurman K, van Tellingen O, Morris AJ, Smyth SS, Moolenaar WH, Ovaa H (2010) Boronic acid-based inhibitor of autotaxin reveals rapid turnover of LPA in the circulation. Proc Natl Acad Sci U S A 107: 7257-7262.

[32] Ferry G, Moulharat N, Pradere JP, Desos P, Try A, Genton A, Giganti A, Beucher-Gaudin M, Lonchampt M, Bertrand M, Saulnier-Blache JS, Tucker GC, Cordi A, Boutin JA (2008) S32826, a nanomolar inhibitor of autotaxin: discovery, synthesis and applications as a pharmacological tool. J Pharmacol Exp Ther 327: 809-819.

[33] Benesch MGK, Tang X, Maeda T, Ohhata A, Zhao YY, Kok BPC, Dewald J, Hitt M, Curtis JM, McMullen TPW, Brindley DN (2014) Inhibition of autotaxin delays breast tumor growth and lung metastasis in mice. FASEB J 28: 2655-2666.

[34] Nishimasu H, Okudaira S, Hama K, Mihara E, Dohmae N, Inoue A, Ishitani R, Takagi J, Aoki J, Nureki O (2011) Crystal structure of autotaxin and insight into GPCR activation by lipid mediators. Nat Struct Mol Biol 18: 205-212.

[35] Fourcade O, Simon MF, Viode C, Rugani N, Leballe F, Ragab A, Fournie B, Sarda L, Chap H (1995) Secretory phospholipase A2 generates the novel lipid mediator lysophosphatidic acid in membrane microvesicles shed from activated cells. Cell 80: 919-927.

[36] Sano T, Baker D, Virag T, Wada A, Yatomi Y, Kobayashi T, Igarashi Y, Tigyi G (2002) Multiple mechanisms linked to platelet activation result in lysophosphatidic acid and sphingosine 1-phosphate generation in blood. J Biol Chem 277: 21197-21206.

[37] Li H, Zhao Z, Wei G, Yan L, Wang D, Zhang H, Sandusky GE, Turk J, Xu Y (2010) Group VIA phospholipase A2 in both host and tumor cells is involved in ovarian cancer development. FASEB J.

[38] Tabchy A, Tigyi G, Mills GB (2011) Location, location, location: a crystal-clear view of autotaxin saturating LPA receptors. Nat Struct Mol Biol 18: 117-118.

[39] Federico L, Pamuklar Z, Smyth SS, Morris AJ (2008) Therapeutic potential of autotaxin/lysophospholipase d inhibitors. Curr Drug Targets 9: 698-708.

[40] Albers HM, Ovaa H (2012) Chemical evolution of autotaxin inhibitors. Chem Rev 112: 2593-2603.

[41] Barbayianni E, Magrioti V, Moutevelis-Minakakis P, Kokotos G (2013) Autotaxin inhibitors: a patent review. Expert Opin Ther Pat 23: 1123-1132.

[42] Clair T, Koh E, Ptaszynska M, Bandle RW, Liotta LA, Schiffmann E, Stracke ML (2005) L-histidine inhibits production of lysophosphatidic acid by the tumor-associated cytokine, autotaxin. Lipids Health Dis 4: 5.

[43] El-Batch M, Ibrahim W, Said S (2011) Effect of histidine on autotaxin activity in experimentally induced liver fibrosis. J Biochem Mol Toxicol 25: 143-150.

[44] Xia Q, Deng AM, Wu SS, Zheng M (2011) Cholera toxin inhibits human hepatocarcinoma cell proliferation in vitro via suppressing ATX/LPA axis. Acta Pharmacol Sin 32: 1055-1062.

[45] Kehlen A, Lauterbach R, Santos AN, Thiele K, Kabisch U, Weber E, Riemann D, Langner J (2001) IL-1 beta-and IL-4-induced down-regulation of autotaxin mRNA and PC-1 in fibroblast-like synoviocytes of patients with rheumatoid arthritis (RA). Clin Exp Immunol 123: 147-154.

[46] Sumida H, Nakamura K, Yanagida K, Ohkawa R, Asano Y, Kadono T, Tamaki K, Igarashi K, Aoki J, Sato S, Ishii S, Shimizu T, Yatomi Y (2013) Decrease in circulating autotaxin by oral administration of prednisolone. Clin Chim Acta 415: 74-80.

[47] Kremer AE, van Dijk R, Leckie P, Schaap FG, Kuiper EM, Mettang T, Reiners KS, Raap U, van Buuren HR, van Erpecum KJ, Davies NA, Rust C, Engert A, Jalan R, Oude Elferink RP, Beuers U (2012) Serum autotaxin is increased in pruritus of cholestasis, but not of other origin, and responds to therapeutic interventions. Hepatology 56: 1391-1400.

[48] Baker DL, Fujiwara Y, Pigg KR, Tsukahara R, Kobayashi S, Murofushi H, Uchiyama A, Murakami-Murofushi K, Koh E, Bandle RW, Byun HS, Bittman R, Fan D, Murph M, Mills GB, Tigyi G (2006) Carba analogs of cyclic phosphatidic acid are selective

inhibitors of autotaxin and cancer cell invasion and metastasis. J Biol Chem 281: 22786-22793.

[49] Kakiuchi Y, Nagai J, Gotoh M, Hotta H, Murofushi H, Ogawa T, Ueda H, Murakami-Murofushi K (2011) Antinociceptive effect of cyclic phosphatidic acid and its derivative on animal models of acute and chronic pain. Mol Pain 7: 1744-8069.

[50] Zhang H, Xu X, Gajewiak J, Tsukahara R, Fujiwara Y, Liu J, Fells JI, Perygin D, Parrill AL, Tigyi G, Prestwich GD (2009) Dual activity lysophosphatidic acid receptor pan-antagonist/autotaxin inhibitor reduces breast cancer cell migration in vitro and causes tumor regression in vivo. Cancer Res 69: 5441-5449.

[51] Xu X, Prestwich GD (2010) Inhibition of tumor growth and angiogenesis by a lysophosphatidic acid antagonist in an engineered three-dimensional lung cancer xenograft model. Cancer 116: 1739-1750.

[52] Schleicher SM, Thotala DK, Linkous AG, Hu R, Leahy KM, Yazlovitskaya EM, Hallahan DE (2011) Autotaxin and LPA receptors represent potential molecular targets for the radiosensitization of murine glioma through effects on tumor vasculature. PLoS One 6: e22182.

[53] Nikitopoulou I, Kaffe E, Sevastou I, Sirioti I, Samiotaki M, Madan D, Prestwich GD, Aidinis V (2013) A metabolically-stabilized phosphonate analog of lysophosphatidic acid attenuates collagen-induced arthritis. PLoS One 8: e70941.

[54] Park GY, Lee YG, Berdyshev E, Nyenhuis S, Du J, Fu P, Gorshkova IA, Li Y, Chung S, Karpurapu M, Deng J, Ranjan R, Xiao L, Jaffe HA, Corbridge SJ, Kelly EA, Jarjour NN, Chun J, Prestwich GD, Kaffe E, Ninou I, Aidinis V, Morris AJ, Smyth SS, Ackerman SJ, Natarajan V, Christman JW (2013) Autotaxin production of lysophosphatidic Acid mediates allergic asthmatic inflammation. Am J Respir Crit Care Med 188: 928-940.

[55] Oikonomou N, Mouratis MA, Tzouvelekis A, Kaffe E, Valavanis C, Vilaras G, Karameris A, Prestwich GD, Bouros D, Aidinis V (2012) Pulmonary autotaxin expression contributes to the pathogenesis of pulmonary fibrosis. Am J Respir Cell Mol Biol 47: 566-574.

[56] Bhave SR, Dadey DY, Karvas RM, Ferraro DJ, Kotipatruni RP, Jaboin JJ, Hallahan AN, Dewees TA, Linkous AG, Hallahan DE, Thotala D (2013) Autotaxin Inhibition with PF-8380 Enhances the Radiosensitivity of Human and Murine Glioblastoma Cell Lines. Front Oncol 3: 00236.

[57] Venkatraman G, Benesch MGK, Tang X, Dewald J, McMullen TPW, Brindley DN (2014) Lysophosphatidate signalling stabilizes Nrf2 and increases the expression of genes involved in drug resistance and oxidative stress responses: Implications for cancer treatment. FASEB J: Under Review.

[58] Saga H, Ohhata A, Hayashi A, Katoh M, Maeda T, Mizuno H, Takada Y, Komichi Y, Ota H, Matsumura N, Shibaya M, Sugiyama T, Nakade S, Kishikawa K (2014) A nov-

el highly potent autotaxin/ENPP2 inhibitor produces prolonged decreases in plasma lysophosphatidic acid formation in vivo and regulates urethral tension. PLoS One 9: e93230.

[59] Nguyen D, Nguyen O, Zhang H, Prestwich GD, Murph MM (2011) A Bromophosphonate Analogue of Lysophosphatidic Acid Surpasses Dacarbazine in Reducing Cell Proliferation and Viability of MeWo Melanoma Cells. In: Murph MM, editor. Research on Melanoma-A Glimpse into Current Directions and Future Trends: InTech.

[60] Jiang G, Madan D, Prestwich GD (2011) Aromatic phosphonates inhibit the lysophospholipase D activity of autotaxin. Bioorg Med Chem Lett 21: 5098-5101.

[61] North EJ, Howard AL, Wanjala IW, Pham TC, Baker DL, Parrill AL (2010) Pharmacophore development and application toward the identification of novel, small-molecule autotaxin inhibitors. J Med Chem 53: 3095-3105.

[62] Ferguson CG, Bigman CS, Richardson RD, van Meeteren LA, Moolenaar WH, Prestwich GD (2006) Fluorogenic phospholipid substrate to detect lysophospholipase D/autotaxin activity. Org Lett 8: 2023-2026.

[63] Saunders LP, Ouellette A, Bandle R, Chang WC, Zhou H, Misra RN, De La Cruz EM, Braddock DT (2008) Identification of small-molecule inhibitors of autotaxin that inhibit melanoma cell migration and invasion. Mol Cancer Ther 7: 3352-3362.

[64] Parrill AL, Echols U, Nguyen T, Pham TC, Hoeglund A, Baker DL (2008) Virtual screening approaches for the identification of non-lipid autotaxin inhibitors. Bioorg Med Chem 16: 1784-1795.

[65] Mize CD, Abbott AM, Gacasan SB, Parrill AL, Baker DL (2011) Ligand-based autotaxin pharmacophore models reflect structure-based docking results. J Mol Graph Model 31: 76-86.

[66] Kawaguchi M, Okabe T, Okudaira S, Nishimasu H, Ishitani R, Kojima H, Nureki O, Aoki J, Nagano T (2013) Screening and X-ray crystal structure-based optimization of autotaxin (ENPP2) inhibitors, using a newly developed fluorescence probe. ACS Chem Biol 8: 1713-1721.

[67] Fells JI, Lee SC, Norman DD, Tsukahara R, Kirby RJ, Nelson S, Seibel W, Papoian R, Patil R, Miller DD, Parrill AL, Pham T-C, Baker DL, Bittman R, Tigyi G (2013) Targeting the Hydrophobic Pocket of Autotaxin with Virtual Screening of Inhibitors Identifies a Common Aromatic Sulfonamide Structural Motif. FEBS Journal 281: 1017-1028.

[68] Fells JI, Lee SC, Fujiwara Y, Norman DD, Lim KG, Tsukahara R, Liu J, Patil R, Miller DD, Kirby RJ, Nelson S, Seibel W, Papoian R, Parrill AL, Baker DL, Bittman R, Tigyi G (2013) Hits of a high-throughput screen identify the hydrophobic pocket of autotaxin/lysophospholipase D as an inhibitory surface. Mol Pharmacol 84: 415-424.

[69] Nam SW, Clair T, Kim YS, McMarlin A, Schiffmann E, Liotta LA, Stracke ML (2001) Autotaxin (NPP-2), a metastasis-enhancing motogen, is an angiogenic factor. Cancer Res 61: 6938-6944.

[70] Bachner D, Ahrens M, Betat N, Schroder D, Gross G (1999) Developmental expression analysis of murine autotaxin (ATX). Mech Dev 84: 121-125.

[71] Kishi Y, Okudaira S, Tanaka M, Hama K, Shida D, Kitayama J, Yamori T, Aoki J, Fujimaki T, Arai H (2006) Autotaxin is overexpressed in glioblastoma multiforme and contributes to cell motility of glioblastoma by converting lysophosphatidylcholine to lysophosphatidic acid. J Biol Chem 281: 17492-17500.

[72] Yukiura H, Hama K, Nakanaga K, Tanaka M, Asaoka Y, Okudaira S, Arima N, Inoue A, Hashimoto T, Arai H, Kawahara A, Nishina H, Aoki J (2011) Autotaxin regulates vascular development via multiple lysophosphatidic acid (LPA) receptors in zebrafish. J Biol Chem 286: 43972-43983.

[73] Moolenaar WH, Houben AJ, Lee SJ, van Meeteren LA (2013) Autotaxin in embryonic development. Biochim Biophys Acta 1831: 13-19.

[74] Yuelling LW, Waggener CT, Afshari FS, Lister JA, Fuss B (2012) Autotaxin/ENPP2 regulates oligodendrocyte differentiation in vivo in the developing zebrafish hindbrain. Glia 60: 1605-1618.

[75] Lai SL, Yao WL, Tsao KC, Houben AJ, Albers HM, Ovaa H, Moolenaar WH, Lee SJ (2012) Autotaxin/Lpar3 signaling regulates Kupffer's vesicle formation and left-right asymmetry in zebrafish. Development 139: 4439-4448.

[76] Rother E, Brandl R, Baker DL, Goyal P, Gebhard H, Tigyi G, Siess W (2003) Subtype-selective antagonists of lysophosphatidic Acid receptors inhibit platelet activation triggered by the lipid core of atherosclerotic plaques. Circulation 108: 741-747.

[77] Rancoule C, Attane C, Gres S, Fournel A, Dusaulcy R, Bertrand C, Vinel C, Treguer K, Prentki M, Valet P, Saulnier-Blache JS (2013) Lysophosphatidic acid impairs glucose homeostasis and inhibits insulin secretion in high-fat diet obese mice. Diabetologia 56: 1394-1402.

[78] Ferry G, Tellier E, Try A, Gres S, Naime I, Simon MF, Rodriguez M, Boucher J, Tack I, Gesta S, Chomarat P, Dieu M, Raes M, Galizzi JP, Valet P, Boutin JA, Saulnier-Blache JS (2003) Autotaxin is released from adipocytes, catalyzes lysophosphatidic acid synthesis, and activates preadipocyte proliferation. Up-regulated expression with adipocyte differentiation and obesity. J Biol Chem 278: 18162-18169.

[79] Federico L, Ren H, Mueller PA, Wu T, Liu S, Popovic J, Blalock EM, Sunkara M, Ovaa H, Albers HM, Mills GB, Morris AJ, Smyth SS (2012) Autotaxin and its product lysophosphatidic acid suppress brown adipose differentiation and promote diet-induced obesity in mice. Mol Endocrinol 26: 786-797.

[80] Nishimura S, Nagasaki M, Okudaira S, Aoki J, Ohmori T, Ohkawa R, Nakamura K, Igarashi K, Yamashita H, Eto K, Uno K, Hayashi N, Kadowaki T, Komuro I, Yatomi

Y, Nagai R (2014) ENPP2 contributes to adipose tissue expansion in diet-induced obesity. Diabetes: doi: 10.2337/db2313-1694.

[81] Rancoule C, Dusaulcy R, Treguer K, Gres S, Attane C, Saulnier-Blache JS (2014) Involvement of autotaxin/lysophosphatidic acid signaling in obesity and impaired glucose homeostasis. Biochimie 96: 140-143.

[82] Dusaulcy R, Rancoule C, Gres S, Wanecq E, Colom A, Guigne C, van Meeteren LA, Moolenaar WH, Valet P, Saulnier-Blache JS (2011) Adipose-specific disruption of autotaxin enhances nutritional fattening and reduces plasma lysophosphatidic acid. J Lipid Res 52: 1247-1255.

[83] Mazereeuw-Hautier J, Gres S, Fanguin M, Cariven C, Fauvel J, Perret B, Chap H, Salles JP, Saulnier-Blache JS (2005) Production of lysophosphatidic acid in blister fluid: involvement of a lysophospholipase D activity. J Invest Dermatol 125: 421-427.

[84] Tokumura A, Taira S, Kikuchi M, Tsutsumi T, Shimizu Y, Watsky MA (2012) Lysophospholipids and lysophospholipase D in rabbit aqueous humor following corneal injury. Prostaglandins Other Lipid Mediat 97: 83-89.

[85] Masuda K, Haruta S, Orino K, Kawaminami M, Kurusu S (2013) Autotaxin as a novel, tissue-remodeling-related factor in regressing corpora lutea of cycling rats. FEBS J 280: 6600-6612.

[86] Grisanti L, Rezza A, Clavel C, Sennett R, Rendl M (2013) Enpp2/Autotaxin in dermal papilla precursors is dispensable for hair follicle morphogenesis. J Invest Dermatol 133: 2332-2339.

[87] Mebarek S, Abousalham A, Magne D, Do le D, Bandorowicz-Pikula J, Pikula S, Buchet R (2013) Phospholipases of mineralization competent cells and matrix vesicles: roles in physiological and pathological mineralizations. Int J Mol Sci 14: 5036-5129.

[88] Evseenko D, Latour B, Richardson W, Corselli M, Sahaghian A, Cardinal S, Zhu Y, Chan R, Dunn B, Crooks GM (2013) Lysophosphatidic acid mediates myeloid differentiation within the human bone marrow microenvironment. PLoS One 8: e63718.

[89] Awada R, Rondeau P, Gres S, Saulnier-Blache JS, Lefebvre d'Hellencourt C, Bourdon E (2012) Autotaxin protects microglial cells against oxidative stress. Free Radic Biol Med 52: 516-526.

[90] Awada R, Saulnier-Blache JS, Gres S, Bourdon E, Rondeau P, Parimisetty A, Orihuela R, Harry GJ, d'Hellencourt CL (2014) Autotaxin Downregulates LPS-Induced Microglia Activation and Pro-Inflammatory Cytokines Production. Journal of Cellular Biochemistry: doi: 10.1002/jcb.24889.

[91] Umemoto E, Hayasaka H, Bai Z, Cai L, Yonekura S, Peng X, Takeda A, Tohya K, Miyasaka M (2011) Novel regulators of lymphocyte trafficking across high endothelial venules. Crit Rev Immunol 31: 147-169.

[92] Bai Z, Cai L, Umemoto E, Takeda A, Tohya K, Komai Y, Veeraveedu PT, Hata E, Sugiura Y, Kubo A, Suematsu M, Hayasaka H, Okudaira S, Aoki J, Tanaka T, Albers HM, Ovaa H, Miyasaka M (2013) Constitutive lymphocyte transmigration across the basal lamina of high endothelial venules is regulated by the autotaxin/lysophosphatidic acid axis. J Immunol 190: 2036-2048.

[93] Zhang Y, Chen YC, Krummel MF, Rosen SD (2012) Autotaxin through lysophosphatidic acid stimulates polarization, motility, and transendothelial migration of naive T cells. J Immunol 189: 3914-3924.

[94] Nakasaki T, Tanaka T, Okudaira S, Hirosawa M, Umemoto E, Otani K, Jin S, Bai Z, Hayasaka H, Fukui Y, Aozasa K, Fujita N, Tsuruo T, Ozono K, Aoki J, Miyasaka M (2008) Involvement of the lysophosphatidic acid-generating enzyme autotaxin in lymphocyte-endothelial cell interactions. Am J Pathol 173: 1566-1576.

[95] van Meeteren LA, Moolenaar WH (2007) Regulation and biological activities of the autotaxin-LPA axis. Prog Lipid Res 46: 145-160.

[96] Budd DC, Qian Y (2013) Development of lysophosphatidic acid pathway modulators as therapies for fibrosis. Future Med Chem 5: 1935-1952.

[97] Lee S, Lynch KR (2005) Brown recluse spider (Loxosceles reclusa) venom phospholipase D (PLD) generates lysophosphatidic acid (LPA). Biochem J 391: 317-323.

[98] Borchani L, Sassi A, Ben Gharsa H, Safra I, Shahbazzadeh D, Ben Lasfar Z, El Ayeb M (2013) The pathological effects of Heminecrolysin, a dermonecrotic toxin from Hemiscorpius lepturus scorpion venom are mediated through its lysophospholipase D activity. Toxicon 68: 30-39.

[99] van Meeteren LA, Frederiks F, Giepmans BN, Pedrosa MF, Billington SJ, Jost BH, Tambourgi DV, Moolenaar WH (2004) Spider and bacterial sphingomyelinases D target cellular lysophosphatidic acid receptors by hydrolyzing lysophosphatidylcholine. J Biol Chem 279: 10833-10836.

[100] Krishnamoorthy S, Honn KV (2006) Inflammation and disease progression. Cancer Metastasis Rev 25: 481-491.

[101] Dvorak HF (1986) Tumors: wounds that do not heal. Similarities between tumor stroma generation and wound healing. N Engl J Med 315: 1650-1659.

[102] Allavena P, Garlanda C, Borrello MG, Sica A, Mantovani A (2008) Pathways connecting inflammation and cancer. Curr Opin Genet Dev 18: 3-10.

[103] Chopra M, Riedel SS, Biehl M, Krieger S, von Krosigk V, Bauerlein CA, Brede C, Jordan Garrote AL, Kraus S, Schafer V, Ritz M, Mattenheimer K, Degla A, Mottok A, Einsele H, Wajant H, Beilhack A (2013) Tumor necrosis factor receptor 2-dependent homeostasis of regulatory T cells as a player in TNF-induced experimental metastasis. Carcinogenesis 34: 1296-1303.

[104] Germano G, Allavena P, Mantovani A (2008) Cytokines as a key component of cancer-related inflammation. Cytokine 43: 374-379.

[105] Grivennikov SI (2013) Inflammation and colorectal cancer: colitis-associated neoplasia. Semin Immunopathol 35: 229-244.

[106] Wu JM, Xu Y, Skill NJ, Sheng H, Zhao Z, Yu M, Saxena R, Maluccio MA (2010) Autotaxin expression and its connection with the TNF-alpha-NF-kappaB axis in human hepatocellular carcinoma. Mol Cancer 9: 71.

[107] Benesch MGK, Ko YM, McMullen TPW, Brindley DN (2014) Autotaxin in the crosshairs: Taking aim at cancer and other inflammatory conditions. FEBS Letters 588: 2712-2727.

[108] Euer N, Schwirzke M, Evtimova V, Burtscher H, Jarsch M, Tarin D, Weidle UH (2002) Identification of genes associated with metastasis of mammary carcinoma in metastatic versus non-metastatic cell lines. Anticancer Res 22: 733-740.

[109] Bollen M, Gijsbers R, Ceulemans H, Stalmans W, Stefan C (2000) Nucleotide pyrophosphatases/phosphodiesterases on the move. Crit Rev Biochem Mol Biol 35: 393-432.

[110] Debies MT, Welch DR (2001) Genetic basis of human breast cancer metastasis. J Mammary Gland Biol Neoplasia 6: 441-451.

[111] Brindley DN (2004) Lipid phosphate phosphatases and related proteins: signaling functions in development, cell division, and cancer. J Cell Biochem 92: 900-912.

[112] Moolenaar WH, van Meeteren LA, Giepmans BN (2004) The ins and outs of lysophosphatidic acid signaling. Bioessays 26: 870-881.

[113] Gendaszewska-Darmach E (2008) Lysophosphatidic acids, cyclic phosphatidic acids and autotaxin as promising targets in therapies of cancer and other diseases. Acta Biochim Pol 55: 227-240.

[114] Liu S, Murph M, Panupinthu N, Mills GB (2009) ATX-LPA receptor axis in inflammation and cancer. Cell Cycle 8: 3695-3701.

[115] Panupinthu N, Lee HY, Mills GB (2010) Lysophosphatidic acid production and action: critical new players in breast cancer initiation and progression. Br J Cancer 102: 941-946.

[116] Houben AJ, Moolenaar WH (2011) Autotaxin and LPA receptor signaling in cancer. Cancer Metastasis Rev 30: 557-565.

[117] Gotoh M, Fujiwara Y, Yue J, Liu J, Lee S, Fells J, Uchiyama A, Murakami-Murofushi K, Kennel S, Wall J, Patil R, Gupte R, Balazs L, Miller DD, Tigyi GJ (2012) Controlling cancer through the autotaxin-lysophosphatidic acid receptor axis. Biochem Soc Trans 40: 31-36.

[118] Peyruchaud O, Leblanc R, David M (2013) Pleiotropic activity of lysophosphatidic acid in bone metastasis. Biochim Biophys Acta 1831: 99-104.

[119] Samadi N, Bekele R, Capatos D, Venkatraman G, Sariahmetoglu M, Brindley DN (2011) Regulation of lysophosphatidate signaling by autotaxin and lipid phosphate phosphatases with respect to tumor progression, angiogenesis, metastasis and chemo-resistance. Biochimie 93: 61-70.

[120] So J, Wang FQ, Navari J, Schreher J, Fishman DA (2005) LPA-induced epithelial ovarian cancer (EOC) in vitro invasion and migration are mediated by VEGF receptor-2 (VEGF-R2). Gynecol Oncol 97: 870-878.

[121] Baker DL, Morrison P, Miller B, Riely CA, Tolley B, Westermann AM, Bonfrer JM, Bais E, Moolenaar WH, Tigyi G (2002) Plasma lysophosphatidic acid concentration and ovarian cancer. JAMA 287: 3081-3082.

[122] Murph MM, Hurst-Kennedy J, Newton V, Brindley DN, Radhakrishna H (2007) Lysophosphatidic acid decreases the nuclear localization and cellular abundance of the p53 tumor suppressor in A549 lung carcinoma cells. Mol Cancer Res 5: 1201-1211.

[123] Liu S, Umezu-Goto M, Murph M, Lu Y, Liu W, Zhang F, Yu S, Stephens LC, Cui X, Murrow G, Coombes K, Muller W, Hung MC, Perou CM, Lee AV, Fang X, Mills GB (2009) Expression of autotaxin and lysophosphatidic acid receptors increases mammary tumorigenesis, invasion, and metastases. Cancer Cell 15: 539-550.

[124] Popnikolov NK, Dalwadi BH, Thomas JD, Johannes GJ, Imagawa WT (2012) Association of autotaxin and lysophosphatidic acid receptor 3 with aggressiveness of human breast carcinoma. Tumour Biol 33: 2237-2243.

[125] Hanahan D, Weinberg RA (2011) Hallmarks of cancer: the next generation. Cell 144: 646-674.

[126] Zhao C, Fernandes MJ, Prestwich GD, Turgeon M, Di Battista J, Clair T, Poubelle PE, Bourgoin SG (2008) Regulation of lysophosphatidic acid receptor expression and function in human synoviocytes: implications for rheumatoid arthritis? Mol Pharmacol 73: 587-600.

[127] Nikitopoulou I, Oikonomou N, Karouzakis E, Sevastou I, Nikolaidou-Katsaridou N, Zhao Z, Mersinias V, Armaka M, Xu Y, Masu M, Mills GB, Gay S, Kollias G, Aidinis V (2012) Autotaxin expression from synovial fibroblasts is essential for the pathogenesis of modeled arthritis. J Exp Med 209: 925-933.

[128] Hartman ZC, Poage GM, den Hollander P, Tsimelzon A, Hill J, Panupinthu N, Zhang Y, Mazumdar A, Hilsenbeck SG, Mills GB, Brown PH (2013) Growth of triple-negative breast cancer cells relies upon coordinate autocrine expression of the proinflammatory cytokines IL-6 and IL-8. Cancer Research 73: 3470-3480.

[129] Kehlen A, Englert N, Seifert A, Klonisch T, Dralle H, Langner J, Hoang-Vu C (2004) Expression, regulation and function of autotaxin in thyroid carcinomas. Int J Cancer 109: 833-838.

[130] Kawagoe H, Stracke ML, Nakamura H, Sano K (1997) Expression and transcriptional regulation of the PD-Ialpha/autotaxin gene in neuroblastoma. Cancer Res 57: 2516-2521.

[131] Farina AR, Cappabianca L, Ruggeri P, Di Ianni N, Ragone M, Merolle S, Sano K, Stracke ML, Horowitz JM, Gulino A, Mackay AR (2012) Constitutive autotaxin transcription by Nmyc-amplified and non-amplified neuroblastoma cells is regulated by a novel AP-1 and SP-mediated mechanism and abrogated by curcumin. FEBS Lett 586: 3681-3691.

[132] Singh AD, Sisley K, Xu Y, Li J, Faber P, Plummer SJ, Mudhar HS, Rennie IG, Kessler PM, Casey G, Williams BG (2007) Reduced expression of autotaxin predicts survival in uveal melanoma. Br J Ophthalmol 91: 1385-1392.

[133] Jankowski M (2011) Autotaxin: its role in biology of melanoma cells and as a pharmacological target. Enzyme Res 8: 194857.

[134] Braeuer RR, Zigler M, Kamiya T, Dobroff AS, Huang L, Choi W, McConkey DJ, Shoshan E, Mobley AK, Song R, Raz A, Bar-Eli M (2012) Galectin-3 contributes to melanoma growth and metastasis via regulation of NFAT1 and autotaxin. Cancer Res 72: 5757-5766.

[135] Samadi N, Gaetano C, Goping IS, Brindley DN (2009) Autotaxin protects MCF-7 breast cancer and MDA-MB-435 melanoma cells against Taxol-induced apoptosis. Oncogene 28: 1028-1039.

[136] Samadi N, Bekele RT, Goping IS, Schang LM, Brindley DN (2011) Lysophosphatidate induces chemo-resistance by releasing breast cancer cells from taxol-induced mitotic arrest. PLoS One 6: e20608.

[137] Vidot S, Witham J, Agarwal R, Greenhough S, Bamrah HS, Tigyi GJ, Kaye SB, Richardson A (2010) Autotaxin delays apoptosis induced by carboplatin in ovarian cancer cells. Cell Signal 22: 926-935.

[138] Hooks SB, Callihan P, Altman MK, Hurst JH, Ali MW, Murph MM (2010) Regulators of G-Protein signaling RGS10 and RGS17 regulate chemoresistance in ovarian cancer cells. Mol Cancer 9: 289.

[139] Brindley DN, Lin FT, Tigyi GJ (2013) Role of the autotaxin-lysophosphatidate axis in cancer resistance to chemotherapy and radiotherapy. Biochim Biophys Acta 1831: 74-85.

[140] Schneider G, Sellers ZP, Abdel-Latif A, Morris AJ, Ratajczak MZ (2014) Bioactive Lipids, LPC and LPA, are Novel Pro-metastatic Factors and Their Tissue Levels Increase

in Response to Radio/Chemotherapy. Mol Cancer Res: doi: 10.1158/1541-7786.MCR-1114-0188.

[141] Prestwich GD, Gajewiak J, Zhang H, Xu X, Yang G, Serban M (2008) Phosphatase-resistant analogues of lysophosphatidic acid: agonists promote healing, antagonists and autotaxin inhibitors treat cancer. Biochim Biophys Acta 1781: 588-594.

Chapter 13

RAGE and Its Ligands in Melanoma

Estelle Leclerc

Additional information is available at the end of the chapter

http://dx.doi.org/10.5772/59172

1. Introduction

Melanoma is a complex disease with both genetic and epigenetic components [1-3]. Once melanoma has formed distant metastases, melanoma patients have generally poor prognoses; less than 10% of these patients will survive 10 years [4]. For many years, treatment with the cytotoxic drug dacarbazine was the standard treatment for patients with metastatic melanoma, but the response rates were low and varied from 5-20% [4]. Intense research efforts on understanding the molecular mechanisms of melanoma progression led to the discovery and the approval by the FDA of two new drugs in 2011, vemurafenib and ipilimumab, which raised great hopes among melanoma patients [5-12]. Although treatment with vemurafenib has resulted in high overall responses rates [11], resistance against the drug appeared in treated melanoma patients within a year of treatment, leading to tumor regrowth [13-16]. On the other hand, treatment with ipilimumab does not result in resistance but can produce life threatening autoimmune adverse effects [17]. In addition, ipilimumab works best in patients whose tumors present abundant tumor infiltrated immune cells [18]. It is therefore essential to identify new therapeutic targets in melanoma.

One potential therapeutic target is the receptor for advanced glycation end products (RAGE). A possible role of RAGE in melanoma is emerging and has been the topic of a growing number of studies in the past decade [19-25]. These studies will be reviewed here and we will also discuss the RAGE ligands that play important roles in melanoma progression.

2. The Receptor for Advanced Glycation End Products (RAGE)

2.1. RAGE function

RAGE is an immunoglobulin-like cell-surface receptor that is involved in a large number of pathologies, including Alzheimer's disease, cancer, infectious diseases and complications of diabetes [31-38]. The ligands of RAGE are numerous (Table 1) and belong to distinct families of molecules. However, they also share structural features such as the propensity to form oligomers [39]. It is believed that RAGE recognizes similar structural elements or patterns within its numerous ligands and therefore RAGE is described as a pattern recognition receptor [40, 41].

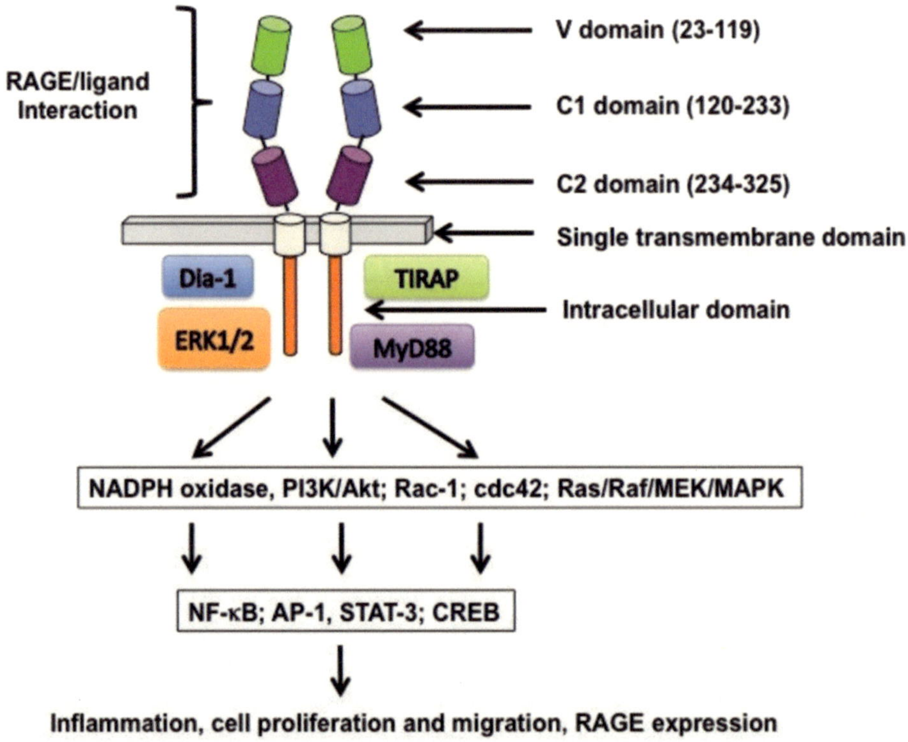

Figure 1. Schematic representation of RAGE. The extracellular part of RAGE is composed of three distinct immunoglobulin-like domains (V, C1 and C2). The V and C1 domains form a structural and functional unit [26]. Most ligands interact with the V-C1 domain. Four adaptor molecules have been suggested to bind to the intracellular domain of RAGE: ERK1/2 [27], diaphanous-1 (Dia-1) [28], TIRAP and MyD88 [29]. Following activation of RAGE by its ligands, multiple signaling pathways (MAPK, PI3K/Akt) or molecules (NADPH oxidase, Rac-1, cdc42) are activated and lead to the transcription of genes related to inflammation, cell proliferation and migration, and to the expression of RAGE itself, resulting in a positive feedback loop [30].

The physiological role of RAGE is not yet fully understood. Studies have shown that RAGE plays a role in the innate but not adaptive immunity and has been shown to play an important function in peripheral nerve repair [42-44]. A characteristic of RAGE is that it is expressed at low basal level in most tissues except in lungs where it has been suggested to exert a protective effect [45-48]. RAGE has also been shown to modulate the auditory system in mice [49].

Several spliced isoforms of RAGE have been described. Besides full-length RAGE, presented in Figure 1, RAGE exists as a soluble form (sRAGE) lacking the intracellular and transmembrane domains. The soluble form can result either from a splicing event or from the action of a metalloprotease such as ADAM 10 [50-58]. Other major identified spliced isoforms lack the N-terminal domain or present a deletion in the intracellular domain, resulting in abnormal ligand interaction and cell signaling activities, respectively [51, 56, 59]. sRAGE has been used in many animal experiments to validate the role of RAGE in various diseases such as Alzheimer's disease, atherosclerosis or encephalomyelitis [60-62]. Two different models explaining the mechanism of action of sRAGE have been proposed. The "classic" mechanism suggests that sRAGE acts as a decoy receptor and interacts with circulating RAGE ligands, which results in the absence of RAGE/ligand complex formation and RAGE activation. Recently, the group of Fritz has proposed a second mechanism of action for sRAGE: Fritz et al. suggest that sRAGE could form a complex with the extracellular part of another full-length receptor and that this receptor complex would not be functional because it possesses only one intracellular domain [63]. According to this hypothesis, RAGE can only transmit a signal if two intracellular domains form a dimer [63].

The role of sRAGE as biomarker has also been investigated in many diseases but has resulted in contradictory data for certain pathologies. In Alzheimer's disease patients, the circulating plasma levels of sRAGE have been shown to be significantly reduced compared to healthy individuals [64]. A more detailed immunohistological examination of AD brain showed that the reduction in sRAGE was more pronounced in the hippocampus of AD brains than normal brains [65]. Systemic low levels of sRAGE have also been found in patients with emphysema, a form of chronic obstructive pulmonary disease (COPD) and sRAGE is suggested to be a biomarker for this lung disease [66, 67]. However, in diabetes, the situation is more complex and in different studies the levels of sRAGE have been either positively or negatively correlated with the disease (reviewed and discussed in [68])

In cancer, an association between sRAGE and the progression of cancer has also been shown. Significantly lower levels of sRAGE have been found in lung, breast, liver or pancreatic cancer patients than in normal individuals [69-72]. Our study of 40 melanoma human samples also showed significantly lower transcript levels of the spliced form of RAGE in 90% of melanoma stage III and stage IV tissue samples compared to normal samples [73].

2.2. RAGE structure and signaling

RAGE is a single transmembrane receptor with a large extracellular part comprising of three domains that share structural features with immunoglobulin domains: a variable type (V) domain (residues 23-119), and two constant type domains (C1: residues 120-233, and C2: residues 234-325) (Figure 1) [74]. The V and C1 domains form a structural and functional unit and are the site of binding of most ligands [26].

Recent studies have suggested that RAGE structure is as complex as RAGE signaling is, and multiple conformational forms of RAGE in complex with its ligands have been proposed [75]. Recent evidence suggests that RAGE exists as a dimer on the surface of cells, in the absence of ligand [76, 77]. It has been suggested that the interaction of RAGE with its ligands occurs mainly through electrostatic interactions between the positive charges present on the V and C1 domains of RAGE and the negative charges present on RAGE ligands [39, 63]. Because both RAGE and its ligands can form oligomers, several oligomeric models of RAGE in complex with its ligands have been proposed to reflect the possible RAGE/ligand interactions [39, 63, 75-79]. RAGE oligomerization could occur through contacts between the V domain [80], C1 domain [80], [77] or C2 domain, [75, 79], in a ligand dependent manner [79].

RAGE signaling is complex and RAGE/ligand interaction results in the activation of multiple signaling pathways that are ligand and tissue specific (Figure 1) [34, 81-84]. In general, RAGE engagement by its ligand leads to the activation of key elements of the PI3K/Akt pathways or the mitogen-activated protein (MAP) kinase signaling pathways which include ERK1/2, p38 and JNK. Small GTPases such as p21-Ras, Rac-1 or cdc42 can also be activated as a result of RAGE activation [28, 81, 85-87]. In many cases, RAGE activation by its ligands leads to the initiation of, and sustained inflammation through the activation of the transcription factor NF-κB, but also AP-1, STAT-3 and CREB (Figure 1) [36-38, 68, 88].

2.3. RAGE in melanoma

A role of RAGE in melanoma progression was first suggested by Huttunen et al [19]. In their study, the authors generated tumors in mice using the mouse melanoma B16F10 cell-line expressing either full-length RAGE or a form of RAGE lacking the cytoplasmic domain [19]. Comparison of the number of metastases formed in the two groups of mice revealed that mice that were implanted with cells expressing the mutant form of RAGE generated significantly less tumors than mice implanted with cells expressing full-length RAGE. In a different study, Abe et al. showed that the growth of xenograft tumor in mice could be reduced using anti-RAGE antibodies [21]. We showed that RAGE overexpression in the WM115 human melanoma cell line resulted in a significant decrease in cell proliferation, but also in a significant increase in cell migration and invasion suggesting that RAGE can modulate different aspects of cancer [24]. We demonstrated that the decrease in cell proliferation was accompanied with a decrease in the activity of ERK1/2 [24] and p38 (Meghnani et al. 2014, International Journal of Biochemistry and Cell Biology, in press). The recent report of Popa et al. also suggests the presence of different oligomeric forms of RAGE with different roles and subcellular location during melanoma progression [25].

Studies in human melanoma tissue samples have shown that RAGE was not present in all melanoma samples but rather in a subset of samples. Hsieh et al. showed that only 20% tissue samples showed RAGE staining [20]. Our analysis of 40 samples of human melanoma tissue samples also showed large variations in RAGE transcripts levels, with up to 50-fold differences between samples [22].

Other studies have identified RAGE ligands as important elements in melanoma development. S100B has been studied in details and its role as a diagnostic marker for melanoma patients is well established (see section 3.1.1 on S100B). Abe et al. showed that AGEs could promote the proliferation of melanoma cells in culture [21]. Saha et al. showed that S100A8/A9 could attract B16F10 melanoma cells to a metastatic site, in a RAGE dependent manner [23]. In addition, our recent study showed a strong correlation between the expression of RAGE and that of its S100 protein ligands, in mouse xenograft melanoma tumors (Meghnani et al. 2014, International Journal of Biochemistry and Cell Biology, in press).

3. RAGE ligands

Since the identification of AGEs as ligands of RAGE, the list of RAGE ligands has grown to more than ten ligands or groups of ligands (Table 1). In this section, we will discuss the current knowledge on ligands that have been shown to play a role in melanoma progression, with a focus on S100 proteins.

RAGE ligand	Examples of disease where the ligand is involved	References
Advanced glycation end products	Inflammation, cancer, Alzheimer's disease, atherosclerosis, aging	[74, 89-92]
S100 proteins	Inflammation, cancer, aging, neurodegenerative disorders	[82, 93-95]
High mobility group box 1 (HMGB-1)	Cancer, inflammation, aging	[34, 96-99]
Alzheimer's β-peptide	Alzheimer's disease	[32, 60]
Transthyretin	Transthyretin amyloidosis	[100]
Prion	Prion's disease	[101, 102]
Mac-1	Diseases of the immune system	[40, 103]
Complement proteins C3a and C1q	Diseases of the immune system	[104, 105]
Phophatidylserine	Diseases of apoptosis	[106, 107]
Heparan sulfate	Cancer, inflammation, developmental disorder	[78, 108, 109]
DNA, RNA	Infectious diseases, autoimmune disorders	[110]

Table 1. Non-exhaustive list of the different ligands of RAGE. The S100 proteins that are ligands of RAGE will be described in details in section 3.1

3.1. S100 proteins

Members of the S100 protein family have amino-acid sequence and structure similarities [111, 112]. They are small calcium binding proteins and belong to the superfamily of EF-hand proteins [111]. Restricted to vertebrates, S100 proteins show strong tissue and cell specificity [111, 113]. Most S100 genes (S100A1 to S100A16) are located on chromosome 1 in a region that is prone to chromosomal rearrangement, linking these S100 proteins to cancer [113]. The presence of EF-hands within the structure of S100 proteins enable them to bind calcium with moderate micromolar affinity [111, 112, 114, 115]. In addition to calcium, S100 proteins can also bind zinc and copper [116, 117]. For most S100 proteins, binding to calcium results in conformational rearrangements that allow the S100 proteins to interact with their targets [115, 117, 118]. Certain target proteins are S100 specific whereas others are shared among multiple S100s (Reviewed in [119]).

Most S100 target proteins are intracellular [111, 112, 120]. An example of such target that plays a role in cancer is the tumor suppressor p53 protein [121-126]. Several members of the S100 protein family (S100B, S100A1, S100A2, S100A4, S100A6 and S100A10] bind to p53 but the outcome of this interaction differs depending of the S100 [121-126]. S100 proteins can also be secreted into the extracellular space through mechanisms that are not clearly understood [127, 128]. When secreted, many S100 proteins have been shown to interact with RAGE [82, 93, 129].

Many S100 proteins are found in cells constituting the epidermis [130]. S100B and S100A6 have been found in both melanocytes and Langerhan's cells [131-133]. S100A2, A7, A10, A11, A12 and S100A15 have been described in normal keratinocytes [131-138]. In pathophysiological conditions, such as in inflamed keratinocytes and melanoma, many S100 proteins have been found overexpressed [130, 136]. The next section will describe the role of these S100 proteins in melanoma.

3.1.1. S100B

S100B is used as a prognostic marker for stage IV malignant melanoma patients [139-141]. Serum concentration of S100B increases during the disease and high levels of S100B in the serum is indicative of a poor prognosis [139-141]. In melanoma tumors, melanoma cells are the main cells responsible for secreting S100B [141]. Within the cells, the role of S100B is not clearly understood but the main target of S100B appears to be the tumor suppressor p53 protein. Indeed, several studies from the group of Weber have shown that S100B interacts with p53 in melanoma cells and tumors, resulting in p53 inhibition and increased expression of S100B, in a negative feedback loop [142-144]. His group is currently investigating small interfering antisense RNA inhibitors of S100B as inhibitors of melanoma tumor growth [145].

Other intracellular target proteins of S100B could also contribute to increases in cellular proliferation and tumor growth in melanoma. For example, S100B interacts with and activates the glycolytic enzyme fructose-1,6-biphosphate aldolase, [146]. Consequences of this activation could be an increase in melanoma cell metabolism and glycolysis. Inhibiting melanoma cell metabolism and glycolysis is currently been considered in clinical trials [147, 148]. Inhibiting S100B/ fructose-1,6-biphosphate aldolase could be an approach to further reduce glycolytic activity in melanoma cells. S100B also interacts with many components of the cytoskeleton such as tubulin [149, 150], the actin binding protein caldesmon [151] or the small GTPase Rac1 and the cdc42 effector IQGAP1 [152]. All these proteins play important function in malignant melanoma [153-155] and increases in S100B levels could therefore favor increases in cell proliferation, migration and invasion through their modulation. S100B could also play a role in melanoma cell growth through the activation of the Nuclear Dbf2 related (ndr) kinase [156-158] and the interaction with the phosphoprotein AHNAK/desmoyokin [159-161].

As mentioned earlier, S100B is secreted from melanoma cells. The mechanisms of S100B secretion are still poorly understood but recent studies have suggested that RAGE participates in the translocation and secretion of several S100s including S100B [127, 128]. Similarly, the role of RAGE/S100B in melanoma is slowly being unraveled. S100B has been shown to signal through RAGE in a large number of diseases (reviewed in [162]) and we studied in details the *in vitro* interaction of RAGE with S100B [26, 81, 163]. For example, we showed that not only dimeric S100B but also tetrameric and hexameric S100B could interact with RAGE and signal in cells [163]. In addition, we recently showed that overexpression of RAGE, in human WM115 melanoma cells, was accompanied by the up-regulation of S100B in these cells [24], suggesting a strong association between RAGE and S100B in melanoma. When the RAGE transfected WM115 cells were implanted in mice as xenografts, we also observed higher levels of S100B in the serum of these animals, compared to animals implanted with control WM115 cells (Meghnani et al. 2014, International Journal of Biochemistry and Cell Biology, in press).

3.1.2. S100A2

S100A2 is mainly located in the nuclei of cells [164]. The function of S100A2 in cancer is not clear. In certain cancers such as prostate, oral, lung and breast cancers, S100A2 has been shown to play the role of tumor suppressor [22, 165-169], whereas in other cancers such as esophageal squamous carcinoma, gastric, and ovarian cancer, studies indicate that it acts as tumor promoter [170-172]. In addition, in certain cancers, such as in non-small cell lung cancer (NSCLC), studies are contradictory since both down-and up-regulation of S100A2 have been reported [173-175].

In melanoma, most studies reported that S100A2 plays the role of tumor suppressor [130, 132, 165, 176]. We also showed a significant reduction in S100A2 mRNA level in both stage III and stage IV melanoma patients samples compared to control samples [22]. Additional evidences of a tumor suppressor effect of S100A2 comes from several studies that show positive correlations between the levels of S100A2 and anti-proliferative effects of chemotherapeutic agents in melanoma cells [177, 178]. However, our most recent study shows that xenograft melanoma tumors overexpressing RAGE, presented a growth advantage over control tumors, and exhibited significant higher levels of S100A2 than control tumors (Meghnani et al. 2014, International Journal of Biochemistry and Cell Biology, in press). We observed that S100A2 was up-regulated, both at the transcript and protein levels, in the RAGE overexpressing tumors (Meghnani et al. unpublished results). These data suggest a complex role of S100A2 in promoting or suppressing melanoma tumor growth.

As mentioned above, S100A2 is located in the nuclei of cells and has been shown to interact with the tumor suppressor p53, in two oral cancer cell lines (FADU and SCC-25), thereby modulating the transcriptional activity of p53 [123]. *In vitro* binding studies have confirmed the interaction between S100A2 and p53 and has shown differences in binding of p53 to S100B and S100A2; for example, although both S100B and S100A2 could bind to the monomeric form of p53, only S100B was able to disrupt the oligomerization of p53, suggesting different mode of transcriptional modulation of p53 by the S100 proteins [124, 126]. In addition to interacting with p53, S100A2 transcriptional activity is regulated by other members of the large p53 family, such as p63 and p73, suggesting an additional level of complexity of the S100A2/p53 regulation [179-181]. In breast cancer tissues and cells, it was shown that both the p53 homologue Np63, and BRCA1 were important for the transcriptional activity of S100A2 [182]. These recent data could have a large impact in understanding the molecular mechanism of melanoma because positive correlations have been found between the BRCA1 associated protein (BAP1] and malignant uveal and cutaneous melanoma [183-185].

We recently demonstrated that *in vitro*, S100A2 could interact with RAGE [22] and our recent study showed an association between RAGE overexpression and the levels of S100A2 in melanoma xenograft tumors (Meghnani et al. 2014, International Journal of Biochemistry and

Cell Biology, in press). However, a direct interaction of S100A2/RAGE in melanoma cells and tissue has yet to be demonstrated.

3.1.3. S100A4

S100A4 was initially identified from metastatic cells and was hence named metastasin [186]. Overexpression of S100A4 in multiple cell lines has been shown to increase cancer cell invasiveness and motility [187, 188]. The role of S100A4 in cancer was further demonstrated in S100A4$^{-/-}$mice that showed delayed tumor growth, compared to control mice, when implanted with highly metastatic mammary carcinoma cells [189, 190].

In melanoma, the role of S100A4 is complex and appears to vary during the progression of the disease. An early study showed no significant differences in S100A4 mRNA levels between melanoma tissue samples and control samples [165]. Our analysis of 40 samples of stage III and stage IV melanoma tissue samples showed a significantly reduction of S100A4 mRNA in stage IV compared to control samples [22]. Another study also reported different correlation between the levels of S100A4 and patient survival rates during the progression of melanoma: high levels of S100A4 in primary melanoma tumors were associated with low patient survival rates whereas high S100A4 levels in metastatic tumors were not associated with differences in patient survival rates, suggesting a role of S100A4 at a early stage of the disease [191].

S100A4 exerts both intra-and extracellular functions (reviewed in [192]). Inside the cells, S100A4 can be found in the nuclei and cytoplasm [192]. S100A4 has been shown to interact with p53 and, as described for S100B, to disrupt p53 oligomerization [193, 194]. *In vivo*, interaction of S100A4 with p53 has been shown to promote degradation of p53, resulting in increases in tumor growth [195]. In the cytoplasm, S100A4 interacts with a large number of proteins of the cytoskeleton such as non-muscle myosin II [196] and tropomyosin [197], resulting in cytoskeletal reorganization, which occurs during cell migration and invasion [198, 199].

An important property of S100A4 is that it has been found secreted in the extracellular medium of cells and is present in the milieu of many tumor types such as breast cancer [200], ovarian carcinoma [201], osteosarcoma [202] or adenocarcinoma tumors [203]. Many cells from normal tissues and from tumors have been shown to release S100A4. These cells include fibroblasts, leukocytes, and endothelial cells [192, 204]. Extracellular S100A4 has been shown to promote tumor growth and metastasis [192], neovascularization and angiogenesis [205-207].

Two main targets of extracellular S100A4 with relevance to tumor growth and metastasis have been identified: Annexin II and RAGE [208, 209]. Interaction of S100A4 with annexin II has been associated with increased mechanisms of angiogenesis such as the formation of capillary-like tubes by endothelial cells [208]. S100A4 has been shown to enhance motility of pulmonary artery smooth muscle cells in a RAGE dependent manner [210]. Similarly, S100A4 was shown to promote prostate and colorectal cancer tumorigenesis and metastasis in a RAGE dependent manner [211, 212]. In melanoma, a recent study has demonstrated that S100A4 derived from macrophages could promote lung colonization of B16F10 melanoma cells in mice, in a RAGE dependent manner as well [213]. We have also observed that RAGE overexpression in the

WM115 melanoma cells resulted in the up-regulation of S100A4, by the melanoma cells, in xenograft tumors implanted in mice (Meghnani et al. 2014, International Journal of Biochemistry and Cell Biology, in press).

3.1.4. S100A6

S100A6 is another member of the S100 family with a link to cancer. S100A6 was identified from melanoma tissue samples by comparing melanocytic lesions from normal nevi [214]. S100A6 is most abundant in epithelial cells and fibroblasts but is also found, in smaller amounts, in other cell-types such as neurons, glial cells, smooth muscle cells, cardiac myocytes, platelets and lymphocytes [215, 216](reviewed in [217]). S100A6 has been found elevated in a large number of cancer types which include colorectal cancer, pancreatic, hepato-cellular carcinoma, melanoma, lung cancer and gastric cancer [165, 218-224](reviewed in [217]). In melanoma tumor samples, a positive correlation was found between the levels of S100A6 transcripts and the severity of the disease [165]. In animal models, S100A6 was found to correlate with the metastatic behavior of the melanoma cells [214, 225]. We also observed higher levels of S1006, at the transcript level, in 43% of stage III melanoma samples examined, compared to control samples [22]. In agreement with our study, examination of another set of melanoma tissue samples showed that 33% of the samples stained positive for S100A6 [133]. However, examination of melanoma tumor biopsies by immunohistochemistry often shows that the expression of S100A6 is weak and patchy, and that other non-melanoma cutaneous lesions also stain positive for S100A6, making it difficult to use S100A6 as a diagnostic marker for melanoma [176, 226, 227].

S100A6 has been shown to interact with both nuclear and cytoplasmic proteins. S100A6 interacts with the tumor suppressor p53 but this interaction is different than the interaction of p53 with S100B, suggesting different regulation of the transcriptional activity of p53 by the two S100 proteins [124, 228]. S100A6 was shown to interact with a peptide derived from cell membrane associated annexin I, but the physiological relevance of this interaction has yet to be demonstrated [229]. We showed that S100A6 could interact with both the VC1 and the C2 domain of RAGE, but that in human neuroblastoma, signaling was transduced through the C2 domain [81]. The interaction of the C3S mutant form of S100A6 with the V domain of RAGE has recently been studied in details [230]. Similarly to what we observed with S100B, S100A2 and S100A4, RAGE overexpression in the WM115 melanoma cells resulted in the up-regulation of S100A6, by the melanoma cells, when the cells were forming xenograft tumors in nude mice, compared to control tumors (Meghnani et al. 2014, International Journal of Biochemistry and Cell Biology, in press).

3.1.5. S100A8/A9

S100A8 and S100A9 are mainly expressed by cells of myeloid origin such as monocytes and macrophages, and were first described as cytokine-like proteins for their up-regulation in inflamed tissues and inflammatory disorders [231]. Recent studies have also shown that they play significant roles in cancer where they promote tumor growth and metastasis in a large number of cancers such as in breast, prostate and pancreatic cancer [232-238]. In tumors, recent studies have shown that S100A8/A9 regulates the accumulation of myeloid-derived suppressor cells (MDSC), and also promote the expansion of these cells, resulting in increased tumor growth [239-243].

Neither S100A8 nor S100A9 is present in significant amounts in the cells of a normal epidermis, including melanocytes [130, 244]. Although a study described that S100A8/A9 was absent from melanocytic lesions [244], other studies have suggested that they participate in melanoma progression. S100A9 has been shown to promote melanoma metastases formation in a mouse model [245]. In a different mouse model of melanoma, the levels of MDSCs correlated with the levels of S100A9, [246]. In addition, Saha et al. recently demonstrated that tail-vein injected B16F10 melanoma cells, that do not express S100A8 or S100A9, could migrate to S100A8/A9-abondant lungs of uteroglobin-knockout mice [23]. The migration of the B16F10 cells occurred along a concentration gradient of S100A8/A9, and resulted in the formation of secondary tumors in the lungs [23].

S100A8/A9 mediates their effect through the interaction with cell surface receptors or molecules. The two pattern recognition receptors, toll-like receptor 4 (TLR-4) and RAGE, have been shown to transmit RAGE signaling [23, 247, 248]. In certain conditions, signaling through RAGE has been shown to require carboxylated glycans that are covalently attached to RAGE [249, 250]. The importance of RAGE glycosylation for RAGE signaling has also been demonstrated for another member of the S100 protein family, S100A12 [251]. S100A8/A9 has been shown to interact with other glycans, such as heparin or heparin sulfate glycosaminoglycans [137]. In addition, S100A9 has also been shown to interact with and transmit signal through EMMPIRIN [245].

3.1.6. Other S100 proteins

Other S100 proteins are found in cells of the epidermis (reviewed by [130]), and their association with melanoma will be briefly described in this paragraph.

S100A7 or "psoriasin" has been linked to psoriasis because of its up-regulation in this disease [252, 253]. Although no direct role of S100A7 in melanoma has been described yet, in one study, significantly higher levels of S100A7 were found in the urine of melanoma patients compared to that of healthy patients [254].

S100A10 has been found expressed at various levels in melanoma tumor samples and melanocytes [22, 244]. Our recent study where we compared the levels of S100 proteins in WM115 xenografts, generated from either control WM115 cells or from RAGE overexpressing WM115 cells, showed that S100A10 was up-regulated in the RAGE overexpressing tumors (unpublished data). Comparison of the WM115-RAGE cells with control cells did not reveal any difference in S100A10 levels between the two cell lines, suggesting that RAGE overexpression was responsible for the up-regulation of S100A10 in the tumors. S100A10 could therefore play a role in melanoma progression.

S100A11 can either promote tumor growth or play the role of tumor suppressor, depending of the type of cancer (reviewed in [255]). S100A11 has been suggested to play a role in uveal melanoma, but has not yet been linked to cutaneous melanoma [256].

3.2. Other ligands of RAGE

3.2.1. Advanced Glycation End products (AGEs)

Among RAGE ligands, AGEs were the first group of ligands to be identified [89]. AGEs form a group of very heterogeneous compounds since they are the result of condensation and oxidation reactions between proteins and sugars [257]. Although the term AGE was initially reserved for brown, fluorescent and cross-linked structures that were produced during the Maillard reaction, such as those found in glycated collagen, it is now used to describe other types of modifications and AGEs now include proteins containing carboxymethyllysine, carboxymethyl hydroxylysine or pyrraline [257]. Since many types of sugars (glucose, ribose…) can modify many proteins, the number of different structures produced by glycation is very large. The large heterogeneity in AGE compounds renders the comparison among studies also very difficult. When comparing the results of studies involving AGEs, it is therefore important to know the type of AGEs used in the study.

Melanoma cells have been shown to produce high levels of reactive carbonyl species such as glyoxal, methylglyoxal and malondialdehyde, which all can lead to the glycation of proteins, and which have been implicated in melanoma cell proliferation and formation of metastases [258-260]. Abe et al. investigated the effects of different AGEs (glucose-derived AGE, glyceraldehyde-derived AGE, glycoaldehyde AGE, methylglyoxal-AGE, glyoxal-AGE and carboxymethyllysine-AGE) on melanoma cell proliferation, migration and invasion, and showed that all these AGEs were strongly present in human melanoma specimen whereas they were hardly detected in melanocytes [21]. However, the same authors showed that only certain types of AGE compounds (glyceraldehyde-derived AGE and glycoaldehyde AGE) could stimulate the proliferation, migration and invasion of G361 metastatic human melanoma cells *in vitro*. The role of RAGE in the *in vitro* AGE-dependent proliferation was demonstrated with anti-RAGE antibodies [21]. In addition, the authors showed that treatment of mice carrying G361 melanoma tumors, with anti-RAGE antibodies, resulted in reduced tumor growth and formation of lungs metastases [21]. These results strongly suggested a role of AGE/RAGE in the development of melanoma tumors by the G361 human melanoma cell line [21]. Our detailed study on melanoma cell proliferation of a panel of 20 glycated proteins showed that many factors influenced the proliferation, such as the extent of lysine modification, the percentage of β-sheet and the oligomerization state of the glycated proteins [261]. We showed that glycated proteins that demonstrated higher percentage of oligomeric forms, β-sheet content and modification of lysine, promoted stronger cell proliferation that proteins that contained lower levels of oligomers, β-sheet or lysine modification.

3.2.2. High Mobility Group Box 1 protein (HMGB1)

HMGB-1 is present in most eukaryotic cells (reviewed by [97]). It functions both as a nuclear protein, where it binds to DNA and assists in the transcription of multiple genes, and as an extracellular protein, where it binds to the pattern recognition receptors TLR-2, TLR-4 and TLR-9 as well as to RAGE, thereby promoting inflammation, mediating response to infection and injury as well as promoting cell proliferation, migration or invasion [98, 262-266]. HMGB-1 is also described as an alarmin or damage-associated molecular pattern [267]. HMGB-1 interacts directly with a large number of transcription factors that are relevant in cancer, and include the tumor suppressor p53, p73, the retinoblastoma protein (RB), the p50 subunit of NF-κB and the estrogen receptor (reviewed by [268]). The release of HMGB-1 has been shown to be triggered by necrosis or apoptosis, such as following treatment of tumors with a chemotherapeutic agent [264, 266, 267].

HMGB-1 has also been shown to be released from necrotic or apoptotic melanoma cells [269]. A recent study showed that HMGB-1 could be released from keratinocytes in culture, or from murine skin, following exposure to UV light [270]. Using a genetically engineered mouse model of melanoma, Bald et al. showed that UV exposure also promoted metastasis and angiogenesis, through HMGB-1, and TLR-4 signaling [271]. In a different mouse model, Tang et al. showed the role of the HMGB-1/RAGE axis in promoting melanoma tumor growth [272]. In melanoma patients, HMGB-1 levels have also been shown to predict patient survival rates [273].

3.2.3. Glycosaminoglycans, β2 integrin Mac-1 and phosphatidylserine

RAGE has been shown to interact with various glycosaminoglycans such as chondroitin sulfate, dermatan sulfate and heparin sulfate [108]. Many of these glycosaminoglycans are abundantly present in tumor stroma and have been shown to be key players of melanoma progression and metastasis formation [274, 275]. RAGE also interacts with β2 integrin Mac-1 on leukocytes and has been shown to promote leukocyte recruitment at the site of inflammation [40]. The interaction between RAGE and Mac-1 is dependent of the presence of cations, and has been shown to be significantly augmented by the presence of S100B. In a different study, S100A9 has also been shown to activate β2 integrin Mac-1 on neutrophils suggesting that other S100 proteins could also participate to the complex between Mac-1 and RAGE [276]. Leukocyte recruitment at tumor sites is an important process that allows cytotoxic T-cells to infiltrate tumors and to help in the elimination of cancer cells [277]. In melanoma, success of the therapy with interleukin-2 (IL-2) is based on the infiltration of cytotoxic T-cells to the interior of the tumor [277]. The involvement of S100 proteins and RAGE in leukocyte recruitment suggests that therapeutic approaches targeting RAGE should be carefully evaluated to avoid inhibiting the recruitment of cytotoxic T-cells at the site of melanoma tumors. On the other hand, targeting RAGE could also result in suppressing the recruitment of MDSCs, another form of leukocyte expressing β2 integrin Mac-1 [278], at the tumor site, which would be beneficial for patients [279, 280].

RAGE has also been shown to interact with the negatively charged phospholipid phosphatidylserine (PS) [106]. This interaction has direct relevance in melanoma because PS has been shown to be exposed to the outer leaflet of the plasma membrane of cells forming melanoma metastases [281]. An association between malignancy of melanoma and PS exposure has also been described [281]. Further studies would be necessary to determine whether RAGE/PS could be targeted in melanoma.

4. Conclusion and therapeutic approaches

In the last two decades, RAGE has emerged as a new therapeutic target in a large number of diseases. Because of the large number of ligands of RAGE that are relevant in melanoma, targeting RAGE/ligand appears to be a promising approach. Several molecules could be used as inhibitors and include the soluble form of the receptor (sRAGE), antibodies against RAGE or small molecules. Both soluble RAGE and anti-RAGE antibodies have been used to demonstrate the role of RAGE in experimental models of a large number of diseases such as atherosclerosis, Alzheimer's disease or melanoma [21, 60, 282-286]. Two small molecule inhibitors of RAGE are currently available. One compound PFS-ZM1 has been recently used in an experimental model of Alzheimer's disease [287]. This inhibitor interacts with the V domain of RAGE and blocks the interaction of amyloid β-peptide with the receptor. The second compound (TPP488) has been evaluated for safety and efficacy, in a phase 2 study, in mild to moderate Alzheimer's disease patients. However, because of the large variation in the levels of RAGE observed in melanoma tumor samples, it is currently not known whether targeting RAGE would be efficacious in all melanoma tumors or only in the subset of tumors where it is overexpressed. Additional studies would be necessary to answer this important question.

Acknowledgements

The author was supported by the NDSU College of Pharmacy, Nursing and Allied Sciences and in part by the NDSU Advance FORWARD program sponsored by NSF HRD-0811239 and ND EPSCoR through grant #EPS-0814442.

Author details

Estelle Leclerc*

Address all correspondence to: Estelle.Leclerc@ndsu.edu

North Dakota State University/Department of Pharmaceutical Sciences, USA

References

[1] Howell PM, Jr., Liu S, Ren S, Behlen C, Fodstad O, Riker AI. Epigenetics in human melanoma. Cancer Control. 2009;16(3):200-18.

[2] Patino WD, Susa J. Epigenetics of cutaneous melanoma. Adv Dermatol. 2008;24:59-70.

[3] Palmieri G, Capone M, Ascierto ML, Gentilcore G, Stroncek DF, Casula M, et al. Main roads to melanoma. J Transl Med. 2009;7:86.

[4] Bhatia S, Tykodi SS, Thompson JA. Treatment of metastatic melanoma: an overview. Oncology (Williston Park). 2009;23(6):488-96.

[5] Eggermont AM, Robert C. Melanoma in 2011: A new paradigm tumor for drug development. Nat Rev Clin Oncol. 2012.

[6] Hodi FS, Oble DA, Drappatz J, Velazquez EF, Ramaiya N, Ramakrishna N, et al. CTLA-4 blockade with ipilimumab induces significant clinical benefit in a female with melanoma metastases to the CNS. Nat Clin Pract Oncol. 2008;5(9):557-61.

[7] Nelson AL, Dhimolea E, Reichert JM. Development trends for human monoclonal antibody therapeutics. Nat Rev Drug Discov. 2010;9(10):767-74.

[8] Robert C, Mateus C. [Anti-CTLA-4 monoclonal antibody: a major step in the treatment of metastatic melanoma]. Med Sci (Paris). 2011;27(10):850-8.

[9] Trinh VA, Hagen B. Ipilimumab for advanced melanoma: A pharmacologic perspective. J Oncol Pharm Pract. 2012.

[10] Wang T, Somasundaram R, Herlyn M. Combination therapy of immunocytokines with ipilimumab: a cure for melanoma? J Invest Dermatol. 2013;133(3):595-6.

[11] Chapman PB, Hauschild A, Robert C, Haanen JB, Ascierto P, Larkin J, et al. Improved survival with vemurafenib in melanoma with BRAF V600E mutation. N Engl J Med. 2011;364(26):2507-16.

[12] Luke JJ, Hodi FS. Vemurafenib and BRAF inhibition: a new class of treatment for metastatic melanoma. Clin Cancer Res. 2012;18(1):9-14.

[13] Flaherty KT, Puzanov I, Kim KB, Ribas A, McArthur GA, Sosman JA, et al. Inhibition of mutated, activated BRAF in metastatic melanoma. N Engl J Med. 2010;363(9): 809-19.

[14] Nazarian R, Shi H, Wang Q, Kong X, Koya RC, Lee H, et al. Melanomas acquire resistance to B-RAF(V600E) inhibition by RTK or N-RAS upregulation. Nature. 2010;468(7326):973-7.

[15] Wagle N, Emery C, Berger MF, Davis MJ, Sawyer A, Pochanard P, et al. Dissecting therapeutic resistance to RAF inhibition in melanoma by tumor genomic profiling. J Clin Oncol. 2011;29(22):3085-96.

[16] Poulikakos PI, Persaud Y, Janakiraman M, Kong X, Ng C, Moriceau G, et al. RAF inhibitor resistance is mediated by dimerization of aberrantly spliced BRAF(V600E). Nature. 2011;480(7377):387-90.

http://dx.doi.org/10.5772/59172

[17] Wolchok JD, Neyns B, Linette G, Negrier S, Lutzky J, Thomas L, et al. Ipilimumab monotherapy in patients with pretreated advanced melanoma: a randomised, double-blind, multicentre, phase 2, dose-ranging study. Lancet Oncol. 2010;11(2):155-64.

[18] Quail DF, Joyce JA. Microenvironmental regulation of tumor progression and metastasis. Nat Med. 2013;19(11):1423-37.

[19] Huttunen HJ, Fages C, Kuja-Panula J, Ridley AJ, Rauvala H. Receptor for advanced glycation end products-binding COOH-terminal motif of amphoterin inhibits invasive migration and metastasis. Cancer Res. 2002;62(16):4805-11.

[20] Hsieh HL, Schafer BW, Sasaki N, Heizmann CW. Expression analysis of S100 proteins and RAGE in human tumors using tissue microarrays. Biochem Biophys Res Commun. 2003;307(2):375-81.

[21] Abe R, Shimizu T, Sugawara H, Watanabe H, Nakamura H, Choei H, et al. Regulation of human melanoma growth and metastasis by AGE-AGE receptor interactions. J Invest Dermatol. 2004;122(2):461-7.

[22] Leclerc E, Heizmann CW, Vetter SW. RAGE and S100 protein transcription levels are highly variable in human melanoma tumors and cells. Gen Physiol Biophys. 2009;28 Spec No Focus:F65-75.

[23] Saha A, Lee YC, Zhang ZJ, Chandra G, Su SB, Mukherjee AB. Lack of an Endogenous Anti-inflammatory Protein in Mice Enhances Colonization of B16F10 Melanoma Cells in the Lungs. Journal of Biological Chemistry. 2010;285(14):10822-31.

[24] Meghnani V, Vetter SW, Leclerc E. RAGE overexpression confers a metastatic phenotype to the WM115 human primary melanoma cell line. Biochim Biophys Acta. 2014;1842(7):1017-27.

[25] Popa I, Ganea E, Petrescu SM. Expression and subcellular localization of RAGE in melanoma cells. Biochem Cell Biol. 2014;92(2):127-36.

[26] Dattilo BM, Fritz G, Leclerc E, Kooi CW, Heizmann CW, Chazin WJ. The extracellular region of the receptor for advanced glycation end products is composed of two independent structural units. Biochemistry. 2007;46(23):6957-70.

[27] Ishihara K, Tsutsumi K, Kawane S, Nakajima M, Kasaoka T. The receptor for advanced glycation end-products (RAGE) directly binds to ERK by a D-domain-like docking site. FEBS Lett. 2003;550(1-3):107-13.

[28] Hudson BI, Kalea AZ, Del Mar Arriero M, Harja E, Boulanger E, D'Agati V, et al. Interaction of the RAGE cytoplasmic domain with diaphanous-1 is required for ligand-stimulated cellular migration through activation of Rac1 and Cdc42. J Biol Chem. 2008;283(49):34457-68.

[29] Sakaguchi M, Murata H, Yamamoto K, Ono T, Sakaguchi Y, Motoyama A, et al. TIRAP, an adaptor protein for TLR2/4, transduces a signal from RAGE phosphorylated upon ligand binding. PLoS One. 2011;6(8):e23132.

[30] Schmidt AM, Yan SD, Yan SF, Stern DM. The multiligand receptor RAGE as a progression factor amplifying immune and inflammatory responses. J Clin Invest. 2001;108(7):949-55.

[31] Schmidt AM, Yan SD, Yan SF, Stern DM. The biology of the receptor for advanced glycation end products and its ligands. Biochim Biophys Acta. 2000;1498(2-3):99-111.

[32] Yan SD, Bierhaus A, Nawroth PP, Stern DM. RAGE and Alzheimer's disease: a progression factor for amyloid-beta-induced cellular perturbation? J Alzheimers Dis. 2009;16(4):833-43.

[33] Bierhaus A, Nawroth PP. Multiple levels of regulation determine the role of the receptor for AGE (RAGE) as common soil in inflammation, immune responses and diabetes mellitus and its complications. Diabetologia. 2009;52(11):2251-63.

[34] Sparvero LJ, Asafu-Adjei D, Kang R, Tang D, Amin N, Im J, et al. RAGE (Receptor for Advanced Glycation Endproducts), RAGE ligands, and their role in cancer and inflammation. J Transl Med. 2009;7:17.

[35] van Zoelen MA, Achouiti A, van der Poll T. RAGE during infectious diseases. Front Biosci (Schol Ed). 2011;3:1119-32.

[36] Sims GP, Rowe DC, Rietdijk ST, Herbst R, Coyle AJ. HMGB1 and RAGE in Inflammation and Cancer. Annual Review of Immunology. 2010;28:367-88.

[37] Ramasamy R, Yan SF, Schmidt AM. Receptor for AGE (RAGE): signaling mechanisms in the pathogenesis of diabetes and its complications. Ann N Y Acad Sci. 2011;1243:88-102.

[38] Park S, Yoon SJ, Tae HJ, Shim CY. RAGE and cardiovascular disease. Front Biosci. 2011;16:486-97.

[39] Fritz G. RAGE: a single receptor fits multiple ligands. Trends Biochem Sci. 2011;36(12):625-32.

[40] Chavakis T, Bierhaus A, Al-Fakhri N, Schneider D, Witte S, Linn T, et al. The pattern recognition receptor (RAGE) is a counterreceptor for leukocyte integrins: a novel pathway for inflammatory cell recruitment. J Exp Med. 2003;198(10):1507-15.

[41] Lin L. RAGE on the Toll Road? Cellular & molecular immunology. 2006;3(5):351-8.

[42] Liliensiek B, Weigand MA, Bierhaus A, Nicklas W, Kasper M, Hofer S, et al. Receptor for advanced glycation end products (RAGE) regulates sepsis but not the adaptive immune response. J Clin Invest. 2004;113(11):1641-50.

[43] Rong LL, Trojaborg W, Qu W, Kostov K, Yan SD, Gooch C, et al. Antagonism of RAGE suppresses peripheral nerve regeneration. Faseb J. 2004;18(15):1812-7.

[44] Rong LL, Yan SF, Wendt T, Hans D, Pachydaki S, Bucciarelli LG, et al. RAGE modulates peripheral nerve regeneration via recruitment of both inflammatory and axonal outgrowth pathways. Faseb J. 2004;18(15):1818-25.

[45] Brett J, Schmidt AM, Yan SD, Zou YS, Weidman E, Pinsky D, et al. Survey of the distribution of a newly characterized receptor for advanced glycation end products in tissues. Am J Pathol. 1993;143(6):1699-712.

[46] Queisser MA, Kouri FM, Konigshoff M, Wygrecka M, Schubert U, Eickelberg O, et al. Loss of RAGE in pulmonary fibrosis: molecular relations to functional changes in pulmonary cell types. Am J Respir Cell Mol Biol. 2008;39(3):337-45.

[47] Ramsgaard L, Englert JM, Tobolewski J, Tomai L, Fattman CL, Leme AS, et al. The role of the receptor for advanced glycation end-products in a murine model of silicosis. PLoS One. 2010;5(3):e9604.

[48] Buckley ST, Ehrhardt C. The receptor for advanced glycation end products (RAGE) and the lung. J Biomed Biotechnol. 2010:in press.

[49] Sakatani S, Yamada K, Homma C, Munesue S, Yamamoto Y, Yamamoto H, et al. Deletion of RAGE causes hyperactivity and increased sensitivity to auditory stimuli in mice. PLoS One. 2009;4(12):e8309.

[50] Ohe K, Watanabe T, Harada S, Munesue S, Yamamoto Y, Yonekura H, et al. Regulation of alternative splicing of the receptor for advanced glycation endproducts (RAGE) through G-rich cis-elements and heterogenous nuclear ribonucleoprotein H. J Biochem. 2010;147(5):651-9.

[51] Hudson BI, Carter AM, Harja E, Kalea AZ, Arriero M, Yang H, et al. Identification, classification, and expression of RAGE gene splice variants. Faseb J. 2008;22(5): 1572-80.

[52] Galichet A, Weibel M, Heizmann CW. Calcium-regulated intramembrane proteolysis of the RAGE receptor. Biochem Biophys Res Commun. 2008;370(1):1-5.

[53] Raucci A, Cugusi S, Antonelli A, Barabino SM, Monti L, Bierhaus A, et al. A soluble form of the receptor for advanced glycation endproducts (RAGE) is produced by proteolytic cleavage of the membrane-bound form by the sheddase a disintegrin and metalloprotease 10 (ADAM10). Faseb J. 2008;22(10):3716-27.

[54] Zhang L, Bukulin M, Kojro E, Roth A, Metz VV, Fahrenholz F, et al. Receptor for advanced glycation end products is subjected to protein ectodomain shedding by metalloproteinases. J Biol Chem. 2008;283(51):35507-16.

[55] Ding Q, Keller JN. Splice variants of the receptor for advanced glycosylation end products (RAGE) in human brain. Neurosci Lett. 2005;373(1):67-72.

[56] Yonekura H, Yamamoto Y, Sakurai S, Petrova RG, Abedin MJ, Li H, et al. Novel splice variants of the receptor for advanced glycation end-products expressed in human vascular endothelial cells and pericytes, and their putative roles in diabetes-induced vascular injury. Biochem J. 2003;370(Pt 3):1097-109.

[57] Park IH, Yeon SI, Youn JH, Choi JE, Sasaki N, Choi IH, et al. Expression of a novel secreted splice variant of the receptor for advanced glycation end products (RAGE) in human brain astrocytes and peripheral blood mononuclear cells. Mol Immunol. 2004;40(16):1203-11.

[58] Kalea AZ, Reiniger N, Yang H, Arriero M, Schmidt AM, Hudson BI. Alternative splicing of the murine receptor for advanced glycation end-products (RAGE) gene. FASEB J. 2009;23(6):1766-74.

[59] Jules J, Maiguel D, Hudson BI. Alternative splicing of the RAGE cytoplasmic domain regulates cell signaling and function. PLoS One. 2013;8(11):e78267.

[60] Deane R, Du Yan S, Submamaryan RK, LaRue B, Jovanovic S, Hogg E, et al. RAGE mediates amyloid-beta peptide transport across the blood-brain barrier and accumulation in brain. Nat Med. 2003;9(7):907-13.

[61] Park L, Raman KG, Lee KJ, Lu Y, Ferran LJ, Jr., Chow WS, et al. Suppression of accelerated diabetic atherosclerosis by the soluble receptor for advanced glycation end-products. Nat Med. 1998;4(9):1025-31.

[62] Yan SS, Wu ZY, Zhang HP, Furtado G, Chen X, Yan SF, et al. Suppression of experimental autoimmune encephalomyelitis by selective blockade of encephalitogenic T-cell infiltration of the central nervous system. Nat Med. 2003;9(3):287-93.

[63] Koch M, Chitayat S, Dattilo BM, Schiefner A, Diez J, Chazin WJ, et al. Structural basis for ligand recognition and activation of RAGE. Structure. 2010;18(10):1342-52.

[64] Emanuele E, D'Angelo A, Tomaino C, Binetti G, Ghidoni R, Politi P, et al. Circulating levels of soluble receptor for advanced glycation end products in Alzheimer disease and vascular dementia. Arch Neurol. 2005;62(11):1734-6.

[65] Nozaki I, Watanabe T, Kawaguchi M, Akatsu H, Tsuneyama K, Yamamoto Y, et al. Reduced expression of endogenous secretory receptor for advanced glycation end-products in hippocampal neurons of Alzheimer's disease brains. Arch Histol Cytol. 2007;70(5):279-90.

[66] Cheng DT, Kim DK, Cockayne DA, Belousov A, Bitter H, Cho MH, et al. Systemic soluble receptor for advanced glycation endproducts is a biomarker of emphysema and associated with AGER genetic variants in patients with chronic obstructive pulmonary disease. Am J Respir Crit Care Med. 2013;188(8):948-57.

[67] Miniati M, Calugi S, Rucci P, Shear MK, Benvenuti A, Santoro D, et al. Predictors of response among patients with panic disorder treated with medications in a naturalistic follow-up: the role of adult separation anxiety. J Affect Disord. 2012;136(3):675-9.

[68] Yan SF, Ramasamy R, Schmidt AM. Soluble RAGE: therapy and biomarker in unraveling the RAGE axis in chronic disease and aging. Biochem Pharmacol. 2010;79(10): 1379-86.

[69] Jing R, Cui M, Wang J, Wang H. Receptor for advanced glycation end products (RAGE) soluble form (sRAGE): a new biomarker for lung cancer. Neoplasma. 2010;57(1):55-61.

[70] Tesarova P, Kalousova M, Jachymova M, Mestek O, Petruzelka L, Zima T. Receptor for advanced glycation end products (RAGE)--soluble form (sRAGE) and gene polymorphisms in patients with breast cancer. Cancer Invest. 2007;25(8):720-5.

[71] Moy KA, Jiao L, Freedman ND, Weinstein SJ, Sinha R, Virtamo J, et al. Soluble receptor for advanced glycation end products and risk of liver cancer. Hepatology. 2013;57(6):2338-45.

[72] Jiao L, Weinstein SJ, Albanes D, Taylor PR, Graubard BI, Virtamo J, et al. Evidence that serum levels of the soluble receptor for advanced glycation end products are inversely associated with pancreatic cancer risk: a prospective study. Cancer Res. 2011;71(10):3582-9.

[73] Leclerc E, Heizmann CW, Vetter SW. RAGE and S100 protein transcription levels are highly variable in human melanoma tumors and cells. General Physiology and Biophysics. 2009;28(Focus Issue):F65-F75.

[74] Neeper M, Schmidt AM, Brett J, Yan SD, Wang F, Pan YC, et al. Cloning and expression of a cell surface receptor for advanced glycosylation end products of proteins. J Biol Chem. 1992;267(21):14998-5004.

[75] Yatime L, Andersen GR. Structural insights into the oligomerization mode of the human receptor for advanced glycation end-products. FEBS J. 2013;280(24):6556-68.

[76] Zong H, Madden A, Ward M, Mooney MH, Elliott CT, Stitt AW. Homodimerization is essential for the receptor for advanced glycation end products (RAGE)-mediated signal transduction. J Biol Chem. 2010;285(30):23137-46.

[77] Xie J, Reverdatto S, Frolov A, Hoffmann R, Burz DS, Shekhtman A. Structural basis for pattern recognition by the receptor for advanced glycation end products (RAGE). J Biol Chem. 2008;283:27255-69.

[78] Xu D, Young JH, Krahn JM, Song D, Corbett KD, Chazin WJ, et al. Stable RAGE-Heparan Sulfate Complexes Are Essential for Signal Transduction. ACS Chem Biol. 2013;8(7):1611-20.

[79] Wei W, Lampe L, Park S, Vangara BS, Waldo GS, Cabantous S, et al. Disulfide bonds within the C2 domain of RAGE play key roles in its dimerization and biogenesis. PLoS One. 2012;7(12):e50736.

[80] Xu D, Young J, Song D, Esko JD. Heparan sulfate is essential for high mobility group protein 1 (HMGB1) signaling by the receptor for advanced glycation end products (RAGE). J Biol Chem. 2011;286(48):41736-44.

[81] Leclerc E, Fritz G, Weibel M, Heizmann CW, Galichet A. S100B and S100A6 differentially modulate cell survival by interacting with distinct RAGE (receptor for advanced glycation end products) immunoglobulin domains. J Biol Chem. 2007;282(43): 31317-31.

[82] Donato R. RAGE: a single receptor for several ligands and different cellular responses: the case of certain S100 proteins. Curr Mol Med. 2007;7(8):711-24.

[83] Logsdon CD, Fuentes MK, Huang EH, Arumugam T. RAGE and RAGE ligands in cancer. Curr Mol Med. 2007;7(8):777-89.

[84] Soman S, Raju R, Sandhya VK, Advani J, Khan AA, Harsha HC, et al. A multicellular signal transduction network of AGE/RAGE signaling. J Cell Commun Signal. 2013;7(1):19-23.

[85] Lander HM, Tauras JM, Ogiste JS, Hori O, Moss RA, Schmidt AM. Activation of the receptor for advanced glycation end products triggers a p21(ras)-dependent mitogen-activated protein kinase pathway regulated by oxidant stress. J Biol Chem. 1997;272(28):17810-4.

[86] Huttunen HJ, Fages C, Rauvala H. Receptor for advanced glycation end products (RAGE)-mediated neurite outgrowth and activation of NF-kappaB require the cytoplasmic domain of the receptor but different downstream signaling pathways. J Biol Chem. 1999;274(28):19919-24.

[87] Brozzi F, Arcuri C, Giambanco I, Donato R. S100B Protein Regulates Astrocyte Shape and Migration via Interaction with Src Kinase: IMPLICATIONS FOR ASTROCYTE DEVELOPMENT, ACTIVATION, AND TUMOR GROWTH. J Biol Chem. 2009;284(13):8797-811.

[88] Bierhaus A, Stern DM, Nawroth PP. RAGE in inflammation: a new therapeutic target? Curr Opin Investig Drugs. 2006;7(11):985-91.

[89] Schmidt AM, Vianna M, Gerlach M, Brett J, Ryan J, Kao J, et al. Isolation and characterization of two binding proteins for advanced glycosylation end products from bovine lung which are present on the endothelial cell surface. J Biol Chem. 1992;267(21): 14987-97.

[90] Basta G, Schmidt AM, De Caterina R. Advanced glycation end products and vascular inflammation: implications for accelerated atherosclerosis in diabetes. Cardiovasc Res. 2004;63(4):582-92.

[91] Yan SF, Ramasamy R, Schmidt AM. The receptor for advanced glycation endproducts (RAGE) and cardiovascular disease. Expert Rev Mol Med. 2009;11:e9.

[92] Srikanth V, Maczurek A, Phan T, Steele M, Westcott B, Juskiw D, et al. Advanced glycation endproducts and their receptor RAGE in Alzheimer's disease. Neurobiol Aging. 2011;32(5):763-77.

[93] Hofmann MA, Drury S, Fu C, Qu W, Taguchi A, Lu Y, et al. RAGE mediates a novel proinflammatory axis: a central cell surface receptor for S100/calgranulin polypeptides. Cell. 1999;97(7):889-901.

[94] Donato R, Cannon BR, Sorci G, Riuzzi F, Hsu K, Weber DJ, et al. Functions of S100 proteins. Curr Mol Med. 2013;13(1):24-57.

[95] Chen H, Xu C, Jin Q, Liu Z. S100 protein family in human cancer. Am J Cancer Res. 2014;4(2):89-115.

[96] Hori O, Brett J, Slattery T, Cao R, Zhang J, Chen JX, et al. The receptor for advanced glycation end products (RAGE) is a cellular binding site for amphoterin. Mediation of neurite outgrowth and co-expression of rage and amphoterin in the developing nervous system. J Biol Chem. 1995;270(43):25752-61.

[97] Huttunen HJ, Rauvala H. Amphoterin as an extracellular regulator of cell motility: from discovery to disease. J Intern Med. 2004;255(3):351-66.

[98] Lotze MT, Tracey KJ. High-mobility group box 1 protein (HMGB1): nuclear weapon in the immune arsenal. Nat Rev Immunol. 2005;5(4):331-42.

[99] Enokido Y, Yoshitake A, Ito H, Okazawa H. Age-dependent change of HMGB1 and DNA double-strand break accumulation in mouse brain. Biochem Biophys Res Commun. 2008;376(1):128-33.

[100] Sousa MM, Yan SD, Stern D, Saraiva MJ. Interaction of the receptor for advanced glycation end products (RAGE) with transthyretin triggers nuclear transcription factor kB (NF-kB) activation. Lab Invest. 2000;80(7):1101-10.

[101] Sasaki N, Takeuchi M, Chowei H, Kikuchi S, Hayashi Y, Nakano N, et al. Advanced glycation end products (AGE) and their receptor (RAGE) in the brain of patients with Creutzfeldt-Jakob disease with prion plaques. Neurosci Lett. 2002;326(2):117-20.

[102] Natale G, Ferrucci M, Lazzeri G, Paparelli A, Fornai F. Transmission of prions within the gut and towards the central nervous system. Prion. 2011;5(3):142-9.

[103] Bullard DC, Hu X, Schoeb TR, Axtell RC, Raman C, Barnum SR. Critical requirement of CD11b (Mac-1) on T cells and accessory cells for development of experimental autoimmune encephalomyelitis. J Immunol. 2005;175(10):6327-33.

[104] Ruan BH, Li X, Winkler AR, Cunningham KM, Kuai J, Greco RM, et al. Complement C3a, CpG oligos, and DNA/C3a complex stimulate IFN-alpha production in a receptor for advanced glycation end product-dependent manner. J Immunol. 2010;185(7): 4213-22.

[105] Ma W, Rai V, Hudson BI, Song F, Schmidt AM, Barile GR. RAGE binds C1q and enhances C1q-mediated phagocytosis. Cell Immunol. 2012;274(1-2):72-82.

[106] He M, Kubo H, Morimoto K, Fujino N, Suzuki T, Takahasi T, et al. Receptor for advanced glycation end products binds to phosphatidylserine and assists in the clearance of apoptotic cells. EMBO Rep. 2011;12(4):358-64.

[107] Fischer U, Schulze-Osthoff K. New approaches and therapeutics targeting apoptosis in disease. Pharmacol Rev. 2005;57(2):187-215.

[108] Mizumoto S, Sugahara K. Glycosaminoglycans are functional ligands for receptor for advanced glycation end-products in tumors. FEBS J. 2013;280(10):2462-70.

[109] Lindahl U, Kjellen L. Pathophysiology of heparan sulphate: many diseases, few drugs. J Intern Med. 2013;273(6):555-71.

[110] Sirois CM, Jin T, Miller AL, Bertheloot D, Nakamura H, Horvath GL, et al. RAGE is a nucleic acid receptor that promotes inflammatory responses to DNA. J Exp Med. 2013;210(11):2447-63.

[111] Heizmann CW, Fritz G, Schäfer BW. S100 proteins: structure, functions and pathology. Front Biosci. 2002;7:d1356-68.

[112] Donato R. Intracellular and extracellular roles of S100 proteins. Microsc Res Tech. 2003;60(6):540-51.

[113] Marenholz I, Lovering RC, Heizmann CW. An update of the S100 nomenclature. Biochim Biophys Acta. 2006;1763(11):1282-3.

[114] Heizmann CW, Ackermann GE, Galichet A. Pathologies involving the S100 proteins and RAGE. Subcell Biochem. 2007;45:93-138.

[115] Zimmer DB, Weber DJ. The Calcium-Dependent Interaction of S100B with Its Protein Targets. Cardiovasc Psychiatry Neurol. 2010;2010.

[116] Moroz OV, Wilson KS, Bronstein IB. The role of zinc in the S100 proteins: insights from the X-ray structures. Amino Acids 2010:in press.

[117] Fritz G, Heizmann CW. 3D Structures of the Calcium and Zinc Binding S100 Proteins. In: Sons JW, editor. Encyclopedia of Inorganic and Bioinorganic Chemistry: Wiley Online Library; 2011.

[118] Nelson MR, Thulin E, Fagan PA, Forsen S, Chazin WJ. The EF-hand domain: a globally cooperative structural unit. Protein Sci. 2002;11(2):198-205.

[119] Leclerc E, Heizmann CW. The importance of Ca2+/Zn2+signaling S100 proteins and RAGE in translational medicine. Frontiers in Biosciences. 2011;S3:1232-62.

[120] Santamaria-Kisiel L, Rintala-Dempsey AC, Shaw GS. Calcium-dependent and-independent interactions of the S100 protein family. Biochem J. 2006;396(2):201-14.

[121] Baudier J, Delphin C, Grunwald D, Khochbin S, Lawrence JJ. Characterization of the tumor suppressor protein p53 as a protein kinase C substrate and a S100b-binding protein. Proc Natl Acad Sci U S A. 1992;89(23):11627-31.

[122] Wilder PT, Lin J, Bair CL, Charpentier TH, Yang D, Liriano M, et al. Recognition of the tumor suppressor protein p53 and other protein targets by the calcium-binding protein S100B. Biochim Biophys Acta. 2006;1763(11):1284-97.

[123] Mueller A, Schäfer BW, Ferrari S, Weibel M, Makek M, Hochli M, et al. The calcium-binding protein S100A2 interacts with p53 and modulates its transcriptional activity. J Biol Chem. 2005;280(32):29186-93.

[124] Fernandez-Fernandez MR, Rutherford TJ, Fersht AR. Members of the S100 family bind p53 in two distinct ways. Protein Sci. 2008;17(10):1663-70.

[125] van Dieck J, Teufel DP, Jaulent AM, Fernandez-Fernandez MR, Rutherford TJ, Wyslouch-Cieszynska A, et al. Posttranslational modifications affect the interaction of S100 proteins with tumor suppressor p53. J Mol Biol. 2009;394(5):922-30.

[126] van Dieck J, Fernandez-Fernandez MR, Veprintsev DB, Fersht AR. Modulation of the oligomerization state of p53 by differential binding of proteins of the S100 family to p53 monomers and tetramers. J Biol Chem. 2009;284(20):13804-11.

[127] Hsieh HL, Schäfer BW, Weigle B, Heizmann CW. S100 protein translocation in response to extracellular S100 is mediated by receptor for advanced glycation endproducts in human endothelial cells. Biochem Biophys Res Commun. 2004;316(3):949-59.

[128] Perrone L, Peluso G, Melone MA. RAGE recycles at the plasma membrane in S100B secretory vesicles and promotes Schwann cells morphological changes. J Cell Physiol. 2008;217(1):60-71.

[129] Leclerc E, Fritz G, Vetter SW, Heizmann CW. Binding of S100 proteins to RAGE: an update. Biochim Biophys Acta. 2009;1793(6):993-1007.

[130] Eckert RL, Broome AM, Ruse M, Robinson N, Ryan D, Lee K. S100 proteins in the epidermis. Journal of Investigative Dermatology. 2004;123(1):23-33.

[131] Ito M, Kizawa K. Expression of calcium-binding S100 proteins A4 and A6 in regions of the epithelial sac associated with the onset of hair follicle regeneration. J Invest Dermatol. 2001;116(6):956-63.

[132] Boni R, Burg G, Doguoglu A, Ilg EC, Schafer BW, Muller B, et al. Immunohistochemical localization of the Ca2+binding S100 proteins in normal human skin and melanocytic lesions. Br J Dermatol. 1997;137(1):39-43.

[133] Ribe A, McNutt NS. S100A6 protein expression is different in Spitz nevi and melanomas. Mod Pathol. 2003;16(5):505-11.

[134] Zhang T, Woods TL, Elder JT. Differential responses of S100A2 to oxidative stress and increased intracellular calcium in normal, immortalized, and malignant human keratinocytes. J Invest Dermatol. 2002;119(5):1196-201.

[135] Deshpande R, Woods TL, Fu J, Zhang T, Stoll SW, Elder JT. Biochemical characterization of S100A2 in human keratinocytes: subcellular localization, dimerization, and oxidative cross-linking. J Invest Dermatol. 2000;115(3):477-85.

[136] Broome AM, Ryan D, Eckert RL. S100 protein subcellular localization during epidermal differentiation and psoriasis. Journal of Histochemistry & Cytochemistry. 2003;51(5):675-85.

[137] Robinson MJ, Tessier P, Poulsom R, Hogg N. The S100 family heterodimer, MRP-8/14, binds with high affinity to heparin and heparan sulfate glycosaminoglycans on endothelial cells. J Biol Chem. 2002;277(5):3658-65.

[138] Mirmohammadsadegh A, Tschakarjan E, Ljoljic A, Bohner K, Michel G, Ruzicka T, et al. Calgranulin C is overexpressed in lesional psoriasis. Journal of Investigative Dermatology. 2000;114(6):1207-8.

[139] Balch CM, Gershenwald JE, Soong SJ, Thompson JF, Atkins MB, Byrd DR, et al. Final version of 2009 AJCC melanoma staging and classification. J Clin Oncol. 2009;27(36): 6199-206.

[140] Ghanem G, Loir B, Morandini R, Sales F, Lienard D, Eggermont A, et al. On the release and half-life of S100B protein in the peripheral blood of melanoma patients. Int J Cancer. 2001;94(4):586-90.

[141] Harpio R, Einarsson R. S100 proteins as cancer biomarkers with focus on S100B in malignant melanoma. Clin Biochem. 2004;37(7):512-8.

[142] Lin J, Blake M, Tang C, Zimmer D, Rustandi RR, Weber DJ, et al. Inhibition of p53 transcriptional activity by the S100B calcium-binding protein. J Biol Chem. 2001;276(37):35037-41.

[143] Lin J, Yang Q, Wilder PT, Carrier F, Weber DJ. The calcium-binding protein S100B down-regulates p53 and apoptosis in malignant melanoma. J Biol Chem. 2010;285(35):27487-98.

[144] Lin J, Yang Q, Yan Z, Markowitz J, Wilder PT, Carrier F, et al. Inhibiting S100B restores p53 levels in primary malignant melanoma cancer cells. J Biol Chem. 2004;279(32):34071-7.

[145] Cavalier M, Wilder PT, Coop A, MacKerell A, Weber DJ, editors. Inhibitors of S100B (SBiXs) in malignant melanoma. AACR-NCI-EORTC International Conference: Molecular Targets and Cancer Therapeutics; 2013; Boston, MA: Mol Cancer Ther.

[146] Zimmer DB, Van Eldik LJ. Identification of a molecular target for the calcium-modulated protein S100. Fructose-1,6-bisphosphate aldolase. J Biol Chem. 1986;261(24):11424-8.

[147] Hersey P, Watts RN, Zhang XD, Hackett J. Metabolic approaches to treatment of melanoma. Clin Cancer Res. 2009;15(21):6490-4.

[148] Xu RH, Pelicano H, Zhou Y, Carew JS, Feng L, Bhalla KN, et al. Inhibition of glycolysis in cancer cells: a novel strategy to overcome drug resistance associated with mitochondrial respiratory defect and hypoxia. Cancer Res. 2005;65(2):613-21.

[149] Donato R. Calcium-independent, pH-regulated effects of S-100 proteins on assembly-disassembly of brain microtubule protein in vitro. J Biol Chem. 1988;263(1):106-10.

[150] Ferguson PL, Shaw GS. Human S100B protein interacts with the Escherichia coli division protein FtsZ in a calcium-sensitive manner. J Biol Chem. 2004;279(18):18806-13.

[151] Skripnikova EV, Gusev NB. Interaction of smooth muscle caldesmon with S-100 protein. FEBS Lett. 1989;257(2):380-2.

[152] Mbele GO, Deloulme JC, Gentil BJ, Delphin C, Ferro M, Garin J, et al. The zinc-and calcium-binding S100B interacts and co-localizes with IQGAP1 during dynamic rearrangement of cell membranes. J Biol Chem. 2002;277(51):49998-50007.

[153] Koganehira Y, Takeoka M, Ehara T, Sasaki K, Murata H, Saida T, et al. Reduced expression of actin-binding proteins, h-caldesmon and calponin h1, in the vascular smooth muscle inside melanoma lesions: an adverse prognostic factor for malignant melanoma. Br J Dermatol. 2003;148(5):971-80.

[154] Wang Z, Chen J, Wang J, Ahn S, Li CM, Lu Y, et al. Novel tubulin polymerization inhibitors overcome multidrug resistance and reduce melanoma lung metastasis. Pharm Res. 2012;29(11):3040-52.

[155] Jameson KL, Mazur PK, Zehnder AM, Zhang J, Zarnegar B, Sage J, et al. IQGAP1 scaffold-kinase interaction blockade selectively targets RAS-MAP kinase-driven tumors. Nat Med. 2013;19(5):626-30.

[156] Bhattacharya S, Large E, Heizmann CW, Hemmings B, Chazin WJ. Structure of the Ca2+/S100B/NDR kinase peptide complex: insights into S100 target specificity and activation of the kinase. Biochemistry. 2003;42(49):14416-26.

[157] Bichsel SJ, Tamaskovic R, Stegert MR, Hemmings BA. Mechanism of activation of NDR (nuclear Dbf2-related) protein kinase by the hMOB1 protein. J Biol Chem. 2004;279(34):35228-35.

[158] Millward TA, Heizmann CW, Schafer BW, Hemmings BA. Calcium regulation of Ndr protein kinase mediated by S100 calcium-binding proteins. Embo J. 1998;17(20):5913-22.

[159] Gentil BJ, Delphin C, Mbele GO, Deloulme JC, Ferro M, Garin J, et al. The giant protein AHNAK is a specific target for the calcium-and zinc-binding S100B protein: po-

tential implications for Ca2+homeostasis regulation by S100B. J Biol Chem. 2001;276(26):23253-61.

[160] Shtivelman E, Bishop JM. The human gene AHNAK encodes a large phosphoprotein located primarily in the nucleus. J Cell Biol. 1993;120(3):625-30.

[161] Fedida-Metula S, Elhyany S, Tsory S, Segal S, Hershfinkel M, Sekler I, et al. Targeting lipid rafts inhibits protein kinase B by disrupting calcium homeostasis and attenuates malignant properties of melanoma cells. Carcinogenesis. 2008;29(8):1546-54.

[162] Donato R, Sorci G, Riuzzi F, Arcuri C, Bianchi R, Brozzi F, et al. S100B's double life: intracellular regulator and extracellular signal. Biochim Biophys Acta. 2009;1793(6): 1008-22.

[163] Ostendorp T, Leclerc E, Galichet A, Koch M, Demling N, Weigle B, et al. Structural and functional insights into RAGE activation by multimeric S100B. Embo J. 2007;26(16):3868-78.

[164] Glenney JR, Jr., Kindy MS, Zokas L. Isolation of a new member of the S100 protein family: amino acid sequence, tissue, and subcellular distribution. J Cell Biol. 1989;108(2):569-78.

[165] Maelandsmo GM, Florenes VA, Mellingsaeter T, Hovig E, Kerbel RS, Fodstad O. Differential expression patterns of S100A2, S100A4 and S100A6 during progression of human malignant melanoma. Int J Cancer. 1997;74(4):464-9.

[166] Gupta S, Hussain T, MacLennan GT, Fu P, Patel J, Mukhtar H. Differential expression of S100A2 and S100A4 during progression of human prostate adenocarcinoma. J Clin Oncol. 2003;21(1):106-12.

[167] Suzuki F, Oridate N, Homma A, Nakamaru Y, Nagahashi T, Yagi K, et al. S100A2 expression as a predictive marker for late cervical metastasis in stage I and II invasive squamous cell carcinoma of the oral cavity. Oncol Rep. 2005;14(6):1493-8.

[168] Feng G, Xu X, Youssef EM, Lotan R. Diminished expression of S100A2, a putative tumor suppressor, at early stage of human lung carcinogenesis. Cancer Res. 2001;61(21):7999-8004.

[169] Lee SW, Tomasetto C, Swisshelm K, Keyomarsi K, Sager R. Down-regulation of a member of the S100 gene family in mammary carcinoma cells and reexpression by azadeoxycytidine treatment. Proc Natl Acad Sci U S A. 1992;89(6):2504-8.

[170] Imazawa M, Hibi K, Fujitake S, Kodera Y, Ito K, Akiyama S, et al. S100A2 overexpression is frequently observed in esophageal squamous cell carcinoma. Anticancer Res. 2005;25:1247-50.

[171] El-Rifai W, Moskaluk CA, Abdrabbo MK, Harper J, Yoshida C, Riggins GJ, et al. Gastric cancers overexpress S100A calcium-binding proteins. Cancer Res. 2002;62(23): 6823-6.

[172] Hough CD, Cho KR, Zonderman AB, Schwartz DR, Morin PJ. Coordinately up-regulated genes in ovarian cancer. Cancer Res. 2001;61(10):3869-76.

[173] Smith SL, Gugger M, Hoban P, Ratschiller D, Watson SG, Field JK, et al. S100A2 is strongly expressed in airway basal cells, preneoplastic bronchial lesions and primary non-small cell lung carcinomas. Br J Cancer. 2004;91(8):1515-24.

[174] Strazisar M, Mlakar V, Glavac D. The expression of COX-2, hTERT, MDM2, LATS2 and S100A2 in different types of non-small cell lung cancer (NSCLC). Cell Mol Biol Lett. 2009;14(3):442-56.

[175] Bulk E, Sargin B, Krug U, Hascher A, Jun Y, Knop M, et al. S100A2 induces metastasis in non-small cell lung cancer. Clin Cancer Res. 2009;15(1):22-9.

[176] Nonaka D, Chiriboga L, Rubin BP. Differential expression of S100 protein subtypes in malignant melanoma, and benign and malignant peripheral nerve sheath tumors. J Cutan Pathol. 2008;35(11):1014-9.

[177] Gollob JA, Sciambi CJ. Decitabine up-regulates S100A2 expression and synergizes with IFN-gamma to kill uveal melanoma cells. Clin Cancer Res. 2007;13(17):5219-25.

[178] Klopper JP, Sharma V, Bissonnette R, Haugen BR. Combination PPARgamma and RXR Agonist Treatment in Melanoma Cells: Functional Importance of S100A2. PPAR Res. 2010;2010:729876.

[179] Tan M, Heizmann CW, Guan K, Schafer BW, Sun Y. Transcriptional activation of the human S100A2 promoter by wild-type p53. FEBS Lett. 1999;445(2-3):265-8.

[180] Lapi E, Iovino A, Fontemaggi G, Soliera AR, Iacovelli S, Sacchi A, et al. S100A2 gene is a direct transcriptional target of p53 homologues during keratinocyte differentiation. Oncogene. 2006;25(26):3628-37.

[181] Kirschner RD, Sanger K, Muller GA, Engeland K. Transcriptional activation of the tumor suppressor and differentiation gene S100A2 by a novel p63-binding site. Nucleic Acids Res. 2008;36(9):2969-80.

[182] Buckley NE, D'Costa Z, Kaminska M, Mullan PB. S100A2 is a BRCA1/p63 coregulated tumour suppressor gene with roles in the regulation of mutant p53 stability. Cell death & disease. 2014;5:e1070.

[183] Harbour JW, Onken MD, Roberson ED, Duan S, Cao L, Worley LA, et al. Frequent mutation of BAP1 in metastasizing uveal melanomas. Science. 2010;330(6009):1410-3.

[184] Carbone M, Ferris LK, Baumann F, Napolitano A, Lum CA, Flores EG, et al. BAP1 cancer syndrome: malignant mesothelioma, uveal and cutaneous melanoma, and MBAITs. J Transl Med. 2012;10:179.

[185] Njauw CN, Kim I, Piris A, Gabree M, Taylor M, Lane AM, et al. Germline BAP1 inactivation is preferentially associated with metastatic ocular melanoma and cutaneous-ocular melanoma families. PLoS One. 2012;7(4):e35295.

[186] Ebralidze A, Tulchinsky E, Grigorian M, Afanasyeva A, Senin V, Revazova E, et al. Isolation and characterization of a gene specifically expressed in different metastatic cells and whose deduced gene product has a high degree of homology to a Ca^{2+}-binding protein family. Genes Dev. 1989;3(7):1086-93.

[187] Takenaga K, Nakamura Y, Endo H, Sakiyama S. Involvement of S100-related calcium-binding protein pEL98 (or mts1) in cell motility and tumor cell invasion. Japanese journal of cancer research : Gann. 1994;85(8):831-9.

[188] Jenkinson SR, Barraclough R, West CR, Rudland PS. S100A4 regulates cell motility and invasion in an in vitro model for breast cancer metastasis. Br J Cancer. 2004;90(1): 253-62.

[189] Grum-Schwensen B, Klingelhofer J, Berg CH, El-Naaman C, Grigorian M, Lukanidin E, et al. Suppression of tumor development and metastasis formation in mice lacking the S100A4(mts1) gene. Cancer Res. 2005;65(9):3772-80.

[190] Ambartsumian N, Grigorian M, Lukanidin E. Genetically modified mouse models to study the role of metastasis-promoting S100A4(mts1) protein in metastatic mammary cancer. J Dairy Res. 2005;72 Spec No:27-33.

[191] Andersen K, Nesland JM, Holm R, Florenes VA, Fodstad O, Maelandsmo GM. Expression of S100A4 combined with reduced E-cadherin expression predicts patient outcome in malignant melanoma. Mod Pathol. 2004;17(8):990-7.

[192] Boye K, Maelandsmo GM. S100A4 and metastasis: a small actor playing many roles. Am J Pathol. 2010;176(2):528-35.

[193] Fernandez-Fernandez MR, Veprintsev DB, Fersht AR. Proteins of the S100 family regulate the oligomerization of p53 tumor suppressor. Proc Natl Acad Sci U S A. 2005;102(13):4735-40.

[194] Berge G, Maelandsmo GM. Evaluation of potential interactions between the metastasis-associated protein S100A4 and the tumor suppressor protein p53. Amino Acids. 2010:in press.

[195] Orre LM, Panizza E, Kaminskyy VO, Vernet E, Graslund T, Zhivotovsky B, et al. S100A4 interacts with p53 in the nucleus and promotes p53 degradation. Oncogene. 2013;32(49):5531-40.

[196] Ford HL, Zain SB. Interaction of metastasis associated Mts1 protein with nonmuscle myosin. Oncogene. 1995;10(8):1597-605.

[197] Takenaga K, Nakamura Y, Sakiyama S, Hasegawa Y, Sato K, Endo H. Binding of pEL98 protein, an S100-related calcium-binding protein, to nonmuscle tropomyosin. J Cell Biol. 1994;124(5):757-68.

[198] Li ZH, Bresnick AR. The S100A4 metastasis factor regulates cellular motility via a direct interaction with myosin-IIA. Cancer Res. 2006;66(10):5173-80.

[199] Kriajevska M, Bronstein IB, Scott DJ, Tarabykina S, Fischer-Larsen M, Issinger O, et al. Metastasis-associated protein Mts1 (S100A4) inhibits CK2-mediated phosphorylation and self-assembly of the heavy chain of nonmuscle myosin. Biochim Biophys Acta. 2000;1498(2-3):252-63.

[200] Cabezon T, Celis JE, Skibshoj I, Klingelhofer J, Grigorian M, Gromov P, et al. Expression of S100A4 by a variety of cell types present in the tumor microenvironment of human breast cancer. Int J Cancer. 2007;121(7):1433-44.

[201] Kikuchi N, Horiuchi A, Osada R, Imai T, Wang C, Chen X, et al. Nuclear expression of S100A4 is associated with aggressive behavior of epithelial ovarian carcinoma: an important autocrine/paracrine factor in tumor progression. Cancer Sci. 2006;97(10): 1061-9.

[202] Pedersen KB, Andersen K, Fodstad O, Maelandsmo GM. Sensitization of interferon-gamma induced apoptosis in human osteosarcoma cells by extracellular S100A4. BMC Cancer. 2004;4:52.

[203] Schmidt-Hansen B, Klingelhofer J, Grum-Schwensen B, Christensen A, Andresen S, Kruse C, et al. Functional significance of metastasis-inducing S100A4(Mts1) in tumor-stroma interplay. J Biol Chem. 2004;279(23):24498-504.

[204] Gibbs FE, Barraclough R, Platt-Higgins A, Rudland PS, Wilkinson MC, Parry EW. Immunocytochemical distribution of the calcium-binding protein p9Ka in normal rat tissues: variation in the cellular location in different tissues. J Histochem Cytochem. 1995;43(2):169-80.

[205] Ambartsumian N, Klingelhofer J, Grigorian M, Christensen C, Kriajevska M, Tulchinsky E, et al. The metastasis-associated Mts1(S100A4) protein could act as an angiogenic factor. Oncogene. 2001;20(34):4685-95.

[206] Ochiya T, Takenaga K, Endo H. Silencing of S100A4, a metastasis-associated protein, in endothelial cells inhibits tumor angiogenesis and growth. Angiogenesis. 2014;17(1):17-26.

[207] Schmidt-Hansen B, Ornas D, Grigorian M, Klingelhofer J, Tulchinsky E, Lukanidin E, et al. Extracellular S100A4(mts1) stimulates invasive growth of mouse endothelial cells and modulates MMP-13 matrix metalloproteinase activity. Oncogene. 2004;23(32):5487-95.

[208] Semov A, Moreno MJ, Onichtchenko A, Abulrob A, Ball M, Ekiel I, et al. Metastasis-associated protein S100A4 induces angiogenesis through interaction with Annexin II and accelerated plasmin formation. J Biol Chem. 2005;280(21):20833-41.

[209] Kiryushko D, Novitskaya V, Soroka V, Klingelhofer J, Lukanidin E, Berezin V, et al. Molecular mechanisms of Ca^{2+}signaling in neurons induced by the S100A4 protein. Mol Cell Biol. 2006;26(9):3625-38.

[210] Spiekerkoetter E, Guignabert C, de Jesus Perez V, Alastalo TP, Powers JM, Wang L, et al. S100A4 and bone morphogenetic protein-2 codependently induce vascular

smooth muscle cell migration via phospho-extracellular signal-regulated kinase and chloride intracellular channel 4. Circ Res. 2009;105(7):639-47, 13 p following 47.

[211] Dahlmann M, Okhrimenko A, Marcinkowski P, Osterland M, Herrmann P, Smith J, et al. RAGE mediates S100A4-induced cell motility via MAPK/ERK and hypoxia signaling and is a prognostic biomarker for human colorectal cancer metastasis. Oncotarget. 2014;5(10):3220-33.

[212] Siddique HR, Adhami VM, Parray A, Johnson JJ, Siddiqui IA, Shekhani MT, et al. The S100A4 Oncoprotein Promotes Prostate Tumorigenesis in a Transgenic Mouse Model: Regulating NFkappaB through the RAGE Receptor. Genes & cancer. 2013;4(5-6):224-34.

[213] Haase-Kohn C, Wolf S, Herwig N, Mosch B, Pietzsch J. Metastatic potential of B16-F10 melanoma cells is enhanced by extracellular S100A4 derived from RAW264.7 macrophages. Biochem Biophys Res Commun. 2014;446(1):143-8.

[214] Weterman MA, van Muijen GN, Bloemers HP, Ruiter DJ. Expression of calcyclin in human melanocytic lesions. Cancer Res. 1993;53(24):6061-6.

[215] Kuznicki J, Kordowska J, Puzianowska M, Wozniewicz BM. Calcyclin as a marker of human epithelial cells and fibroblasts. Exp Cell Res. 1992;200(2):425-30.

[216] Kuznicki J, Filipek A, Heimann P, Kaczmarek L, Kaminska B. Tissue specific distribution of calcyclin--10.5 kDa Ca2+-binding protein. FEBS Lett. 1989;254(1-2):141-4.

[217] Lesniak W, Slomnicki LP, Filipek A. S100A6-new facts and features. Biochem Biophys Res Commun. 2009;390(4):1087-92.

[218] Komatsu K, Andoh A, Ishiguro S, Suzuki N, Hunai H, Kobune-Fujiwara Y, et al. Increased expression of S100A6 (Calcyclin), a calcium-binding protein of the S100 family, in human colorectal adenocarcinomas. Clin Cancer Res. 2000;6(1):172-7.

[219] Nedjadi T, Kitteringham N, Campbell F, Jenkins RE, Park BK, Navarro P, et al. S100A6 binds to annexin 2 in pancreatic cancer cells and promotes pancreatic cancer cell motility. Br J Cancer. 2009;101(7):1145-54.

[220] De Petris L, Orre LM, Kanter L, Pernemalm M, Koyi H, Lewensohn R, et al. Tumor expression of S100A6 correlates with survival of patients with stage I non-small-cell lung cancer. Lung Cancer. 2009;63:410-7.

[221] Ohuchida K, Mizumoto K, Yu J, Yamaguchi H, Konomi H, Nagai E, et al. S100A6 is increased in a stepwise manner during pancreatic carcinogenesis: clinical value of expression analysis in 98 pancreatic juice samples. Cancer Epidemiol Biomarkers Prev. 2007;16(4):649-54.

[222] Yang YQ, Zhang LJ, Dong H, Jiang CL, Zhu ZG, Wu JX, et al. Upregulated expression of S100A6 in human gastric cancer. J Dig Dis. 2007;8(4):186-93.

[223] Vimalachandran D, Greenhalf W, Thompson C, Luttges J, Prime W, Campbell F, et al. High nuclear S100A6 (Calcyclin) is significantly associated with poor survival in pancreatic cancer patients. Cancer Res. 2005;65(8):3218-25.

[224] Li Z, Tang M, Ling B, Liu S, Zheng Y, Nie C, et al. Increased expression of S100A6 promotes cell proliferation and migration in human hepatocellular carcinoma. Journal of molecular medicine. 2014;92(3):291-303.

[225] Weterman MA, Stoopen GM, van Muijen GN, Kuznicki J, Ruiter DJ, Bloemers HP. Expression of calcyclin in human melanoma cell lines correlates with metastatic behavior in nude mice. Cancer Res. 1992;52(5):1291-6.

[226] Fullen DR, Garrisi AJ, Sanders D, Thomas D. Expression of S100A6 protein in a broad spectrum of cutaneous tumors using tissue microarrays. J Cutan Pathol. 2008;35 Suppl 2:28-34.

[227] Puri PK, Elston CA, Tyler WB, Ferringer TC, Elston DM. The staining pattern of pigmented spindle cell nevi with S100A6 protein. J Cutan Pathol. 2011;38(1):14-7.

[228] Slomnicki LP, Nawrot B, Lesniak W. S100A6 binds p53 and affects its activity. Int J Biochem Cell Biol. 2009;41(4):784-90.

[229] Streicher WW, Lopez MM, Makhatadze GI. Annexin I and annexin II N-terminal peptides binding to S100 protein family members: specificity and thermodynamic characterization. Biochemistry. 2009;48(12):2788-98.

[230] Mohan SK, Gupta AA, Yu C. Interaction of the S100A6 mutant (C3S) with the V domain of the receptor for advanced glycation end products (RAGE). Biochem Biophys Res Commun. 2013;434(2):328-33.

[231] Roth J, Vogl T, Sorg C, Sunderkotter C. Phagocyte-specific S100 proteins: a novel group of proinflammatory molecules. Trends Immunol. 2003;24(4):155-8.

[232] Yin C, Li H, Zhang B, Liu Y, Lu G, Lu S, et al. RAGE-binding S100A8/A9 promotes the migration and invasion of human breast cancer cells through actin polymerization and epithelial-mesenchymal transition. Breast Cancer Res Treat. 2013;142(2): 297-309.

[233] Grebhardt S, Muller-Decker K, Bestvater F, Hershfinkel M, Mayer D. Impact of S100A8/A9 expression on prostate cancer progression in vitro and in vivo. J Cell Physiol. 2014;229(5):661-71.

[234] Khammanivong A, Wang C, Sorenson BS, Ross KF, Herzberg MC. S100A8/A9 (calprotectin) negatively regulates G2/M cell cycle progression and growth of squamous cell carcinoma. PLoS One. 2013;8(7):e69395.

[235] Kwon CH, Moon HJ, Park HJ, Choi JH, Park do Y. S100A8 and S100A9 promotes invasion and migration through p38 mitogen-activated protein kinase-dependent NF-kappaB activation in gastric cancer cells. Mol Cells. 2013;35(3):226-34.

[236] Ehrchen JM, Sunderkotter C, Foell D, Vogl T, Roth J. The endogenous Toll-like receptor 4 agonist S100A8/S100A9 (calprotectin) as innate amplifier of infection, autoimmunity, and cancer. J Leukoc Biol. 2009;86(3):557-66.

[237] Ghavami S, Chitayat S, Hashemi M, Eshraghi M, Chazin WJ, Halayko AJ, et al. S100A8/A9: a Janus-faced molecule in cancer therapy and tumorgenesis. Eur J Pharmacol. 2009;625(1-3):73-83.

[238] Ang CW, Nedjadi T, Sheikh AA, Tweedle EM, Tonack S, Honap S, et al. Smad4 loss is associated with fewer S100A8-positive monocytes in colorectal tumors and attenuated response to S100A8 in colorectal and pancreatic cancer cells. Carcinogenesis. 2010;31(9):1541-51.

[239] Sinha P, Okoro C, Foell D, Freeze HH, Ostrand-Rosenberg S, Srikrishna G. Proinflammatory S100 proteins regulate the accumulation of myeloid-derived suppressor cells. J Immunol. 2008;181(7):4666-75.

[240] Srikrishna G. S100A8 and S100A9: new insights into their roles in malignancy. Journal of innate immunity. 2012;4(1):31-40.

[241] Wang L, Chang EW, Wong SC, Ong SM, Chong DQ, Ling KL. Increased myeloid-derived suppressor cells in gastric cancer correlate with cancer stage and plasma S100A8/A9 proinflammatory proteins. J Immunol. 2013;190(2):794-804.

[242] Basso D, Fogar P, Plebani M. The S100A8/A9 complex reduces CTLA4 expression by immature myeloid cells: Implications for pancreatic cancer-driven immunosuppression. Oncoimmunology. 2013;2(6):e24441.

[243] Burke M, Choksawangkarn W, Edwards N, Ostrand-Rosenberg S, Fenselau C. Exosomes from myeloid-derived suppressor cells carry biologically active proteins. J Proteome Res. 2014;13(2):836-43.

[244] Petersson S, Shubbar E, Enerback L, Enerback C. Expression patterns of S100 proteins in melanocytes and melanocytic lesions. Melanoma Res. 2009;19(4):215-25.

[245] Hibino T, Sakaguchi M, Miyamoto S, Yamamoto M, Motoyama A, Hosoi J, et al. S100A9 is a novel ligand of EMMPRIN that promotes melanoma metastasis. Cancer Res. 2013;73(1):172-83.

[246] Meyer C, Sevko A, Ramacher M, Bazhin AV, Falk CS, Osen W, et al. Chronic inflammation promotes myeloid-derived suppressor cell activation blocking antitumor immunity in transgenic mouse melanoma model. Proc Natl Acad Sci U S A. 2011;108(41):17111-6.

[247] Vogl T, Tenbrock K, Ludwig S, Leukert N, Ehrhardt C, van Zoelen MA, et al. MRP8 and MRP14 are endogenous activators of Toll-like receptor 4, promoting lethal, endotoxin-induced shock. Nat Med. 2007;13(9):1042-9.

[248] Ghavami S, Rashedi I, Dattilo BM, Eshraghi M, Chazin WJ, Hashemi M, et al. S100A8/A9 at low concentration promotes tumor cell growth via RAGE ligation and MAP kinase-dependent pathway. J Leukoc Biol. 2008;83(6):1484-92.

[249] Turovskaya O, Foell D, Sinha P, Vogl T, Newlin R, Nayak J, et al. RAGE, carboxylated glycans and S100A8/A9 play essential roles in colitis-associated carcinogenesis. Carcinogenesis. 2008;29:2035-43.

[250] Srikrishna G, Panneerselvam K, Westphal V, Abraham V, Varki A, Freeze HH. Two proteins modulating transendothelial migration of leukocytes recognize novel carboxylated glycans on endothelial cells. J Immunol. 2001;166(7):4678-88.

[251] Srikrishna G, Nayak J, Weigle B, Temme A, Foell D, Hazelwood L, et al. Carboxylated N-glycans on RAGE promote S100A12 binding and signaling. J Cell Biochem. 2010;110(3):645-59.

[252] Hagens G, Masouye I, Augsburger E, Hotz R, Saurat JH, Siegenthaler G. Calcium-binding protein S100A7 and epidermal-type fatty acid-binding protein are associated in the cytosol of human keratinocytes. Biochemical Journal. 1999;339:419-27.

[253] Semprini S, Capon F, Tacconelli A, Giardina E, Orecchia A, Mingarelli R, et al. Evidence for differential S100 gene over-expression in psoriatic patients from genetically heterogeneous pedigrees. Hum Genet. 2002;111(4-5):310-3.

[254] Brouard MC, Saurat JH, Ghanem G, Siegenthaler G. Urinary excretion of epidermal-type fatty acid-binding protein and S100A7 protein in patients with cutaneous melanoma. Melanoma Res. 2002;12(6):627-31.

[255] He H, Li J, Weng S, Li M, Yu Y. S100A11: diverse function and pathology corresponding to different target proteins. Cell Biochem Biophys. 2009;55(3):117-26.

[256] Van Ginkel PR, Gee RL, Walker TM, Hu DN, Heizmann CW, Polans AS. The identification and differential expression of calcium-binding proteins associated with ocular melanoma. Biochim Biophys Acta. 1998;1448(2):290-7.

[257] Reddy S, Bichler J, Wells-Knecht KJ, Thorpe SR, Baynes JW. N epsilon-(carboxymethyl)lysine is a dominant advanced glycation end product (AGE) antigen in tissue proteins. Biochemistry. 1995;34(34):10872-8.

[258] Thornalley PJ. Advances in glyoxalase research. Glyoxalase expression in malignancy, anti-proliferative effects of methylglyoxal, glyoxalase I inhibitor diesters and S-D-lactoylglutathione, and methylglyoxal-modified protein binding and endocytosis by the advanced glycation endproduct receptor. Crit Rev Oncol Hematol. 1995;20(1-2): 99-128.

[259] Wondrak GT, Jacobson MK, Jacobson EL. Antimelanoma activity of apoptogenic carbonyl scavengers. J Pharmacol Exp Ther. 2006;316(2):805-14.

[260] Sander CS, Hamm F, Elsner P, Thiele JJ. Oxidative stress in malignant melanoma and non-melanoma skin cancer. Br J Dermatol. 2003;148(5):913-22.

[261] Indurthi VS, Leclerc E, Vetter SW. Interaction between glycated serum albumin and AGE-receptors depends on structural changes and the glycation reagent. Arch Biochem Biophys. 2012;528(2):185-96.

[262] Bianchi ME, Beltrame M, Paonessa G. Specific recognition of cruciform DNA by nuclear protein HMG1. Science. 1989;243(4894 Pt 1):1056-9.

[263] Wang H, Bloom O, Zhang M, Vishnubhakat JM, Ombrellino M, Che J, et al. HMG-1 as a late mediator of endotoxin lethality in mice. Science. 1999;285(5425):248-51.

[264] Scaffidi P, Misteli T, Bianchi ME. Release of chromatin protein HMGB1 by necrotic cells triggers inflammation. Nature. 2002;418(6894):191-5.

[265] Tian J, Avalos AM, Mao SY, Chen B, Senthil K, Wu H, et al. Toll-like receptor 9-dependent activation by DNA-containing immune complexes is mediated by HMGB1 and RAGE. Nat Immunol. 2007;8(5):487-96.

[266] Dong Xda E, Ito N, Lotze MT, Demarco RA, Popovic P, Shand SH, et al. High mobility group box I (HMGB1) release from tumor cells after treatment: implications for development of targeted chemoimmunotherapy. J Immunother. 2007;30(6):596-606.

[267] Bianchi ME. DAMPs, PAMPs and alarmins: all we need to know about danger. J Leukoc Biol. 2007;81(1):1-5.

[268] Tang D, Kang R, Zeh HJ, 3rd, Lotze MT. High-mobility group box 1 and cancer. Biochim Biophys Acta. 2010;1799(1-2):131-40.

[269] Ito N, DeMarco RA, Mailliard RB, Han J, Rabinowich H, Kalinski P, et al. Cytolytic cells induce HMGB1 release from melanoma cell lines. J Leukoc Biol. 2007;81(1): 75-83.

[270] Johnson KE, Wulff BC, Oberyszyn TM, Wilgus TA. Ultraviolet light exposure stimulates HMGB1 release by keratinocytes. Archives of dermatological research. 2013;305(9):805-15.

[271] Bald T, Quast T, Landsberg J, Rogava M, Glodde N, Lopez-Ramos D, et al. Ultraviolet-radiation-induced inflammation promotes angiotropism and metastasis in melanoma. Nature. 2014;507(7490):109-13.

[272] Tang Q, Li J, Zhu H, Li P, Zou Z, Xiao Y. Hmgb1-IL-23-IL-17-IL-6-Stat3 axis promotes tumor growth in murine models of melanoma. Mediators of inflammation. 2013;2013:713859.

[273] Li Q, Li J, Wen T, Zeng W, Peng C, Yan S, et al. Overexpression of HMGB1 in melanoma predicts patient survival and suppression of HMGB1 induces cell cycle arrest and senescence in association with p21 (Waf1/Cip1) up-regulation via a p53-independent, Sp1-dependent pathway. Oncotarget. 2014;5(15):6387-403.

[274] O'Connell MP, Weeraratna AT. A spoonful of sugar makes the melanoma go: the role of heparan sulfate proteoglycans in melanoma metastasis. Pigment Cell Melanoma Res. 2011;24(6):1133-47.

[275] Nikitovic D, Mytilinaiou M, Berdiaki A, Karamanos NK, Tzanakakis GN. Heparan sulfate proteoglycans and heparin regulate melanoma cell functions. Biochim Biophys Acta. 2014;1840(8):2471-81.

[276] Newton RA, Hogg N. The human S100 protein MRP-14 is a novel activator of the beta 2 integrin Mac-1 on neutrophils. J Immunol. 1998;160(3):1427-35.

[277] Carlos TM. Leukocyte recruitment at sites of tumor: dissonant orchestration. J Leukoc Biol. 2001;70(2):171-84.

[278] Gabrilovich DI, Nagaraj S. Myeloid-derived suppressor cells as regulators of the immune system. Nat Rev Immunol. 2009;9(3):162-74.

[279] Mahnke K, Skorokhod A, Grabbe S, Enk AH. Opening a niche for therapy: local lymphodepletion helps the immune system to fight melanoma. J Invest Dermatol. 2014;134(7):1794-6.

[280] Najjar YG, Finke JH. Clinical perspectives on targeting of myeloid derived suppressor cells in the treatment of cancer. Frontiers in oncology. 2013;3:49.

[281] Riedl S, Rinner B, Asslaber M, Schaider H, Walzer S, Novak A, et al. In search of a novel target-phosphatidylserine exposed by non-apoptotic tumor cells and metastases of malignancies with poor treatment efficacy. Biochim Biophys Acta. 2011;1808(11):2638-45.

[282] Bro S, Flyvbjerg A, Binder CJ, Bang CA, Denner L, Olgaard K, et al. A neutralizing antibody against receptor for advanced glycation end products (RAGE) reduces atherosclerosis in uremic mice. Atherosclerosis. 2008;201(2):274-80.

[283] Taguchi A, Blood DC, del Toro G, Canet A, Lee DC, Qu W, et al. Blockade of RAGE-amphoterin signalling suppresses tumour growth and metastases. Nature. 2000;405(6784):354-60.

[284] Bierhaus A, Humpert PM, Morcos M, Wendt T, Chavakis T, Arnold B, et al. Understanding RAGE, the receptor for advanced glycation end products. J Mol Med. 2005;83(11):876-86.

[285] Hudson BI, Bucciarelli LG, Wendt T, Sakaguchi T, Lalla E, Qu W, et al. Blockade of receptor for advanced glycation endproducts: a new target for therapeutic intervention in diabetic complications and inflammatory disorders. Arch Biochem Biophys. 2003;419(1):80-8.

[286] Oldfield MD, Bach LA, Forbes JM, Nikolic-Paterson D, McRobert A, Thallas V, et al. Advanced glycation end products cause epithelial-myofibroblast transdifferentiation

via the receptor for advanced glycation end products (RAGE). J Clin Invest. 2001;108(12):1853-63.

[287] Deane R, Singh I, Sagare AP, Bell RD, Ross NT, LaRue B, et al. A multimodal RAGE-specific inhibitor reduces amyloid beta-mediated brain disorder in a mouse model of Alzheimer disease. J Clin Invest. 2012;122(4):1377-92.

Chapter 14

Gangliosides and Antigangliosides in Malignant Melanoma

Corina-Daniela Ene (Nicolae) and Ilinca Nicolae

Additional information is available at the end of the chapter

http://dx.doi.org/10.5772/59176

1. Introduction

Cutaneous malignant melanoma is the most agressive skin cancer with rising incidence in the last years [1]. Nowadays, the only treatment to cure melanoma is the early diagnosis and surgical removal of the primer tumor. New research directions developed in order to discover markers for early detection and therapeutic response of melanoma, treatments that could improve the survival rate. Recent studies showed that melanoma is a heterogeneous group of complex molecular disorders [2-16]. The diversity of these alterations sustain the importance of, on one hand, an individualized diagnosis, prognosis and treatment of melanoma patients, and, on the other hand, the detection of new biomarkers and therapeutic approaches in these patients.

The development of new research and investigation techniques in the last years, offered information regarding pathogenesis of melanoma. The skin is considered a hypoxic organ and the low level of oxygen induces the transcription of some hypoxic markers. The cells respond to hypoxia by stimulating the synthesis of some heterodimeric factors, composed by alpha inductible subunit (hypoxia inducible factor alpha-HIF alpha) and beta subunit (aryl hydrocarbon receptor nuclear transducer ARNT). Cutaneous melanocytes, from the dermic-epidermic junction, lay in a low oxygen medium [16, 17]. Tissue hypoxia can modify cellular behavior by direct influence on: cell cycle, cellular metabolism, differentiation, proliferation and survival, degradation and remodeling of extracellular matrix, tumor migration, invasion and metastasis, angiogenesis, apoptosis, cells sensitivity to antitumor therapy (Table 1) [16-29]. Cells ability to adapt to hypoxia is mediated by several transcription factors. A major role in cells response to hypoxia is played by HIF 1 alpha. Its expression and tissue distribution are influnenced by many factors [3, 30-38]: modulators of cellular degradation (EPF, UCP, VDU2, Sumoylation, DeSUMOylation, Prolyl hydroxylases, PVLH, OS-9, SSAT 1, SSAT 2, GSK3 beta,

FOXO 4, Calcineurin A), modulators of translation (RNA-binding protein, PTB and HuR, PtdIns3k and MAPK pathways, IRES-mediated translation, calcium signaling bng, miRNA).

Function	Gene
Cell metabolism	**Iron** - Erythropoietin (EPO); Transferrin; Transferrin receptor (TfR); Ceruloplasmin **pH** - Carbonic anhydrase-9, 12 **Nucleotide** - Adenylate kinase; Ecto-5-nucleotidase **Aminoacids** - Transglutaminase 2; **Glucose** - Adenylate kinase; Aldolase A,C (ALDA,C); Carbonic anhydrase-9,-12; Enolase- 1 (ENO1); Glucose transporter-,1,3 (GLU1,3); Glyceraldehyde phosphate dehydrogenase (GAPDH); Hexokinase1,2 (HK1,2); Lactate dehydrogenase-A (LDHA); Pyruvate kinase M (PKM); Phosphofructokinase L (PFKL); Phosphoglycerate kinase 1(PGK1); 6-phosphofructo-2-kinase/fructose-2,6-bisphosphonate-3 (PFKFB3). **Lipids-**Sphingosine kinase 1 (Sphk 1); Lpin 1.
Matrix metabolism	Matrix metalloproteinases (MMPs) ; Plasminogen activator receptors and inhibitors (PAIs); Collagen prolyl hidroxylase .
Cytoskeletal structure	Keratin 14,18,19 (KRT 14,18,19); Vimentin
Mitochondrial respiration	Pyruvate dehydrogenase kinase1 (PDK1) ; Monocarboxylate transporter (MCT4) ; Cytochrome c oxidase (COX1-4).
Transcriptional regulation	Differentiated embryo-chondrocyte exppressed gene 1,2 (DEC1,20; Nuclear receptor 77 (NUR77); v-ets erythroblastosis virus E26 oncogene homolog1 (ETS1).
Vascular tone	Nitric oxide synthase2 (NOS2); Heme oxigenase ; Endothelin 1 (ET1) ; Adrenomedullin (ADM); Alpha-,beta-adrenergic receptor
Stem cells	KLF4; Nanog; Oct-3/4; Oct-4A,SOX2; Wnt/beta-catenin.
Cell proliferation/ survival	Insulin-like growth factor-2 (IGF2) ; IGF-factor binding protein 1,2,3 (IGF-BP1,2,3); Adrenomedulin (ADM); Coiled-coil-DIX1 (CCD1); Transforming growth factor alpha,beta (TGF alpha,beta); Cyclin G2; Survivin ; Notch-1; Nitric oxide synthase 2 (NOS2); P21; Erythropoietin.
Cell differentiation	Notch signal activation; Tertiary complex p300/HIF1/STAT3/ROR gamma; Multistructural complex Foxp3/pVHLE3/HIF1/nUb
Cell migration/invasion	Collagen V; Autocrine motility factor/ glucose-6-phosphate isomerase (AMF/GPI); Cathepsin D(CATHD); Integrin-linked kinase; Integrins; Lysyloxidase (LOX); Plasminogen activator receptor and inhibitor1 (PAI1); LDL receptor-related protein1 (LRP1); Microneme protein2/ CD99 (MIC2/CD99); Fibronectin; Urokinase plasminogen activator receptor (UPAR); Proto-oncogenes c-MET; Chemokine receptor type4 (CXCR4) ; MMP2
Angiogenesis	**Proangiogenic** - Vascular endothelial growth factor/receptors (VEGF, Flt-1 /VEGfF-R1, Kdr/VEGF-R2); Endocrine-gland-derived VEGF (EG-VEGF); Leptin (LEP); Transforming growth factor –beta 3 (TGF-beta3); Angiopoietin 1,2 (Ang-1,2); TEK- tyrosine kinase endothelial (Tie-2); Adrenomedullin (ADM) ; Fibroblast growth factor (FGFs) ; Placenta

Function	Gene
	growth factor (PLGF); Plateled-derived growth factor- beta (PDGF); Stem cell factor (SCF); Osteopontin; Plasminogen activator receptor and inhibitor -1 (PAI-1); Matrix metalloproteinases (MMPs); Tissue inhibitor of metalloproteinases (TIMPs); Nitric oxide synthase (NOS2); Cyclo-oxigenase-2 (COX-2); Endoglin; Alpha, beta-Adrenergic receptor; Endothelin-1; Semaphorin-4D; Integrins; Leptin; Endosialin; Adenosine A2A receptor ; Oxygen regulated protein-150; Stromal derived growth factor-1 (SDF-1); Interleukins (IL 1, 2, 4, 6, 8, 10). **Antiangiogenic** - Delta-like ligand 1-4 (DLL1-4); Carbonic anhydrase-9; Vasohibin-1; Thrombospondin-1; Regulator of G-protein signaling 5; Angiostatin; Endostatin; Canstatin; Interferons (alpha, beta, gamma). **Neovessel formation** - FGFs/FGFRs; PDGF-B/PDGFR; PLGF/VEGFR1(Flt-1); Thrombospondin-1/CD36,CD47,integrins; Integrins/Extracellular matrix; SDF-1/CXCR4L SCF/c-kit; DLL1-4/Notch; Interleukins/Interleukin receptors; Wnt/beta-catenin. **Cell maturation** - Vasohibin-1/vasohibin receptors; Endothelin receptors(Et-A,Et-B); Angiopoietin1/Tie-2; PDGF-B/PDGFR
Cell apoptosis	Bcl2/adenovirus EIB19KD-interacting protein3 (BNip3); Nip3-like protein X(NIX); Regulated in development and DNA damage responses1 (RTP801/REDD1); Redox factor-1 (Ref-1); Nuclear factor kappa B (NFKB); Heat shock protein 70 (HSP70); P53; Bax; Puma/ Bax; Bcl-2-Interacting Domain (BID).
Metastasis	Twist upregulation; CXC chemokine CCL2/ JE/MCP-1; HGF-R/c-MET; CTGF/CCN2; ZEB1; TCF-3/E2A; Snail; MKP-1; MMPs upregulation; E-cadherin downregulation.
Drug metabolism	Multidrug resistance gene/P-glycoprotein (MDR!/P-GP); Multidrug resistance – associated protein1 (MRP!).

Table 1. Representative target genes of Hypoxia-Inducible Factor1 (HIF1) and their functions [17-29].

Post-translational changes (polyubiquitination by PVHL-signaling for degradation, lysine acetylation by ARD1-facilitating PVHL binding) influence HIF activity. Biological disponibility of HIF 1 alpha might be altered by enviromental regulators (nickel, cobalt, arsenite, chromium, cadmium, desferroxamine, cigarette smoking, UVB, cytokines, hormones, oncogenes). Alterations in HIF-signaling pathways have major role in initiation and progression of malignant tumors (Table 1) [17-38]. Recent studies confirmed that HIF 1 alpha controls the expression of some genes involved in melanoma biology [39, 40]. Changes in lipids biochemistry associated with HIF overexpression were described in different types of neoplastic cells. Hypoxia promotes synthesis of free fatty acids, cholesterol, phospholipids, hormones, prostaglandins, leucotriens, sphingolipids. Cellular lipid uptake is increased in hypoxic conditions due to the interactions between lipids and hypoxia signaling pathways [41, 42]. These imbalances induce alteration of cell cycle, cellular proliferation, apoptosis, signal transduction, or alteration of antigenic structure of cellular membranes. Some studies reported the expression of an extensive adipose gene in pVHL cancer, in which HIF is constitutively activated [43]. Hypoxia inducible genes influence lipid droplet formation (hypoxia-inducible protein 2), prostaglandin biosynthesis (cyclooxygenase 2), lipid signaling systems (lipoxygenase 12-lox, sphingosine kinase, SphK1) and synthetic processes (stearoyl-CoA desaturase-1, a rate-limiting enzyme in the biosynthesis of monounsaturated fatty acids) [44-47]. Some of these genes are direct targets of HIF, while others are up-regulated by transcriptional factors HIF-dependent. Hypoxia interacts with transcriptional networks involved in lipid metabolism, including sterol response element binding proteins (SREBPs), DEC1/2 and GATA2/3 [9-11, 48-52].

Gangliosides form lipoproteic domains in cells membrane and affect series of fundamental biological processes like cell signal transduction, cell growth and differentiation, imune responses, cell transformation and degradation. Reference researches about gangliosides system in malignant tumors offer new data, useful for a better understanding of melanoma biology. Melanoma development needs high levels of oxygen and substances over the offer of the existent blood vessels. Angiogenesis is promoted under these conditions [10, 51]. The main stimuli of the angiogenic switch are: HIF 1alfa, low ph, hypoglycemia, presence of reactive oxygen/nitrogen species, inflammation. In hypoxic conditions, melanoma cells release proangiogenesis (VEGFs, FGFs, PDGF, HGF, TGF, TNF, PGF, Ang-1, IL8) and antiagiogenesis (trombospondin, angiostatin, endostatin, Ang2, IFNs, IL12, fibronectin, TIMPs, PAI-1, dopamine, retinoic acid, vitamin D) factors [56-58]. These molecules interact with RTKs signaling pathway from melanoma cells, endothelial cells, pericytes, immune cells. Gangliosides and their degradation products could influence angiogenesis in malignant melanoma by multiple mechanisms [59-61]. Monosialogangliosides and gangliosides in b series counteract the effects of proangiogenic growth factors, while complex gangliosides control endothelial cell response to the action of proangiogenic factors. Lisogangliosides and sphingosine inhibit the activity of protein-kinase associated growth factors, GM1 and GM3 inactivate PDGFR, GD1a and GD1b inactivate PKC, GM3 inhibits EGFR, GD1a and GQ1b intensify the activity of calcium/calmoduline dependent kinase [54, 61].

Gangliosides control cell differentiation and proliferation [62-64]. Monosialogangliosides suppress cell growth (GM1-MMP9, GM1-PDGF, GM1-NGF, GM3-EGF, GM3-IGFs, GM2-pFAK), while polisialogangliosides stimulate cell growth (GD3 binding integrin, p-FAK, pp130Cas, p=paxilin, p-Yes or GD2 binding p-FAK, p-p38, c-Met) [65]. The transduction mechanism is complex including complex signaling pathways (p38-MAPK, Erk1/2, p13k/AKT, JNK1/2/3) [65-70]. Gangliosides act as inhibitors or promoters of cell apoptosis in melanoma [71, 72]. GD3 induces apoptosis by activating caspases and stimulates production of reactive oxygen species (ROS). GD3 acetylation cancels apoptotic effect of GD3, conferring resistance to antitumor therapy [73, 74]. GM3 induces apoptosis by intracellular accumulation of ceramide; GM1 stimulates apoptosis by disrupting the flow of intramitochondrial calcium [73-75].

GD1b, GT1b, GQ1b have inhibitor effects on adenylate cyclase in peripheral T cells and suppress the production of cytokines, controlling humoral immune response (IL4, IL5) [76]. GM1 and GD1a inhibit the activity of protein-kinases involved in the immune response. GQ1b promotes production of immunoglobulins [74, 77, 78]. Anti-GD2 antibodies modify integrin conformation through signaling pathways FAK, ERK, p38/MAPK [74, 77, 78].

Gangliosides influence anticancerous therapy through several mechanisms [51, 79-85] i) overexpression of proangiogenic factors; ii) functional mutations in tumor suppression genes; iii) overexpression of some oncogenes conferring resistance to hypoxia, and though instability of genes and inhibition of apoptosis; iv) impaired detoxification and DNA repair mechanisms; v) mutations of endothelial cells; vi) selective activation of genes associated with melanoma resistance to apoptosis; vii) cells inability to accumulate sphingosine, sphingaanine and ceramide; viii) ability of melanoma cells to acetylate gangliosides.

In a recent study the authors showed that malignant fenotype was associated with overexpression of ganglioside sialic acid on the membranes of melanoma cells. The tissue level of ganglioside sialic acid was correlated with histological markers of melanoma (Breslow index, Clark level, presence/absence of ulceration) [53]. The gangliosides identified in melanoma were complex (Fig. 1) and they could be used as a differentiation marker between normal and malignant tissue [55]. The model of membranous gangliosides was characteristic for a cell type and for a tumor stage. The observed gangliosides in malignant melanoma were: *GD3>GM3>GD2>GM2>O-Ac GD3>GD1a>GT1b>GD1b>GQ1b>GM1*; in dysplastic nevi: *GD3>GM3>GD2>GM2>GM1*; in healthy tissue around the tumor: *GM3>GM2>GD3>GD2>GM1*. The transition from radial to vertical growth of melanoma was followed by high synthesis of polisialogangliosides [53].

The compositional analysis of gangliosides in melanocytic tumors showed that aberant glycosilation of sphingolipids could stimulate or inhibate invasion and metastasis of malignant tumor cells. High levels of monosialogangliosides could be found in benign tumors with slight evolution and in healthy tissue. Polisialogangliosides had high levels in malignant proliferations with quick and irregular evolution. A special attention was given to gangliosides acetylation in malignant melanoma. Acetylated gliocsphigolipids were determined only in melanoma cells with vertical development. O-acetylation was selectively on disialogangliosides and was associated with metastasis of malignant melanoma [53].

Another research subject was the immunogenic potential of melanoma-associated gangliosides. Several tumor gangliosides induced the synthesis of antiganglioside antibodies in melanoma patients [9, 85-92]. The role of these antibodies is a subject of great current interest in medical research [9, 10, 78, 90, 93]. The data regarding endogenous immune response against gangliosides in melanoma patients and its pathophysiological relevance in management of melanoma were the main interests of the authors.

The **objective** of the study was to evaluate the role of gangliosides and antiganglioside antibodies in detection, staging and progression of cutaneous malignant melanoma. We aimed to determine the status of serum gangliosides and antiganglioside antibodies in patients with untreated malignant melanoma compared with patients with dysplastic nevi and control, their variation with surgical removal of the tumor and the relation between these parameters and some histological/biochemical factors used for melanoma staging (accepted by American Joint Committee of Cancer).

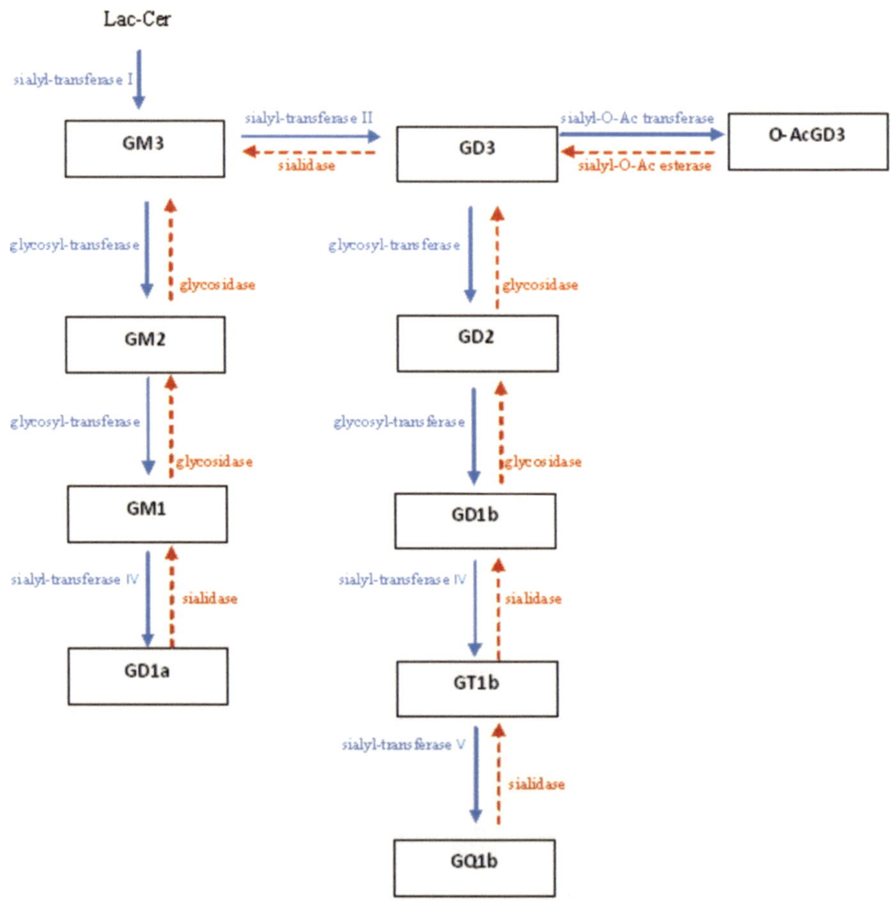

Figure 1. Metabolism of gangliosides in malignant melanoma. **GM1**=Gal-3GalNAc-4(Neu5Ac-3)Gal-4GlcCer; **GM2**=GalNAc-4(Neu5Ac-3)Gal-4GlcCer; **GM3**=Neu5Ac-3Gal-4GlcCer; **GD1a**=Neu5Ac-3Gal-3GalNAc-4(Neu5Ac-3)Gal-4GlcCer; **GD1b**=Gal-3GalNAc-4(Neu5Ac-8Neu5Ac-3)Gal-4GlcCer; **GD2**=GalNAc-4(Neu5Ac-8Neu5Ac-3)Gal-4GlcCer; **GD3**=Neu5Ac-8Neu5Ac-3Gal-4GlcCer; **GT1b**=Neu5Ac-3Gal-3GalNAc-4(Neu5Ac-8Neu5Ac-3)Gal-4GlcCer; **GQ1b**=Neu5Ac-8Neu5Ac-3Gal-3GalNAc-4(Neu5Ac-8Neu5Ac-3)Gal-4GlcCer; **O-acetyl-GD3**=Acetyl-O-Neu5Ac-8Neu5Ac-3Gal-4Glc1Cer; Glc=glucose; Gal=galactose; GalNAc=N-acetyl-galactosamine; NeuAc=neuraminic-acid; Cer=ceramide; NANA=N-acetyl-neuraminic-acid.

2. Materials and method

The study lasted five years and was based on the prospective-observational analysis of patients with melanocytic lesions. All the patients in the study signed the informed consent accordind with the Declaration from Helsinki in 1964. Our study included three groups: malignant melanoma group (128 adult patients diagnosed with malignant melanoma, with adequate nutritional status, without associated diseases, with no treatment for melanoma before the inclusion in the study), dysplastic nevi group (48 adult patients with dysplastic nevi without associated diseases) and control group (48 healthy subjects). The groups were similar for age, sex and nutritional characteristics.

http://dx.doi.org/10.5772/59176

No patients with age under 18 years, pregnancy, alcoholism or drug dependence, with any hormonal, antidepressive, antioxidant, with MAO inhibitors or blockers of dopaminergic receptors treatment or with associated diseases (neurological, psychiatric, digestive, endocrine, cardiovascular, hepatic, renal, pulmonary, metabolic, autoimmune disorders, chronic infections/inflammation, others neoplastic diseases) were included in the study.

The diagnosis protocol was based on clinical examination, common haematological and biochemical determinations for all the patients in the study. The histological and immunohistochemical analysis were made for the patients with malignant melanoma and dysplastic nevi. After the diagnosis, in malignant melanoma and nevi groups the tumors were surgically removed. In all the patients included in the study we determined molecular markers that could indicate melanoma progression (lactate dehydrogenase, interleukin 8, C reactive protein); gangliosides and antigangliosides.

In nevi and melanoma groups, the variations of these factors were evaluated in six moments: T0-when included in the study; T1 – 8 weeks after surgical removal of the tumour, at 3(T2), 6 (T3), 12 (T4), 18 (T5) and 36 (T6) months after surgical removal of the tumour. In melanoma group, the variations of gangliosides and antigangliosides were analysed in relation to serum factors – lactate dehydrogenase, interleukin 8, C reactive proteins and histological factors – Breslow index, Clark level, presence/absence of ulceration.

2.1. Clinical and biological characteristics of melanoma patients

The clinical examination showed the following localization of cutaneous malignant melanoma: 64% on trunk, 21% on limbs, less than 10% on head and neck (Fig. 2). By histological characteristics, we found nodular melanoma in 60 patients (47%), superficial melanoma in 22 patients (17%), acral lenticular melanoma in 9 patients (7%) and unclassified melanoma in 22 patients (17%) (Fig. 3).

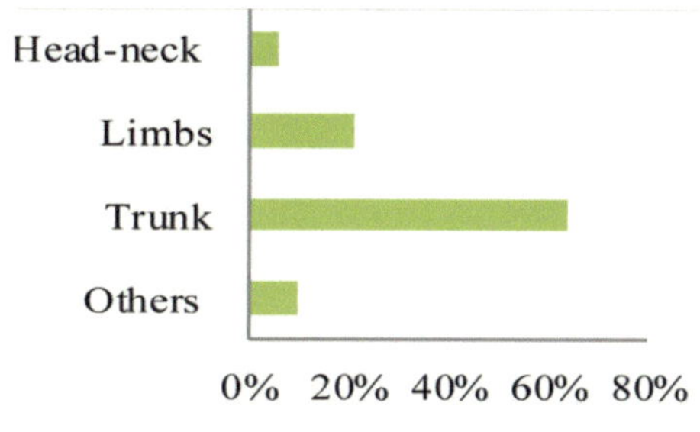

Figure 2. Anatomical site of melanomas

From patients with melanoma, 28 cases (22%) had Clark II, 47 cases (37%) had Clark III, 36 cases (28%) had Clark IV, 17 cases (13%) had Clark V. None of the patients included in the study had Clark I melanoma. From the patients with melanoma, 20.68% had Breslow under 1.00mm, 24.82% Breslow 1.01-2.0mm, 19.71% Breslow 2.01-3.0mm, 18.49% Breslow over 3.01mm. The ulceration was present in 12.5% patients with melanoma. After staging melano-

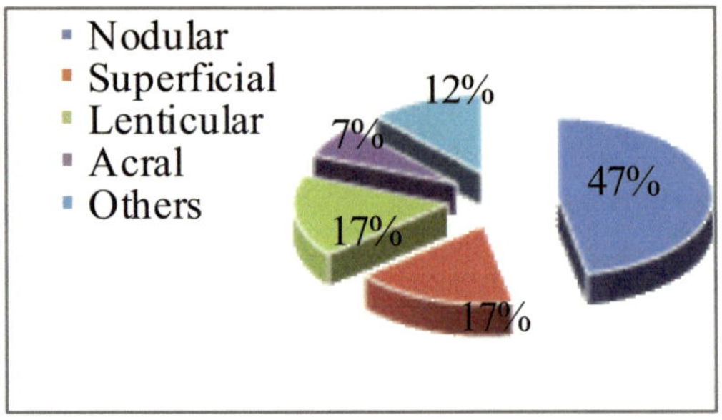

Figure 3. Histological features of melanomas

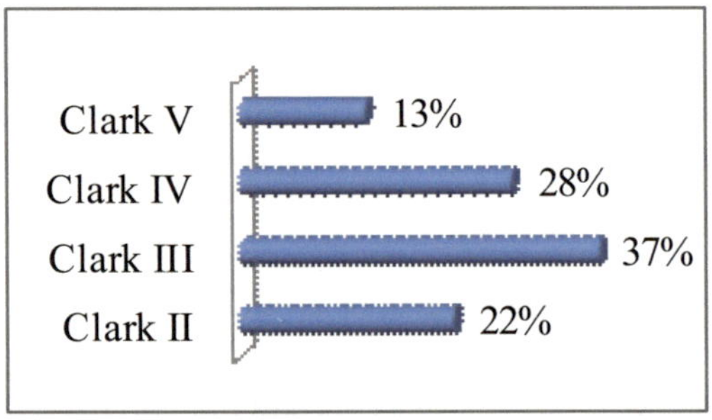

Figure 4. Melanomas Clark levels

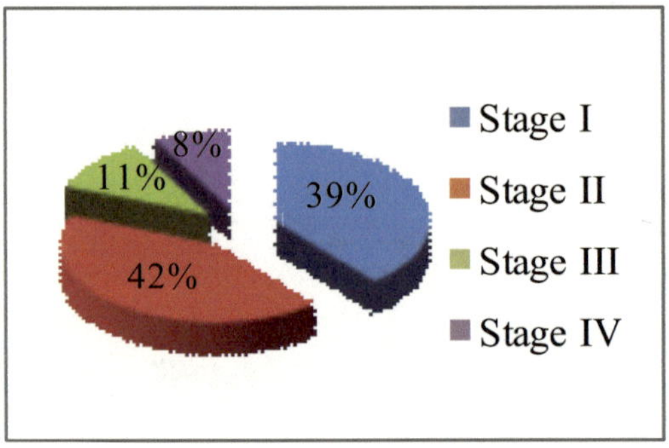

Figure 5. Clinical stages of melanomas

ma, we identified melanoma stage I – 51 cases, stage II – 54 cases, stage III – 54 cases, stage IV – 9 cases (Fig. 5).

The researchers in melanoma field considered lactatdehydeogenase (LDH), C reactive protein (CRP), interleukin 8 (IL8) useful for melanoma follow-up. High serum levels of those markers indicate the progression of melanoma. We presented their levels in the studied groups in Table 2.

http://dx.doi.org/10.5772/59176

Groups	LDH (U/L)	CRP (mg/dl)	IL8 (pg/ml)
Melanoma	389±217	1.07±0.88	68.9±17.2
Dysplastic nevi	241±88	0.26±0.23	28.7±13.3
Control	207±82	0.12±0.12	10.9±4.6

Table 2. Serum level of LDH, CRP and IL8 in melanoma, dysplastic nevi and control groups

In melanoma group, LDH had the following levels at T0: in 0.5% cases smaller than 120U/L, in 73% between 120 and 450 U/L and in 26.5% over 450U/L. In dysplastic nevi patients and in control group, LDH level varied between 120 and 450 U/L. We considered the interval 120-450U/L as normal values for LDH. CRP was in 19% patients between 0 and 0.30mg/dl, in 47%patients between 0.30-0.60mg/dl and in 33% over 0.60mg/dl. We considered the interval 0.30-0.60mg/dl as normal level for CRP. IL8 is a marker of angiogenesis. We considered the normal level for IL8 5-42pg/ml. In melanoma group, IL8 had the following levels: in 16% patients under 15pg/ml, in 22% patients between 15 and 42pg/ml, and in 62% over 42pg/ml.

2.2. Statistical analysis

All the results were analysed using SPSS, a soft for statistic determinations. The results were presented as mean±standard deviation. The variations between groups were determined using t test or ANOVA test. The correlations between groups were calculated using linear regression and Pearson coefficient. $p<0.05$ was considered with statistical significance. We evaluated the relapse-free survival using Kaplan-Meier curves.

2.3. Laboratory methods

Serum determination of gangliosides. The assessment of gangliosidic acid (LASA) had the following steps: 50 microliters serum were diluted with 150 microliters of cold distilled water and the solution was shacked. There were added 3 ml of choloroform:methanol (v/v) 2:1, at 4-5 celsius degrees. The extraction and partition was finished after adding 0.5ml of cold distilled water. After separating the phases by centrifugation, sialic acid was titred with resorcinol-chlorhidric acid [94].

Sialic acid assessment by resorcinol method. Sialic acid, after the cleavage from glicoconjugates through acid hydrolysis, reacted with resorcinol in acid solution, in the presence of divalent cooper ions. Thus, it formed a blue-violet complex. The complex was evaluated by photometric determination at 580nm, after extraction in a mixture of butanol-acetate and butyl-acetate [95, 96].

Serum assessment of antiganglioside antibodies. Antiganglioside antibodies were assessed using Euroline kits, by Immunoblot, a technique for in vivo determination (serum or plasma) of human antiganglioside antibodies Ig G and IgM type. We evaluated the immune response against seven types of ganglioside: GM1, GM2, GM3, GD1a, GD1b, GT1b and GQ1b. The test kit contained strips coated with parallel lines of purified antigens [97].

3. Results

3.1. Serum profile of gangliosides

Serum gangliosides had increased levels in melanoma and nevi patients compared with control, before the surgical removal of the tumours. In metastatic melanoma, gangliosides levels were statistically significant higher than in melanoma without metastasis (Table 3). Serum gangliosides had a statistically significant decrease after the surgical removal of the tumour in patients with primary melanoma (39.82± 21.13 vs 57.29±17.61mg/dl, $p<0.05$). In patients with metastatic melanoma, respectively, dysplastic nevi, no statistically significant variations were determined with surgical removal of the tumour.

Groups	Gangliosides (mg/dL)	p_1	p_2
Control	18.02±2.78	-	1
Dysplastic nevi	18.86±3.27	1	0.88
Malignant melanoma	57.29±17.61	0.04	0.03
Metastatic melanoma	80.14±19.26	0.00	0.00

p_1-melanoma, metastasis vs dysplastic nevi, p_2-melanoma, metastasis, dysplastic nevi vs control group

Table 3. Serum levels of gangliosides in melanoma, dysplastic nevi and control groups

Serum gangliosides were analyzed in relation to age, sex, histological characteristics of melanoma (Breslow index, Clark level, histological type of the tumor, presence/absence of ulceration) (Table 4). Serum gangliosides did not vary significantly with age and sex, with tumor localization. Serum gangliosides had statistically significant increased values in patients with high Breslow index, respectively high Clark level. We analyzed serum level of gangliosides for the same Clark level in relation to Breslow index and histological type of melanoma (Fig 6).

Parameters	Serum gangliosides (mg/dl)	P
Women	19.06±2.66	p_1=0.18
Men	18.17±2.85	
Tumor localization		
Head-neck	49.20±6.23	
Trunk	77.31±19.42	p_2=0.30
Limbs	66.81±12.51	
Histological type		
Nodular melanoma	81.61±27.43	
Extensive in surface melanoma	36.42±18.55	p_3=0.03
Lenticular malignant melanoma	72.53±27.51	

http://dx.doi.org/10.5772/59176

Parameters	Serum gangliosides (mg/dl)	P
Acral lenticular malignant melanoma	44.17±16.51	
Breslow index		
0-1.0 mm	32.67±9,23	
1.01-2.0 mm	50.88±9.74	p_4=0.02
2.01 – 3.0mm	73.12±23.19	
3.01-4.0mm	89.15±2.31	
Clark level		
II	25.92±8.93	
III	33.42±16.75	p_5=0.01
IV	62.37±20.91	
V	78.01±20.66	
Ulceration		
Melanoma with ulceration	55.87±13.11	p_6=0.04
Melanoma without ulceration	39.72±12.33	

p<0,05 was considered with statistically significance for IC=95%. p_1-women vs men, p_2-trunk vs limbs, p_3-nodular melanoma vs extensive in surface melanoma, p_4-Breslow<1.0mm vs Breslow>3.01mm, p_5-Clark II vs Clark V, p_6-ulcerated melanoma vs melanoma without ulceration

Table 4. Serum gangliosides in relation to clinical and histological features of melanoma

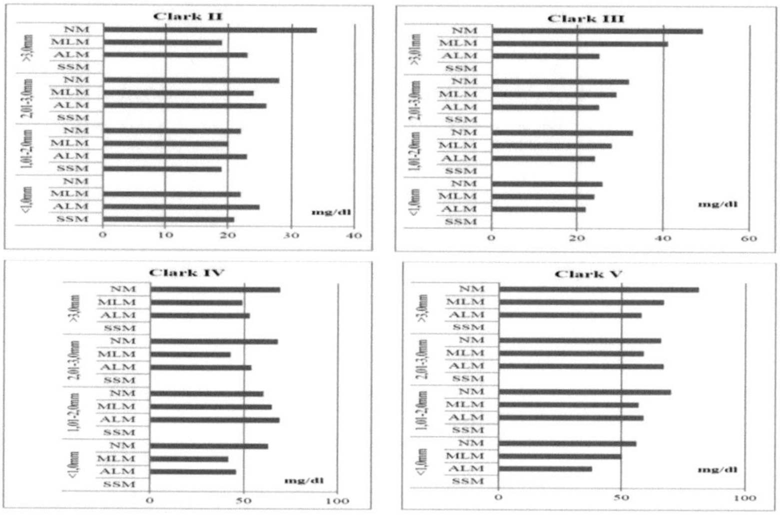

Figure 6. Graphical representation of serum levels of gangliosides in melanoma for the same Clark level in relation to Breslow index (p<0.05) and histological type of tumour (p>0.05) NM-nodular melanoma, MLM-lenticular melanoma, ALM-acral lenticular melanoma, SSM-extensive in surface melanoma

The correlation coefficient showed a positive relation between ganglioside levels and Clark level (r=0.60, CI=0.30-0.90, p<0.05), respectively, Breslow index (r=0.31, CI=0.19-0.58, p<0.05). For the same Clark level and Breslow index, the production of gangliosides was higher in nodular melanoma and in lentigous acral malignant melanoma compared with lenticular acral melanoma and extensive in surface melanoma (Figure 6).

3.2. Serum profile of antiganglioside antibodies

The immune response against gangliosides GM1, GM2, GM3, GD1a, GD1b, GT1b, GQ1b was evaluated by antiganglioside antibodies IgG and IgM type, before the surgical removal of the tumor. The types of antiganglioside antibodies in melanoma, dysplastic nevi and control group will be presented in this section only for moment 0. We considered antiganglioside antibodies negative when signal intensity was undetectable (0-5) or low (5-10) and positive when signal intensity was medium (11-50) or high (>50).

3.2.1. Anti-GM1 prevalence in studied groups

In patients with malignant melanoma, antiganglioside antibodies anti-GM1 IgG type were undetectable in 90.62% patients, with low intensity of the signal in 4.69% patients, with medium intensity of the signal in 4.68% patients. In dysplastic nevi group, 91.64% patients had undetectable IgG antibodies, in 8.33% the signal was low. In the control group we did not detect any positive anti-GM1 of IgG type. 72.65% patients with melanoma had signal of anti-GM1 IgM class negative, 11.71% low signal,13.29% medium signal and 2.34% high signal. 88.33% patients with dysplastic nevi had negative IgM anti-GM1 signal, in 10.42% the signal intensity was low, in 6.25% medium. In 93.75% healthy patients IgM antibodies had negative signal, in 4.17% the signal was low, in 2.08% medium. In melanoma patients anti-GM1 IgG type were positive in 4.68% cases and IgM in 15.63% cases. No statistical differences were observed in anti-GM1 IgG class status between melanoma, dysplastic nevi and control group. Anti-GM1 IgM class varied significantly between the studied groups (Table 5).

Groups	Antibodies type	Positive	Negative	P
Melanoma	IgG	6	122	NS
	IgM	20	108	0.00
Dysplastic nevi	IgG	0	48	NS
	IgM	3	45	NS
Control	IgG	0	48	1
	IgM	1	47	1

p-melanoma vs control, dysplastic vs control, NS=no statistical significance

Table 5. Anti-GM1 IgG and IgM class in patients with malignant melanoma, dysplastic nevi and control

http://dx.doi.org/10.5772/59176

Due to its statistically significant variation, we analysed IgM status in relation to clinical and histological features of melanoma. Anti-GM1 status was analyzed in relation to age, sex, histological characteristics of the tumor (Breslow index, Clark level, histological type of the tumor, presence/absence of ulceration) (Table 6).The intensity of the signal did not vary with sex and age. Anti-GM1 varied with histological type: in patients with nodular melanoma the intensity signal was significantly increased compared with acral lenticular melanoma ($p<0.05$), extensive in surface melanoma ($p<0.05$) or lenticular melanoma ($p<0.05$).

Parameters	IgM intensity signal	P
Sex		
Women	8.96±18.28	p_1=0.14
Men	5.14±11.09	
Tumor site		
Head-neck	13.28±9.86	
Trunk	8.87±17.30	p_2=0.02
Limbs	0.88±1.24	
Histological type		
Nodular melanoma	13.26±19.28	
Extensive in surface melanoma	0.82±1.11	p_3=0.00
Lenticular melanoma	0.77±0.97	
Acral lenticular melanoma	1.31±0.65	
Breslow index		
0-1.0 mm	0.82±1.11	
1.01-2.0 mm	2.53±1.15	
2.01 – 3.0mm	9.18±6.82	p_4=0.00
>3.01 mm	13.65±15.59	
Clark level		
II	1.07±1.30	
III	1.07±0.97	
IV	12.61±14.85	p_5=0.00
V	18.38±27.59	
Ulceration		
Melanoma with ulceration	36.43±23.86	p_6=0.00
Melanoma without ulceration	2.46±4.39	

$p<0.05$ was considered with statistically significance for IC=95%. p_1-women vs men, p_2-trunk vs limbs, p_3-nodular melanoma vs extensive in surface melanoma, p_4-Breslow<1.0mm vs Breslow>3.01mm, p_5-Clark II vs Clark V, p_6-ulcerated melanoma vs melanoma without ulceration

Table 6. Anti-GM1 antibodies IgM class in relation to clinical and histological features of melanoma

Anti-GM1 IgM intensity signal was significantly increased in melanoma on head and neck, compared with melanoma on trunk ($p<0.05$), respectively on limbs ($p<0.05$) (Table 6). Anti-GM1 signal varied statistically significant with Breslow index and Clark level. Compared with Breslow <1.0mm, signal intensity was significantly higher in patients with Breslow 2.01-3.0mm ($p<0.05$), respectively Breslow>3.01mm ($p<0.05$). Compared with Clark II, signal intensity was significantly higher in patients with Clark IV ($p<0.05$), respectively, Clark V ($p<0.05$). Signal intensity of anti-GM1 IgM type antibodies was statistically significant increased in melanoma with ulceration compared with melanoma without ulceration ($p<0.05$).

3.2.2. Anti-GM2 prevalence in studied groups

In patients with malignant melanoma, signal of antiganglioside antibodies anti-GM2 IgG type was undetectable in 96.87% patients, with low intensity in 1.57% patients, with medium intensity in 1.56% patients. In dysplastic nevi group, signal of antiganglioside antibodies anti-GM2 IgG type was undetectable in 97.92% cases, with low signal in 2.08% cases. In patients with malignant melanoma, signal of antiganglioside antibodies anti-GM2 IgM type was undetectable in 58.59% patients, with low intensity in 21.10% patients, with medium intensity in 4.68% patients and high intensity in 15.63% patients. In dysplastic nevi group, signal of antiganglioside antibodies anti-GM2 IgM type was undetectable in 70.83% cases, with low signal in 25.12% cases, and with medium intensity in 4.17% cases. In control group, anti-GM2 IgM type was undetectable in 91.67% volunteers, with weak signal in 6.25% and with medium signal in 2.08% volunteers. Only anti-GM2 IgM class varied significantly between the studied groups, therefore we analyzed IgM status by clinical and histological features of melanoma.

Groups	Antibodies type	Positive	Negative	P
Melanoma	IgG	2	126	NS
	IgM	26	102	<0.05
Dysplastic nevi	IgG	0	48	NS
	IgM	2	46	NS
Control	IgG	0	48	1
	IgM	1	47	1

p-melanoma vs control, dysplastic vs control, NS=no statistical significance

Table 7. Anti-GM2 IgG and IgM class in patients with malignant melanoma, dysplastic nevi and control

Anti-GM2 IgM status was analyzed in relation to age, sex, histological characteristics of the tumor (Breslow index, Clark level, histological type of the tumor, presence/absence of ulceration) (Table 8). The intensity level did not vary with sex and age, with anatomical site of tumor or histological type of melanoma, Breslow index, Clark level, respectively presence/absence of ulceration.

Parameters	IgM signal intensity	p
Sex		
Women	19.24±28.46	p_1=0.14
Men	12.51±23.70	
Tumor site		
Head-neck	13.00±24.96	p_2=0.35
Trunk	15.12±25.39	
Limbs	22.92±32.36	
Histological type		
Nodular melanoma	14.91±24.38	p_3=0.51
Extensive in surface melanoma	12.47±20.84	
Lenticular melanoma	14.51±26.60	
Acral lenticular melanoma	23.77±37.34	
Breslow index		
0-1.0 mm	12.13±20.41	p_4=0.30
1.01-2.0 mm	21.02±31.78	
2.01 – 3.0mm	11.93±22.99	
>3.01mm	18.80±28.25	
Clark level		
II	13.14±21.31	p_5=0.63
III	18.48±30.80	
IV	17.63±26.57	
V	17.23±26.56	
Ulceration		
Melanoma with ulceration	13.43±21.73	p_6=0.56
Melanoma without ulceration	16.91±27.43	

$p<0.05$ was considered with statistically significance for IC=95%. p_1-women vs men, p_2-trunk vs limbs, p_3-nodular melanoma vs extensive in surface melanoma, p_4-Breslow<1.0mm vs Breslow>3.01mm, p_5-Clark II vs Clark V, p_6-ulcerated melanoma vs melanoma without ulceration

Table 8. Anti-GM2 antibodies IgM class by clinical and histological features of melanoma

3.2.3. Anti-GM3 prevalence in studied groups

In patients with malignant melanoma, signal of antiganglioside antibodies anti-GM3 IgG type was undetectable in 96.10% patients, with low intensity in 3.12% patients, with medium intensity in 0.78% patients. In dysplastic nevi group, signal of antiganglioside antibodies anti-

GM3 IgG type was undetectable in 87.50% cases, with low signal in 12.25% cases. IgG did not vary significantly between groups. In patients with malignant melanoma, signal of antiganglioside antibodies anti-GM3 IgM type was undetectable in 74.22% patients, with low intensity in 8.59% patients, with medium intensity in 13.28% patients and high intensity in 3.91% patients. In dysplastic nevi group, signal of antiganglioside antibodies anti-GM3 IgM type was undetectable in 77.08% cases, with low signal in 18.75% cases, and with medium intensity in 4.17% cases. Anti-GM3 IgM class varied significantly between the studied groups (Table 9).

Groups	Antibodies type	Positive	Negative	P
Melanoma	IgG	1	127	NS
	IgM	6	122	<0.05
Dysplastic nevi	IgG	0	48	NS
	IgM	2	46	NS
Control	IgG	0	48	1
	IgM	0	48	1

p-melanoma vs control, dysplastic vs control, NS=no statistical significance

Table 9. Anti-GM3 IgG and IgM class in patients with malignant melanoma, dysplastic nevi and control

Anti-GM3 IgM status was analyzed in relation to age, sex, histological characteristics of the tumor (Table 10). The intensity level did not vary with sex and age, anatomical site or histological type of tumor, Breslow index or Clark level. Anti-GM3 antibodies had statistically significant higher intensity in ulcerated melanoma compared with melanoma without ulceration (Table 10).

Parameters	IgM signal intensity	p
Sex		
Women	10.42±19.74	p_1=0.08
Men	10.88.±19.57	
Tumor site		
Head-neck	11.85±15.87	
Trunk	9.43±18.08	p_2=0.68
Limbs	15.01±25.07	
Histological type		
Nodular melanoma	7.73±12.84	p_3=0.57
Extensive in surface melanoma	14.81±24.57	

http://dx.doi.org/10.5772/59176

Lenticular melanoma	12.13±25.81	
Acral lenticular melanoma	10.75±16.50	
Breslow index		
0,0-1.0 mm	15.72±25.48	
1.01-2.0 mm	11.94±22.79	p_4=0.13
2.01 – 3.0mm	12.37±15.93	
>3.01mm	7.71±14.22	
Clark level		
II	13.11±23.58	
III	12.80±23.34	p_5=0.09
IV	9.13±13.89	
V	4.66±8.56	
Ulceration		
Melanoma with ulceration	2.81±2.31	p_6=0.00
Melanoma without ulceration	11.82±20.66	

$p<0.05$ was considered with statistically significance for IC=95%. p_1-women vs men, p_2-trunk vs limbs, p_3-nodular melanoma vs extensive in surface melanoma, p_4-Breslow<1.0mm vs Breslow>3.01mm, p_5-Clark II vs Clark V, p_6-ulcerated melanoma vs melanoma without ulceration

Table 10. Anti-GM3 antibodies IgM class by clinical and histological features

3.2.4. Anti-GD1a prevalence in studied groups

In patients with malignant melanoma, signal of antiganglioside antibodies anti-GD1a IgG type was undetectable in 89.06% patients, with low intensity in 10.16% patients, with medium intensity in 0.78% patients. In dysplastic nevi group, signal of antiganglioside antibodies anti-GD1a IgG type was undetectable in 95.83% cases, with low signal in 4.17% cases. No positive anti-GD1a IgG type were detected in nevi or control groups. In patients with malignant melanoma, signal of antiganglioside antibodies anti-GD1a IgM type was undetectable in 57.81% patients, with low intensity in 28.12% patients, with medium intensity in 3.12% patients and high intensity in 10.94% patients. In dysplastic nevi group, signal of antiganglioside antibodies anti-GD1a IgM type was undetectable in 77.08% cases, with low signal in 16.67% cases, and with medium intensity in 6.25% cases. No positive anti-GD1a IgM type were detected in nevi or control groups. No statistical differences were observed in anti-GD1a IgG class status between melanoma, dysplastic nevi and control group. Anti-GD1a IgM class varied significantly between the studied groups (Table 11). Due to this variation, we analyzed IgM status in relation to clinical and histological features of melanoma. In melanoma patients anti-GD1a IgG type were positive in 0,78% cases and IgM in 14,06% cases.

Groups	Antibodies type	Positive	Negative	P
Melanoma	IgG	1	127	NS
	IgM	18	110	<0.05
Dysplastic nevi	IgG	0	48	NS
	IgM	3	45	NS
Control	IgG	0	48	1
	IgM	0	48	1

p-melanoma vs control, dysplastic vs control, NS=no statistical significance

Table 11. Anti-GD1a IgG and IgM class in patients with malignant melanoma, dysplastic nevi and control

Anti-GD1a IgM status was analyzed in relation to age, sex, histological characteristics of the tumor (Breslow index, Clark level, histological type of the tumor, presence/absence of ulceration) (Table 12). The intensity level did not vary with sex and age or histological type of melanoma. The antibodies varied with tumor site: the highest intensity was determined in melanoma situated on trunk ($p<0.05$), followed by melanomas on head and neck ($p<0.05$) compared with melanomas on limbs. High intensity of anti-GD1a were observed in melanoma with Breslow 2.01-3.0mm ($p<0.05$), respectively Breslow>3.01mm ($p<0.05$) compared with Breslow 0.0-1.0mm. Increased intensity of anti-GD1a were determined in Clark IV ($p<0.05$), respectively Clark V ($p<0.05$) compared with Clark II melanomas. Anti-GD1a signal intensity varied significantly with ulceration, with higher levels in ulcerated melanomas ($p<0.05$) (Table 12).

Parameters	IgM signal intensity	p
Sex		
Women	12.96±24.08	$p_1=0.93$
Men	13.32±23.34	
Tumor site		
Head-neck	10.42±8.31	
Trunk	16.26±6.65	$p_2=0.03$
Limbs	2.38±83.22	
Histological type		
Nodular melanoma	25.25±30.38	
Extensive in surface melanoma	2.37±1.76	$p_3=0.70$
Lenticular melanoma	2.54±1.76	
Acral lenticular melanoma	2.33±1.38	
Breslow index		
0,0-1.0 mm	2.45±1.71	
1.01-2.0 mm	2.41±1.74	$p_4=0.03$
2.01 – 3.0mm	8.93±5.48	

Parameters	IgM signal intensity	p
> 3.01 mm	25.01±35.92	
Clark level		
II	2.40±1.71	p_5=0.01
III	4.57±10.34	
IV	19.55±26.08	
V	38.66±36.54	
Ulceration		
Melanoma with ulceration	46.65±38.07	p_6=0.00
Melanoma without ulceration	8.33±16.16	

$p<0.05$ was considered with statistically significance for IC=95%. p_1-women vs men, p_2-trunk vs limbs, p_3-nodular melanoma vs extensive in surface melanoma, p_4-Breslow<1.0mm vs Breslow>3.01mm, p_5-Clark II vs Clark V, p_6-ulcerated melanoma vs melanoma without ulceration

Table 12. Anti-GD1a antibodies IgM class in relation to clinical and histological features of melanoma

3.2.5. Anti-GD1b prevalence in studied groups

In patients with malignant melanoma, signal of antiganglioside antibodies anti-GD1b IgG type was undetectable in 61.71% patients, with low intensity in 34.37% patients, with medium intensity in 3.12% patients. In dysplastic nevi group, signal of antiganglioside antibodies anti-GD1b IgG type was undetectable in 81.25% cases, with low signal in 18.75% cases. In patients with malignant melanoma, signal of antiganglioside antibodies anti-GD1b IgM type was undetectable in 64.84% patients, with low intensity in 25.10% patients, with medium intensity in 4.68% patients and high intensity in 5.46% patients (Table 13).

Groups	Antibodies type	Positive	Negative	p
Melanoma	IgG	4	124	NS
	IgM	13	115	<0.05
Dysplastic nevi	IgG	0	48	NS
	IgM	2	46	NS
Control	IgG	0	48	1
	IgM	0	48	1

p-melanoma vs control, dysplastic vs control, NS=no statistical significance

Table 13. Anti-GD1b IgG and IgM class in patients with malignant melanoma, dysplastic nevi and control

In dysplastic nevi group, signal of anti-GD1b IgM type was undetectable in 81.25% cases, with low signal in 5.46% cases, and with medium intensity in 1.56% cases. No positive anti-GD1b IgM type were detected in nevi or control groups. In melanoma patients anti-GD1b IgG type were positive in 3.12% cases, while IgM in 10.14% cases. Anti-GD1b IgG class had no significant variations between groups, while, IgM class modified significantly (Table 13).

Anti-GD1b IgM status was analyzed in relation to age, sex, histological characteristics of the tumor (Breslow index, Clark level, histological type of the tumor, presence/absence of ulceration) (Table 14). We did not determine significant variations of anti-GD1b except with the histological type of melanoma. Compared with nodular melanoma, we detected statistically increased intensity in extensive in surface melanoma ($p<0.05$) and acral lentiguos melanoma ($p<0.05$).

Parameters	IgM signal intensity	P
Sex		
Women	7.67±12.57	$p_1=0.52$
Men	9.36±16.02	
Tumor site		
Head-neck	10.57±21.36	
Trunk	6.74±12.44	$p_2=0.14$
Limbs	14.30±20.88	
Histological type		
Nodular melanoma	6.00±11.40	
Extensive in surface melanoma	13.72±18.44	$p_3=0.00$
Lenticular melanoma	7.36±15.95	
Acral lenticular melanoma	16.55±19.00	
Breslow index		
0-1.0 mm	13.72±18.49	
1.01-2.0 mm	11.52±18.17	$p_4=0.14$
2.01 – 3.0mm	6.43±14.07	
>3.01 mm	5.65±8.33	
Clark level		
II	12.44±16.85	
III	9.29±15.93	$p_5=0.35$
IV	6.44±13.88	
V	5.88±7.22	
Ulceration		
Melanom with ulceration	4.56±6.19	$p_6=0.23$
Melanom without ulceration	3.92±5.36	

$p<0.05$ was considered with statistically significance for IC=95%. p_1-women vs men, p_2-trunk vs limbs, p_3-nodular melanoma vs extensive in surface melanoma, p_4-Breslow<1,0mm vs Breslow>3,01mm, p_5-Clark II vs Clark V, p_6-ulcerated melanoma vs melanoma without ulceration

Table 14. Anti-GD1b antibodies IgM class in relation to clinical and histological features of melanoma

3.2.6. *Anti-GT1b prevalence in studied groups*

In patients with malignant melanoma, signal of anti-GT1b IgG type was undetectable in 83.59% patients, with low intensity in 16.40% patients. In dysplastic nevi group, signal of anti-GT1b

IgG type was undetectable in 85.41% cases, with low signal in 14.58% cases. In patients with malignant melanoma, signal of anti-GT1b IgM type was undetectable in 53.24% patients, with low intensity in 33.59% patients, with medium intensity in 10.93% patients and high intensity in 3.12% patients. In dysplastic nevi group, signal of anti-GT1b IgM type was undetectable in 68.75% cases, with low signal in 27.08% cases, and with medium intensity in 4.16% cases. No positive anti-GT1b IgM or IgG type were detected in control group. The statistical analysis showed that IgM antibodies varied significantly between the studied groups (Table 15). We analyzed IgM status in relation to clinical and histological features of melanoma.

Groups	Antibodies type	Positive	Negative	p
Melanoma	IgG	0	128	NS
	IgM	18	110	<0.05
Dysplastic nevi	IgG	0	48	NS
	IgM	2	46	NS
Control	IgG	0	48	1
	IgM	0	48	1

p-melanoma vs control, dysplastic vs control, NS=no statistical significance

Table 15. Anti-GT1b IgG and IgM class in patients with malignant melanoma, dysplastic nevi and control

Anti-GT1b status was analyzed in relation to age, sex, histological characteristics of the tumor (Breslow index, Clark level, histological type of the tumor, presence/absence of ulceration) (Table 16). We did not determine significant variations of anti-GD1b except with the tumor site of melanoma. Compared with melanomas on head-neck, we detected statistically increased intensity in melanomas on trunk ($p<0.05$) or on limbs ($p<0.05$).

Parameters	IgM signal intensity	p
Sex		
Women	8.59±13.30	$p_1=0.53$
Men	9.23±14.97	
Tumor site		
Head-neck	2.85±2.79	
Trunk	7.36±13.46	$p_2=0.02$
Limbs	16.15±19.12	

Histological type		
Nodular melanoma	6.61±14.96	
Extensive in surface melanoma	13.27±17.92	p_3=0.10
Lenticular melanoma	6.31±4.84	
Acral lenticular melanoma	16.33±16.62	
Breslow index		
0-1.0 mm	13.27±17.92	
1.01-2.0 mm	11.47±11.04	p_4=0.07
2.01 – 3.0mm	2.75±2.04	
>3.01 mm	7.85±16.35	
Clark level		
II	12.18±16.28	
III	9.74±10.76	p_5=0.28
IV	5.33±13.25	
V	9.44±19.85	
Ulceration		
Melanom with ulceration	2.75±1.69	p_6=0.23
Melanom without ulceration	9.86±15.03	

p<0.05 was considered with statistically significance for IC=95%. p_1-women vs men, p_2-trunk vs limbs, p_3-nodular melanoma vs extensive in surface melanoma, p_4-Breslow<1.0mm vs Breslow>3.01mm, p_5-Clark II vs Clark V, p_6-ulcerated melanoma vs melanoma without ulceration

Table 16. Anti-GT1b antibodies IgM class in relation to clinical and histological features of melanoma

3.2.7. Anti-GQ1b prevalence in studied groups

In all patients with malignant melanoma, dysplastic nevi and control group, antiganglioside antibodies anti-GQ1b IgG type were negative. In patients with malignant melanoma, signal of antiganglioside antibodies anti-GQ1b IgM type was undetectable in 90.62% patients, with low intensity in 4.68% patients, with medium intensity in 3.90% patients and high intensity in 0.78% patients. No positive anti-GT1b IgM type were detected in dysplastic nevi, respectively, control groups. No statistical differences were observed in anti-GQ1b IgG class status between melanoma, dysplastic nevi and control group. Anti-GQ1b IgM class varied significantly between the studied groups (Table 17). We analyzed IgM status by clinical and histological features of melanoma.

Groups	Antibodies type	Positive	Negative	p
Melanoma	IgG	0	128	NS
	IgM	6	122	<0,05
Dysplastic nevi	IgG	0	48	NS
	IgM	0	48	NS
Control	IgG	0	48	1
	IgM	0	48	1

p-melanoma vs control, dysplastic vs control, NS=no statistical significance

Table 17. Anti-GQ1b IgG and IgM class in patients with malignant melanoma, dysplastic nevi and control

Anti-GQ1b IgM status was analyzed in relation to age, sex, histological characteristics of the tumor (Breslow index, Clark level, histological type of the tumor, presence/absence of ulceration) (Table 18) The intensity level did not vary with sex and age, tumor site or histological type of melanoma, Clark level, Breslow index, presence/absence of ulceration.

Parameters	IgM signal intensity	p
Sex		
Women	4.69±8.91	p_1=0.32
Men	4.84±10.27	
Tumor site		
Head-neck	2.00±1.52	
Trunck	4.60±7.61	p_2=0.30
Limbs	6.69±16.76	
Histological type		
Nodular melanoma	3.45±5.94	
Extensive in surface melanoma	6.81±17.13	p_3=0.16
Lenticular melanoma	5.90±9.64	
Acral lenticular melanoma	9.77±12.22	
Breslow index		
0-1.0 mm	6.81±17.13	p_4=0.70

1.01-2.0 mm	4.44±7.03	
2.01 – 3.0mm	2.81±1.72	
>3.01 mm	5.03±8.92	
Clark level		
II	5.66±15.60	
III	5.68±8.64	p_5=0.60
IV	2.97±1.62	
V	4.72±10.68	
Ulceration		
Melanoma with ulceration	2.87±1.78	p_6=0.82
Melanoma without ulceration	5.05±10.33	

$p<0.05$ was considered with statistically significance for IC=95%. p_1-women vs men, p_2-trunk vs limbs, p_3-nodular melanoma vs extensive in surface melanoma, p_4-Breslow<1.0mm vs Breslow>3.01mm, p_5-Clark II vs Clark V, p_6-ulcerated melanoma vs melanoma without ulceration

Table 18. Anti-GQ1b antibodies IgM class in relation to clinical and histological features of melanoma

3.3. The relationship between gangliosidic system and biochemical factors used for melanoma staging

In this section we will present the statistical correlations between LDH, CRP and IL8 in melanoma patients, before the surgical removal of the tumor, and also, the relation between the biochemical factors and serum gangliosides/antigangliosides in melanoma patients (Table 19).

	LDH	**CRP**	**IL8**
IL8	r=0.36 p=0.00	r=0.92 p=0.00	-
CRP	r=0.40 p=0.00	-	-
Serum gangliosides (LASA)	r=0.44 p=0.00	r=0.43 p=0.00	r=0.47 p=0.00

Table 19. The correlations between gangliosidic system and staging factors in malignant melanoma patients

http://dx.doi.org/10.5772/59176

In melanoma group positive statistical significant correlations were determined between LDH and Il8, LDH and CRP, respectively, CRP and IL8. A strong positive correlation was detected between serum gangliosides and LDH, CRP and IL8 in melanoma group.

	LDH	CRP	IL8
Anti-GM1	r=0.75 p=0.00	r=0.33 p=0.00	r=0.37 p=0.00
Anti-GM2	r=0.07 p=0.38	r= - 0.06 p=0.47	r= - 0.03 p=0.67
Anti-GM3	r= - 0.12 p=0.16	r= - 0.17 p=0.05	r= - 0.15 p=0.02
Anti-GD1a	r=0.140 p=0.00	r=0.45 p=0.00	r=0.53 p=0.00
Anti-GD1b	r= - 0.15 p=0.06	r= - 0.24 p=0.00	r= - 0.22 p=0.00
Anti-GT1b	r= - 0.16 p=0.05	r= - 0.29 p=0.00	r= - 0.25 p=0.00
Anti-GQ1b	r= - 0.02 p=0.81	r= - 0.13 p=0.11	r= - 0.15 p=0.09

Table 20. The correlations between antigangliosides and staging factors in malignant melanoma patients

Anti-GM1 correlated positive, statistically significant with LDH, CRP and IL8. Anti-GM2 IgM type correlated weakly, statistically insignificant with the markers used for melanoma staging. Anti-GM3 was negatively associated before surgical intervention, with the markers that indicate the progression of melanoma: statistically insignificant with LDH, statistically significant with CRP respectively, IL8. Anti-GD1a was strongly positive associated with the markers for melanoma staging, before surgical intervention. The b serie of antiganglioside antibodies correlated weakly, negatively, with LDH, CRP and IL8.

3.4. Variation of gangliosidic system in melanoma patients after surgical intervention

From the 128 patients with malignant melanoma, we selected 30 cases with the same clinical stage (I or II), that were monitored for 36 months using the same investigation protocol. The decision to continue monitoring without receiving any treatment was based on oncologist decision, no signs of melanoma evolution, and also on patients attitude/agreement. The moments of evaluation were: T0-when included in the study; T1 – 8 weeks after surgical removal of the tumor, at 3(T2), 6 (T3), 12 (T4), 18 (T5) and 36 (T6) months after surgical removal of the tumor (Table 21).

	T1	T2	T3	T4	T5	T6
LASA	40.73±28.40	41.86±28.49	42.30±30.55	44.60±32.22	45.53±34.54	53.11±41.26(1)
Anti-GM1	8.14±12.16	7.80±11.40	6.22±7.12	8.15±9.30	9.33±7.24	13.10±10.25(1)
Anti-GM2	14.35±7.85	10.26±8.20	12.15±5.12	9.37±8.75	10.6±6.25	5.22±6.10
Anti-GM3	10.66±12.37	6,15±10.27(1)	4.06±3.86(1)	6.04±9.05(1)	4.60±8.15(1)	3.90±5.10(1)
Anti-GD1a	17.42±18.32	14,05±9.61	20.10±16.10	21.17±9.25	18.00±10.82	23.10±11.50(1)
Anti-GD1b	11.15±9,10	17.10±6.33	15.16±5.15	11,10±8.32	9.11±8.17	8.30±6.25
Anti-GT1b	11.15±18.10	16.22±17.02	10.61±8.33	8.62±6.55	7.14±8.09(1)	8.32±10.12
Anti-GQ1b	4.10±6,44	6.22±5.17	8.77±10.21(1)	9.40±7.25(1)	6.18±7.35	10.40±7.35

1)=statistically significant variation compared with moment 1

Table 21. Variation of serum gangliosides and antiganglioside antibodies after surgical removal of melanoma

LASA increased after surgical intervention, having the biggest level at T6, its variation being statistically significant ($p<0.05$). Anti-GM1 decreased in the first six months after surgical removal of melanoma, afterwards its level increased, at T6 being statistically significant higher compared with its level at T1 ($p<0.05$). Anti-GM2 decreased during the 36 months of evaluation, but its variation was not statistically significant ($p>0.05$). Anti-GM3 decreased significantly at T2, T3, T4, T5, and respectively, at T6 compared with T1. Anti-GD1a increased significantly during the 36 months of evaluation compared with its level at T1. Antigangioside antibodies from b series had a sinuous variation during evaluation: anti-GD1b increased in the first 12 months after surgical removal of the tumor, afterwards, its intensity decreased compared with T1; anti-GT1b increased at T2, and then, its intensity decreased during evaluation; anti-GQ1b increased during evaluation.

After surgical removal of melanoma we detected anti-GM3 IgM type in 12 patients, data that could indicate the regression of melanoma. High pathological levels of serum gangliosides and detectable levels of anti-GD1a IgM were determined in 11 patients, data that could be associated with progression of melanoma and possible metastasis. The increase of serum gangliosides, during evaluation and the absence of antiganglioside antibodies in 7 patients suggest tumoral recurrence.

3.5. Determination of relapse-free survival in malignant melanoma patients

We determined the relapse free survival using Kaplan-Meier curves, in patients with operated malignant melanoma, monitored for 36 months. Survival rate was assessed in relation to serum levels of gangliosides, anti-GM3 IgM type and anti-GD1a IgM type. We choose a cut-off value suitable for estimating the prognosis.

Biological parameters		Free-relapse survival (months)	p
Serum gangliosides (mg/dl)	≤25	22.15±1.19	1
	>25	16.33±1.72	0.01
Anti-GM3/IgM	≤14.20	17.82±0.94	1
	>14.20	21.32±1.53	0.04
Anti-GD1a/IgM	≤15.35	21.67±1.04	1
	>15.35	13.85±1.37	0.00

p –statistical significance

Table 22. Free-relapse survival in patients with malignant melanoma

The relapse-free survival curves in relation to serum gangliosides showed an increase in survival in patients with serum gangliosides lower than 25mg/dl compared with those that had gangliosides over 25mg/dl (22.15±1.19 versus 16.33±1.72 months, $p<0.05$) (Table 22). The relapse-free survival curves in relation to serum anti-GM3 IgM type showed an increase in survival in patients with signal intensity over 14,20 compared with patients with lower anti-GM3 intensity signal (21.31±1.53 versus 17.82±0.94 months, $p<0.05$) (Table 22). The relapse-free survival curves in relation to serum anti-GD1a IgM type showed an increase in survival in patients with signal intensity under 15.35 compared with patients with higher anti-GM3 intensity signal (13.85±1.37 versus 21.67±1.04 months, $p<0.05$) (Table 22).

4. Discussions

There is little information about quantitative variations of serum gangliosides, their origin and progression of malignant melanoma in medical literature. Serum gangliosides are derived on one hand, from tumor microenvironment, and, on the other hand, from membranous components turn-over. The ability of melanoma cells to synthetize and release gangliosides in extracellular space are sustained by the results of this study.

Though, in systemic circulation, we detected high levels of gangliosides in patients with primary melanoma and metastatic melanoma compared with dysplastic nevi and control groups. The patients with metastatic melanoma had significantly increased levels of gangliosides compared with patients with primary tumor. The serum levels of gangliosides were similar in nevi and control group.

Important data regarding the origin of serum gangliosides were obtained by analyzing their levels before and after surgical removal of melanocytic tumors. The levels of serum gangliosides varied statistically significant with surgical intervention in patients with localized melanoma, and without statistical significance in patients with metastatic melanoma, respectively, dysplastic nevi. Therefore, serum concentration of gangliosides could give important data about tumor mass, tumor volume or tumor progression. We consider that low levels of gangliosides in multiple determinations after surgical removal of the tumor could indicate a correct surgical treatment of melanoma, while high levels in the same conditions could mean a progression of melanoma.

Our study showed a strong association between increased serum gangliosides and high Breslow index or high Clark level and presence of ulceration. Serum gangliosides correlated strong and positive with biological factors used for melanoma staging – LDH, CRP, IL8. High levels of LDH, CRP, IL8 are markers for melanoma progression. These correlations show that the principle elements involved in melanoma progression are vascularization and neoangiogenesis.

Therefore, the levels of serum gangliosides could become a useful marker for clinical staging of melanoma, but its usage is limited by the lack of satisfactory criteria for interpretation. The problem becomes more complex, because there are multiple sources of serum gangloside, being difficult to know if the exact source are the tumoral cells or the host organism. This statement is sustained by the variability in composition of serum gangliosides and altered immunologic reactivity of melanoma patients. In the model of serum gangliosides before and after surgical treatment, we observed a tendency of the body to adjust the biosynthesis of gangliosides, mainly by normalizing glycosyltransferase activity in melanoma patients. To demonstrate a possible link between ganglioside system and prognosis of patients with cutaneous malignant melanoma, we calculated relapse-free survival of the disease according to serum levels of gangliosides. Based on this analysis, the authors found that low levels of circulating gangliosides are positive prognosis factors, in terms of increasing the relapse free survival in patients with malignant melanoma. These results justify the role of serum gangliosides as potential biomarkers in the management of patients with melanoma, a finding that supports previous researches [10, 11, 53, 102, 103].

Data in literature about the involvement of gangliosides in tumor processes are controversial. Some studies claim that overexpression of gangliosides on cells membrane and their accumulation in intercellular space and in serum of patients with cancer may play a role in tumor growth, neovascularization, and lack of immune response. Gangliosides influence tumor metastasis and angiogenesis by modulating the autocrine production of growth factors and thereby, protect the tumor from the host's immune system [67, 98, 100, 101,104, 105, 106].

In this sense, the relationship between ganglioside, tumor growth and progression have been the subject of several studies. A number of in vivo and in vitro studies have shown that gangliosides are involved in tumor suppression. Gangliosides metabolic products such as ceramides may be involved in apoptosis. Other studies argue that metastatic melanoma produces a variety of growth factors and interleukins that induce cell proliferation. Gangliosides can alter the growth of metastatic melanoma by modulation the activity of some growth factors, by regulating cAMP and some signaling pathways. Recently it has been demonstrated that gangliosides of human melanoma promote differentiation of dendritic cells from monocytes, maturation of Langerhans cells in the epidermis, and induce apoptosis of both cell types. Melanoma cells release active chemo attractants and other mediators to stimulate the migration and activation of macrophages, monocytes, granulocytes, keratinocytes, fibroblasts, platelets, and other components of the native immunity. Metastatic melanoma release these molecules in the tumor microenvironment [52, 82, 99, 107, 108, 109, 110, 111, 112, 113, 114, 115, 116, 117].

Other studies claim that metastatic melanoma produces a number of growth factors such as interleukin-8, alpha protein that regulates the growth/the activity of melanocytes. It has been suggested that gangliosides could alter the growth of metastatic melanoma by modulating the production of an autocrine growth factor and by adjusting the 3 '5'adenozin cyclic monophosphate (cAMP) and its corresponding signaling paths. Other studies have suggested that soluble gangliosides could be involved in tumor-induced immunosuppression [98, 111, 112, 115, 116, 117, 118, 119].

Melanoma cells, especially those of metastatic melanoma overexpress a variety of gangliosides. Aberrant gangliosides and their high level could be a marker of malignancy. Serum levels of compounds with sialic acid did not vary in patients with precancerous pigmentary lesions. We observed that in early diagnosed melanoma serum level of gangliosides was not significantly increased. Low levels of gangliosides in melanoma patients without ulceration or metastasis were associated with an increased relapse-free survival after surgical removal of the tumor. High levels of gangliosides in patients with metastatic melanoma were associated with progression of the disease and a decrease in relapse-free survival after surgical intervention [49, 53, 103].

The presence in the body of glicosphingolipids antigens, recognized by the immune system as nonself, determines the proliferation of some lymphocitary clones, that promote the synthesis of antibodies against these molecules. Glicosphigolipids associated with tumors, induce also, the synthesis of antibodies against gangliosides by a complex mechanism. It was accepted the idea of genetic similarity between some exogenous antigens and some components of nervous cells.

The umoral immune response in adult patients with untreated malignant melanoma, in dysplastic nevi and healthy volunteers was evaluated by the assessment of antigangliosides of IgG and IgM type against GM1, GM2, GM3, GD1a, GD1b, GT1b, GQ1b. In healthy individuals, antigangliosides antibodies IgG and IgM type were negative, in dysplastic nevi group, antibodies IgG type were absent, with the exception of anti-GM1 that were present in 4.17% cases. Antibodies IgM type had the following distribution: 6.25% anti-GM1; 4.17% anti-GM2; 4.17% anti-GM3; 6.25% anti-GD1a; 4.17% anti-GD1b; 4.17% anti-GT1b; 0% anti-GQ1b. In melanoma group, IgG antibodies had the following distribution: 4.68% anti-GM1; 1.56% anti-GM2; 0.78% anti-GM3; 0.78% anti-GD1a; 3.12% anti-GD1b, while the positive IgM were 15.63% anti-GM1; 20.31% anti-GM2; 17.19% anti-GM3; 14.06% anti-GD1a; 10,16% anti-GD1b; 14.06% anti-GT1b; 4.69% anti-GQ1b. No statistical differences were observed in IgG status between the studied groups. Significant variations of IgM antibodies were determined between melanoma and nevi, respectively control group.

Based on these results, we can appreciate that gangliosides expressed on melanoma cells induced the synthesis of antiganglioside antibodies. The presence of antiganglioside antibodies was associated with oncogenic transformation of melanocytes, but the moment of antibodies synthesis could not be determined. The antibodies identified in melanoma patients were mostly of IgM type.

To evaluate if the presence of IgM antibodies was associated with melanoma development, we determined their relation to clinical, histological and biological factors recommended by AJCC for melanoma staging. Anti-GM1 varied significantly with tumor site, histological site of melanoma, Breslow index, Clark level, presence of ulceration, anti-GM2 did not vary with histological characteristics of melanoma, anti-GM3 varied significantly with Clark level and presence of ulceration and anti-GD1a was influnced significanlty by tumor site, Breslow index, Clark level and presence of ulceration. Anti-GD1b was influenced significantly by histological type of melanoma, anti-GT1b only by tumor site, while anti-GQ1b was not influenced by histological characteristics of melanoma.

Positive correlation with statistical significance were determined between anti-GM1 and LDH, CRP, respectively, IL8, between anti-GD1a and LDH, CRP, respectively, IL8. Negative significant correlations were observed between anti-GM3, anti-GT1b and LDH, CRP, respectively, IL8. The transition from radial to vertical growth of melanoma marked by high levels of LDH, CRP and IL8 was associated with an increase in anti-GM1, anti-GD1a and a decrease in anti-GM3, anti-GM2 antibodies of IgM type. Therefore, the IgM antibodies against GM1 and GD1a might be useful in malignant melanoma staging and diagnosis. Also, they could facilitate tumor growth by promoting neovascularization, inflammation and angiogenesis.

Other important findings of our study are the potential protective role of anti-GM2 and anti-GM3 antibodies of IgM type in melanoma patients. Anti-GM2 and anti-GM3 could affect gangliosides expression on melanoma cells, and though, might influence indirectly cell proliferation, transmembrane signaling and cells interaction. IgM antibodies against GD1b, GT1b, GQ1b offered no data about melanoma progression in relation to analyzed histological factors. Their negative correlation with IL8, LDH and CRP suggest that they could suppress tumor growth and angiogenesis indirectly.

Ganglioside and antiganglioside antibodies could be used for melanoma staging and though, they could increase the precision of the outcome. High levels of gangliosides and anti-GM1 and GD1a before the surgical removal of the tumor were associated with advanced melanoma and poor prognosis. The presence of anti-GM2,-GM3,-GD1b,-GT1b,-GQ1b in patients with dysplastic nevi could be suggestive of malignant transformation. Assessment of gangliosides and antigangliosides before the surgical intervention could be an important item for the post-surgical follow-up.

Other studies in patients with prostate cancer or soft tissue sarcoma showed that anti-GM1 antibodies had no value for diagnose and prognosis. In patients with thyroid cancer well differentiated, the level of anti-GM1 IgG and IgM type was associated with carcinogenesis, with no diagnose value in thyroid cancer [120, 121, 122]. In a big cohort of patients with lupus systemic erythematous the presence of both anti-GM1 IgM and IgG type were associated with neuro-psychiatric disorders and depression. Anti-GM1 were identified in the serum of patients with chronic idiopathic hepatitis, in systemic infections, autoimmune disorders with neurological involvement (encephalopathy, HIV neuropathy) and after parenteral administration of gangliosides [123, 124, 125, 126, 127, 128, 129, 130].

Manipulation of cellular growth dependent of GD1b, GT1b, GQ1b gangliosides was demonstrated in several cellular systems. In vitro growth of human metastatic melanoma WM266-4 was inhibited by GD1b, GT1b, GQ1b, while other gangliosides (GM 1, GM2, GM3, GD1a, GD2 and GD3) had no effect. The action of gangliosides from b series was inhibited by IL8. This phenomena could be antagonized by exogenous anti-IL8. No other growth factor (regulating of oncogene alpha growth factor, platelet regulating growth factor, interleukin 6) influenced melanoma evolution. A possible mechanism through which GD1b, GT1b and GQ1b inhibit melanoma growth could be the suppression of IL8 secretion, of ARNm expression and activation. Other studies suggest that GD1b could determine melanoma progression in vivo by stimulating angiogenesis. GT1b also influenced growth and motility of endothelial cells, while GM3 had an angiostatic effect. Multiple results proved the role of anti-GD1b,-GT1b,-GQ1b IgM type in soft tissue sarcoma Erlich subcutaneous solid tumor, Erlich carcinoma with ascitis [76, 121, 131, 132, 133, 134].

The ability of the human organism to promote an anti-GM1,-GM2,-GM3,-GD1a,-GD1b-GT1b,-GQ1b immune response could influence the evolution of patients with malignant tumors. Taking into account the immunogenic capacity of gangliosides in malignant melanoma and their effect on tumor development, we consider that an action on gangliosides metabolism could be a strategy of reducing tumor angiogenesis. Low gangliosides and increased antibodies against gangliosides from melanoma cells confer an advantage in survival of melanoma patients compared with patients without antiganglioside antibodies. Based on our results regarding gangliosides and antigangliosides profile in patients with cutaneous malignant melanoma, the authors consider that pharmacological modulation of ganglioside-antiganglioside system could be a way to control melanoma development.

Author details

Corina-Daniela Ene (Nicolae)[1*] and Ilinca Nicolae[2]

*Address all correspondence to: koranik85@yahoo.com

1 University of Medicine and Pharmacy, Carol Davila, Bucharest, Romania

2 Victor Babes Hospital of Tropical and Infectious Diseases, Research in Dermatology, Bucharest, Romania

References

[1] Liu ZJ, Herlyn M., DeVita VT Jr, Hellman S, Rosenberg SA, Cancer: principles and practice of oncology. 7th ed.Philadelphia: Lippincott,Williams&Wilkins 2005. p1745-1824.

[2] Lomas J, Martin-Duque P, Pons M, Quintanilla M. The genetics of malignant melanoma. Front Biosci. 2008; 13 5071-5093.

[3] Gogas H, EggermontA M M, Hauschild A, Hersey P, Mohr P, Schadendorf D, Spatz A, Dummer R, Biomarkers in melanoma. Ann Oncol. 2009; 20(6) vi8-vi13.

[4] Markovic NS, Erickson AL, RaoDR., Weening HR., Pockaj AB. Malignant melanoma in the 21st century, part 1: epidemiology, risk factors, screening, prevention and diagnosis. Mayo Clin. Proc. 2007; 82(3) 364 –380.

[5] Nicolae (Ene) CD. Rolul unor factori moleculari în aprecierea răspunsului terapeutic la pacienţii cu melanom malign cutanat, PhD thesis. Carol Davila University of Medicine and Pharmacy, Bucharest 2014.

[6] Nicolae I. Metabolismul lipidelor in melanom malign. PhD thesis. University of Bucharest 1998.

[7] Ene (Nicolae) CD, Nicolae I, Musetescu A, Tampa M, Matei C, Georgescu SR. Exposure to Heavy Metals in Plastics Industry and Dyes-Risk Factor in the Development of Skin Cancer, Plastic Materials 2014; 51(2) 176-180.

[8] Nicolae I, Nicolae CD, Coman O. Ganglioside serum levels-prognostic significance in melanoma patients survival, CCLM. 2011; 49, 261.

[9] Nicolae, CD, Nicolae I. Antibodies against GM1 gangliosides associated with metastatic melanoma. Acta Dermatovenerol Croat. 2013; 21(2) 86-92.

[10] Nicolae I, Nicolae CD, Coman OA, Stefanescu M, Coman L, Ardeleanu C. Serum total ganglioside level: clinical prognostic implication. Rom J MorpholEmbryol. 2011; 52(4) 1277-1281.

[11] Nicolae I, Caragheorgheopol A, Schipor S, Nicolae C, Paun D, Coman O, Benea V. Gangliosides and sex hormones in human melanoma. Acta Endo. 2011; 7(3) 337-344.

[12] Nicolae C, Nicolae I, Tampa M, Matei C, Georgescu SR. Butyrylcholinesterase in UV Reactions. Rev Chim. 2013; 64(6) 654-658.

[13] Ene (Nicolae) CD, Tampa M, Georgescu SR, Tudose I, Grigore M, Matei C, Benea V, Nicolae I. Cholinergic stimulation in skin cancer. Medicine in Evolution 2013; 19(4) 647-654.

[14] Nicolae C, Coman OA, Nicolae I, Fulga I, Monitoring therapeutic response to ferrum in cutaneous melanoma patients with secondary anemia. Medicina Moderna 2012, XIX(3) 200-204.

[15] Nicolae C, Coman OA, Nicolae I, Fulga I, Anemia in melanomul malign-incidenta, severitate, aspecte fiziopatologice. Medicina Moderna 2011; XVIII(4) 183-188.

[16] Bedogni, B, Warneke JA, Nickoloff BJ, Giaccia AJ, Powell MB. Notch1 is an effector of Akt and hypoxia in melanoma development. J Clin Invest. 2008; 118(11) 3660-3670.

[17] Masson, N, Ratcliffe PJ. Hypoxia signaling pathways in cancer metabolism: the importance of co-selecting interconnected physiological pathways. Cancer Metab. 2014; 2(1) 3. doi:10.1186/2049-3002-2-3.

[18] Liu W, Shen S, Zhao M, X Y, Chen G Q. Targeted genes and interacting proteins of hypoxia inducible factor-1. Int J Biochem Mol Biol 2012; 3(2) 165-168.

[19] Krock BL, Skuli N, Simon MC. Hypoxia-Induced Angiogenesis Good and Evil. Genes Cancer. 2011; 2(12) 1117-1133.

[20] Ke Q, Costa M. Hypoxia-inducible factor-1 (HIF-1). Mol Pharmacol. 2006; 70(5) 1469-1480.

[21] Weidemann A, Johnson R S. Biology of HIF-1α. Cell Death Diff. 2008; 15(4) 621-627.

[22] Dang EV, Barbi J, Yang H Y, Jinasena D, Yu H, Zheng Y, Pan F. Control of T< sub> H</sub> 17/T< sub> reg</sub> Balance by Hypoxia-Inducible Factor 1. Cell 2011; 146(5) 772-784.

[23] Gunaratnam L, Bonventre J V. HIF in kidney disease and development. J Am Soc Nephrol. 2009; 20(9) 1877-1887.

[24] Leek RD, Talks K L, Pezzella F, Turley H, Campo L, Brown NS, Harris AL. Relation of hypoxia-inducible factor-2α (HIF-2α) expression in tumor-infiltrative macrophages to tumor angiogenesis and the oxidative thymidine phosphorylase pathway in human breast cancer. Cancer Res. 2002; 62(5) 1326-1329.

[25] Song G, Cai Q F, Mao YB, Ming YL, Bao SD, Ouyang GL. Osteopontin promotes ovarian cancer progression and cell survival and increases HIF-1α expression through the PI3-K/Akt pathway. Cancer Sci. 2008; 99(10) 1901-1907.

[26] Zhang T, Du G. Gysregulated lipid metabolism in cancer, World J Biol Chem 2012; 3(8) 167-174.

[27] Mylonis I, Sembongi H, Befani C, Liakos P, Siniossoglou S, Simos G. Hypoxia causes triglyceride accumulation by HIF-1-mediated stimulation of lipin 1 expression. J Cell Sci. 2012; 125(14) 3485-3493.

[28] Li G, Lu WH, Ai R, Yang, J H. Chen F, Tang Z Z. The relationship between serum hypoxia-inducible factor 1α and coronary artery calcification in asymptomatic type 2 diabetic patients. Cardiovasc Diabetol 2014; 13(1) 52 doi: 10.1186/1475-2840-13-52

[29] Ji Z, Long H, Hu Y, Qiu X, Chen X, Li Z, Fan Q. Expression of MDR1, HIF-1a and MRP1 in sacral chordoma and chordoma cell line CM-319. J Exp Clin Cancer Res. 2010; (17569966) 29 doi: 10.1186/1756-9966-29-158

[30] Jing Y, Liu LZ, Jiang Y, Zhu Y, Guo N L, Barnett J, Jiang B H. Cadmium increases HIF-1 and VEGF expression through ROS, ERK, and AKT signaling pathways and induces malignant transformation of human bronchial epithelial cells. Toxicol Sci. 2012; 125(1) 10-19.

[31] Guo L, Li L, Wang W, Pan Z, Zhou Q, Wu Z. Mitochondrial reactive oxygen species mediates nicotine-induced hypoxia-inducible factor-1α expression in human non-small cell lung cancer cells. Biochimica et Biophysica Acta (BBA).Molecular Basis of Disease 2012; 1822(6) 852-861.

[32] Li Y, Bi Z, Yan B, Wan Y. UVB radiation induces expression of HIF-1alpha and VEGF through the EGFR/PI3K/DEC1 pathway. Int J Mol Med. 2006; 18(4) 713-719.

[33] Koh MY, Spivak-Kroizman TR, Powis G. HIF-1 regulation: not so easy come, easy go. Trends Biochem Sci. 2008; 33(11) 526-534.

[34] Antoniou X, Sclip A, Ploia C, Colombo A, Moroy G, Borsello T. JNK contributes to Hif-1α regulation in hypoxic neurons. Molecules. 2009; 15(1) 114-127.

[35] BelAiba RS, Bonello S, Zähringer C, Schmidt S, Hess J, Kietzmann T, Görlach A. Hypoxia up-regulates hypoxia-inducible factor-1α transcription by involving phosphatidylinositol 3-kinase and nuclear factor κB in pulmonary artery smooth muscle cells. Mol Biol Cell 2007; 18(12) 4691-4697.

[36] Cavadas MA, Nguyen LK, Cheong A. Hypoxia-inducible factor (HIF) network: insights from mathematical models. Cell Commun Signal. 2013; 11(1) 42 doi: 10.1186/1478-811X-11-42.

[37] Lim W, Cho J, Kwon HY, Park Y, Rhyu M R, Lee Y. Hypoxia-inducible factor 1α activates and is inhibited by unoccupied estrogen receptor β. FEBS Lett. 2009; 583(8) 1314-1318.

[38] Barfeld S, Itkonen H, Urbanucci A, Mills I. Androgen-regulated metabolism and biosynthises in prostate cancer. Endocr Relat Canc 2014; ERC-13-0515 T57-66.

[39] Mills CN, Joshi SS, Niles RM. Expression and function of hypoxia inducible factor-1 alpha in human melanoma under non-hypoxic conditions. Mol Cancer. 2009; 8(104) 49, doi:10.1186/1476-4598-8-104.

[40] Trisciuoglio D, Gabellini C, Desideri M, Ziparo E, Zupi G, Del Bufalo D. Bcl-2 regulates HIF-1α protein stabilization in hypoxic melanoma cells via the molecular chaperone HSP90 2010; PLoS One, 5(7), e11772. doi: 10.1371/journal.pone.0011772.

[41] Ader I, Brizuela L, Bouquerel P, Malavaud B, Cuvillier O. Sphingosine kinase 1: a new modulator of hypoxia inducible factor 1alpha during hypoxia in human cancer cells. Cancer Res 2008; 68(20) 8635-8642.

[42] Widmer DS, Hoek K S, Cheng PF, Eichhoff OM, Biedermann T, Raaijmakers MI, Levesque MP. Hypoxia Contributes to Melanoma Heterogeneity by Triggering HIF1α-Dependent Phenotype Switching. J Invest Dermatol. 2013; 133(10) 2436-2443.

[43] Tun HW, Marlow LA, von Roemeling CA, Cooper SJ, Kreinest P, Wu K, Luxon BA, Sinha M, Anastasiadis PZ, Copland JA: Pathway signature and cellular differentia-

tion in clear cell renal cell carcinoma. PLoS One 2010, 5:e10696 doi: 10.1371/journal.pone.0010696..

[44] Kaidi A, Qualtrough D, Williams AC, Paraskeva C. Direct transcriptional up-regulation of cyclooxygenase-2 by hypoxia-inducible factor (HIF)-1 promotes colorectal tumor cell survival and enhances HIF-1 transcriptional activity during hypoxia. Cancer Res. 2006; 66(13) 6683-6691.

[45] Gimm T, Wiese M, Teschemacher B, Deggerich A, Schödel J, Knaup KX, Hackenbeck T, Hellerbrand C, Amann K, Wiesener MS, Höning S, Eckardt KU, Warnecke C. Hypoxia-inducible protein 2 is a novel lipid droplet protein and a specific target gene of hypoxia-inducible factor-1. FASEB J 2010; 24(11) 4443-4458.

[46] Zhang Y, Wang H, Zhang J, Lv J, Huang Y. Positive feedback loop and synergistic effects between hypoxia-inducible factor-2alpha and stearoyl-CoA desaturase-1 promote tumorigenesis in clear cell renal cell carcinoma. Cancer Sci. 2013; 104(4) 416-422.

[47] Krishnamoorthy S, Honn KV. Eicosanoids and other lipid mediators and the tumor hypoxic microenvironment. Cancer Metastasis Rev. 2011; 30(3-4) 613-618.

[48] Furuta E, Pai SK, Zhan R, Bandyopadhyay S, Watabe M, Mo YY, Hirota S, Hosobe S, Tsukada T, Miura K, Kamada S, Saito K, Iiizumi M, Liu W, Ericsson J, Watabe K. Fatty acid synthase gene is up-regulated by hypoxia via activation of Akt and sterol regulatory element binding protein-1. Cancer Res. 2008; 68(4) 1003-1011.

[49] Nicolae I, Miscalencu D, Mailat F, Diaconu J. Lipid bound sialic acid – biological markers in human melanoma. J Med Biochem. 1998; 2(3) 261–266.

[50] Hakomori S. Glycosylation defining cancer malignancy: New wine in old bottle. Proc Natl Acad Sci. 2002; 99(16) 10231-10233.

[51] Anghel A, Nicolae I, Georgescu SR, Diaconu JD. Interleukin 8 serum levels evaluation in cutaneous melanoma. Medicina Moderna. 2011; 18(2) 98-103.

[52] Ribatti D, Annese T, Longo V. Angiogenesis and Melanoma. Cancers. 2010; 2(1) 114-132.

[53] Nicolae C, Nicolae I. Heterogeneity of gangliosides in melanocytic tumors. Acta Endocrinol. 2012; VIII(1) 17-26.

[54] Lenggenhager D, Curioni A, Storz M, Shakhova O, Sommer L, Widmer D, Seifert B, Moch H, Dummer R, Mihic D. An aggressive hypoxia related subpopulation of melanoma cells in TRP-2 negativ, Transl Oncol 2014; 7(2) 206-212.

[55] Shi D, Guo W, Chen W, Fu L, Wang J, Tian Y, Deng W. Nicotine promotes proliferation of human nasopharyngeal carcinoma cells by regulating α7AChR, ERK, HIF-1α and VEGF/PEDF signaling. PloS one 2012; 7(8) e43898. doi: 10.1371/journal.pone.0043898.

[56] Basu S, Sarkar C, Chakroborty D, Nagy J, Mitra, R B, Dasgupta PS, Mukhopadhyay D. Ablation of Peripheral Dopaminergic Nerves StimulatesFactor/Vascular Endothe-

lial Growth Factor-Mediated Malignant Tumor Growth by Inducing Vascular Permeability Angiogenesis. Cancer Res. 2004; 64(16) 5551-5555.

[57] Basu B, Biswas S, Wrigley J, Sirohi B, Corrie P. Angiogenesis in cutaneous malignant melanoma and potential therapeutic strategies. Expert Rev Anticancer The. 2009; 9(11) 1583-1598.

[58] Shome S, Rana T, Ganguly S, Basu B, Choudhury SC, Sarkar C, Basu S. Dopamine regulates angiogenesis in normal dermal wound tissues. PloS one 2011; 6(9) e25215. doi: 10.1371/journal.pone.0025215.

[59] Gammous MV, Lucas R,Dean R, Coupland S E, Oltean S, Bates DV. Targeting SPRK1 to control VEGF-mediated tumour angiogenesis in metastatic melanoma, Br J Cancer. 2014; 111(3) 477-485.

[60] Alessandri G, Cornaglia-Ferraris P, Gullino PM. Angiogenic and angiostatic microenvironment in tumors-role of gangliosides. Acta Oncol. 1997; 36(4) 383–387.

[61] Mukherjee P, Faber AC, Shelton LM, Baek RC, Chiles TC, Seyfried TN. Ganglioside GM3 suppresses the proangiogenic effects of vascular endothelial growth factor and ganglioside GD1a. J Lipid Res. 2008; 49(5) 929–938.

[62] Ferrari G, Anderson BL, Stephens RM, Kaplan DR, Greene LA. Prevention of apoptotic neuronal death by GM1 ganglioside. Involvement of Trk neurotrophin receptors. J Biol Chem. 1995; 270(7) 3074–3080.

[63] Rusnati M, Urbinati C, Tanghetti E, Dell'Era P, Lortat-Jacob H, Presta M. Cell membrane GM1 ganglioside is a functional coreceptor for fibroblast growth factor 2. Proc Natl Acad Sci USA. 2002; 99(7) 4367–4372.

[64] Julien S, Bobowski M, Steenackers A, Le Bourhis X, Delannoy P. How Do Gangliosides Regulate RTKs Signaling?. Cells. 2013, 2(4) 751-767.

[65] Chung T, Kim S, Choi H, Kim K, Kim M, Kim S, Lee H, Ko J, Lee Y, Suzuki A, Kim C. Ganglioside GM3 inhibits VEGF/VEGFR-2-mediated angiogenesis: direct interaction of GM3 with VEGFR-2. Glycobiology. 2009; 19(3) 229–239.

[66] Dyatlovitskaya EV, Kandyba AG. Sphingolipids in tumor metastases and angiogenesis. Biochemistry 2006; 71(4) 347–353.

[67] Bar-Eli M. Role of interleukin 8 in tumor growth and metastasis of human melanoma. Pathobiology 1999; 67(1) 12-18.

[68] Seyfried TN, Mukherjee P. Ganglioside GM3 Is Antiangiogenic in Malignant Brain Cancer. J Oncol. 2010; 961243. doi: 10.1155/2010/961243.

[69] Cazet A, Bobowski M, Rombouts Y, Lefebvre J, Steenackers A, Popa I, Guérardel Y, Le Bourhis X, Tulasne D, Delannoy P. The ganglioside G(D2) induces the constitutive activation of c-Met in MDA-MB-231 breast cancer cells expressing the G(D3) synthase. Glycobiology 2012; 22(6) 806–816.

[70] Ma Y, Shurin GV, Peiyuan Z, Shurin MR. Dendritic Cells in the Cancer Microenvironment. J Cancer. 2013; 4(1) 36-44.

[71] Huang S, Mills L, Mian B, Tellez C, McCarty M, Yang XD, Gudas JM, Bar-Eli M. Fully humanized neutralizing antibodies to interleukin-8 (ABX-IL8) inhibit angiogenesis, tumor growth, and metastasis of human melanoma. Am J Pathol. 2002; 161(1) 125-134.

[72] Todeschini AR, Hakomori SI. Functional role of glycosphingolipids and gangliosides in control of cell adhesion, motility, and growth, through glycosynaptic microdomains. Biochim Biophys Acta. 2008; 1780(3) 421-433.

[73] Bennaceur K, Popa I, Portoukalian J, Berthier-Vergnes O, Peguet-Navarro J. Melanoma-derived gangliosides impair migratory and antigen-presenting function of human epidermal Langerhans cells and induce their apoptosis. Int Immunol. 2006; 18(6) 879-886.

[74] Peguet-Navarro J. Melanoma-derived gangliosides impair migratory and antigen-presenting function of human epidermal Langerhans cells and induce their apoptosis. Int Immunol. 2006; 18(6) 18879-18886.

[75] Yuan J, d'Azzo A, Tessitore A, Sano R. Gangliosides as apoptotic signals in ER stress response. Cell Death Diff. 2006; 13(3) 13404–13414.

[76] Kanda N, Watanabe S. Gangliosides GD1b, GT1b, and GQ1b enhance IL-2 and IFN-gamma production and suppress IL-4 and IL-5 production in phytohemagglutinin-stimulated human T cells. J Immunol. 2001; 166(1) 72-80.

[77] Deng W, Li R, Ladisch S. Influence of cellular ganglioside depletion on tumor formation. J Natl Cancer Inst. 2000; 92(11) 912-917.

[78] Barreca T, Picciotto A, Franceschini R, Varagona G, Garibaldi A, Valle F, Cataldi A, D'Agostino S, Rolandi E. Sex hormones and sex-hormone binding globulin in males with chronic viral hepatitis during recombinant interferon-alpha 2b therapy. J Interferon Res. 1993;13(3) 209-211.

[79] Kichina JV, Rauth S, Das Gupta TK, Gudkov AV. Melanoma cells can tolerate high levels of transcriptionally active endogenous p53 but are sensitive to retrovirus-transduced p53. Oncogene. 2003; 22(31) 4911-4917.

[80] LiA, Varney ML, Valasek J. Autocrine role of interleukine 8 induction of endothelial cells proliferation, survival, migration and MMP-2 production and angiogenesis. Angiogenesis. 2005; 8(1) 63-71.

[81] Yu J, Zhang L. The transcriptional targets of p53 in apoptosis control. Biochem Biophys Res Commun. 2005; 331(3) 851-858.

[82] Tilan J, Kitlinska J. Sympathetic Neurotransmitters and Tumor Angiogenesis-Link-between Stress and Cancer Progression. J Oncol. 2010; 539706. doi: 10.1155/2010/539706.

[83] Rodríguez MI, Peralta-Leal A, Gonzalez-Flores A, López L, Rodríguez-Manzaneque JC, Fernández R, Del Moral RG, De Almodóvar JM, Oliver FJ. PARP-1 Regulates Metastatic Melanoma through Modulation of Vimentin-induced Malignant Transformation. PLoS Genet 2012; 9(6) e1003531. doi: 10.1371/journal.pgen.1003531.

[84] Iyengar B. Hormone expression in melanomas related to tumor angiogenesis. Journal of Solid Tumors 2012; 2(6) 36-45.

[85] Hoon DS, Kaback MM, Lim-Steele J, Tsuchida T, Morton DL, Irie RF. Ganglioside GM2 levels in human melanoma cells: Inverse correlation with lysosomal beta-hexosaminidase A activity. Biochem Int. 1992; 27(2) 343–352.

[86] Freimer ML, McIntosh K, Adams RA, Alving CR, Drachman DB. Gangliosides elicit a T-cell independent antibody response. J Autoimmun. 1993; 6(3) 281-289.

[87] Irie RF, Hachida M. Cancer therapy with monoclonal antibody. Tanpakushitsu Kakusan Koso 1986; 31(14) 1501-1510.

[88] Irie A, Takedachi S, Katayama Y, Matsuyama T, Harano YNihon Rinsho. Measurement and pathophysiology of Tamm-Horsfall glycoprotein (THP) Nihon Rinsho. 1989; 48 135-137.

[89] Ravindranath MH, Morton DL, Irie RF. An epitope common to gangliosides O-acetyl-GD3 and GD3 recognized by antibodies in melanoma patients after active specific immunotherapy. Cancer Res. 1989; 49(14) 3891–3897.

[90] Ravindranath MH, Vijayalakshmi, Hindupur K, Anandatheerthavarada, Susarla KS. Xenobiotic metabolism in human brain—presence of cytochrome P-450 and associated mono-oxygenases. Brain Res. 1989; 496(1) 331-335.

[91] Morton DL, Wen DR, Wong J H, Economou JS, Cagle LA, Storm FK, Cochran AJ. Technical details of intraoperative lymphatic mapping for early stage melanoma. Arch Surg. 1992; 127(4) 392-399.

[92] Agostino M, Yuriev E, Ramsland PA. Antibody Recognition of Cancer-Related Gangliosides and Their Mimics Investigated Using in silico Site Mapping. PLoS ONE. 2012; 7(4) e35457:1-12.

[93] Ravindranath MH, Muthugounder S, Ye X, Morton DL. Innate immune response to gangliosides of primary melanoma favors danger hypothesis. Proc Amer Assoc Cancer Res. 2004; 45 164-168.

[94] Katopodis N, Stock C. Improved method to determine lipid bound sialic acid in plasma or serum-Res. Commun Chem Pathol Pharmacol. 1980; 30(1) 171-180.

[95] Ariga T,Blaine GM, Yoshino H, Dawson G, Kanda T, Zeng GC, Kasama T, Kushi Y,Yu RK. Glycosphingolipid composition of murine neuroblastoma cells: O-acetyles-

terase gene downregulates the expression of O-acetylated GD3. Biochemistry. 1995, 34 (36) 11500-11507.

[96] Svennerholm L. Quantitative estimation of sialic acid II: a resorcinol-hydrochloric acid method. Biochim Biophys. 1957; 24(3) 611-618.

[97] Meyer W, Schneider B, Nobile Orazio E, Klotz M, Schlumberger W, Stocker W, EUROLINE Anti-Ganglioside-Profile. A new membrane test for detection of antibodies against gangliosides. Autoimmun Rev. 2002; 1 69-71.

[98] Bennaceur K, Popa I, Chapman JA, Migdal C, Peguet-Navarro J, Touraine JL, Portoukalian J. Different mechanisms are involved in apoptosis induced by melanoma gangliosides on human monocyte-derived dendritic cells. Glycobiology. 2009; 19(6) 576-582.

[99] Schipor S, Caragheorgheopol A, Nicolae CD, Nicolae I,Paun D-Serum level of VEGF in cutaneous malignant melanoma. CCLM. 2011; 40 267

[100] Fredman P, Hedberg K, Brezicka T. Gangliosides as Therapeutic Targets for Cancer. Biodrugs. 2003; 17(3) 155-167.

[101] Fernandez LE, Gabri MR, Guthmann MD, Gomez RE, Gold S, Fainboim L, Gomez DE, Alonso DF. NGcGM3 ganglioside: a privileged target for cancer vaccines. Clin Dev Immunol 2010; 814397.

[102] Zigler M, Villares GJ, Lev DC, Melnikova VO, Bar-Eli M. Tumor immunotherapy in melanoma: strategies for over-coming mechanisms of resistance and escape. Am J Clin Dermatol 2008; 9 (5) 307–311.

[103] Ria R, Reale A, Vacca A. Role of Angiogenesis and Microenvironment in Melanoma Progression. Research on melanoma 2011; 15 311-335.

[104] Kolter T, Sandhoff K. Sphingolipids: their metabolic pathways and the pathobiochemistry of neurodegenerative diseases. Angew Chem Int Ed. 1999; 38 4000-4036.

[105] Kanda N, Nakai K, Watanabe S. Gangliosides GD1b, GT1b, and GQ1b suppress the growth of human melanoma by inhibiting interleukin-8 production: the inhibition of adenylate cyclase. J Invest Dermatol. 2001; 117(2) 284–293.

[106] Thaker PH, Han LY, Kamat AA, Arevalo JM, Takahashi R, Lu C, Sood AK. Chronic stress promotes tumor growth and angiogenesis in a mouse model of ovarian carcinoma. Nat Med. 2006; 12(8) 939–944.

[107] Mitsuzuka K, Handa K, Satoh M. A specific microdomain ("glycosynapse 3") controls phenotypic conversion and reversion of bladder cancer cells through GM3-mediated interaction of alpha3beta1 integrin with CD9. J Biol Chem 2005; 280 35545-35553.

[108] De Cristan G, Morbidelli L, Alessandri G. Synergism between gangliosides and basic fibroblastic growth factor in favouring survival, growth, and motility of capillary endothelium. J Cell Physiol. 1990;144 505-510.

[109] Ravindranath MH, Tsuchida MH, Morton DL, Irie RF. Ganglioside GM3: GD3 ratio as an index for the management of melanoma. Cancer. 1991; 67 (12) 3029-3035.

[110] Ranes MK, El-Abbadi M, Manfredi MG. N-butyldeoxynojirimycin reduces growth and ganglioside content of experimental mouse brain tumours. Br Jcancer. 2001; 84 1107-1114.

[111] McKallip R, Li R, Landisch S. Tumor gangliosides inhibit the tumor-specific immune response. J Immunol. 1999; 163 3718-3726.

[112] Heitger A, Ladisch S. Gangliosides block antigen presentation by human monocytes. Biochem. Biophys Acta 1996: 1303:161.

[113] Melnikova VO, Bar-Eli M. Inflammation and melanoma metastasis. Pigment Cell Melanoma Res 2009; 22(3) 257–267.

[114] Weiss M, Hettmer S, Smith P. Inhibition of melanoma tumor growth by a novel inhibitor of glucosylceramide synthase. Cancer Res 2003; 63 3654-3658.

[115] Portoukalian J, Zwingelstein G, Abdul-Malak N, Doré JF. Alteration of gangliosides in plasma and red cells of humans bearing melanoma tumors. Biochem Biophys Res Commun 1978; 85(3) 916–920.

[116] Ladisch S, Gillard B, Wong C, Ulsh L. Shedding and immunoregulatory activity of YAC-1 lymphoma cell gangliosides. Cancer Res 1983; 43(8) 3808–3813.

[117] Bernhard H, Meyer zum Büschenfelde KH, Dippold WG. Ganglioside GD3 shedding by human malignant melanoma cells. Int J Cancer 1989; 44(1) 155–160.

[118] Abate LE, Mukherjee P, Seyfried T N. Gene-linked shift in ganglioside distribution influences growth and vascularity in a mouse astrocytoma. J Neurochem 2006; 98 1973-1984.

[119] Zeng G, Gao L, Birklem S. Suppression of ganglioside GD3 expression in a rat F-11 tumor cell line reduces tumor growth, angiogenesis, and vascular endothelial growth factor production. Cancer Res 2000; 60 6670-6676.

[120] Ravindranath MH, Muthugounder S, Presser N, Ye X, Brosman S, Morton DL. Endogenous immune response to gangliosides in patients with confined prostate cancer. Int J Cancer 2005; 116(3) 368–377.

[121] Perez CA, Ravindranath MH, Soh D, Gonzales A, Ye W, Morton DL. Serum anti-ganglioside IgM antibodies in soft tissue sarcoma: clinical prognostic implications. Cancer J 2002; 8(5) 384-394.

[122] Lewartowska A, Pacuszka T, Adler G, Panasiewicz M, Wojciechowska W. Ganglioside reactive antibodies of IgG and IgM class in sera of patients with differentiated thyroid cancer. Immunology Lett. 2002; 80(2) 129-132.

[123] Galleazzi M, Annunziata P, Sebastiani GD, Bellisai F, Campanella V, Ferrara GB, Font J, Houssianu F, De Ranon G, Fernandez-Nebro A, Bracci L, Scorza R, Puddu P,

Jedryka-Goral A, Smolen J, Tincani A, Carcassi C, Morozzi G, Marcolongo R. Anti-ganglioside antibodies in a large cohort of European patients with systemic lupus erythematosus: clinical, serological, and HLA class II gene associations. European Concerted Action on the Immunogenetics of SLE. Rheumatol. 2000; 27(1) 135-41.

[124] Van der Kruijk RA, Affourtit MJ, Endtz HPh, Arts WFM. Campylobacter jejuni gastroenteritis and acute encephalopathy. J Infect 1994; 28 99-100.

[125] Sorice M, Griggi T, Circella A, Nicodemo G, Ciarardi M, Mastroianani CM, Sorice F. Cerebrospinal fluid antiganglioside antibodies in patients with AIDS. Infection 1995; 23(5) 288-291.

[126] Illa I, Ortiz N, Gallard E, Juarez C, Grau JM, Dalakas MC. Acute axonal Guillain-Barré syndrome with IgG antibodies against motor axons following parenteral gangliosides. Ann Neurol 1995; 38 218-224.

[127] Barka N, Shen G-Q, Shoenfeld Y, Alosachie I J, Gershwin M E, Reyes H, Peter JB. Multireactive pattern of serum autoantibodies in asymptomatic individuals with immunoglobulin A deficiency. Clin Diagn Lab Immunol 1995; 2 469-472.

[128] McCombe PA, Wilson R, Prentice RL. Results of testing for anti-GM1 antibodies. J Clin Neurosci 2000; 7 209-12.

[129] Terryberry J, Sutjita M, Shoenfeld Y. Myelin-and microbe-specific antibodies in Guillain-Barré syndrome. J Clin Lab Anal. 1995.

[130] [130] Livingston PO, Ritterr G, Calves MJ. Antibody response after immunization with the gangliosides GM1, GM2, GM3, GD2 and GD3 in the mouse. Cancer Immunol. Immunoth. 1989; 29(3) 179-184.

[131] Hettmer S, Ladisch S, Kaucic K. Low complex ganglioside expression characterizes human neuroblastoma cell lines. Cancer Lett. 2005; 225(1) 141-149.

[132] Wang XQ, Sun P, Paller AS. Inhibition of integrin-linked kinase/protein kinase B/Akt signaling: Mechanism for ganglioside-induced apoptosis. J Biol Chem 2001; 276 44504-44511.

[133] Sahal S, Mondal S. Supression of Ehrlich subcutaneous solid tumor growth by immunization with ganglioside GT1b of its origin, its IgM antibody or anti-idiotype antibody. J Exp Clin Cancer Res 2001; 20(1) 75.

[134] Mondal B, Sahal S. Inhibition of subcutaneous growth of Ehrilch ascites carcinoma (EAC), tumor by post-immunization with EAC-cells gangliosides and its anti-idiotype antibody in relation to tumor angiogenesis, apoptosis, cell cycle and infiltration of CD4+, CD8+lymphocites, NK cells, suppressor cells and APC-cells in tumor. Indian J Exp Biol 2011; 49 574-584.